Studies in Inherited
Metabolic Disease

Prenatal and Perinatal Diagnosis

Studies in Inherited Metabolic Disease

Prenatal and Perinatal Diagnosis

Proceedings of the 26th Annual
Symposium of the SSIEM,
Glasgow, UK,
September 1988

The combined supplements of *Journal of Inherited Metabolic Disease* Volume 12 (1989)

edited by G. M. Addison,
J. M. Connor, R. A. Harkness
and R. J. Pollitt

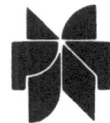

KLUWER ACADEMIC PUBLISHERS
DORDRECHT / BOSTON / LONDON

Distributors

for the United States and Canada: Kluwer Academic Publishers,
PO Box 358, Accord Station, Hingham, MA 02018-0358, USA
for all other countries: Kluwer Academic Publishers Group,
Distribution Center, PO Box 322, 3300 AH Dordrecht, The
Netherlands

ISBN-13:978-94-010-6970-0   e-ISBN-13:978-94-009-1069-0
DOI:10.1007/978-94-009-1069-0

Contents

Author Index

Title Index

J. Inher. Metab. Dis. 12 Suppl. 1 (1989)

Preface

With improved control of most environmental causes of disease, genetic illness has assumed a primary importance in the causation of handicap and mortality in all age groups. At present, effective therapy is available for relatively few genetic conditions and prenatal diagnosis is an important option for couples at high risk. The task of providing prenatal diagnosis for these couples requires a team approach between clinicians and scientists, and is complicated by the large number of diverse conditions and by the rapid developments in the field, both obstetric in relation to imaging and tissue sampling methods and genetic in relation to techniques for analysis. Against this background, the aim of the Symposium was to provide an overview of the current status of prenatal and perinatal diagnosis of inborn errors of metabolism.

The format consisted of the usual mixture of specific invited overviews and free communications in either oral or poster form. The invited overviews, as can be seen from this publication, covered a wide range, from accepted methods for neonatal diagnosis and screening to newer techniques for prenatal diagnosis and likely future developments with respect to gene therapy. Similarly, the oral communications included reviews of experience with biochemical analysis of chorionic villus sampling from major centres, more specific examples of progress towards the basic defect in Batten's disease and Canavan's disease, and prospects for effective therapy in Menkes' disease and a lipid myopathy. In addition, 175 posters were displayed and few if any inborn errors of metabolism were neglected. The SSIEM award was presented to Professor Reuben Matalon for his work on the characterization of the enzyme defect (aspartoacylase) in Canavan's disease, a possibility already indicated by Divry at last year's SSIEM meeting. This presentation was made by Dr Simon Garrod whose great-grandfather's brother was Sir Archibald Garrod. Dr Garrod gave an illuminating insight into his remarkable forebears and this complemented the presidential address by Professor Scriver, which was based on Sir Archibald's less well-known book *Inborn Factors in Disease*. The essential message expressed in this book is that genetic factors are involved in most disorders by rendering certain individuals more susceptible to environmental agents. This message is still true today and the new developments in recombinant DNA have provided a means to investigate this genetic contribution and so extend the future remit of the SSIEM.

The minisymposium on Neurotransmitters and Inherited Metabolic Disease was organized by Dr King.

The administration of the remainder of the 16th Symposium was in the hands of Prof. Cockburn, Prof. Connor, Mr Donaghy, Dr Glass, Dr Logan, Mr Kennedy, Mrs Rae, Mrs Thomson, the SSIEM secretary Mrs Anne Green and the assistant secretary Mr Griffiths. Invaluable secretarial help was provided by Mrs Barr and useful help at the meeting by Mr Irwin. The expert secretarial help in the production of this publication and the necessary editorial assistance are gratefully acknowledged. The Society was also grateful for the generous financial support from Scientific Hospital Supplies.

G. M. Addison, J. M. Connor, R. A. Harkness and R. J. Pollitt

1

Journal of Inherited Metabolic Disease. ISSN 0141–8955. Copyright © SSIEM and Kluwer Academic Publishers, PO Box 55, Lancaster, UK.

J. Inher. Metab. Dis. 12 Suppl. 1 (1989) 2–8

Perspectives

Family Influences on A. E. Garrod's Thinking

S. C. GARROD
Reader in Psychology, University of Glasgow, Glasgow, UK

The author of *Inborn Errors of Metabolism* and *Inborn Factors in Disease* had a somewhat unexceptional early career. Born in London in 1857, he received a first class degree at Cambridge in Natural Sciences before entering St. Bartholomew's Hospital to become qualified in medicine in 1884. Apart from a stimulating year spent in Vienna where he learned about some of the new scientific techniques in medicine, he spent the next 7 years working in his father's West End practice. But Archibald Garrod soon became dissatisfied with general medicine and at the age of 35 took up an appointment as Assistant Physician to the Hospital for Sick Children at Great Ormond Street. It was at this time that he began his work on rare childhood diseases such as alkaptonuria and struck up an important friendship with Gowland Hopkins, one of the most distinguished biochemists of the day. Eventually at the age of 55, 3 years after the publication of his *Croonian Lectures on Inborn Errors*, Archibald was made a consultant physician at St. Batholomew's. But it was not long before his career was to be interrupted by the First World War.

Although the War took all three of his sons, Archibald himself had a distinguished military career. Initially, he was gazetted a major and stationed in London at the General Hospital in Camberwell. Then in 1915 he embarked for Malta to serve as a Consultant Physician in the hospital at Gozo. Between then and 1918 he was mentioned six times in despatches and eventually, as Colonel Sir Archibald Garrod, appointed to be a Knight Commander of St. Michael and St. George. On his return from the war, he was finally appointed to head the new medical professorial unit at St. Bartholomew's and within barely a year had been appointed Regius Professor of Medicine at Oxford at the age of 63. In his final years at Oxford, Archibald published his last book on *Inborn Factors in Disease* (Figure 1).

Looking back on this career it seems surprising that a physician of the late 19th century – a time when practical medicine was preoccupied with the treatment of infectious diseases – should have been capable of such insights in biochemical genetics. His thinking was unconventional by the standards of his time in at least two respects: first he looked for medical explanations at the level of the body's biochemistry and second, he was prepared to entertain genetic origins for conditions such as alkaptonuria when others still presumed them to be infectious childhood diseases (Bearn, 1976). But the bare bones of his curriculum vitae disguise the fact that Archibald was brought up in a rather special intellectual environment. Both the biochemical and genetic influences on his thinking can be traced in some form

Journal of Inherited Metabolic Disease. ISSN 0141–8955. Copyright © SSIEM and Kluwer Academic Publishers, PO Box 55, Lancaster, UK.

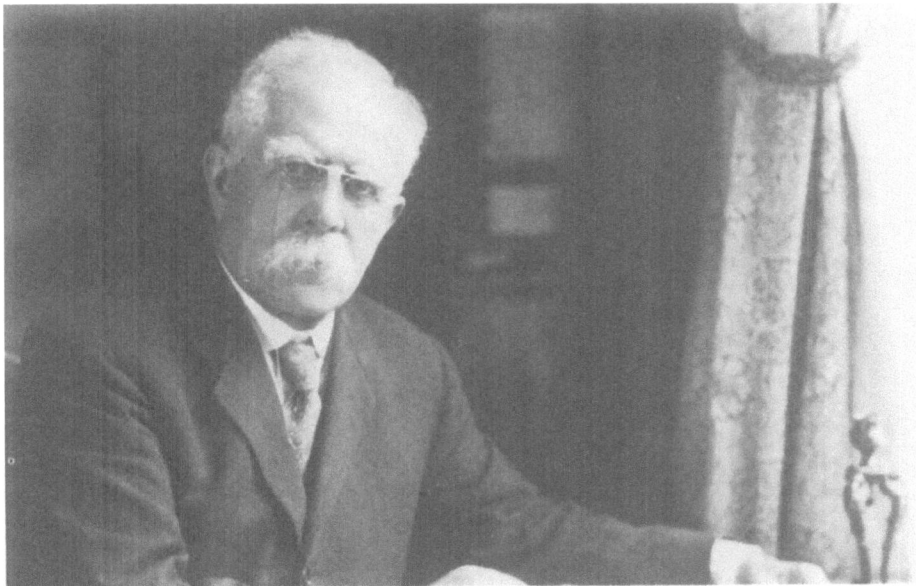

Figure 1 Archibald when Regius Professor at Oxford, at the time when *Inborn Factors in Disease* was published

right back to his early days as part of a family heavily involved in the biomedical scientific revolution of the latter part of the century.

Archibald was the youngest son of the physician Alfred Baring Garrod, FRS (1819–1907), who is now recognized as one of the pioneers of scientific medicine (Figure 2). A. B. Garrod's main contribution was to produce a scientific classification of the various rheumatic diseases at a time when most physicians were still working according to the mysticism of ancient humoralistic theory. Alfred began by developing chemical techniques to assess the exact concentration of sodium urate in serum, as compared to urine, and other techniques to identify the compound in joints and connective tissue. This enabled him to differentiate gout from the other rheumatic diseases, and then construct a modern classification. By 1847 Garrod senior was able to report that gout 'would appear to depend on a loss (temporary or permanent) of the uric-acid-excreting function of the kidneys . . . any undue formation of this compound (sodium urate) would favour occurrence of the disease, and hence the connection between gout and uric acid, gravel and calculi, and hence the influence of high living, wine, porter, want of exercise, etc. in inducing it'. This early work led him to establish that in the other forms of rheumatism (simply distinguished at the time as acute [rheumatic fever] and subacute [rheumatic gout]) there was no such chemical evidence. By 1859 Garrod had published a classic book on *The Nature and Treatment of Gout and Rheumatic Gout* in which he coined the term Rheumatoid Arthritis – 'Although unwilling to add to the number of names, I cannot help expressing a desire that a name might be found for this disease [*Rheumatic Gout*], not implying any necessary relation between it and either gout

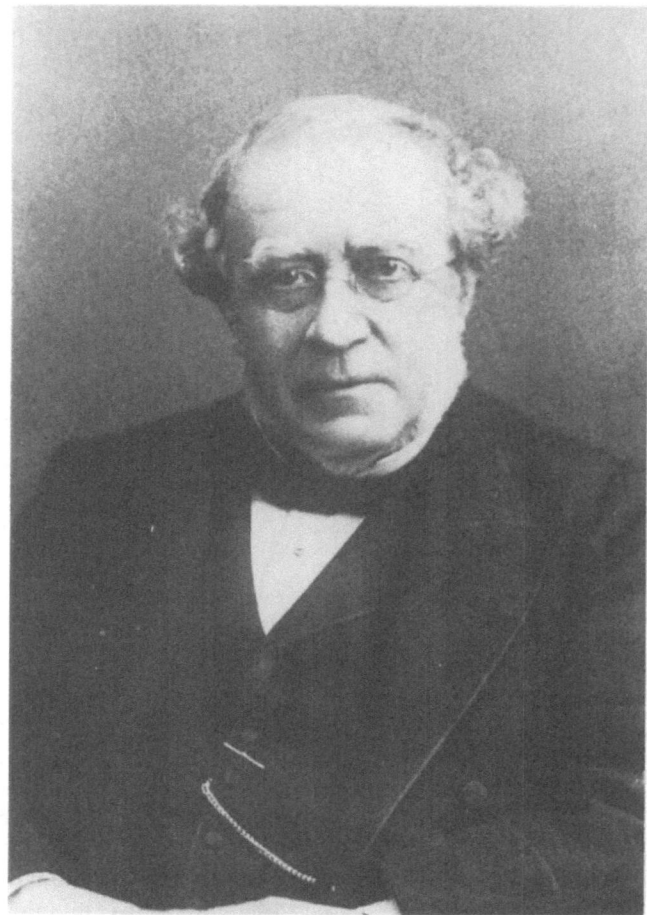

Figure 2   Garrod's father, Alfred Baring Garrod

or rheumatism. Perhaps *Rheumatoid Arthritis* would answer the object, by which term I should wish to imply an inflammatory affection of the joints, not unlike rheumatism in some of its characters but differing materially from it.' By a combination of careful clinical observation and perceptive biochemical experiment, Alfred Garrod had been able to lay the foundations for the modern classification of the rheumatic diseases and, in recognition of the historical significance of this work, he is now hailed as the 'Father of modern Rheumatology' (*J. Am. Med. Assoc.*, 1973)

So Archibald was born into a family already clearly identified with the new scientific developments in medicine to a father who has been described as the very first practical biochemist. That his father influenced Archibald's own work is beyond doubt. In the first place, he took his Natural Sciences degree at Cambridge in Chemistry, before taking up medicine and this always remained one of his great interests, eventually expressed in the establishment of the Biochemistry Department at Oxford University. Apart from engendering a general interest in chemistry, A. B. Garrod also directly influenced his son's early work in medicine which revolved around the study of the rheumatic diseases. In Archibald's first book entitled *A Treatise on Rheumatism and Rheumatoid Arthritis*, he was able to differentiate osteoarthritis from both gout and rheumatoid arthritis and so help to complete the modern classification of these diseases.

Thus Archibald followed in his father's footsteps as a physician with an overriding interest in chemical explanations for disease, so much so that some of his contemporaries thought of him more as a chemical pathologist than a physician. This is clearly illustrated in a passage from Sir Francis Fraser's obituary where he says 'his was the mind of a true scientist and often one wondered and he wondered also, how he had come to be a practising physician. He was almost an onlooker when he applied himself to the daily task of seeing patients and treating them. The daily task was something that had to be done, a price that had to be paid for the privilege of contact with the numerous intriguing puzzles which he found and set himself to solve. Often he would spend all morning at the window of a ward testing urine that presented an unusual colour or smell. The morning's round could be left to others' (Fraser, 1936) (Figure 3).

So one can discern a clear influence on Garrod's biochemical approach to

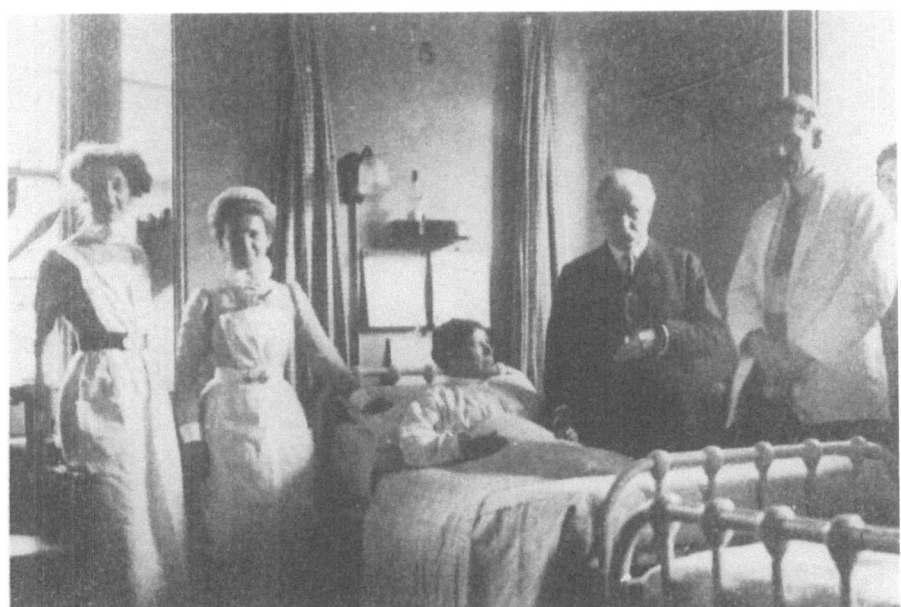

Figure 3 Archibald Garrod on a ward round at St. Batholomew's

medicine from his father's work. It is also possible to find a more diffuse influence on Garrod's thinking from another member of his immediate family. Archibald's eldest brother, Alfred Henry Garrod, FRS (1846–79), was one of the leading zoologists of the day (Figure 4). At the time of his premature death at 33 years of age, A. H. Garrod had published 75 scientific papers, held two Professorships, was

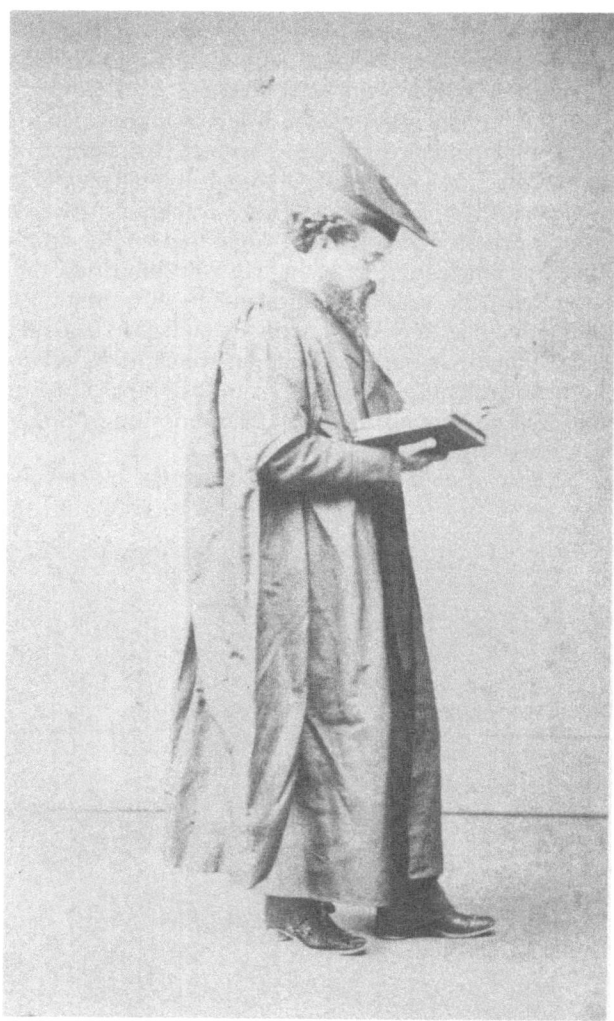

Figure 4   Garrod's brother, Alfred Henry Garrod

Prosector of the London Zoo and Fellow of the Royal Society. His own work ranged from pioneering studies of the physiology of the circulation to the definitive anatomical classification of the passerine birds. Sadly this extraordinarily talented brother died of tuberculosis when Archibald was only 22. Yet it is clear that he must have exerted a formative influence on his younger brother. For instance, the young Archibald demonstrated an interest in natural history and genetics from a very early age. At 12 he was an avid collector and classifier of butterflies and at the same age was writing his second childhood book on *The Tiger*, where he reports the following, 'There has been an instance of a lion being the father and a tigress the mother, of cubs. The lion was born in captivity and the tiger was captured at a very early age. The cub had the head of the lion but tigerene stripes on the body' (Bearn, 1976). This looks like just the sort of information an elder brother, about to be appointed Prosector of the London Zoo, might supply.

What is certain is that Archibald would have been exposed to the major figures of the day in both the Zoological Society of London and the Royal Society. Alfred had presented papers with Francis Darwin and was acquainted with a number of key figures of the time, including Francis's father Charles as well as T. H. R. Huxley. This might well help to explain how Archibald could have been aware of the Mendelian laws and the importance of consanguinity in the inheritance of recessive genetic diseases as early as 1902, a fact pointed out to him by his friend the botanist William Bateson (Garrod, 1902; Bateson and Saunders, 1902). It also might account for A. E. Garrod's interest in promoting a broad scientific education for medical students (Garrod, 1912–13), at a time when English medical education was very different from today.

So it is fair to say that A. E. Garrod's ideas and approach to scientific medicine were strongly influenced by an immediate family who afforded him both hereditary and environmental advantages. In the words of Gowland Hopkins (1936), 'A vivid interest in the chemical aspects of medicine was innate in Archibald Garrod, and remained with him to the last. It is of interest to remember that his father Sir Alfred Garrod made in 1848 what his son liked to recall as the first biochemical observation on the living human body.' But at the same time, like his father, Archibald was very much a clinician, as Hopkins also pointed out, 'With all his predilections for experimental science Garrod remained first and foremost a clinician, with a deep sense of the dignity and importance of that calling. When speaking, as he often did, of the help that modern medicine receives from science, he was always concerned to emphasize that this is but a repayment of the debt that science has owed medicine. He held that all research with direct clinical bearings should be inspired by the clinician, who must always be the final judge as to its justification and value.' It is possible to discern in both Archibald Garrod and his father a very modern view of the clinical scientist, concerned with advancing scientific knowledge but in the service of the practical treatment of disease.

REFERENCES

Bateson, W. and Saunders, E. R. Report of the Evolution Committee of the Royal Society (London) No. 1, 1902, p. 133

Bearn, A. G. Inborn errors of metabolism. 1. Archibald Garrod and the birth of an idea. *Lettsomian Lectures*, Feb. 9th, 1976

Fraser, F. R. Sir Archibald Garrod. Obituary. *Lancet* 1 (1936) 807

Garrod, A. B. Observations on certain pathological conditions of the blood and urine in gout, rheumatism and Bright's disease. *Med. Chir. Trans.* 31 (1848) 83–97

Garrod, A. B. *The Nature and Treatment of Gout and Rheumatic Gout*, Walton and Maberly, London, 1859

Garrod, A. E. *A Treatise on Rheumatism and Rheumatoid Arthritis*, Charles Griffin & Co. Ltd., London, 1890

Garrod, A. E. The incidence of alkaptonuria; a study in chemical individuality. *Lancet* 2 (1902) 1616

Garrod, A. E. *Inborn Errors of Metabolism*, Frowde, Hodder and Stoughton, London, 1909

Garrod, A. E. The scientific spirit in medicine: inaugural sessional address to the Abernethian Society. *St. Bart's Hosp. J.* 20 (1912–13) 19

Garrod, A. E. *The Inborn Factors in Disease: An Essay*, Clarendon Press, Oxford, 1931

Hopkins, G. Obituary to Archibald Garrod. *Br. Med. J.* 4th April, 1936

J. Am. Med. Assoc. Cover Story: Sir Alfred Baring Garrod, FRS. In Primer on the Rheumatic Diseases, *J. Am. Med. Assoc.*, Suppl., 30 April 224 (1973) No. 5.

J. Inher. Metab. Dis. 12 Suppl. 1 (1989) 9–24

Perspectives

The Salience of Garrod's 'Molecular Groupings' and 'Inborn Factors in Disease'*

C. R. SCRIVER

deBelle Laboratory for Biochemical Genetics, McGill University–Montreal Children's Hospital Research Institute, Montreal, Quebec, Canada H3H 1P3

Summary: Garrod's important second book, *Inborn Factors in Disease* (1931), was about inherited predisposition to disease. Chemical and metabolic individuality, which are the modalities of predisposition, originated in 'molecular groupings' (proteins) in Garrod's view of life. Such 'groupings' as interlocus molecular hybrids, allelic complementation and expressions of modifier genes, can assume variant expression in heterozygotes. Here, it is shown that genetic variation in such 'molecular groupings' has clinical relevance, for example (1) in reproductive counselling for thalassaemia; (2) in heterozygosity where the affected enzymes are normally homopolymeric; (3) in clinical severity of 'monogenic' disease (e.g. familial hypercholesterolaemia and muscular dystrophy) when variation is not explained by allelic heterogeneity. The associated chemical individuality in each case can be used to identify risk and thus as a mode of predictive medicine.

Sir Archibald E. Garrod, the founder of human biochemical genetics, attempted to interpret the whole organism's phenotype while dealing with its chemical parts. In using his particular form of reductionist science, he faced an old yet continuing problem in biology, the problem of 'emergence' (Mayr, 1982). Emergence is the biological equivalent of the uncertainty principle and it says that one cannot know the whole organism by studying its parts in isolation. The molecular geneticists face the same problem now. Meantime, we admire still the man who found the larger message of chemical individuality in the 'inborn error of metabolism' (Garrod, 1909) and in its extension – 'the inborn factor in disease' (Garrod, 1931). No harm then to spend a few moments with Garrod and his second book before going on to examine the modern salience of those extraordinarily clear ideas about chemical individuality (Childs, 1970; Burgio, 1986), their more mystical counterparts, the 'molecular groupings' (Scriver and Childs, 1989), and our predisposition to health or disease therein.

Although Garrod was trained as a physician he apparently escaped the potentially limiting vision of that formal education. We cannot know the precise influences on him that gave rise to the novel vision he had of health and disease, but among them

---

*From a talk delivered, while I was President, to the 26th Annual Meeting of the Society for the Study of Inborn Errors of Metabolism.

Journal of Inherited Metabolic Disease. ISSN 0141–8955. Copyright © SSIEM and Kluwer Academic Publishers, PO Box 55, Lancaster, UK.

must be at least three: the eldest brother (Herbert)†, distinguished zoologist and Fellow of the Royal Society, who could have conveyed Darwinian ideas to the younger brother in terms unfamiliar to most contemporary students and teachers of medicine; Frederick Gowland Hopkins (Needham, 1962), to whom Garrod turned for advice and preceptorship (and whose three obituary notices on Garrod (Hopkins, 1936a, 1936b, 1938) are an indication of the respect one had for the other); and Bateson with whom Garrod corresponded on the significance of consanguinity in alkaptonuria families (Bearn and Miller, 1979). From such influences and from the observations he made himself on patients came the great hypothesis: 'The inborn error of metabolism'. Underlying it was Garrod's special idea of human chemical individuality (Childs, 1970) and it informed nearly all of the important lectures he gave after the Croonian Lectures of 1908. Nevertheless, the concept of chemical individuality evolved slowly but perceptibly into a modified version which Garrod called 'inborn factors in disease'. In this form it became the title of the second book (Garrod, 1931) but initially, in the Huxley lecture (Garrod, 1927), it was called 'diathesis'. Garrod saw diathesis – 'an old idea impaired by a lack of knowledge' – as inherited predisposition expressed as chemical individuality in forms more subtle than those so obvious in the inborn errors of metabolism. The Table of Contents for *Inborn Factors in Disease* shows the breadth of Garrod's late vision in this context (Table 1).

Table 1   The Table of Contents of Garrod's *Inborn Factors in Disease* (Oxford University Press, 1931)[a]

[a]Barton Childs (1985) used this same Table of Contents to show how Garrod went beyond pathways and blocks to consider chemical individuality as a general theme in medicine, with implications for individuality in response to 'attacking agents' and resistance or susceptibility to disease

†I thank Simon Garrod, PhD, Reader in Psychology, Glasgow University and great grand-nephew of Sir Archibald Garrod, for enhancing my knowledge of his ancestor. Alex Bearn (see references) gave me the Garrod pedigree and other useful information.

J. Inher. Metab. Dis. 12 Suppl. 1 (1989)

Garrod's penetrating view of medicine was not perceived that way when *Inborn Factors* was published. First, Garrod himself had only a dim idea about the nature of genes and genes remained abstractions for him and his readers. Second, there was no way to identify persons at particular risk who might become sick patients, there being no technology to see genes. Third, the physicians of his day were preoccupied with diseases whose causes were patently extrinsic to the patient and the usual question – what is the disease my patient has? – was by force of practice the dominant one. Accordingly, Garrod's concern for inborn factors in common disease sputtered in the wind and, in due course, his second book sank from sight and along with it his insights. Few copies of the book can be found today even in major medical libraries and few of us have read it. Meanwhile, the circumstances of medicine have changed. The heritability of disease, that is the relative importance of the genetic causes of diseases, has increased; we know more about genes and we have methods to analyse ultimate forms of chemical individuality residing in the variation of nucleotide sequences in DNA. For such reasons Garrod's second book is now salient and it will once again be available to read (Scriver and Childs, 1989).

PHYSIOLOGICAL GENETICS: WHAT DO WE MEAN?

Molecular genetics is a powerful way to solve biological problems and most of us, myself included, willingly join the cadre of reductionists who use 'reverse genetics' as an interpretive paradigm in biology (Childs, 1988). But in some ways molecular genetics is a welcome respite from the difficult task of dealing with phenotype paradigms. All phenotypes in whole organisms have complex determinants since they reflect in varying degrees the expression of major and modifier genes and their interactions with constitutional factors and experience (Childs and Scriver, 1986). Hence it is not surprising that normal individuals have 'private' phenotypes – even for example, plasma amino acid values (Scriver *et al.*, 1985) – as evidence of their chemical individuality and it is a normal phenomenon (Williams, 1963). When it comes to explaining disease the answers are again likely to be complex, since its manifestations (phenotype) are the outcome of processes (pathogenesis) which originated in a cause. The cause has either overwhelmed or undermined, usually both, the mechanisms of homeostasis responsible for the normal phenotype and the resistance or susceptibility to disease will be a matter of the endowment the person has to maintain homeostasis. Health is the counterpart, in which the experiences are tolerated and the intrinsic determinants (genes) maintain the central tendencies of the homeostatic systems (Scriver, 1982a; Murphy and Pyeritz, 1986). From this point of view the usual question in medicine – What is the disease my patient has? – is not the central question. The proper one is: Why does my patient have this disease now? (King, 1982), and its corollary is: Who is the patient with the disease? Geoffrey Rose (1985) thought the latter one important; he said it could explain sick cases (who reflect causes) and it set them apart from sick populations (which tell us about incidence).

This form of medical thinking is not trivial nor is it a diversion from the main business of medicine. It was in fact Garrod's principal concern that we find the answers to questions of this nature; in this he was reflecting perhaps the influence of his brother, if that man did indeed encourage Garrod to reflect on what has since been referred to as the evolutionary implications in disease (Scriver, 1984). Although Garrod's brother could not have understood disease in quite that way, we know now that selection acts only on a property (a phenotype) of the organism whereas the object selected is the gene which confers the phenotype (Sober, 1984). Thus it becomes clear why Garrod's concern for chemical individuality and the modern ability to pursue 'reverse genetics' are simply different faces of the same coin, the coin that Garrod minted and which has become the common currency of physiological genetics.

CHEMICAL INDIVIDUALITY IN 'MOLECULAR GROUPINGS'

In the 1909 version of his hypothesis, Garrod's vision of individuality was reflected in the composition of metabolites in body fluids. In the 1931 version he refers to 'molecular groupings', by which he apparently meant proteins (Scriver and Childs, 1989). Others working later and independently, but echoing Garrod while incorporating new knowledge, perceived that 'every individual is a [chemical] deviant in one way or another' (Williams, 1963), and that a gene encodes an enzyme (or polypeptide) (Beadle, 1959). From the vantage point of the phenotype paradigm, where DNA makes RNA makes protein, we begin to understand the origin and variety of chemical individuality. Here I try to illustrate Garrod's concept of diathesis as chemical individuality in terms of 'molecular (protein) groupings'. The associated phenotypes are less categorical than inborn errors of metabolism and more like 'inborn factors' (see Childs, 1985) but under certain conditions they could become disadaptive and therefore they are relevant to our understanding of 'diathesis'. More important, they represent subtle rather than discontinuous deviations from normal distributions (homeostasis) with significance for diagnosis and counselling; in brief, they are relevant to the practice of medicine and they are the essence of 'physiological genetics' (Scriver, 1987).

Effects of coordinate expression of interlocus hybrid products

The inborn errors of metabolism fixed our attention on solitary genes whose products control metabolism. The corresponding metabolic phenotypes tend to be recessive but can be dominant if the gene in question encodes a major determinant of the homeostatic pathway or network (Kacser and Burns, 1981; Scriver, 1985). Since a person is heterozygous at many loci and has many multimeric protein assemblies often comprising interlocus molecular hybrids, it is relevant to consider how coordinate expression of alleles at the independent loci encoding such assemblies might affect the associated phenotype. Harris and colleagues (1977) noticed that heteropolymeric assemblies were less often polymorphic than homopolymers and monomers and they suggested that selection pressures to achieve heterozygosity were weaker at loci that encoded interlocus hybrids. Haemoglobin, an obvious exception to the Harris hypothesis, is the prototype of an interlocus hybrid and the coordinate expression of α- and β-thalassaemia genes provides us with the opportunity to measure an effect of interlocus variation on phenotype and to show how this form of variant 'molecular grouping' can be relevant in genetic counselling.

Following World War II (and several other wars) uprooted citizens of Mediterranean and Asian countries immigrated to Quebec and with them came their genes. Thalassaemia is now an important disease in our province and, in an effort to reduce its burden, our group established a carrier screening and counselling programme for thalassaemia in the province (Scriver *et al.*, 1984).The frequency of β-thalassaemia heterozygosity is about 7% among Greeks living in Quebec and about 3% in Italians. However, you do not have to be a recent immigrant to be at risk of thalassaemia because about 1% of long-established French Canadians in Portneuf County are heterozygous for β-thalassaemia (Prévost *et al.*, 1988). (The origin of thalassaemia mutation(s) in the French Canadian population is a matter of great interest (Kaplan *et al.*, 1988), as is the origin of any mutation in any settled population.) The frequency of α-thalassaemia heterozygosity in Quebec populations has also been determined (Akerman, 1987; Akerman *et al.*, 1987) and it can be as high as 12% in some social groups in the province. Accordingly, the likelihood exists that we will encounter individuals doubly heterozygous for α- and β-thalassaemia genes in our thalassaemia counselling programme.

We found such persons by molecular screening of β-thalassaemia heterozygotes and we investigated the effect of coordinate expression of α- and β-thalassaemia mutations on two informative erythrocyte parameters (mean corpuscular volume, MCV (fl) and haemoglobin A_2, HbA_2 (%)) (Zannis-Hadjopoulos *et al.*, 1977; Scriver *et al.*, 1984). Simple heterozygotes for β-thalassaemia have low MCV values (<80 fl on electronic counters) and elevated HbA_2 values (>3%). Simple heterozygotes for α-thalassaemia have low MCV values but normal HbA_2 values.

The appropriate molecular analysis of α-globin genes distinguishes the number of α-globin genes expressed in the α-thalassaemia heterozygote; it could be 2 (α-/α-), 3 (α-/αα) or 5 (ααα/αα), the normal number being 4 (αα/αα). In our study (Akerman, 1987; Akerman *et al.*, 1987) 11 of 74 β-thalassaemia heterozygotes had co-existent α-thalassaemia genotypes. In these double heterozygotes expression of fewer α-globin genes was associated with a trend toward more normal erythrocyte parameters (Figure 1). This finding has been reported by others for MCV values alone (Kanavakis *et al.*, 1982; Rosatelli *et al.*, 1984; Weatherall *et al.*, 1989) but it has not been recorded for MCV and HbA_2 values together. The finding has an explanation. Imbalance in the chain ratio is the origin of the erythrocyte phenotype in isolated β-thalassaemia (Weatherall *et al.*, 1989) and chain ratio is normalized in the α-/α-, β/thal double heterozygote (Table 2).

The finding has real significance when counselling couples at risk of having an offspring affected with β-thalassaemia. The occasional person who is doubly heterozygous will be wrongly classified as a non-carrier on the basis of normalized erythrocyte parameters and the likelihood of encountering such a person in the high-risk populations of Quebec could approach 0.00075 among Italians, and 0.00196 among Greeks, for example. Although not high, the very existence of such risk imposes uncertainty on our interpretation of every thalassaemia screening test.

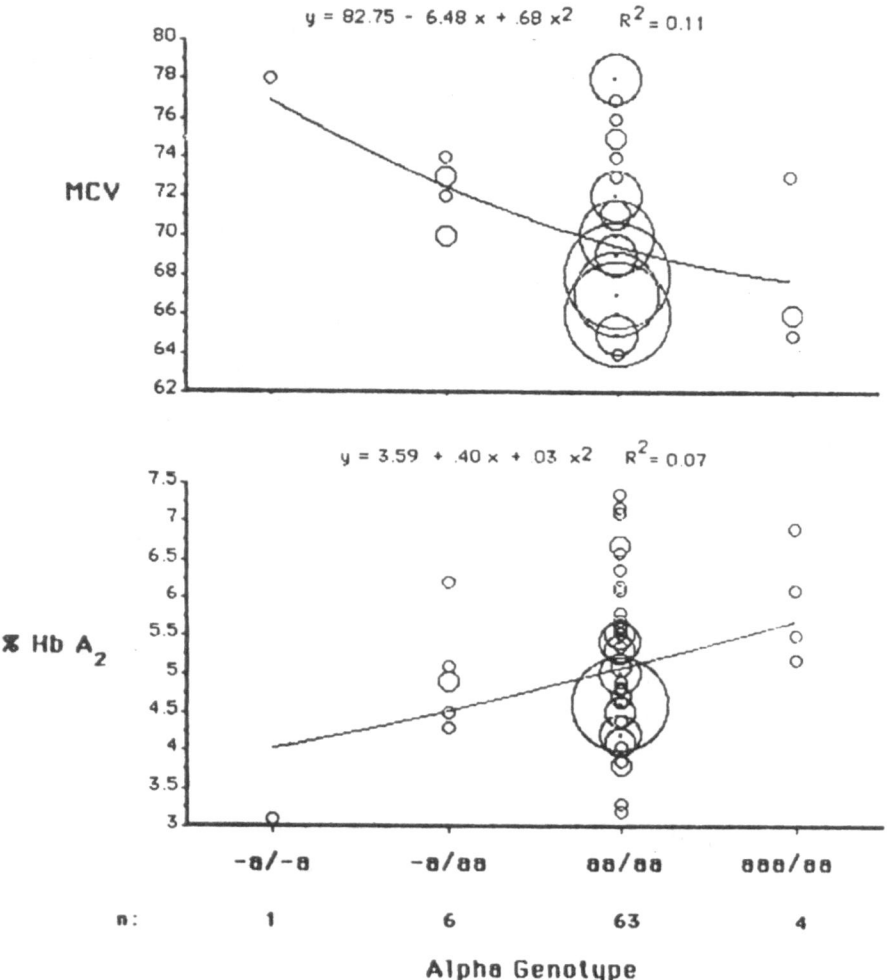

Figure 1 Polynomial regression of α-globin genotype (abscissae) on erythrocyte parameters (ordinates). Density of measurements is proportional to symbol area. Source population was 74 persons heterozygous for a β-thalassaemia mutation among which were 11 with α-thalassaemia genotypes. (Individuals with a *cis* α-thalassaemia mutation ($\alpha--/\alpha\alpha$) were not ascertained by the appropriate molecular analysis and therefore may have been classified as normal); Top: effect of gene and chain ratios on mean cell volume (MCV, fl); bottom: effect of gene and chain ratios on haemoglobin A_2 (% HbA_2) (from Akerman, 1987)

Accordingly, we must change our policy for reproductive counselling and carry out DNA analysis of globin genes to determine genotype in every couple seeking advice. The variant 'molecular grouping' here predisposes to disease (thalassaemia) yet the 'chemical individuality' associated with the corresponding coordinate gene expression (erythrocyte values) obscures the true (genetic) individuality of the

Table 2   Cordinate gene expression and formation of variant interlocus hybrids (haemoglobins) for thalassaemia mutations in double heterozygotes

Genotype	Gene ratio (normal genes)	Chain ratio (relative to normal)
Variant		
ααα/αα, βthal/β	5α : 1β	2.5
αα/αα, βthal/β	4α : 1β	2.0
–α/αα, βthal/β	3α : 1β	1.5
–α/–α, βthal/β	2α : 1β	1.0
Normal		
αα/αα, β/β	4α : 2β	—

consultands. Much is at stake (the life of a fetus) in this circumstance and its subtlety would, no doubt, have been appreciated by Garrod.

Effects of intralocus allele product interaction

An exaggerated gene dosage effect in the heterozygote is usually attributed to negative allelic complementation (Kaufman *et al.*, 1975; Harris, 1980). Here, the 'measured heterozygous genotype' is found in enzyme activity which is significantly below half the mean value for the homozygous normal phenotype. When one considers how prevalent heterozygosity is, one might ask: Could a severely deviant gene dosage effect be of functional significance and might it explain some of our predisposition to disease? The answer to that question is important and some investigators have begun to examine the costs to health of heterozygosity at some major autosomal loci (Vogel, 1984). Meanwhile there are new examples of negative allelic complementation that do not appear in Harris' original discussion of the phenomenon (Harris, 1980), with its counterparts in the 'dominant negative mutation' (Herskowitz, 1987) and 'metabolic interference' (Johnson, 1980).

In Canada, we screen systematically for mutations causing hyperphenylalaninaemia that are not at the phenylalanine hydroxylases locus (Scriver, 1982b). A Chinese infant with neonatal hyperphenylalaninaemia and an abnormal urine neopterin : biopterin ratio was identified in the Canadian programme. He had severely deficient 6-pyruvoyl tetrahydropterin synthase activity (Scriver *et al.*, 1987a). His parents had only 20% normal 6-pyruvoyl tetrahydropterin synthase activity in their erythrocytes and, upon further investigation, a deviant gene dosage effect proved to be the rule and not the exception among obligate heterozygotes for 6-pyruvoyl tetrahydropterin synthase deficiency (Scriver *et al.*, 1987a). We observed further that some 6-pyruvoyl tetrahydropterin synthase deficient heterozygotes had mildly impaired biopterin homeostasis as measured by urine biopterin values (Figure 2). The finding implies that 6-pyruvoyl tetrahydropterin synthase is a principal determinant of the flux through the pathway leading to synthesis of tetrahydrobiopterin and it suggests that some heterozygotes for 6-pyruvoyl tetrahydropterin synthase deficiency perhaps live on the edge of trouble if there is any correlation between brain and urine biopterin values. Meantime, the deviant gene dosage effect must be taken into account in the interpretation of 6-pyruvoyl tetrahydropterin synthase activity in amniocytes when it is measured for purposes of prenatal diagnosis, because the distinction between mutant homozygosity and heterozygosity by 6-pyruvoyl tetrahydropterin synthase assay is not as clean as one needs for accurate diagnosis of genotype (Scriver *et al.*, 1987a).

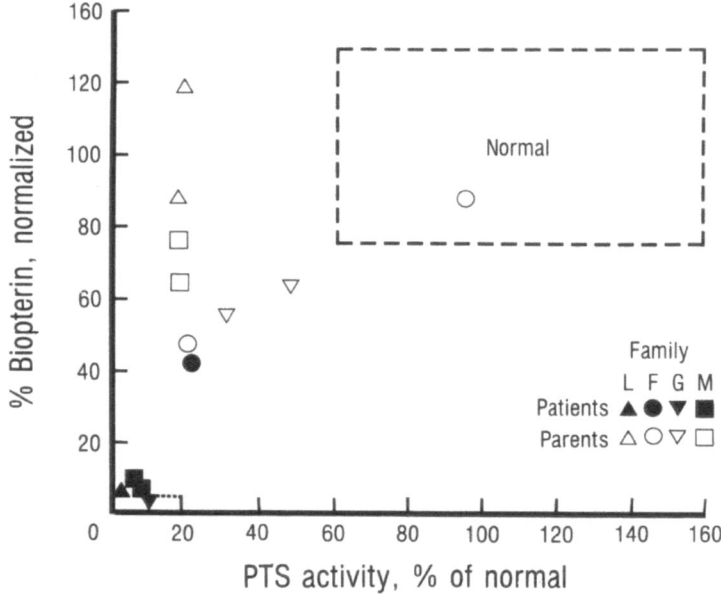

Figure 2 Urine biopterin (normalized for age) related to erythrocyte 6-pyruvoyl tetrahydropterin synthase activity in obligate heterozygotes (open symbols) and their offspring (closed symbols). Deviant gene dosage effect on 6-pyruvoyl tetrahydropterin synthase activity is associated with low urine biopterin excretion (implying impaired tetrahydrobiopterin synthesis) in some heterozygotes (adapted from Scriver *et al.*, 1987a)

6-Pyruvoyl tetrahydropterin synthase is a multimeric enzyme, it is a homotetramer (Takikawa *et al.*, 1986) and, if one assumes the heteropolymeric forms ($\alpha3\alpha'1$, $\alpha2\alpha'2$, $\alpha1\alpha'3$ where α and α' are normal and mutant forms of subunit) have reduced or no catalytic activity, then enzyme activity in heterozygotes with CRM positive mutations will be less than half normal and will be proportional to the amount of normal homotetramer formed.

In Table 3 are other examples – the list is not comprehensive – of deviant gene dosage effect with a putative 'dominant negative' phenotype. The deviant phenotype is manifest under standard conditions of assay in some forms; others require a permissive condition and, even though the phenotype is demonstrated *in vitro*, the corresponding *in vivo et situ* catalytic activity is mostly unknown. The deviant metabolic phenotype in 6-pyruvoyl tetrahydropterin synthase heterozygotes implies they, at least, have a deviant dosage effect on function *in vivo et situ*.

Since intralocus negative (allelic) complementation is observed with enzymes

Table 3   Some examples in humans of putative negative allelic complementation[a] expressed as deviant gene dosage effect on enzyme activity in the heterozygote

Variant phenotype	Enzyme[b] (no. of subunits) (Activity in heterozygote % normal)	Reference
Homocystinuria	cystathionine β-synthase (2) (25%)	Fleischer *et al.*, 1973; McGill, Mettler, and Scriver, unpub. data, 1988
Aspartylglucosaminuria	aspartylglycosylamine amido hydrolase (2?) (17%)	Aula *et al.*, 1973
Non-phenylketonuria hyperphenylalaninaemia	ibid. (13%)	Kaufman *et al.*, 1975
Phenylketonuria	Phenylalanine hydroxylase (3 or 4) (14–44%)	Grimm *et al.*, 1977 Bartholomé, 1979 Bartholomé and Dresel, 1982
Malignant hyperphenyl-alaninaemia	dihydropteridin reductase (2) (11–41%)	Milstien *et al.*, 1976 Firgaira *et al.*, 1979 Danks *et al.*, 1979 Ponzone *et al.*, 1988
Malignant hyperphenyl-alaninaemia	6-pyruvoyl tetrahydropterin (4) synthase (19–50%)	Scriver *et al.*, 1987a
Sandhoff disease	β-hexosaminidase (Hex B) (4) [↑ heat lability][c]	Lane and Jenkins, 1978 Lowden, 1979
Glutaric acidaemia I	glutaryl CoA dehydrogenase (4) (12–42%)	Goodman and Kohlhoff, 1975 Christensen and Brandt, 1978 Whelan *et al.*, 1979
GABA transaminase deficiency	γ-aminobutyrate transaminase (2) (15–37%)	Gibson *et al.*, 1985
Prolidase deficiency	Peptidase D (2) [↑ heat lability][c]	Boright *et al.*, 1988 Boright, 1988

[a]Discussed by Harris (1980) the phenomenon is considered here as a counterpart of other concepts notably 'dominant negative mutation' (Herskowitz, 1987) and 'metabolic interference' (Johnson, 1980)
[b]These enzymes, in their normal forms, are multimeric homopolymers (identical subunits). In the heterozygote-expressing cross-reacting antigenic materal (CRM positive mutations) there is opportunity to form heteropolymeric and homopolymeric (normal and mutant forms) enzyme species. Activity values in square brackets are means or ranges from publications cited
[c]Under conventional assay conditions activity is about half normal, but under selective conditions (e.g. thermal stress) heterozygotes express excessive gene dosage (e.g. increased thermolability)

that are homopolymeric in the normal state, one presumes that the heterozygote expressing a CRM positive allele forms interallelic molecular hybrids (heteropolymeric enzymes) to account for the deviant gene dosage effect. The putative heteropolymers have not been demonstrated so far in any of the disorders listed in Table 3, to my knowledge. Nonetheless, these experiments of nature provide examples of 'molecular grouping' that may be common enough, since heterozygosity is common, and may have functional and clinical effects. The prevalence of this form of risk will be roughly proportional to the homopolymeric multimers in our 'molecular groupings'. This problem has received little attention up to now and, no doubt, Garrod is urging us to get on with it.

Effects of modifier genes (independent locus co-expression)

Most phenotypes are complex, meaning that they reflect both involvement and expression of more than one locus and interaction with experience. Yet even 'monogenic' (Mendelian) diseases are complex phenotypes; take phenylketonuria as an example. First, interaction with the environment is necessary for disease to occur and to treat it. Second, phenylketonuria patients have about a two-fold interindividual variation in phenylalanine tolerance (Scriver and Rosenberg, 1973). Allelic variation at the phenylalanine hydroxylase locus may be one explanation for this variation but epistatic activity of the additional determinants of phenylalanine homeostasis (which have greater relative importance in the phenylketonuria subject) is another. Net transport of phenylalanine into tissues, a mediated process (Salter *et al.*, 1986), and chemical conversions of the amino acid to other derivatives (Scriver and Rosenberg, 1973) are each controlled by gene products, the relative activities of which will determine metabolic homeostasis in the mutant (phenylketonuria) phenotype just as they do, to a lesser extent, in the normal state. Langenbeck and colleagues (1988) pursuing this line of reasoning sought evidence that the cognitive outcome in untreated phenylketonuria patients was related to the activity of alternative pathways, notably the transamination route, for phenylalanine disposal in phenylketonuria. Whereas the findings are preliminary and may not be confirmed, the hypothesis motivating the study goes to the heart of the problem, in my view.

Langenbeck referred to a study of ours that addressed a corresponding question in Hartnup disorder (Scriver *et al.*, 1987b). Prospective ascertainment of Hartnup probands – by newborn urine screening – discovers largely healthy subjects, whereas retrospective ascertainment yields sick Hartnup patients with pellagra-like illness, impaired development and other manifestations. Accordingly, an explanation of the difference between Hartnup *disorder* (the metabolic phenotype) and Hartnup *disease* is important. The former is an inborn error of amino acid transport which shows allelic heterogeneity (alleles did not explain cases with Hartnup disease in our study). On the other hand, Hartnup disease is multifactorial and is precipitated against a background genotype that predisposes a low (outlier) plasma value for the group of amino acids affected by the Hartnup allele. The combination of 'low' modifier genes and a Hartnup major gene renders the person susceptible to experiences (e.g. change of diet) that are trivial for non-Hartnup persons and Hartnup probands with 'normal' or 'high' modifier genes. The finding encourages one to put aside categorical thinking (e.g. Hartnup probands have a disease) and it explains reasonably well why only about one in ten Hartnup probands are actually at risk of disease manifestations. More importantly, it shows that one can apparently predict, from plasma amino acid values, which Hartnup subject is at increased risk of disease and who should receive prophylactic treatment.

So phenylketonuria and Hartnup disease are both complex phenotypes dependent on a major gene, modifier (epistatic) genes and experience to explain their manifestations. In that sense indeed, they are no different from any other 'genetic' disease (Childs and Scriver, 1986). However, that is not how I used to think about so-called Mendelian disease. Yet, while I am changing my own views, I am merely taking an intellectual journey already charted by Garrod between the publication of his two books.

If a genetically-minded physician scientist can make the transition to believing that even Mendelian diseases are multifactorial, can clinicians make the transition to believe that common multifactorial diseases have important genetic determinants? It would change their view of patients and the causes of their diseases. Here are two further examples – just two of many – to illustrate the theme that the major gene by itself is not necessarily the disease.

Familial hypercholesterolaemia is a cause of atherosclerosis and ischaemic heart disease (Goldstein *et al.*, 1973). It is a disorder of the LDL receptor encoded at a locus on chromosome 19 and several mutant alleles account for loss of LDL receptor function among different pedigrees (Brown and Goldstein, 1986). The associated metabolic phenotype (hypercholesterolaemia) is dominantly inherited and there is a gene dosage effect which indicates the importance of LDL receptor activity in maintaining cholesterol homeostasis. The origin of LDL receptor mutations is a matter of interest (why are there so many?) and in French Canadians, among whom the frequency of familial hypercholesterolaemia is unusually high (≈ 0.005), about 60% of individuals with familial hypercholesterolaemia have one particular allele (Hobbs *et al.*, 1987; Jean Davignon, personal communication, 1988). Founder effect with spread from a centre of diffusion in Kamouraska county (Jomphe *et al.*, 1988; De Braekeleer *et al.*, 1988) explains distribution in the population of the particular allele, which is a 5' deletion affecting promoter and first exon with a null phenotype (Hobbs *et al.*, 1987; Y. Ma, C. Bétard, J. Davignon, A. H. Kessling, unpublished data, 1988). Despite apparent uniformity of the major cause of familial hypercholesterolaemia in the Quebec population, a survey of patients with the homozygous (or compound) familial hypercholesterolaemia phenotype in Quebec (Moorjani *et al.*, 1989) revealed considerable interindividual variation in age at onset and manifestations of their disease. One explanation for this finding might be allelic heterogeneity and indeed 40% of familial hypercholesterolaemia individuals in Quebec do not have the 'Kamouraska' deletion. The presence of additional determinants of phenotype is another and the evidence for it is compelling because even probands genetically homozygous for the Kamouraska deletion show remarkable heterogeneity of the associated clinical phenotype (Hobbs *et al.*, 1987). Accordingly, other genes that control components in the network of cholesterol homeostasis, constitutional factors that set thresholds for atherogenic processes and environmental factors are all real or potential determinants of the clinical phenotype (Table 4). Which determinants are acting in a particular person is of great clinical interest and to know them is to refine prognosis and treatment for the particular person who has inherited a familial hypercholesterolaemia allele.

Table 4   Some determinants of variation in the atherogenic phenotype associated with familial hypercholesterolaemia alleles in French Canadians

Genes	*Constitutional*	*Environmental*
Major		
Familial hypercholesterolaemia$_{Kamouraska}$[a]	age	socioeconomic
Other familial hypercholesterolaemia alleles[b]	sex	status
Modifier	other	education
Normal allele and/or haplotype at familial		occupation
hypercholesterolaemia locus		dietary habits
Apolipoprotein B-100		other habits
Apolipoprotein E polymorphism		geographic region
Activity of HMG CoA reductase and other		migration
catalysts of cholesterol synthesis		other
Lipoprotein (a) (Lp(a))		
HDL level and type		
Mitogens (e.g. PDGF A)		
Genes controlling triglyceride metabolism		
Other		

[a]A 5' deletion (Hobbs *et al.*, 1987) which accounts for 60% of familial hypercholesterolaemia alleles at the LDL receptor locus in French Canadians (Y. Ma, C. Bétard, J. Davignon, A. M. Kessling, unpublished data, 1988)
[b]40% of familial hypercholesterolaemia alleles in French Canadians are not the familial hypercholesterolaemia$_{Kamouraska}$ allele; two or three other alleles apparently account for most of these genes (Y. Ma *et al.*, unpublished data, 1988)

Muscular dystrophy is another illustration of the role of modifier genes. The dystrophin gene at the Xp21 locus has been cloned and alleles causing Duchenne and Becker forms of muscular dystrophy are being characterized. The difference between Duchenne and Becker muscular dystrophy phenotypes proves not to be the difference between frame-shift and in-frame deletions (Malhotra *et al.*, 1988), as others had proposed. Moreover, between families and even within families, similar deletions of exons 3–7 are phenotypically heterogeneous. This finding emphasizes the arbitrary nature of the classification of Duchenne and Becker muscular dystrophies (Malhotra *et al.*, 1988) and the mechanisms of phenotypic heterogeneity have to be found in secondary factors such as genetic background. Further studies of human Duchenne and Becker muscular dystrophies and of its inbred canine counterpart (Cooper *et al.*, 1988), in which there is interindividual variation between and even within litters, are awaited to explain the clinical variation in 'monoallelic' pedigrees.

CONCLUSION

We do not know what Garrod made of his 'molecular groupings' beyond his own commitment to the idea that 'the extreme complexity of the molecules of the proteins . . . makes it possible to imagine how chemical individuality can exist' (p. 44, *Inborn Factors*). About the existence of human 'chemical individuality' there is no longer doubt. That it has genetic determinants is now proven. That it can serve predictive medicine has already been exemplified in newborn screening for hyperphenylalaninaemia, for example. A dazzling array of molecular methods translates Garrod's inborn errors of metabolism, one by one, into phenotypes and genotypes that could not otherwise be known in such detail. Garrod's 'molecular groupings', in variant forms of interlocus hybrids, interallelic complementation and modifier genes acting in the mosaic of cellular reactions and fluxes, are more subtle determinants of chemical deviance than the inborn errors of metabolism. Their effects can be manifestations of heterozygosity which means they are probably prevalent and, if they confer predisposition to disease, they will constitute mechanisms that explain why 'inborn factors in disease' are common. All of which indicates that molecular geneticists and physiological geneticists must ultimately share their views of cause and pathogenesis of disease.

ACKNOWLEDGEMENTS

I thank the SSIEM for providing the occasion for this article and the talk that preceded it. I am grateful also to colleagues, notably Barton Childs, for exchange of ideas, and to Paul Goodyer who suggested 'that some ideas presented long ago at a seminar should be developed further'. Support from various granting agencies and supporters is greatly appreciated, as also is the help of Lynne Prevost in preparing the typescript.

REFERENCES

Akerman, B. Molecular studies of the alpha globin gene in Quebec populations. *MSc Thesis*, McGill University, 1987

Akerman, B. R., Lancaster, G. A. and Scriver, C. R. Alpha-thalassemia mutations are common in Quebec populations and they modify β-thalassemia gene expression. *Am. J. Hum. Genet.* (1987) A93

Aula, P., Nänto, V., Laipio, M.-L. and Autio, S. Aspartylglucosaminuria: deficiency of aspartylglucosaminidase in cultured fibroblasts of patients and their heterozygous parents. *Clin. Genet.* 4 (1973) 297

Bartholomé, K. Genetics and biochemistry of the phenylketonuria – present state. *Hum. Genet.* 51 (1979) 241–245

Bartholomé, K. and Dresel, A. Studies on the molecular defect in phenylketonuria and hyperphenylalaninemia using antibodies against phenylalanine hydroxylase. *J. Inher. Metab. Dis.* 5 (1982) 7–10

Beadle, G. W. Genes and chemical reactions in neurospora. *Science* 129 (1959) 1715–1719

Bearn, A. G. and Miller, E. D. Archibald Garrod and the development of the concept of inborn errors of metabolism. *Bull. Hist. Med.* 53 (1979) 315–328

Boright, A. P. Studies of prolidase deficiency in cultured skin fibroblasts. *Doctoral Thesis*, McGill University, 1988

Boright, A. P., Lancaster, G. A. and Scriver, C. R. A classification of rare alleles causing prolidase deficiency. *Am. J. Hum. Genet.* (1988) A3

Brown, M. S. and Goldstein, J. L. A receptor-mediated pathway for cholesterol homeostasis. *Science* 232 (1986) 34–47

Burgio, G. R. 'Inborn errors of metabolism' and 'chemical individuality', two ideas of Sir Archibald Garrod briefly revisited 50 years after his death. *Eur. J. Pediatr.* 145 (1986) 2–5

Childs, B. Sir Archibald Garrod's conception of chemical individuality: a modern appreciation. *N. Engl. J. Med.* 282 (1970) 71–77

Childs, B. Implications for disease of Sir Archibald Garrod's views on chemical individuality. In Wapnir, R. A. (ed.) *Congenital Metabolic Diseases Diagnosis and Treatment*, Marcel Dekker Inc., New York, 1985, pp. 3–11

Childs, B. Introduction to molecular genetics in medicine. *Progr. Med. Genet.* (new series) 7 (1988) 1–16

Childs, B. and Scriver, C. R. Age at onset and causes of disease. *Perspect. Biol. Med.* 29 (1986) 437–460

Christensen, E. and Brandt, N. J. Studies on glutaryl-CoA dehydrogenase in leucocytes, fibroblasts and amniotic fluid cells. The normal enzyme and the mutant form in patients with glutaric aciduria. *Clin. Chim. Acta.* 88 (1978) 267–276

Cooper, B. J., Winand, N. J., Stedman, H., Valentine, B. A., Hoffman, E. P., Kunkel, L. M., Scott, M.-O., Fischbeck, K. H., Kornegay, J. N., Avery, R. J., Williams, J. R., Schmickel, R. D. and Sylvester, J. E. The homologue of the Duchenne locus is defective in X-linked muscular dystrophy of dogs. *Nature (London)* 334 (1988) 154–156

Danks, D. M., Schlesinger, R., Firgaira, F., Cotton, R. G. H., Watson, B. M., Rembold, H. and Hennings, G. Malignant hyperphenylalaninemia – clinical features, biochemical findings, and experience with administration of biopterins. *Pediatr. Res.* 13 (1979) 1150–1155

De Braekeleer, M., Morgan, K., Jomphe, M., Buchard, G., Davignon, J., Kessling, A., Laberge, C., Moorjani, S., Roy, M. and Scriver, C. R. Familial hypercholesterolemia in French-Canadians: geographical distribution and centre of origin of an LDL-receptor deletion mutation. *SOREP* (Univ. du Qué. à Chicoutimi) (Document No. III-C-60 Oct.), 1988

Firgaira, F. A., Cotton, R. G. H. and Danks, D. M. Dihydropteridine reductase deficiency diagnosis by assay on peripheral blood-cells. *Lancet* 2 (1979) 1260–1263

Fleisher, L. D., Tallan, H. H., Bertis, H. G., Hirschhorn, K. and Gaull, G. E. Cystathionine synthase deficiency: heterozygote detection using cultured skin fibroblasts. *Biochem. Biophys. Res. Comun.* 55 (1973) 38–43

Garrod, A. E. *Inborn Errors of Metabolism:* The Croonian Lectures delivered before the Royal College of Physicians of London in June 1908. Frowde; Hodder and Stoughton, London, 1909

Garrod, A. E. The Huxley Lecture on diathesis. *Lancet* 2 (1927) 1113–1118

Garrod, A. E. *The Inborn Factors in Disease*, Oxford at the Clarendon Press, 1931

Gibson, K. M., Sweetman, L., Nyhan, W. L., Jansen, I. and Jaeken, J. Demonstration of 4-aminobutyric acid aminotransferase deficiency in lymphocytes and lymphoblasts. *J. Inher. Metab. Dis.* 8 (1985) 204–208

Goldstein, J. L., Hazzard, W. R., Schrott, H. G., Bierman, E. L., Motulsky, A. G., Levinski, M. J. and Campbell, E. D. Hyperlipidemia in coronary heart disease. I. Lipid levels in 500 survivors of myocardial infarction. *J. Clin. Invest.* 52 (1973) 1533–1543

Goodman, S. I. and Kohlhoff, J. G. Glutaric aciduria: inherited deficiency of glutaryl-CoA dehydrogenase activity. *Biochem. Med.* 13 (1975) 138–140

Grimm, U., Knapp, A., Schlenzka, K. and Hesse, R. Phenylalaninhydroxylase-aktivatät beiheterozygoten Anlageträgern für das Phenylketonurie-Gen. *Acta Biol. Med. Germ.* 36 (1977) 1179–1182

Harris, H. *The Principles of Human Biochemical Genetics*, 3rd edn, rev., Elsevier, New York, 1980, pp. 246–256

Harris, H., Hopkinson, D. A. and Edwards, Y. H. Polymorphism and the subunit structure of enzymes: a contribution to the neutralist selectionist controversy. *Proc. Natl. Acad. Sci. USA* 74 (1977) 697–701

Herskowitz, I. Functional inactivation of genes by dominant negative mutations. *Nature (London)* 329 (1987) 219–222

Hobbs, H. H., Brown, M. S., Russell, D. W., Davignon, J. and Goldstein, J. L. Deletion in the gene for the low-density-lipoprotein receptor in a majority of French Canadians with familial hypercholesterolemia. *N. Engl. J. Med.* 317 (1987) 734–737

Hopkins, F. G. Obituary – Sir Archibald Garrod. *Br. Med. J.* 1 (1936a) 775–776

Hopkins, F. G. Sir Archibald Garrod, KCMG, FRS. *Nature (London)* May 9 (1936b) 770–771

Hopkins, F. G. Obituaries of A. E. Garrod. *The Royal Society (Obituary Notices)* 2 (1938) 225–228

Johnson, W. G. Metabolic interference and the +-heterozygote. A hypothetical form of simple inheritance which is neither dominant nor recessive. *Am. J. Hum. Genet.* 32 (1980) 374–386

Jomphe, M., Bouchard, G., Davignon, J., De Braekeleer, M., Gradie, M., Kessling, A., Laberge, C., Moorjani, S., Morgan, K., Roy, M. and Scriver, C. R. Familial hypercholesterolemia in French-Canadians: geographical distribution and centre of origin of an LDL-receptor deletion mutation. *Am. J. Hum. Genet.* 43 (1988) A216

Kacser, H. and Burns, J. A. The molecular basis of dominance. *Genetics* 97 (1981) 639–666

Kanavakis, E., Wainscoat, J. S., Wood, W. G., Weatherall, D. J., Cao, A., Furbeta, M., Galanello, R., Georgiou, D. and Sophocleous, T. The interaction of α thalassemia with heterozygous β thalassemia. *Br. J. Haematal.* 52 (1982) 465

Kaplan, F., Akerman, B., Bardanis, M. and Scriver, C. R. The β-globin gene, a β-thalassemia allele and associated RFLP haplotypes in French-Canadians. *Am. J. Hum. Genet.* 43 (1988) A216

Kaufman, S., Max, E. E. and Kang, E. S. Phenylalanine hydroxylase activity in liver biopsies from hyperphenylalaninemia heterozygotes: deviation from proportionality with gene dosage. *Pediatr. Res.* 9 (1975) 632–634

King, L. S. *Medical Thinking. A Historial Preface*, Princeton University Press, Princeton, 1982, pp. 187–203

Lane, A. B. and Jenkins, T. Two variant hexosaminidase β-chain alleles segregating in a South African family. *Clin. Chim. Acta* 87 (1978) 219–228

Langenbeck, U., Lukas, H. D., Mench-Hoinowski, A., Stenzig, K. P. and Lane, J. D. Correlative study of mental and biochemical phenotypes in never treated patients with classic phenylketonuria. *Brain Dysfunction* 1 (1988) 103–110

Lowden, J. A. Evidence for a hybrid hexosaminidase isoenzyme in heterozygotes for Sandhoff disease. *Am. J. Hum. Genet.* 31 (1979) 281–289

Malhotra, S. B., Hart, K. A., Klamut, H. J., Thomas, S. T., Bodrug, S. E., Burghes, A. H. M., Bobrow, M., Harper, P. S., Thompson, M. W., Ray, P. N. and Worton, R. G. Frame-shift deletions in patients with Duchenne and Becker muscular dystrophy. *Science* 242 (1988) 755–759

Mayr, E. *The Growth of Biological Thought*. Harvard University Press, Cambridge, MA, 1982, pp. 63–64

Milstien, S., Holtzman, N. A., O'Flynn, M. E., Thomas, G. H., Butler, I. J. and Kaufman, S. Hyperphenylalaninemia due to dihydropteridine reductase deficiency. *J. Pediatr.* 89 (1976) 763–766

Moorjani, S., Roy, M., Gagné, C., Davignon, J., Brun, D., Toussaint, M., Lambert, M., Campeau, L., Blaichman, S. and Lupien, P. Homozygous familial hypercholesterolemia among French Canadians in Province of Quebec. *Arteriosclerosis* (1989) in press

Murphy, E. A. and Pyeritz, R. E. Homeostasis. VII. A conspectus. *Am. J. Med. Genet.* 24 (1986) 735–751

Needham, J. Frederick Gowland Hopkins. *Perspect. Biol. Med.* 6 (1962) 2–46

Ponzone, A., Guardamagna, O., Ferraris, S., Bracco, G., Niederwieser, A. and Cotton,

R. G. M. The mutations of dihydropteridine reductase deficiency. *Arch. Dis. Child.* 63 (1988) 154–157

Prévost, C., Laframboise, R., Bardanis, M., Clow, C., Lancaster, G., Desjardins, L., Cantin, F. and Scriver, C. R. Le gène de la β-thalassémie au Canada français: relance dans le comté de Portneuf. *L'Union Méd. du Can.* 18 (1988) 141–144

Rosatelli, C., Falchi, A. M., Scalas, M. T., Tuveri, T., Furbetta, M. and Cao, A. Hematological phenotype of double heterozygous state for alpha and beta thalassemia. *Hemoglobin* 8 (1984) 25

Rose, G. Sick individuals and sick populations. *Int. J. Epidemiol.* 14 (1985) 32–38

Salter, M., Knowles, R. G. and Pogson, C. I. Quantification of the importance of individual steps in the control of aromatic amino acid metabolism. *Biochem. J.* 234 (1986) 635–647

Scriver, C. R. Window panes of eternity. Health, disease, and inherited risk. *Yale J. Biol. Med.* 55 (1982a) 487–513

Scriver, C. R. Screening for medical intervention: the PKU experience. In Human Genetics, Part B. Medical aspects. *Prog. Clin. Biol. Res.* 103B (1982b) 437–445

Scriver, C. R. The Canadian Rutherford lecture: an evolutionary view of disease in man. *Proc. R. Soc. Lond. B.* 220 (1984) 273–298

Scriver, C. R. Inborn errors of metabolic homeostasis: Garrod's message revisited. In Wapnir, R. A. (ed.) *Congenital Metabolic Diseases and Treatment*, Marcel Dekker, New York, 1985, pp. 11–40

Scriver, C. R. Presidential Address: Physiological genetics – Who needs it? *Am. J. Hum. Genet.* 40 (1987) 199–211

Scriver, C. R. and Childs, B. *Garrod's Inborn Factors in Disease*, Oxford Monographs in Medical Genetics, 16, Oxford University Press, Oxford, 1989

Scriver, C. R. and Rosenberg, L. E. *Amino Acid Metabolism and its Disorders*, Saunders, Philadelphia, 1973, pp. 290–337

Scriver, C. R., Bardanis, M, Cartier, L., Clow, C. L., Lancaster, G. A. and Ostrowsky, J. T. β-thalassemia disease prevention: genetic medicine applied. *Am. J. Hum. Genet.* 36 (1984) 1024–1038

Scriver, C. R., Gregory, D. M., Sovetts, D. and Tissenbaum, G. Normal plasma free amino acid values in adults: the influence of some common physiological variables. *Metabolism* 34 (1985) 868–873

Scriver, C. R., Clow, C. L., Kaplan, P. and Niederwieser, A. Hyperphenylalaninemia due to deficiency of 6-pyruvoyl tetrahydropterin synthase. Unusual gene dosage effect in heterozygotes. *Hum. Genet.* 77 (1987a) 168–171

Scriver, C. R., Mahon, B., Levy, H. L., Clow, C. L., Reade, T. M., Kronick, J., Lemieux, B. and Laberge, C. The Hartnup phenotype: Mendelian transport disorder, multifactorial disease. *Am. J. Hum. Genet.* 40 (1987b) 401–412

Sober, E. *The Nature of Selection. Evolutionary Theory in Philosophical Focus*, MIT Press, Cambridge, MA, 1984, pp. 278–281

Takikawa, S.-I., Curtius, H.-C., Redweik, U., Leimbacher, W. and Ghisla, S. Biosynthesis of tetrahydrobiopterin. Purification and characterization of 6-pyruvoyl tetrahydropterin synthase from human liver. *Eur. J. Biochem.* 161 (1986) 296–302

Vogel, F. Clinical consequences of heterozygosity for autosomal-recessive diseases. *Clin. Genet.* 25 (1984) 381–415

Weatherall, D. J., Clegg, J. B., Higgs, D. R. and Wood, W. G. The hemoglobinopathies. In Scriver, C. R., Beaudet, A., Sly, W. L. and Valle, D. (eds.) *The Metabolic Basis of Inherited Disease*, 6th edition, McGraw Hill Book Co., New York, 1989, pp. 2281–2340

Whelan, D. T., Hill, R., Ryan, E. D. and Spate, M. L-glutaric acidemia: investigation of a patient and his family. *Pediatrics* 63 (1979) 88–93

Williams, R. J. Biochemical individuality. The basis for the genetotrophic concept. *Science Edition*, J. Wiley and Son, New York, 1963

Zannis-Hadjopoulos, M., Gold, R. J. M., Maag, U. R., Metrakos, J. D. and Scriver, C. R. Improved detection of β-thalassemia carriers by a two-test method. *Hum. Genet* 38 (1977) 315–324

J. Inher. Metab. Dis. 12 Suppl. 1 (1989) 25–41

Clinical Approach to Inherited Metabolic Diseases in the Neonatal Period: A 20-year Survey

J. M. Saudubray[1], H. Ogier[1], J. P. Bonnefont[1], A. Munnich[1],
A. Lombes[1], F. Hervé[1], G. Mitchel[1], B. Poll Thé[1], N. Specola[1],
P. Parvy[2], J. Bardet[2], D. Rabier[2], M. Coudé[2], C. Charpentier[2] and
J. Frézal[1]

[1]*Département de Pédiatrie, Clinique et Unité de Recherches de génétique Médicale, INSERM U-12;* [2]*Laboratoire de Biochimie, P. Kamoun, Hôpital des Enfants-Malades, 149, rue de Sèvres, 75743 Paris Cedex 15, France*

Summary: Every newborn with unexplained neurological deterioration, ketosis, metabolic acidosis or hypoglycaemia should be suspected of having an inherited error of intermediary metabolism. Many of these conditions can be diagnosed clinically with the aid of simple laboratory investigations. Since a substantial number of these diseases respond well to treatment but may otherwise be fatal, and in order to assure adequate prenatal diagnosis in subsequent pregnancies, a high index of suspicion and rapid diagnosis are necessary in the face of the clinical presentations described. According to three major clinical presentations observed in 218 neonates with inborn errors of intermediary metabolism (neurological distress 'intoxication' type, neurological distress 'energy deficiency' type and hypoglycaemia with liver dysfunction) and according to the proper use of few laboratory investigations, we propose a method of diagnosis which groups these children into five categories. Initial therapy, and sophisticated investigations can be planned on the basis of this grouping.

Inherited metabolic diseases have become a major cause of neonatal pathology, as the classical causes of neonatal distress have been markedly diminished by advances in obstetrical, prenatal and perinatal management. Their incidence may well be underestimated as diagnostic errors are frequent. Nevertheless, accurate diagnosis is essential in order to provide genetic counselling and prenatal diagnosis of subsequent pregnancies and especially because some of these conditions have an excellent response to therapy (Saudubray *et al.*, 1984).

Inborn errors of metabolism are individually rare but are collectively numerous. Many of them present early in the neonatal period, have a rapid fatal course and, as a whole, cannot be recognized through systematic screening tests which are too

Published in Czech as a translation in *J. Československá Pediatrie* 44 (1989)

Journal of Inherited Metabolic Disease. ISSN 0141–8955. Copyright © SSIEM and Kluwer Academic Publishers, PO Box 55, Lancaster, UK.

slow, too expensive and unreliable. This makes it an absolute necessity to teach primary care physicians a simple method of clinical screening before making decisions about sophisticated biochemical investigations. Clinical diagnosis of inborn errors of metabolism in the newborn infant may at times be difficult. This is at least partly due to four reasons:

(1) Many physicians think that, because individual inborn errors are rare, they should be considered only after more common conditions like sepsis have been excluded.

(2) In view of the large number of inborn errors, it might appear that their diagnosis requires precise knowledge of a large number of biochemical pathways and their inter-relationships. As a matter of fact an adequate diagnostic approach can be based on the proper use of only a few tests.

(3) The neonate has an apparently limited repertoire of responses to severe overwhelming illness and the predominant clinical signs and symptoms are non-specific: poor feeding, lethargy, failure to thrive, etc. It is certain that many patients with such defects succumb in the newborn period without having received a specific diagnosis, death often having been attributed to sepsis or some other common causes.

(4) Classical autopsy findings in such cases are often non-specific and unrevealing. Infection is often suspected as the cause of the death, whereas sepsis is the common accompaniment of metabolic disorders.

Within the last decade, a number of reviews have attempted to given an overview on diagnosis and management of inborn errors of metabolism in the neonatal period, mostly based on the literature (Ampola, 1976; Nyhan, 1977; Aleck and Shapiro, 1978; Goodman, 1986; Burton and Nadler, 1978; Burton, 1987). Since 1968, a total of 218 newborns with inborn errors of intermediary metabolism, presenting with acute symptoms within the first month of life, have been evaluated by the metabolic and genetics service at Hôpital des Enfants Malades, Paris (Table 1). From this experience, a method of initial clinical evaluation and management has been developed. Acute neonatal forms of inherited errors of intermediary metabolism can be diagnosed or strongly suspected and assigned to one of five schematical bioclinical groups on the basis of the clinical history, physical examination, and readily available laboratory tests. Prospectively this method has proved to be a useful clinical tool in the approach to ill newborns.

'INTOXICATIONS' AND 'ENERGY DEFICIENCIES'

As far as physiopathology is concerned, most inborn errors of intermediary metabolism revealed in the neonatal period fall schematically into the two categories: 'intoxications' and 'energy deficiencies'.

Intoxications: These are diseases which lead to an acute or progressive intoxication secondary to an accumulation of toxic compounds proximal to the metabolic block. Maple syrup urine disease is an intoxication due to branched chain keto-acids and amino acids). Most organic acidurias (methylmalonic, propionic and isovaleric

Table 1 Inborn errors of intermediary metabolism: Hôpital Enfants-Malades 1968-1987

	Neonatal	*Total*	*Group Total*
A. Aminoacidopathies			102
Maple syrup urine disease	26	35	
Non-ketotic hyperglycinaemia	23	24	
Homocystinuria (classic+variants)	5	25	
Sulphite oxidase	8	9	
Others (tyrosinaemia types I and II)	4	9	
B. Organic acidurias			88
Methylmalonic aciduria	20	31	
Propionic aciduria	17	21	
Isovaleric aciduria	12	14	
Multicarboxylase defects	0	11	
Others (glutaric aciduria type I, pyroglutamic aciduria, ketolysis defects)	2	11	
C. Hyperammonaemias			68
Ornithine transcarbamylase deficiency	16	32	
Citrullinaemia	15	16	
Others (arginosuccinate lyase deficiency, carbamyl phosphate synthetase deficiency, triple H syndrome)	16	20	
D. Respiratory chain, hyperlactacidaemias			39
Respiratory chain	18	25	
Others (pyruvate dehydrogenase deficiency, pyruvate carboxylase deficiency, Krebs cycle disorders)	11	14	
E. Glycogenosis–gluconeogenesis (glucose-6-phosphatase deficiency, fructose diphosphatase deficiency, glycogen storage disease types III and VI)	11	27	27
F. Fatty acid oxidation (idiopathic systemic carnitine deficiency, palmitoyl carnitine transferase deficiency, multiple acyl-CoA dehydrogenase deficiency, medium and long-chain acyl-CoA dehydrogenase deficiency)	3	27	27
G. Peroxisomal disorders (Zellweger syndrome and variants, pipecolic acidaemia)	11	15	15
TOTAL	218	326	

acidurias), congenital urea cycle defects (hepatic and cerebral ammonia intoxication), galactosaemia, fructosaemia and tyrosinaemia all belong to this first group. All the conditions in this group present clinical similarities including a symptom-free interval between birth and onset of the illness, clinical signs of 'intoxication' (vomiting, lethargy, coma, liver failure) and frequent humoral disturbances (acidosis, ketosis, hyperammonaemia). Treatment of these disorders requires toxin removal (blood exchange transfusion, peritoneal dialysis, special diets, etc.).

Energy deficiencies: In this second category are the diseases in which symptoms are at least partly due to a deficiency in the energy production or utilization processes arising from defects in liver, myocardium, muscle or brain. Gluconeo-genesis defects, congenital lactic acidaemias (pyruvate carboxylase and pyruvate dehydrogenase deficiencies), fatty acid oxidation defects, mitochondrial respiratory disorders and inborn errors of peroxisomal metabolism belong to this group. These diseases present an overlapping clinical spectrum which sometimes also results, in part, from the accumulation of toxic compounds in addition to the deficiency in energy production. Frequent symptoms common to this group include hyperlactacidaemia, severe generalized hypotonia, cardiomyopathy, failure to thrive, heart failure, circulatory collapse, sudden infant death syndrome and malformations, suggesting that the abnormal processes affect the fetal energy producing pathways. Treatment of these disorders, if one exists, require adequate energy replacement.

IDENTIFICATION OF CHILDREN AT RISK

As already stated, the neonate has a limited repertoire of responses to severe illness and at first glance presents with unspecific symptoms such as a respiratory disorder, hypotonia, poor sucking reflex, vomiting, dehydration, lethargy or seizures – all symptoms easily attributable to infection or some other common cause. Sometimes the severity of vomiting associated with abdominal distension can mimic pyloric stenosis or intestinal obstruction. A family history of unexplained neonatal death may be present as may be a history of parental consanguinity. However, in day-to-day practice this is rather rare. Although most genetic metabolic errors are autoso-mal recessive, a large number of cases appear to be sporadic because of the small size of sibships in developed countries. If present, death of affected siblings may have been falsely attributed to sepsis, heart failure or intraventricular haemorrhage and it will be important to review clinical records and autopsy reports critically when these are available. However, all neonatal sibling deaths should be considered as suspect. A highly typical clinical setting is the course of a full-term baby born after a normal pregnancy and delivery who, after an initial symptom-free period during which he is entirely normal, undergoes a relentless deterioration which has no apparent cause and which is unresponsive to symptomatic therapy. The interval between birth and clinical symptoms may range from hours to weeks, depending on the nature of the metabolic block and environment. In organic acidaemias and urea cycle defects the interval is not necessarily correlated to protein feeding.

The regular investigations in all these sick neonates, including chest X-ray, CSF examination, bacteriological studies and cerebral ultrasound yield normal results. This unexpected and 'mysterious' deterioration of a child after a normal initial period is the most important signal of the presence of an inherited disease of the intoxication type. If present, a careful re-evaluation of the child is warranted. Signs previously interpreted as non-specific manifestations of neonatal hypoxia, infection or other common diagnoses take on new significance in this context.

Neurological deterioration is the main way in which these diseases come to medical attention. The initial symptom-free interval varies in duration amongst the different conditions. Typically the first reported sign is poor sucking and diminished feeding, after which the child sinks into an unexplained coma despite supportive measures. At a more advanced stage neurovegetative problems with respiratory disorders, hiccough, apnoeas, bradycardia and hypothermia can appear. Investigations for common causes of neurological distress are normal. In the comatose state, many of these conditions have characteristic changes in muscle tone and involuntary movements. Generalized hypertonic episodes with opisthotonus are frequent and boxing or pedalling movements as well as slow limb elevations, spontaneous or upon stimulation, are observed. Most non-metabolic causes of coma are associated with hypotonia, and the presence of 'normal' peripheral muscle tone in a comatose child reflects a relative hypertonia. Another suggestive neurological pattern is axial hypotonia and limb hypertonia with large amplitude tremors and myoclonic jerks which are often mistaken for convulsions. In contrast, true convulsions occur late and inconsistently in inborn errors of intermediary metabolism. Newborns with the conditions discussed in this report rarely if ever experience seizures in the absence of pre-existing stupor or coma, or hypoglycaemia. The EEG often shows a periodic pattern in which bursts of intense activity alternate with nearly flat segments.

An abnormal urine and body odour is present in some diseases in which volatile metabolites accumulate. The most important examples are the maple syrup odour of maple syrup urine disease and the sweaty feet odour of isovaleric acidaemia and type II glutaric acidaemia. If one of the preceding risk factors is present, metabolic disorders should be given high diagnostic priority and should be investigated simultaneously with other diagnostic considerations.

In energy deficiency, the clinical presentation is less evocative and displays a more variable severity. In many conditions there is no symptom-free interval. The most frequent symptoms are severe generalized hypotonia, hypertrophic cardiomyopathy, rapidly progressive neurologic deterioration and possible dysmorphia or malformations. However, in contrast to the intoxication group, lethargy and coma are rarely early signs. Hyperlactacidaemia with or without metabolic acidosis is a very frequent symptom.

A last group of patients presents evidence of hypoglycaemia, liver dysfunction and hepatomegaly. This association strongly suggests the diagnosis of gluconeogenesis defects, galactosaemia, fructosaemia in case of fructose containing diet, tyrosinaemia type I or α_1-antitrypsin deficiency.

Initial approach

The initial approach is set out in Table 2. Once clinical suspicion is aroused, general supportive measures and laboratory investigations must be undertaken immediately. Abnormal urine odours can best be detected on a drying filter paper

Table 2 Initial investigations

Urine	Smell
	Acetone
	Reducing substances
	Ketotacids (dinitrophenylhydrazine test)
	Sulphites (Sulfitest, Merck)
	pH
Blood	Blood cell count
	Electrolytes (look for anion gap)
	Calcium
	Glucose
	Blood gases (pH, Pco_2, HCO_3, Po_2)
	Ammonia
	Lactic acid and pyruvic acid
	3-hydroxy butyrate, acetoacetate
	Uric acid
Store at $-20°C$	Urine (as much possible)
	Heparinized plasma, 2–5 mL
	Do not freeze whole blood!
	CSF, 0.5–1.0 mL
Miscellaneous	EEG, bacteriological samples,
	chest X-ray, lumbar puncture,
	cardiac echography,
	cerebral ultrasound

or by opening a container of urine which has been closed and left at room temperature for a few minutes. Although serum ketone bodies reach 0.5–1 mmol L^{-1} in early neonatal life, acetonuria is an important sign of a metabolic disease and is rarely if ever observed in a normal newborn (Settergren *et al.*, 1976; Saudubray *et al.*, 1987). Its presence is always abnormal in neonates. The dinitrophenylhydrazine test screens for the presence of α-keto acids such as are seen in maple syrup urine disease and can be considered significant only in the absence of glucose and acetone in the urine which also react with dinitrophenyl-hydrazine. Hypocalcaemia and elevated or reduced blood glucose are frequently present in metabolic diseases. The physician should be wary of attributing marked neurological dysfunction merely to these findings.

The metabolic acidosis of organic acidurias is usually accompanied by an elevated anion gap. Urine pH should be below 5.5, otherwise renal acidosis is a consideration. Plasma ammonia and lactic acid concentrations should be determined systematically in newborns at risk. An elevated plasma ammonia concentration by itself can induce respiratory alkalosis; hyperammonaemia with ketoacidosis suggests an underlying organic acidaemia. Elevated plasma lactic acid concentrations in the absence of infection or tissue hypoxia are a significant finding. We have often observed moderate elevations (3–6 mmol L^{-1}) in organic acidaemias and in the hyperammonaemias; concentrations of plasma lactate greater than 10 mmol L^{-1} are frequent in hypoxia. A normal blood pH does not exclude hyperlactacidaemia as neutrality is usually maintained until levels of $5\,mmol\,L^{-1}$ are present. It is important to measure as often as necessary lactate, pyruvate, 3-hydroxybutyrate and acetoacetate on a plasma sample immediately deproteinized at the bedside, in order to assess cytoplasmic and mitochondrial redox states through the measurement of lactate:pyruvate and 3-hydroxybutyrate:acetoacetate ratios, respectively. Some organic acidurias induce granulocytopenia and thrombopenia, which may be mistaken for sepsis.

The storage of adequate amounts of plasma, urine and CSF is an important element in diagnosis. The utilization of these precious samples should be carefully planned after taking advice from specialists in inborn errors of metabolism. Although not available in most hospital laboratories, some sophisticated investigations such as amino acid or organic acid chromatography are available in many places. It is important to insist, however, that any reference laboratory used for this purpose should not only provide prompt test results and reference ranges but also provide interpretation of abnormal results (Burton, 1987).

If the child dies, adequate diagnosis is nonetheless important in order to perform adequate genetic counselling. A postmortem protocol for the diagnosis of genetic disease has been proposed by Kronick and colleagues (1983) which includes the taking of urine and serum samples, fibroblast culture (premortem if possible) and muscle and liver biopsies (three or more one centimetre cubes of each, stored frozen on dry ice or in liquid nitrogen).

Once the above clinical and laboratory data have been assembled, specific therapeutic recommendations can be made. This process can be complete within 2 or 3 h and often eliminates long waiting periods for sophisticated diagnostic results. On the basis of this evaluation, most patients can be classified into five groups (Table 3).

CLINICAL PRESENTATION OF METABOLIC DISEASES: APPROACH TO AETIOLOGIES

According to the three major clinical presentations (neurological distress 'intoxication' type, neurological distress 'energy deficiency' type, and hypoglycaemia with liver dysfunction) and according to the proper use of the laboratory data described above most patients can be assigned to one of five schematic syndromes (Table 3). In our experience type I (maple syrup urine disease), type II (organic acidurias), type IVa (urea cycle defects) and non-ketotic hyperglycinaemia (the most common disease in type IVb) make up more than 65% of the newborn infants with inborn errors of intermediary metabolism. The experienced clinician will of course have to interpret the metabolic data carefully especially in relation to the time when they were collected and the treatments which were used. In the following tables most if not all of the biological data were collected before or very early after the beginning of symptomatic treatment (glucose or bicarbonate infusion). It is important to insist on the need to collect at the same time all the biological data listed in Table 2. Some very significant symptoms (such as metabolic acidosis and especially ketosis) can be moderate and transient, largely depending on

Table 3   Five neonatal types of inherited metabolic distress

Types	Clinical symptoms	Acidosis	Ketosis	Hyperlact-acidaemia	Hyperam-monaemia	Most frequent diagnoses
I	Neurological distress	0	+	0	0	Maple syrup urine disease
II	Neurological distress	+	+	0	+	Organic acidurias
III	Neurological distress	+	+	+	0	Congenital lactic acidaemias
IVA	Neurological distress	0	0	0	+	Urea cycle defects
IVB	Neurological distress	0	0	0	0	Non-ketotic hyperglycinaemia, sulphite oxidase deficiency Peroxisomal disorders Respiratory chain defects
V	Hepatomegaly Liver dysfunction Seizures	+	+	+	0	Gluconeogenesis defects Galactosaemia Tyrosinaemia type I α_1-Antitrypsin deficiency

the symptomatic therapy. Conversely, at an advanced state, many non-specific abnormalities (such as respiratory acidosis, severe hyperlactacidaemia and secondary hyperammonaemia) can disturb the primitive purity of the biological pattern.

Type I: Neurological distress 'intoxication' type with ketosis

Maple syrup urine disease is one of the commonest aminoacidopathies (26 of our 218 patients, Table 1). The main symptoms of our patients with maple syrup urine disease are listed in Table 4. After a symptom-free interval of 4 to 5 days, feeding difficulties develop and the child gradually becomes comatose. Generalized hypertonic episodes with opisthotonus and boxing and pedalling movements as well as slow limb elevations are constant. A maple syrup odour is present and the urine dinitrophenylhydrazine test is strongly positive whereas urine tests for acetone may be negative. None of our patients with maple syrup urine disease had an initial blood pH less than 7.30. The diagnosis is confirmed by serum amino acid chromatography which displays an elevation of the branched-chain amino acids leucine (usually higher than $2 \, \text{mmol} \, \text{L}^{-1}$), valine, isoleucine and the presence of alloisoleucine.

Type II: Neurological distress 'intoxication type' with ketoacidosis

The main diseases in this group are methylmalonic acidaemia, propionic acidaemia, and isovaleric acidaemia (Tanaka and Rosenberg, 1983; Rosenberg, 1983; Matsui et al., 1983). We have observed 49 neonates with such diseases, 43 of them are

Table 4 Neonatal neurological distress type I and II: Clinical presentation before treatment in 69 patients

	Maple syrup urine disease (n = 26)	Methyl-malonic aciduria (n = 18)	Propionic aciduria (n = 15)	Isovaleric aciduria (n = 10)
Symptom-free period (days)[ab]	5 (3–8)	2.9 (1.5–6)	2.1 (0.25–4)	3.7 (1–9)
Feeding refusal	100	61	100	100
Coma	100	100	100	100
Hypertonia and abnormal movements	100	100	93	90
Ketosis	100	83	87	100
Dehydration (% loss of body weight)[a]	15 (7%±4)	100 (14%±4)	100 (13%±2)	20 (10%)
Acidosis (pH <7.30)	0	94	87	90
Hyperammonaemia (>100 μmol L^{-1})	19	100	100	100
Actual values in all patients [ab]	118 (89–135)	380 (165–750)	350 (165–810)	360 (145–780)
Hypocalcaemia (<1.7 mmol L^{-1})	0	72	73	70
Actual values in all patients[a]	—	1.53±0.14	1.59±0.2	1.58±0.3

Data are expressed as the percentage of *n* the total number of patients; [a]means (±SD, where shown); [b]ranges in parentheses

presented in Table 4. Between the ages of 1 and 4 days, these children develop feeding difficulties and deteriorate into a coma over hours to days. In contrast to maple syrup urine disease, these patients are acutely ill, dehydrated, acidotic with an increased anion gap and they are often hypothermic. The usual approach to such patients is first to exclude adrenogenital syndrome by carefully checking serum electrolytes, searching for high potassium and low sodium concentrations. Truncal hypotonia and peripheral hypertonia are seen but large amplitude tremors are the dominant abnormal movement. In isovaleric acidaemia, a potent 'sweaty feet' odour is present. The urine in the acute phase is positive for ketones but this highly significant sign can be transient. Neutropenia and thrombocytopenia are also commonly observed and can contribute to the confusion with sepsis. Hyperammon-aemia, sometimes as high as that observed in urea cycle defects, is a constant finding (Cathelineau *et al.*, 1981; MacKenzie, 1983). Moderate hypocalcaemia is also frequent. In some patients we have observed severe hyperglycaemia (greater than 15 mmol L^{-1}) with glycosuria before treatment with glucose. These data associated with dehydration and ketoacidosis can suggest neonatal diabetes. The metabolic acidosis and other humoral disturbances observed in organic acidaemias may have adverse consequences on many different organ systems and may lead to a variety of erroneous diagnoses (Burton, 1987).

In addition to methylmalonic, propionic and isovaleric acidurias, a large number of rare organic acidurias, presenting usually with neurological distress and metabolic acidosis, have been described in recent years as organic acid analysis techniques have become more available and reliable (Chalmers and Lawson, 1982). Among them, glutaric aciduria type II or multiple acyl-CoA dehydrogenase deficiency (Goodman *et al.*, 1987) and hydroxymethylglutaryl-CoA lyase deficiency (Wysocki and Hähnel, 1986) have many similarities with methylmalonic, propionic and isovaleric acidurias except that ketosis is absent and hypoglycaemia is frequent. Patients, with multiple acyl-CoA dehydrogenase deficiency have a 'sweaty feet' odour similar to that seen in isovaleric aciduria, severe lactic acidosis and can have congenital defects (Goodman *et al.*, 1987). Other very rare conditions in this group are succinyl-CoA transferase deficiency (Tildon and Cornblath, 1972; Saudubray *et al.*, 1987), biotin-dependent multiple carboxylase defects due to holoenzyme synthetase deficiency (Burri *et al.*, 1981), short-chain fatty acyl-CoA dehydrogenase deficiency (Amendt *et al.*, 1987), 3-methyl-crotonyl-CoA carboxylase deficiency (Tanaka and Rosenberg, 1983), 3-methylglutaconicuria (Divry *et al.*, 1987) and glycerol kinase deficiency (Francke *et al.*, 1987). On the other hand, from the literature and from our personal experience, organic acidurias such as 3-ketothiolase deficiency (Saudubray *et al.*, 1987), biotin-responsive biotinidase deficiency (Wolf *et al.*, 1983), medium-chain and long-chain acyl-CoA dehydrogenase deficiency and glutaric aciduria type I rarely present, if ever, in the neonatal period (Stanley, 1987; Vianey-Liaud *et al.*, 1987). Pyroglutamic aciduria is a rare condition which can start in the first days of life with a severe metabolic acidosis but without ketosis, or abnormalities of blood glucose, lactate and ammonia. There are no severe neurological signs and the clinical picture mimics renal tubular acidosis.

The final diagnosis of all these organic acidurias is made by identifying specific abnormal metabolites by gas chromatography–mass spectrometry of blood and urine. Free carnitine plasma concentrations are always decreased, with abnormal excretion of specific acylcarnitines. By contrast, plasma and urine amino acid chromatography are often normal or non-specific with, for example, a profile showing a slight increase in glycine.

Type III: Lactic acidosis with neurological distress 'energy deficiency' type

The clinical presentation of these children is very diverse. Unlike the previous disease category in which moderate acidosis is noted during the evaluation of an acutely ill comatose child, the main medical presentation in group III patients is the acidosis itself, which clinically may be surprisingly well tolerated. However, the acidosis can at times be mild. Blood pH is usually normal until lactate concentrations of $5\,\mathrm{mmol\,L^{-1}}$ are reached. An elevated anion gap exists, which can be explained in part by the presence of equimolar amounts of lactic acid in the blood. Often the acidosis recurs soon after bicarbonate therapy, in the absence of adequate treatment.

If a high lactic acid concentration is found, it is urgent to rule out readily treatable causes especially hypoxia. Ketosis is present in most of the primary lactic acidaemias but is absent in acidosis secondary to tissue hypoxia. Biotin-responsive multiple carboxylase deficiency may present as lactic acidosis and biotin therapy is indicated in all patients with lactic acidosis of unknown cause after baseline blood and urine samples are taken. Primary lactic acidoses form a complex group (Robinson and Sherwood, 1984). A definite diagnosis is often elusive and is attempted with specific enzyme assays and by considering metabolite levels, redox potential states and fluxes under fasting and fed conditions. Defects most frequently demonstrated are pyruvate carboxylase deficiency, pyruvate dehydrogenase deficiency, respiratory chain disorders (complex I and IV), and multiple carboxylase deficiency which has already been discussed with group II diseases. Many cases remain unexplained. The pyruvate carboxylase deficiencies which we have investigated have had a stereotypic biochemical pattern with an elevated lactate:pyruvate ratio contrasting with a reduced 3-hydroxybutyrate:acetoacetate ratio, moderate citrullinaemia and hyperammonaemia and hepatic dysfunction. This pattern has been called 'French phenotype' by Robinson (Robinson *et al.*, 1987). Respiratory chain disorders are frequently observed in the neonatal period. Since the early descriptions (Van Biervliet *et al.*, 1977), a number of cases have been described (Di Mauro *et al.*, 1987). During the last 3 years, we have investigated 18 patients with respiratory chain defects in our clinic. The most frequent symptoms were severe generalized hypotonia, cardiomyopathy of hypertrophic type, rapid neurological deterioration, respiratory failure and severe lactic acidaemia. Some patients displayed facial dysmorphia and malformations, as has also been observed in infants with a deficiency of the pyruvate dehydrogenase complex (Nyhan and Sakati, 1987; Clayton and Thompson, 1988).

Type IVa: Neurological distress 'intoxication type' with hyperammonaemia and without ketoacidosis: Urea cycle defects

As mentioned above this group of patients is one of the most important among neonatal inborn errors of metabolism. We have investigated 47 neonates with these disorders, 44 of them are presented in Table 5. Primary hyperammonaemias due to urea cycle defects have a variable symptom-free interval, sometimes only a matter of hours. A brief hypertonic period and hiccoughs may occur, after which a profound hypotonic coma rapidly develops and cardiocirculatory function may be compromised. Coagulation factor depletion, elevated serum aminotransferases and hepatomegaly are frequent. The blood ammonia rises precipitously to levels of $400–2000\,\mu mol\,L^{-1}$ or more. Respiratory alkalosis (pH>7.40) and moderate hyperlactacidaemia are frequently observed. An important diagnostic clue to separate urea cycle defects from organic acidurias with hyperammonaemia is the universal absence of ketonuria.

The two principal urea cycle disorders, which have non-diagnostic amino acid chromatograms are ornithine transcarbamylase deficiency and carbamyl phosphate synthetase deficiency. The former is the only sex-linked congenital hyperammonaemia, the others being autosomal recessive. Massive orotic acid excretion is present and blood citrulline is very low. Carbamyl phosphate synthetase deficiency is initially detected by the negative findings of a non-specific amino acid chromatogram

Table 5 Neonatal neurological distress type IVA: urea cycle defects. Clinical presentation in 41 patients

	Ornithine trans-carbamylase deficiency ($n = 16$)	Carbamyl phosphate synthetase deficiency ($n = 10$)	Citrullinaemia ($n = 15$)
Symptom-free period (days)[a]	2.9	1.9	2.8
	(1.5–7)	(1–3)	(0–8)
Age at diagnosis (days)[a]	4	3	5
	(0.3–15)	(2–4)	(2–10)
Feeding refusal	50	40	53
Coma	100	100	100
Hypertonia and abnormal movements	80	80	60
Seizures	60	100	87
Ketosis	0	0	13
Respiratory alkalosis (pH>7.40)	69	80	73
Hyperlacticacidaemia (>2.5 mmol L^{-1})	69	60	87
Actual elevated plasma lactate values[a]	5	9	7
	(3–8)	(5–17)	(3–13)
Plasma ammonia values (μmol L^{-1})[a]	563	1150	1280
	(247–1200)	(490–2575)	(355–3114)
Interval between first symptom and coma (h)	18	20	29
	(9–24)	(10–30)	(0–72)

Data expressed as percentage of n the total number of patients: [a]means with ranges in parentheses

and the absence of orotic acid excretion. Enzyme diagnosis by liver biopsy is the only definitive diagnostic technique. Citrullinaemia, arginosuccinic aciduria and argininaemia are diagnosed by amino acid chromatography which demonstrates the accumulation of citrulline, arginosuccinate and arginine, respectively (MacKenzie, 1983). In the 'triple H' syndrome, hyperammonaemia, hyperornithinaemia and homocitrullinuria are present. An especially important diagnostic consideration is transient hyperammonaemia of the neonate, in which the patient, often premature and having mild respiratory distress syndrome, develops a deep coma and severe hyperammonaemia, which disappears permanently if initial treatment is successful (Ballard *et al.*, 1978).

Type IVb: Neurological distress 'energy deficiency' type without ketoacidosis and without hyperammonaemia

In our current experience the most frequent diseases in this type are non-ketotic hyperglycinaemia, sulphite oxidase deficiency and inborn errors of peroxisomal metabolism. In addition, some patients with respiratory chain disorders can present in the neonatal period without evidence of lactic acidosis. Beside these four disorders, an increasing number of other rare conditions has been described in recent years and we can assume that the list of disorders of this group will expand dramatically in the near future. A provisional classification of these disorders,

Table 6 Neonatal neurological distress: Provisional classification of type IV B

1. Energy deficiences:
   respiratory chain disorders
   peroxisomal disorders
   fatty acid oxidation disorders

2. Neurotransmitters defects:
   glycine (non-ketotic hyperglycinaemia, D-glyceraciduria)
   GABA (transaminase, 4-hydroxybutyric aciduria)
   DOPA, serotonin (biopterin synthesis deficiencies)

3. Disturbed metabolism of complex lipids:
   plasmalogen (peroxisomal disorders)
   acylcholesterol, dolichol
   mevalonic, 3-hydroxy glutaconic acidurias, cytoplasmic 3-ketothiolase deficiency

4. Intracellular vitamin disturbances:
   folic acid, B_{12}, B_6, etc.

5. Metals
   molybdenum (sulphite oxidase deficiency)
   copper (Menkes disease)

6. Others

based upon their hypothetical physiopathology is presented in Table 6. Non-ketotic hyperglycinaemia displays a very typical, although non-pathognonomic, pattern. It is characterized by coma, hypotonia and myoclonic jerks appearing at birth or after a few hours of age in a child who did not experience perinatal hypoxia. A burst suppression EEG pattern (Mises *et al.*, 1982) is always present. The diagnosis rests upon the demonstration of elevated serum glycine levels and especially an elevated CSF/serum glycine ratio. Our experience on 23 patients is presented in Table 7. The very rare D-glyceric acidaemia shares most of the signs of non-ketotic hyperglycinaemia, including hyperglycinaemia in some cases, whereas others present different patterns with metabolic acidosis.

The clinical spectrum of sulphite oxidase and combined sulphite and xanthine oxidase deficiencies (Wadman *et al.*, 1983) includes hypotonia, seizures, myoclonic jerks, microcephaly and dysmorphic features. Lens dislocation may occasionally be noted as early as the first month of life. This disorder is probably underdiagnosed as its clinical pattern shares many similarities with common acute fetal distress. In combined sulphite and xanthine oxidase deficiencies due to an abnormal molybdenum cofactor, uric acid concentration is very low in plasma and urine which is a very useful tool for diagnosis. In both sulphite oxidase deficiencies, sulphites are found in fresh urine in high concentrations (test with sulfitest, Merck). Amino acid chromatography performed on immediately deproteinized plasma and on fresh urine, shows a specific profile with high sulphite concentrations in the form of sulphocysteine, whereas cystine concentration is close to zero.

Table 7   Non-ketotic hyperglycinaemia: Clinical presentation in 23
patients

Symptom-free period (days)[a]	22(0–72)
Coma	100
Myoclonia	77
Seizures	27
Apnoea	77
Metabolic acidosis	0
Ketosis	0
Hyperammonaemia	0
Hyperlacticacidaemia	0
Glycinaemia (mmol L^{-1})[ab]	1.12(0.28–3.1)
Glycine in CSF (mmol L^{-1})[ab]	0.250 (0.10–0.57)
Glycine CSF:plasma ratio[ab]	0.22 (0.1–1)

Data expressed as the percentage of the total number of patients:
[a]means with ranges in parenthesis
[b]Normal ranges for glycine values (mmol L^{-1}): 0.2–0.4 in plasma;
0.002–0.008 in CSF; CSF:plasma ratio 0.01

The common symptoms of peroxisomal disorders presenting in the neonatal
period are an absence of a symptom-free interval, severe generalized hypotonia,
early onset epileptic seizures and craniofacial dysmorphism (Poll The *et al.*,
1987). Diagnosis requires special investigations including very-long chain fatty acid,
plasmalogen, phytanic, bile acids and pipecolic acid determinations in plasma,
urine and fibroblasts. The most frequent conditions are Zellweger syndrome and
neonatal adrenoleukodystrophy. Many other rare variants have been recently
described. The detailed description of these disorders is beyond the scope of this
paper and is presented in another article in this journal (Schutgens, 1989).
   In most diseases of intermediary metabolism, convulsions are a late manifestation. However, they may be important elements in the clinical presentation of
most patients with non-ketotic hyperglycinaemia sulphite oxidase deficiency, and
peroxisomal disorders described above. They are also the unique symptom in
pyridoxine-dependent convulsions. This rare disorder should be considered with
all refractory seizures in children under 1 year of age. The clinical response to
vitamin B$_6$ administration is the best way of making the diagnosis. If it is available
without delay, an EEG should be done during the injection of pyridoxine; an
immediate improvement in the tracing may be seen (Bankier *et al.* 1983).

Type V: Hypoglycaemia with hepatomegaly and liver dysfunction

The clinical presentation of this group of diseases is different from the preceding
ones. Hypoglycaemic seizures are often the presenting sign and hepatomegaly,
ketosis and lactic acidosis are present. The child has a dramatic improvement with
intravenous glucose administration. The main diseases of this group are glucose-6-
phosphate deficiency (type I glycogen storage disease), glycogenosis type III,
and fructose-1,6-biphosphatase deficiency. Until now, the clinical presentation of
phosphoenolpyruvate carboxykinase deficiency has been poorly defined in the

neonatal period. Marked hepatocellular dysfunction is uncommon but may occur, especially in fructose-1,6-biphosphatase deficiency. In other metabolic conditions such as tyrosinaemia type I, galactosaemia, fructosaemia with a fructose containing diet, and α_1-antitrypsin deficiency, hypoglycaemia is usually an incidental finding in a clinical setting dominated by jaundice or other evidence of liver dysfunction. Discussion of these conditions is beyond the scope of this article.

Gluconeogenesis is active only in the fasting state, thus the patient becomes hypoglycaemic only during fasting, and, unlike the other diseases discussed in this review, is safe from harm if a continuous supply of oral or intravenous glucose is provided. Often, these children become symptomatic only when feeding intervals are increased at several months of age. Exploration of these conditions involves enzyme assays in fibroblasts, blood cells or liver tissue and must often be performed under expert supervision, as precipitous drops in blood glucose are possible.

CONCLUSION

Despite the large number of inborn errors of intermediary metabolism which can be observed in the neonatal period, it is possible to assign most patients to one of the five biochemical syndromes. The above method of doing so is easy to implement and prospectively we have found it very reliable over the past 20 years. It provides considerable cost-benefit advantages over techniques such as mass screening for acute metabolic errors and is much more rapid, allowing specific treatment to be undertaken within hours in these critically ill neonates. Furthermore, because of their relatively simple origins in single gene lesions, our approach to inherited diseases of intermediary metabolism is already starting to benefit from the new developments in molecular biology.

Despite this sophistication of diagnosis and treatment, however, the crucial step of early clinical suspicion and diagnosis lies in the hands of the primary care physician.

ACKNOWLEDGEMENTS

We thank all the French and foreign colleagues from intensive care units for having referred all these patients to us in the last 20 years. We thank Monique Poussière for her skilful assistance.

REFERENCES

Aleck, K. A. and Shapiro, L. J. Genetic metabolic considerations in the sick neonate. *Pediatr. Clin. N. Am.* 25 (1978) 431–451

Amendt, B. A., Greene, C., Sweetman, L., Cloherty, J., Shih, V., Moon, A., Teel, L. and Rhead, W. J. Short chain acyl-CoA dehydrogenase deficiency. Clinical and biochemical studies in two patients. *J. Clin. Invest.* 79 (1987) 1303–1309

Ampola, M. G., (Ed.): Early detection and management of inborn errors. *Clin. Perinatal.* 3 (1976) 1–18

Ballard, R. A., Vinocour, B., Reynolds, J. W., Wennburg, R. P., Merritt, A., Sweetman,

L. and Nyhan, W. L. Transient hyperammonemia of the preterm infant. *N. Engl. J. Med.* 299 (1978) 920–925

Bankier, A., Turner, M. and Hopkins, I. J. Pyridoxine dependent seizures. A wider clinical spectrum. *Arch. Dis. Child.* 58 (1983) 415–418

Burri, B. J., Sweetman, L. and Nyhan, W. L. Mutant holocarboxylase synthetase: evidence for the enzyme defect in early biotin-responsive multiple carboxylase deficiency. *J. Clin. Invest.* 68 (1981) 1491–1495

Burton, B. K. Inborn errors of metabolism: the clinical diagnosis in early infancy. *Pediatrics* 79 (1987) 359–369

Burton, B. K. and Nadler, H. L. Clinical diagnosis of the inborn errors of metabolism in the neonatal period. *Pediatrics* 61 (1978) 398–405

Cathelineau, L., Briand, P., Ogier, H., Charpentier, C., Coude, F. X. and Saudubray, J. M. Occurence of hyperammonemia in the course of 17 cases of methylmalonic aciduria. *J. Pediatr.* 99 (1981) 279–281

Chalmers, R. A. and Lawson, A. H. *Organic Acids in Man*, Chapman and Hall, 1982, Vol. 1

Clayton, P. T. and Thompson, E. Dysmorphic syndrome with demonstrable biochemical abnormalities. *J. Med. Genet.* 25 (1988) 463–472

Di Mauro, S., Bonilla, E., Zeviani, M., Servidei, S., De Vivo, D. C. and Schon, E. A. Mitochondrial myopathies. *J. Inher. Metab. Dis.* 10 Suppl. 1 (1987) 113–128

Divry, P., Vianey-Liaud, C., Mory, O. and Ravussin, S. S. A methylglutaconic aciduria familial neonatal form with fatal onset. *J. Inher. Metab. Dis.* 10 Suppl. 2 (1987) 286–289

Francke, U., Harper, J. F., Darras, B. T., Cowan, J. M., McCabe, E. R. B., Kohlschutter, A., Seltzer, W. K., Saito, F., Goto, J., Harpey, J. P. and Wise, J. E. Congenital adrenal hypoplasia, myopathy, and glycerol kinase deficiency: Molecular genetic evidence for deletions. *Am. J. Hum. Genet.* 40 (1987) 212–227

Goodman, S. I. Inherited metabolic disease in the newborn: approach to diagnosis and treatment. *Adv. Pediatr.* 33 (1986) 197–224

Goodman, S. I., Frerman, F. E. and Loehr, J. P. Recent progress in understanding glutaric acidemias. *Enzyme* 38 (1987) 76–79

Kronick, J. B., Scriver, C. R., Goodyear, P. R. and Kaplan, P. B. A perimortem protocol for suspected genetic disease. *Pediatrics* 71 (1983) 960–963

Mackenzie, W. Urea cycle disorders and other hereditary hyperammonemic syndromes. In Stanbury, J. B. *et al.* (Eds.), *The Metabolic Basis of Inherited Disease*, McGraw-Hill, New York, 1983, pp. 402–438

Matsui, S. M., Mahoney, M. J. and Rosenberg, L. E. The natural history of the inherited methylmalonic acidurias. *N. Engl. J. Med.* 308 (1983) 857–861

Mises, J., Moussalli-Salefranque, F., Laroque, M. L., Ogier, H., Coude, F. X., Charpentier, C. and Saudubray, J. M. EEG findings as an aid to the diagnosis of neonatal nonketotic hyperglycinemia. *J. Inher. Metab. Dis.* 5 Suppl. 2 (1982) 117–120

Nyhan, W. L. An approach to the diagnosis of overwhelming metabolic diseases in early infancy. *Curr. Prob. Pediatr.* 7 (1977) 1–12

Nyhan, W. L. and Sakati, N. A. *Diagnostic Recognition of Genetic Diseases*, Philadelphia, Lea-Febiger, 1987

Poll-The, B. T., Saudubray, J. M., Ogier, J., Lombes, A., Munnich, A. and Frezal, J. Clinical approach to inherited peroxisomal disorders. In Vogel, F. and Sperling, K. (Eds.), *Human Genetics*, Springer-Verlag, Berlin, 1987, pp. 345–351

Robinson, B. H. and Sherwood, W. G. Lactic acidaemia. *J. Inher. Metab. Dis.* 7 Suppl. 1 (1984) 69–73

Robinson, B. H., Oei, J., Saudubray, J. M., Marsac, C., Bartlett, K., Quan, F. and Gravel, R. The French and North American phenotypes of pyruvate carboxylase deficiency, correlation with biotin containing protein by ^{3}H-biotin incorporation, ^{35}S-streptavidin labeling, and Northern blotting with a cloned cDNA probe. *Am. J. Hum. Genet.* 40 (1987) 50–59

Rosenberg, L. A. Disorders of propionate and methylmalonate metabolism. In Stanbury,

J. B. *et al.* (Eds.) *The Metabolic Basis of Inherited Disease*, McGraw-Hill, New York, 1983, pp. 474–497

Saudubray, J. M., Ogier, H., Charpentier, C., Depondt, E., Coude, F. X., Munnich, A., Mitchell, G., Rey, F. and Frezal, J. Neonatal management of organic acidurias. Clinical update. *J. Inher. Metab. Dis.* 7 Suppl. 1 (1984) 2–9

Saudubray, J. M., Specola, N., Middleton, B., Lombes, A., Bonnefont, J. P., Jakobs, C., Vassault, A., Charpentier, C. and Day, R. Hyperketotic states due to inherited defects of ketolysis. *Enzyme* 38 (1987) 80–90

Schutgens, R. B. H., Schrakamp, G., Wanders, R. J. A., Heymans, H. S. A., Tager, J. M. and van den Bosch, U. Prenatal and perinatal diagnosis of peroxisomal disorders. *J. Inher. Metab. Dis.* 12 Suppl. 1 (1989) 118–134

Settergren, G., Lindblad, B. S. and Persson, B. Cerebral blood flow and exchange of oxygen, glucose, ketone bodies, lactate, pyruvate and amino acids in infants. *Acta Paediatr. Scand.* 65 (1976) 343–353

Stanley, C. A. New genetic defects in mitochondrial fatty acid oxidation and carnitine deficiency. *Adv. Pediatr.* 34 (1987) 59–88

Tanaka, K. and Rosenberg, L. Disorders of branched chain aminoacid and organic acid metabolism. In Stanbury, J. B. *et al.* (Eds.) *The Metabolic Basis of Inherited Disease*, McGraw-Hill, New York, 1983, pp. 440–473

Tildon, J. T. and Cornblath, M. Succinyl-CoA: 3-ketoacidosis in infancy. *J. Clin. Invest.* 51 (1972) 493–498

Van Biervliet, J. P. G. M., Bruinvis, L., Ketting, D., De Bree, P. K., Van der Heiden, C., Wadman, S. K., Willems, J. L., Brookelman, H., Van Haelst, U. and Monnens, L. A. H. Hereditary mitochondrial myopathy with lactic acidemia, a DeToni-Fanconi-Debré syndrome and a defective respiratory chain in voluntary muscle. *Pediatr. Res.* 1 (1977) 1088–1093

Vianey-Liaud, C., Divry, P., Gregersen, N., Mathieu, M. The inborn errors of mitochondria fatty acid oxidation. *J. Inher. Metab. Dis.* 10 Suppl. 1 (1987) 159–198

Wadman, S. K., Duran, M., Beemer, F. A., Cats, B. P., Johnson, J. L., Rajagopalan, K. V., Saudubray, J. M., Ogier, H., Charpentier, C., Berger, R., Smit, G. P. A., Wilson, J. and Krywawych, S. Absence of hepatic molybdenum cofactor: an inborn error of metabolism leading to a combined deficiency of sulphite oxidase and xanthine dehydrogenase. *J. Inher. Metab. Dis.* 6 (1983) 78–83

Wolf, B., Grier, R. E., Allen, R. J., Goodman, S. I., Kien, C. L., Parker, W. D., Howell, D. M. and Hurst, D. L. Phenotypic variation in biotinidase deficiency. *J. Pediatr.* 103 (1983) 233–237

Wysocki, S. J., Hahnel, R. 3 hydroxy-3-methylglutaryl-coenzyme A lyase deficiency. A review. *J. Inher. Metab. Dis.* 9 (1986) 225–233

J. Inher. Metab. Dis. 12 Suppl. 1 (1989) 42–54

Acute Metabolic Encephalopathy: A Review of Causes, Mechanisms and Treatment

R. Surtees and J. V. Leonard

Department of Child Health, Institute of Child Health, London, WC1, UK

Summary: Acute encephalopathy is a relatively common problem: one of the causes is metabolic disorders. A detailed history, examination and investigations performed during the acute illness (blood sugar, blood gases, plasma ammonia, blood lactate, plasma ketones, plasma amino acids, liver function tests, and urinary organic acids) should identify those patients in whom a metabolic disorder is likely. More detailed studies may be needed to establish a precise diagnosis.

The mechanism of the acute brain dysfunction is multifactorial. Factors that contribute include changes in blood flow and, initially, a disturbance in neurotransmitter function followed by failure of energy metabolism and cellular depolarization. Treatment of these conditions is largely supportive, with especial attention to the management of cerebral perfusion pressure.

Acute encephalopathy is a rapid decrease in conscious level (over hours or days), not secondary to ictal nor syncopal episodes. The differential diagnosis is wide

Table 1 Differential diagnosis of acute encephalopathy

1. Trauma
2. Infection (meningitis/encephalitis)
3. Space-occupying lesion
4. Ingestion of drugs or toxins (including lead-poisoning)
5. Parainfectious encephalitis and mycoplasma encephalopathy
6. Hypoxia/ischaemia (including near-miss sudden infant death syndrome and migraine)
7. Hypertension
8. Cerebral vasculitis (including haemolytic-uraemic syndrome)
9. Metabolic
10. Others: toxic-shock encephalopathy syndrome
    haemorrhagic shock encephalopathy syndrome
    remote effects of tumour

(Table 1) and includes metabolic disorders. Faced with a sick child it is important to identify any underlying metabolic disorder rapidly. These can be conveniently divided into six broad diagnostic groups (Table 2). There is considerable overlap between these groups, and if patients fall into more than one group this will increase the clinician's suspicions. These categories will be discussed but, although it is recognized that fluid and electrolyte shifts are important in the pathogenesis of

42

Journal of Inherited Metabolic Disease. ISSN 0141–8955. Copyright © SSIEM and Kluwer Academic Publishers, PO Box 55, Lancaster, UK.

Table 2 Metabolic causes of acute metabolic encephalopathy and the initial investigations

Disturbances of glucose homeostasis	glucose (B,U), gases (B)
Metabolic acidosis	gases (B), lactate (P), ketones (U)
Hyperammonaemia	ammonia (P)
Hepatic failure	liver function and enzymes (P) clotting studies (B)
Electrolyte disturbance	urea and electrolytes (P) creatinine (P)
Mitochondrial encephalopathy	lactate (B, U)

B = blood, P = plasma, U = urine. In all cases in which the diagnosis is not certain plasma (5 mL) and urine 20 mL should be deep frozen in aliquots
The investigations listed represent the basic minimum and in many centres other investigations may be able to be done at an early stage

metabolic encephalopathy these will not be considered; discussion will be confined to encephalopathy after the immediate neonatal period.

If a metabolic disorder is suspected it is essential to obtain a detailed past and family history together with the basic investigations listed in Table 2. These represent the bare minimum and both plasma and urine should be deep frozen so that they can be analysed later if necessary.

INVESTIGATION AND DIAGNOSIS

Disorders of glucose homeostasis

Hypoglycaemia: It is widely accepted that hypoglycaemia is defined as a blood glucose concentration of less than $2 \, mmol \, L^{-1}$ although recent electrophysiological studies suggest that the value should be $2.5 \, mmol \, L^{-1}$ (Koh *et al.*, 1988). The possibility of hypoglycaemia should always be considered when conscious level is disturbed, even in the absence of symptoms of adrenergic counter-regulation. Most commonly the disturbance of consciousness is only transient, often secondary to a convulsion. However some disorders may present with encephalopathy (see Table 3) and, regardless of the cause, if there are complications such as cerebral oedema there may be prolonged disturbance of consciousness. The differential diagnosis of acute metabolic encephalopathy and hypoglycaemia can be divided into three broad categories, endocrine, metabolic and hepatic (Table 3). The history and clinical examination may give important clues, for instance endocrine causes might be suggested by the birthweight, micropenis and subsequent growth of the child, while massive hepatomegaly suggests a defect in glycogen metabolism.

The cause of hypoglycaemia should always be sought. The most useful diagnostic information is that obtained from samples taken when the child is hypoglycaemic. These are sent for endocrine (insulin, cortisol, growth hormone) and metabolic tests (blood free fatty acids, β-hydroxybutyrate, lactate and alanine, and urine organic acids) as well as tests of liver function. The results of these may give a precise diagnosis and if not they at least enable a broad category of cause to be identified.

If the results are not helpful or the samples are not collected during the acute

Table 3   Causes of hypoglycaemia and acute encephalopathy

Endocrine
  Hypopituitary coma

Metabolic
  Organic acidaemias:
    Maple syrup urine disease
    Methylmalonic acidaemia
    Acetoacetyl-CoA thiolase deficiency
    Propionic and isovaleric acidaemias (more rarely)

  Fat oxidation defects:
    Medium, long-chain and multiple acyl-CoA dehydrogenase deficiencies
    3-Hydroxy-3-methylglutaryl-CoA lyase deficiency
    Others (defects not fully characterized)

  Drugs and toxins:
    Alcohol
    Oral hypoglycaemic agents
    Salicylates

Hepatic
  Fulminant liver failure
  Reye's syndrome

This table gives the causes of illnesses presenting with acute encephalopathy (as defined above) and hypoglycaemia. Any cause of hypoglycaemia may be responsible for transient symptomatic (or even asymptomatic) central nervous system dysfunction; most commonly this presents as a fit. Regardless of the cause of hypoglycaemia, prolonged symptoms can also result in acute encephalopathy (see, for instance, Leonard and Dunger, 1978) and in this situation the differential diagnosis is much wider

episode, the child should be investigated after recovery by studying the metabolic response to fasting using the same investigations as listed above (Saudubray *et al.*, 1981). Based on the results of the tests, further appropriate studies should be undertaken to determine the precise cause. These are beyond the scope of this article (see Aynsley-Green and Soltesz, 1985; appropriate chapters in Stanbury *et al.*, 1983).

Hyperglycaemia: Diabetes mellitus presenting as acute metabolic encephalopathy should be clear from the history, but it should be noted that hyperglycaemia and glycosuria can also occur with ketoacidosis due to organic acidurias. This may rarely be a presenting feature. However hyperglycaemia is most commonly secondary to high glucose intake given to control metabolic disturbance. We have also seen hyperglycaemia complicating severe illness in organic acidaemias caused by acute pancreatitis (maple syrup urine disease, methylmalonic acidaemia and isovaleric acidaemia; unpublished observations).

Metabolic acidosis

Metabolic acidosis is common in sick children regardless of the cause and in most is secondary to poor tissue perfusion. A metabolic cause is more likely if there have been previous episodes; the acidosis persists after correction of shock; if there is metabolic acidosis without shock; or persistent ketosis. It can be particularly difficult to recognize an underlying metabolic disorder if the patient has other complications such as acute cardiomyopathy. The inherited disorders that may present with acidosis are listed in Table 4.

Table 4   Acute metabolic encephalopathy and metabolic acidosis

Defects in glucose homeostasis:
  Defects of gluconeogenesis (glucose 6-phosphatase and fructose 1,6-bisphosphatase deficiences)

Organic acidaemias:
  Maple syrup urine disease
  Methylmalonic, propionic, 3-methylcrotonyl and isovaleric acidaemias, etc.
  Multiple acyl CoA dehydrogenase deficiency and ethylmalonic–adipic aciduria
  Holocarboxylase synthase deficiency

Defects in ketone body utilisation:
  3-Oxoacid-CoA transferase deficiency
  Acetoacetyl-CoA thiolase deficiency

Congenital lactic acidoses:
  Pyruvate dehydrogenase deficiency
  Deficiencies of the respiratory chain complex

The diagnosis is based on both the clinical findings and the blood glucose, lactate and 3-hydroxybutyrate with the urine organic acids. In some patients, particularly congenital lactic acidoses and ketone body utilization defects, the diagnosis may only be established by studying the metabolic responses to fasting and glucose loading once the child has recovered from the acute illness (Saudubray *et al.*, 1987). The diagnosis should be confirmed by enzyme analysis in fibroblasts or other appropriate tissue.

Hyperammonaemia

In healthy adults and children venous plasma ammonia is usually less than $40 \mu mol \, L^{-1}$, but this may rise to $100 \mu mol \, L^{-1}$ with systemic illness or shock. However, the relationship between plasma ammonia concentrations and neurological symptoms is not good. In patients with inherited disorders encephalopathic symptoms may develop at ammonia concentrations of around $100 \mu mol \, L^{-1}$ but some patients with urea cycle disorders may have no symptoms at much higher concentrations ($200 \mu mol \, L^{-1}$). However as a general guide, at ammonia concentrations of $100-200 \mu mol \, L^{-1}$ vomiting, ataxia and irritability occur. Higher levels of ammonia are usually associated with increasing stupor, often alternating with delirium and progressing to coma.

The differential diagnosis of acute hyperammonaemic encephalopathy is given in Table 5 and the investigations to elucidate the cause can be deduced from this list (Leonard, 1984).

Table 5   Hyperammonaemia and acute encephalopathy

Inherited disorders of the urea cycle:
  Carbamyl phosphate synthase deficiency
  Ornithine carbamoyl transferase deficiency
  Citrullinaemia
  Arginosuccinic aciduria
  Arginase deficiency (rarely)

Organic acidaemias:
  Propionic and methylmalonic acidaemias particularly

Other inherited disorders:
  HHH syndrome
  Hyperlysinaemia
  Fat oxidation defects (medium and long-chain and multiple acyl-CoA dehydrogenase
    defects)

Liver disease:
  Any cause of severe chronic liver disease
  Infective
  Ischaemic
  Drugs and toxins (e.g. valproate therapy, unripe Ackee fruit)
  Wilson's disease
  Reye's syndrome

Other:
  Urinary tract infection with stasis
  Asparaginase therapy
  Leukaemia

Liver disease

Acute hepatic encephalopathy is characterized by confusion, depressed conscious level, prominent motor abnormalities (tremor, asterixis, hyperactive stretch reflexes) and neuro-ophthalmological changes (normal pupils and brisk ocular responses). This may complicate either acute fulminant hepatic disease or acute deterioration in chronic hepatic disease regardless of the underlying cause. Liver disease should be suspected if liver enzymes are markedly raised and liver function deranged (low albumin and fibrinogen, raised bilirubin). The presence of encephalopathy, raised liver enzymes and a normal bilirubin suggests Reye's syndrome; liver biopsy in this disease shows pathognomic changes (Partin *et al.*, 1979). Detailed diagnosis of the other causes is outside the scope of this article (see Russell *et al.*, 1987; Fraser and Arieff, 1985), but of particular importance is acute Wilson's disease in older children which needs to be diagnosed urgently because of the importance of giving specific therapy.

Mitochondrial encephalopathy

Patients with defects in the respiratory chain or of pyruvate dehydrogenase are increasingly recognized, and may occasionally present acutely with encephalopathy. These include Leigh syndrome (Pincus, 1972), Alpers syndrome (Gabreëls *et al.*,

1984) and MELAS (myoclonus epilepsy, lactic acidosis and stroke-like episodes) syndrome (Montagna *et al.*, 1987). Although Leigh and Alpers syndromes can only be diagnosed with certainty at post-mortem it is possible to establish the likely diagnosis in life from the clinical course, raised lactate concentrations (which may only be evident in cerebrospinal fluid) and characteristic changes on computerized tomography or magnetic resonance imaging of the brain (van Erven *et al.*, 1987).

MECHANISMS

The pathogenesis of acute metabolic encephalopathy is probably always multifactorial, with the more global effects of alterations in blood flow and intracranial pressure acting in concert with more specific defects in one or more metabolic pathways. Despite much interest and research, little is known about the interplay of such factors and their impact upon the many different cell types in the central nervous system.

It is likely that the initial symptoms and signs of acute metabolic encephalopathy are caused by disordered neurotransmission and that only in the later stages of the illness by energy failure and depolarization of cell membranes. All forms of acute metabolic encephalopathy, with the exception of the mitochondrial encephalopathies, are probably readily reversible in the early stages but with increasing duration of the encephalopathy or repeated episodes permanent brain damage (Martin and Schlote, 1972; Kendall *et al.*, 1983) becomes more likely. This review concentrates upon the disturbances secondary to hyperammonaemia and hypoglycaemia. Mechanisms of permanent brain cell damage following acute metabolic encephalopathy and secondary structural damage that may complicate treatment (such as central pontine myelinolysis) will not be discussed. The mechanisms that may cause hepatic encephalopathy are also outside the scope of this article, except for the consideration of those applicable to hyperammonaemia.

Hypoglycaemia

The mechanisms of hypoglycaemic encephalopathy are likely to vary depending on the disorder responsible for the reduced blood glucose concentration. Not only is the major substrate for brain energy metabolism reduced but in some disorders 'toxic' metabolites may interfere directly with neurological function.

Cerebral perfusion pressure: Studies in man (della Porta *et al.*, 1964) and animals (Norberg and Siesjö, 1976) show that total cerebral blood flow rises during hypoglycaemia but animal studies also show that there is a regionally selective loss of autoregulation of cerebral blood flow (Ghajar *et al.*, 1982). Therefore a fall in systemic blood pressure during hypoglycaemia may well cause some regional underperfusion. Some causes of hypoglycaemia ('toxic') may lead to cerebral oedema because of accumulation of fatty acids (and possibly organic acids) in the cells and, in theory, the large electrolyte shifts across cell membranes due to hypoglycaemia *per se* may also cause cerebral oedema. Whilst measured fluid shifts have been small in 'isolated' hypoglycaemia, when 'toxic' metabolites are formed cerebral oedema may become a major problem.

Effect on brain energy metabolism: Hypoglycaemia should have marked effects upon cerebral energy metabolism because glucose is the main (and ordinarily the sole) substrate for brain energy metabolism and the brain has high energy requirements but slender substrate stores. In animals (Lewis *et al.*, 1974) and man (Koh *et al.*, 1988) there is a critical blood glucose concentration below which neurological dysfunction occurs.

Hypoglycaemia causes a fall in brain concentrations of glycolytic and tricarboxylic acid cycle intermediates (Norberg and Siesjö, 1976; Lewis *et al.*, 1974) and also a fall in the high energy phosphate nucleotide pools (Chapman *et al.*, 1981). The fall in the high energy phosphate nucleotide pools occurs before a detectable fall in cerebral metabolic rates and may be due to an uncoupling of oxidative phosphorylation, perhaps by accumulation of intramitochondrial free fatty acids. However, energy failure and subsequent generalized cellular depolarization occur only when spontaneous brain electrical activity ceases, and cannot explain the major symptoms of brain dysfunction during hypoglycaemia.

Neurotransmitter metabolism: Hypoglycaemia causing pre-coma results in drastic changes in amino-acid (Lewis *et al.*, 1974), acetyl-choline (Gibson and Blass, 1976) and monoamine (Siesjö, 1988) metabolism. It has been suggested that the symptoms of hypoglycaemia that occur before development of energy failure are due to the disruption of neurotransmission caused by such disordered metabolism (Siesjö and Plum, 1972). In addition, the marked deamination of amino acids to provide carbon skeletons for oxidation during hypoglycaemia causes brain ammonia to rise to levels seen in hyperammonaemic coma (Ghajar *et al.*, 1982); this may further impair synaptic transmission (see below).

Hyperammonaemia

Cerebral perfusion pressure: The effect of hyperammonaemia upon cerebral blood flow seems variable; however, there is an increase in cerebral blood flow (Voorhies *et al.*, 1983) in primates with acute hyperammonaemia, the vasodilation is probably due to a direct effect of ammonia on vascular smooth muscle. However since there is also a rise in intracranial pressure there may be no increase in perfusion pressure. A rise in intracranial pressure and cerebral oedema may complicate hyperammonaemia due to any cause and it has been suggested that this is due to the osmotic effects of the large increase in brain glutamine (Watson *et al.*, 1985). In hepatic encephalopathy, cerebral oedema is found in 80% of deaths (Ware *et al.*, 1979).

Blood–brain barrier: Ammonia crosses the blood–brain barrier by diffusion, and consequently the brain ammonia concentration increases in proportion with that of blood. Hyperammonaemia appears to alter the properties of the blood–brain barrier. In rats there is a selective increase in the uptake of tryptophan (perhaps because of linked glutamine efflux) and a decrease in lysine uptake. The enhanced uptake of tryptophan will increase brain serotonin and may have effects upon some of the vegetative functions of the brain (Mans *et al.*, 1987).

Effect on brain energy metabolism: Many experiments have shown that animals in coma secondary to acute hyperammonaemia have depletion of ATP and phosphocreatine, although this may show marked regional variation (McCandless and Schenker, 1981). The mechanism by which hyperammonaemia depletes energy stores is not well understood, nor is it known why some areas of the brain should be more vulnerable than others.

The brain lacks the urea-cycle enzymes carbamyl phosphate synthase and ornithine carbamoyl transferase; therefore detoxification of ammonia in this organ relies upon the formation of glutamine from glutamate, and ultimately from α-ketoglutarate. One hypothesis, that ammonia interferes with the brain tricarboxylic acid cycle by draining α-ketoglutarate (Bessman and Bessman, 1955), has now been disproved by the demonstration that in acute hyperammonaemia in animals the brain α-ketoglutarate levels are normal or raised. However, in one study in children with urea cycle disorders a negative correlation between plasma α-ketoglutarate and ammonia has been shown (Batshaw *et al.*, 1980).

The adult brain relies upon the oxidation of glucose to carbon dioxide to provide energy and the cytoplasmic NADH produced must be regenerated as NAD^+ by the mitochondrial electron transport chain. Cytoplasmic NADH cannot cross the mitochondrial membrane and instead the reducing equivalents are transported via shuttles. Of particular interest is the malate–aspartate shuttle, because its activity in brain is closely linked to the tricarboxylic cycle and glutamate is an integral part of the shuttle. In acutely hyperammonaemic rats, symptoms, occuring before changes in the high energy phosphate intermediates are noted, are accompanied by changes in the cytosolic and mitochondrial $NADH/NAD^+$ ratio and by decreased aspartate and glutamate with raised pyruvate and alanine (Hindfield *et al.*, 1977). Initial symptoms of hyperammonaemia may be due to decreased shunting of reducing equivalents and a decrease in excitatory neurotransmitters (aspartate and glutamate). Eventually the reduced turnover of the shuttle will cause a slowing of the tricarboxylic cycle and a fall in high energy phosphate intermediates.

Electrophysiology: In addition to the marked biochemical effects of hyperammonaemia there are also effects on the electrophysiological properties of synapses. In theory ammonia should have a potassium-like depolarizing effect upon the axon, but this requires a much higher ammonia concentration than that seen in hyperammonaemic encephalopathy (Alger and Nicoll, 1983). However, marked effects upon central nervous system excitatory and inhibitory synapses are seen at ammonia concentrations more likely to be achieved in encephalopathy (Raabe, 1987). At excitatory synapses ammonia probably exerts its effect by depleting the glutamine within presynaptic vesicles. Glutamine is the source for glutamate in the synaptic vesicles (Bradford and Ward, 1976), and raised ammonia concentrations also inhibit glutaminase activity. At inhibitory synapses ammonia prevents the hyperpolarizing inhibitory potential at the post-synaptic neurone by decreasing the chloride-dependent hyperpolarization triggered by calcium-influx or neuronal depolarization (Raabe and Lin, 1985).

Metabolic acidosis and mitochondrial disorders

Acidosis increases cerebral blood flow, although any benefit from this is offset by the rise in intracranial pressure due to the osmotic effects of the abnormal metabolites. This is further complicated by the fluid loss from the circulation that occurs secondarily to the diuresis induced by the excretion of abnormal metabolites. In methylmalonic acidaemia many patients have a renal concentrating defect which exacerbates the hypovolaemia and dehydration.

Although short-chain fatty acids are known to cause uncoupling of oxidative phosphorylation in brain mitochondria (Ahmed and Schofield, 1961), coma induced by an infusion of these does not seem to be due to impaired cerebral energy metabolism (Walker *et al.*, 1970). It seems likely that disordered neurotransmission is responsible for the initial symptoms and it is known that ketoacids and short-chain fatty acids affect the metabolism of both excitatory and inhibitory amino-acid neurotransmitters (Tashian, 1961; Lopez-Lahoya *et al.*, 1981).

The pathogenesis of acute encephalopathy in mitochondrial disorders is not known. It is possible that increased energy demands exceed the residual activity of the respiratory chain with failure in brain energy metabolism.

TREATMENT

The management of acute metabolic encephalopathy is largely general, with little specific therapy. The general management of acute metabolic encephalopathy is outlined in Table 6.

Table 6   General management of acute metabolic encephalopathy

1. *Supportive*
   Maintain oxygenation
   Maintain circulation
   Maintain normal body temperature
   Prevent agitation

2. *Corrective*
   Electrolyte, calcium and phosphate imbalance
   Acidosis
   Seizures
   Prevent protein and fat catabolism

3. *Reduce raised intracranial pressure*
   Restrict fluids to $\frac{2}{3}$ maintainance
   Intubation and controlled ventilation
   Monitor intracranial pressure
   Intracranial pressure >20 mmHg or cerebral perfusion pressure <40 mmHg use mannitol 0.25–0.5 g kg^{-1} then frusemide 1 mg kg^{-1}
   Consider pentobarbitone or thiopentone

The maintenance of an adequate circulation (with monitoring of the arterial and venous pressures) is of especial importance because cerebral vascular autoregulation is often lost in these disorders. Electrolyte disturbance may be prominent in methylmalonic acidaemia and hepatic failure and hypovolaemia should be corrected – but fluid overload avoided as it can exacerbate cerebral symptoms. It is essential to prevent further protein and fat catabolism which frequently generate the abnormal toxic metabolites in these diseases; this can be achieved by infusing glucose using concentrated solutions at $75–100\,\mathrm{g\,m^{-2}\,day^{-1}}$ ($2.5–3.5\,\mathrm{g\,kg^{-1}\,day^{-1}}$) plus insulin if hyperglycaemia becomes a problem. Acidosis should be corrected with sodium bicarbonate and if this is ineffective or hypernatraemia develops bicarbonate peritoneal dialysis should be instituted (Leonard, 1985).

Patients with inherited metabolic disorders are at particular risk of cerebral oedema and care needs to be taken to reduce the risk of this developing. Fluid overload should be avoided and in general any patient who is seriously ill should be electively intubated and hyperventilated. This is particularly important before any procedure or drugs that may compromise respiratory reserve such as peritoneal dialysis. For any child who is clearly seriously ill, careful thought should be given to monitoring the intracranial pressure before encephalopathy develops. Suspicious signs are a deteriorating level of consciousness despite treatment and, in addition, any of the following: (1) insensibility to pain; (2) extensor hypertonus; (3) sluggishly reacting, dilated pupils; (4) abnormal respiratory pattern; (5) circulatory changes; (6) spontaneous limb cycling. In early stages fluid restriction, elective intubation and hyperventilation may be sufficient. The decision to monitor intracranial pressure is easier now that reliable transducers can be easily inserted at the bedside. Measures to consider to reduce intracranial pressure are summarised in Table 6.

Specific therapy

Hypoglycaemia: Hypoglycaemia should be immediately corrected with a bolus of glucose intravenously (after collecting blood for diagnostic investigations) followed by an infusion. Glucose therapy may need to be continued for some time before improvement of encephalopathy is seen in 'toxic' hypoglycaemia, but may cause a rapid reversal of symptoms in hypoglycaemia due to substrate deficiency. Specific treatment may be used to prevent further episodes including hormone or drug therapy.

Hyperammonaemia: Excretion of ammonia in urea cycle disorders can be enhanced by treatment with sodium benzoate and phenylacetic (or phenylbutyric) acid. Benzoate combines with glycine to form hippuric acid and phenylacetate combines with glutamine to form phenylacetylglutamine, both of these compounds are readily excreted in the urine and therefore reduce the total nitrogen load on the urea cycle. Additionally the urea cycle itself can be primed with arginine, and in arginosuccinic aciduria and citrullinaemia this will reduce plasma ammonia concentrations (Brusilow, 1985; Walter and Leonard, 1988).

Regardless of cause, very high ammonia levels ($500–700\,\mu\mathrm{mol\,L^{-1}}$) or a poor response to therapy indicate that dialysis should be considered, haemodialysis being more effective than peritoneal.

Organic acidaemia: Glycine increases the excretion of isovaleric acid since it is conjugated to form isovalerylglycine which is readily excreted in the urine. Carnitine may increase the efflux of organic or fatty acids from the mitochondria, thereby reducing the toxic effects upon the energy metabolism and promoting their excretion (Wolff *et al.*, 1986). If the toxicity is severe, dialysis will help to reduce the organic acid load and ameliorate the encephalopathy.

Liver disease: Acute Wilson's disease requires prompt therapy to reduce the total copper load of the body. Measures used with some success include albumin infusion and plasmapheresis, and more recently peritoneal dialysis against penicillamine (de Bont *et al.*, 1985) and liver transplantation (Sokol *et al.*, 1985).

In other forms of hepatic encephalopathy attempts to ameliorate the metabolic disturbance have met with rather limited success. The use of branched-chain amino or keto-acids, glutamate and γ-aminobutyric acid antagonists have all been suggested.

CONCLUSIONS

It is important to recognize acute metabolic encephalopathy at the earliest stage possible and to institute treament to prevent permanent neurological damage. Unfortunately, despite the very extensive literature on the mechanisms of acute metabolic encephalopathy, very little of this information has yet been used in the management of patients presenting acutely, and much of the treatment remains supportive rather than specific.

REFERENCES

Ahmed, K. and Schofield, P. G. Studies on fatty acid oxidation 8. The effects of fatty acids on metabolism of rat brain cortex *in vitro. Biochem. J.* 81 (1961) 45–53

Alger, B. E. and Nicoll, R. A. Ammonia does not selectively block IPSPs in rat hippocampal pyramidal cells. *J. Neurophysiol.* 49 (1983) 1381–1391

Aynsley-Green, A. and Soltesz, G. Hypoglycaemia in infancy and childhood. *Current Reviews in Paediatrics*, Vol. 1, Churchill Livingston, Edinburgh and London, 1985, pp. 151–161

Batshaw, M. L., Walser, M. and Brusilow, S. Plasma α-ketoglutarate in urea cycle enzymopathies and its role as harbinger of hyperammonemic coma. *Pediatr. Res.* 14 (1980) 1316–1319

Bessman, S. P. and Bessman, A. N. The cerebral and peripheral uptake of ammonia in liver disease with an hypothesis for the mechanism of hepatic coma. *J. Clin. Invest.* 34 (1955) 622–628

de Bont, B., Moulin, D., Stein, F., van Hoof, F. and Lauwerys, R. Peritoneal dialysis with D-penicillamine in Wilson disease. *J. Pediatr.* 107 (1985) 545–547

Bradford, H. F. and Ward, H. K. On glutaminase activity in mammalian synaptosomes. *Brain. Res.* 110 (1976) 115–125

Brusilow, S. W. Inborn errors of urea synthesis. In Lloyd, J. K. and Scriver, C. R. (Eds.), *Genetic and Metabolic Disease in Paediatrics*, Butterworths, London, 1985, pp. 140–165

Chapman, A. G., Westerberg, E. and Siesjö, B. K. The metabolism of purine and pyrimidine nucleotides in rat cortex during insulin-induced hypoglycaemia and recovery. *J. Neurochem.* 36 (1981) 179–189

van Erven, P. M. M., Cillesen, J. P. M., Eekhoff, E. M. W., Gabreëls, F. J. M., Doesberg, W. H., Lemmens, W. A. J. G., Slooff, J. L., Renier, W. O. and Ruitenbeek, W. Leigh syndrome, a mitochondrial encephalo(myo)opathy. *Clin. Neurol. Neurosurg.* 89 (1987) 217–230

Fraser, C. L. and Arieff, A. I. Hepatic encephalopathy. *N. Engl. J. Med.* 313 (1985) 865–873

Ghajar, J. B. G., Plum, F. and Duffy, T. E. Cerebral oxidative metabolism and blood flow during acute hypoglycaemia and recovery in unanaesthetised rats. *J. Neurochem.* 38 (1982) 397–409

Gabreëls, F. J. M., Prick, M. J. J., Trijbels, J. M. F., Renier, W. O., Jaspar, H. H. J., Jansen, A. J. M. and Sloof, J. L. Defects in citric acid cycle and the electron transport chain in progressive poliodystrophy. *Acta Neurol. Scand.* 70 (1984) 145–154

Gibson, G. E. and Blass, J. P. Impaired synthesis of acetylcholine in brain accompanying mild hypoxia and hypoglycaemia. *J. Neurochem.* 27 (1976) 37–42

Hindfield, B., Plum, F. and Duffy, T. E. Effect of acute ammonia intoxication on cerebral metabolism in rats with portocaval shunts. *J. Clin. Invest.* 59 (1977) 386–396

Kendall, B. E., Kingsley, D. P. E., Leonard, J. V., Lingam, S. and Oberholzer, V. G. Neurological features and computed tomography of the brain in children with ornithine carbamoyl transferase deficiency. *J. Neurol. Neurosurg. Psychiatr.* 46 (1983) 28–34

Koh, T. H. H. G., Aynsley-Green, A., Tarbit, M. and Eyre, J. A. Neural dysfunction during hypoglycaemia. *Arch. Dis. Child.* 63 (1988) 1353–1358

Leonard, J. V. Hyperammonaemia in childhood. In Clayton, B. E. and Round, J. M. (Eds.), *Chemical Pathology and the Sick Child*, Blackwell, Oxford, 1984, pp. 96–119

Leonard, J. V. The early detection and management of inborn errors presenting acutely in the neonatal period. *Eur. J. Pediatr.* 143 (1983) 253–257

Leonard, J. V. and Dunger, D. B. Hypoglycaemia complicating feeding regimes for glycogen storage disease. *Lancet* 2 (1978) 1203–1204

Lewis, L. D., Ljundgren, B., Ratcheson, R. A. and Siesjö, B. K. Changes in the carbohydrate substrates, amino acids and ammonia in the brain during insulin-induced hypoglycaemia. *J. Neurochem.* 23 (1974) 659–671

Lopez-Lahoya, J., Garcìa, M. L., Benavides, J. and Ugarte, M. Inhibition by methylmalonate of glycine uptake by synaptosomes from the rat spinal cord. *J. Neurochem.* 36 (1981) 325–327

McCandless, D. W. and Schenker, S. Effects of acute ammonia intoxication on energy stores in the reticular activating system *Exp. Brain Res.* 44 (1981) 325–330

Mans, A., Biebuyk, J. and Hawkins, R. Brain tryptophan abnormalities in hyperammonaemia and liver disease. In Bender, D. A., Joseph, M. H., Kochen, W. and Steinhart, H. (Eds.), *Progress in Tryptophan and Serotonin Research 1986*, Walter de Guyter, Berlin, 1987, pp. 207–213

Martin, J. J. and Schlote, W. Central nervous system lesions in disorders of amino-acid metabolism: a neuropathological study. *J. Neurol. Sci.* 15 (1972) 49–76

Montagna, P., Gallassi, R., Medori, R., Govone, E., Eeviani, M., di Mauro, S., Lugaresi, E. and Andermann, F. MELAS syndrome: characteristic migrainous and epileptic features and maternal transmission. *Neurology* 38 (1988) 751–754

Norberg, K., Siesjö, B. K. Oxidative metabolism of the cerebral cortex of the rat in severe insulin-induced hypoglycaemia. *J. Neurochem.* 26 (1976) 179–189

Partin, J. C., Bove, K., Partin, J. S. and Schubert, W. K. Liver and muscle ultrastructure in Reye's syndrome. In Crocker, J. F. S. (Ed.), *Reye's Syndrome*, Vol. II Grune and Stratton, New York, 1979, pp. 215–232

Pincus, J. H. Subacute necrotising encephalomyelopathy (Leigh's disease): a consideration of clinical features and etiology. *Dev. Med. Child. Neurol.* 14 (1972) 87–101

della Porta, P., Maiolo, A. T., Negri, V. U. and Rosella, E. Cerebral blood flow and metabolism in therapeutic insulin coma. *Metabolism* 13 (1964) 131–140

Raabe, W. Synaptic transmission in ammonia intoxication. *Neurochem. Pathol.* 67 (1987) 145–166

Raabe, W. and Lin, S. Pathophysiology of ammonia intoxification. *Exp. Neurol.* 87 (1985) 519–532

Russell, G. J., Fitzgerald, J. F. and Clark, J. H. Fulminant hepatic failure. *J. Pediatr.* 111 (1987) 313–319

Saudubray, J. M., Marsac, C., Limal, J. M., Dumurgier, E., Charpentier, C., Ogier, H. and Coudè, F. X. Variation in plasma ketone bodies during a 24-hour fast in normal and in hypoglycaemic children: relationship to age. *J. Pediatr.* 98 (1981) 904–908

Saudubray, J. M., Specola, N., Middleton, B., Lombes, A., Bonnefont, J. P., Jakobs, C., Vassault, A., Charpentier, C. and Day, R. Hyperketotic states due to inherited defects of ketolysis. *Enzyme* 38 (1987) 80–90

Siesjö, B. K. Hypoglycaemia, brain metabolism, and brain damage. *Diabetes Metab. Rev.* 4 (1988) 113–144

Siesjö, B. K. and Plum, F. Pathophysiology of anoxic brain damage. In Gaull, G. E. (Ed.), *Biology of Brain Dysfunction*, Plenum Press, New York, 1972, pp. 319–372

Sokol, R. J., Francis, P. D., Gold, S. H., Ford, D. M., Lum, G. M. and Ambruso, D. R. Orthotopic liver transplantation for acute fulminant Wilson disease. *J. Pediatr.* 107 (1985) 549–552

Stanbury, J. B., Wyngaarden, J. B., Fredrickson, D. S., Goldstein, J. L. and Brown, M. S. (Eds.). *The Metabolic Basis of Inherited Disease*, 5th edn., McGraw-Hill Book Co., New York, 1983

Tashian, R. E. Inhibition of brain glutamic dehydrogenase by phenylalanine, leucine and valine derivatives: a suggestion concerning the neurological defect in phenylketonuria and branched-chain ketoaciduria. *Metabolism* 10 (1961) 393–402

Voorhies, T. M., Ehrlich, M. E., Duffy, T. E., Petito, C. K. and Plum, F. Acute hyperammonaemia in the young primate: physiologic and neuropathologic correlates. *Pediatr. Res.* 17 (1983) 970–975

Walker, C. O., McCandless, D. W., McGarry, J. D. and Shenker, S. Cerebral energy metabolism in short chain fatty acid induced coma. *J. Lab. Clin. Med.* 76 (1970) 569–583

Walter, J. H. and Leonard, J. V. Inborn errors of the urea cycle. *Br. J. Hosp. Med.* 38 (1987) 176–183

Ware, A. J., d'Agostino, A. and Combes, B. Cerebral oedema: a major complication of massive hepatic necrosis. *Gastroenterology* 76 (1979) 123–131

Watson, A. J., Karp, J. E., Walker, W. G., Chamber, T., Risch, V. R. and Brusilow, S. W. Transient idiopathic hyperammonaemia in adults. *Lancet* 2 (1985) 1271–1274

Wolfff, J. A., Caroll, J. E., Thuy, L. P., Haas, R. and Nyhan, W. L. Carnitine reduces fasting ketogenesis in patients with disorders of propionate metabolism. *Lancet* 1 (1986) 289–291

J. Inher. Metab. Dis. 12 Suppl. 1 (1989) 55–63

A Clinician's View of the Mass Screening of the Newborn for Inherited Diseases: Current Practice and Future Considerations

I. B. SARDHARWALLA and J. E. WRAITH
Willink Biochemical Genetics Unit, Royal Manchester Children's Hospital, Pendlebury, Manchester M27 1HA, UK

Summary: The case for or against mass screening for inherited diseases is discussed. There is universal acceptance for mass screening for phenylketonuria and congenital hypothyroidism. The case for mass screening for galactosaemia and for maple syrup urine disease is not very strong; they could be considered under the heading of 'urgent screening of the sick newborn'. It is difficult to find good arguments for mass screening for congenital adrenal hyperplasia. For screening for glucose-6-phosphate dehydrogenase deficiency and sickle cell disease, the established criteria for mass screening do not apply. A simple tool for early detection is now available and the population afflicted with a mutant gene which causes major health problems should receive special attention from its government. It is too early to offer any comment about cystic fibrosis screening; further developments must be awaited.

INTRODUCTION

The development of simple laboratory methods using microsamples of blood has been the key element in the mass screening of newborns and has led to the extension of screening for a number of inherited and other disorders since the screening programme for phenylketonuria was first introduced about 25 years ago. This paper attempts to make a rational examination of arguments for or against such screening programmes.

PHENYLKETONURIA SCREENING

In the late fifties and early sixties, circumstantial evidence was accumulated to show that early introduction of treatment of patients with phenylketonuria with a low phenylalanine diet would prevent mental retardation. In the absence of any reliable clinical parameters which would lead the paediatricians to request laboratory investigation for phenylketonuria in the newborn period, it became obvious that biochemical testing would have to be an essential part of a screening programme. In response to this need a number of reliable biochemical screening

Journal of Inherited Metabolic Disease. ISSN 0141-8955. Copyright © SSIEM and Kluwer Academic Publishers, PO Box 55, Lancaster, UK.

methods for phenylketonuria were developed using microsamples of blood. The aim was to detect increased levels of blood phenylalanine as the testing of urine for phenylalanine by chromatography or phenylpyruvic acid by Phenistix had fallen into disrepute due to the unreliability of these methods. With the availability of blood methods, the newborn screening programme became a reality.

The concept of mass screening of all newborn infants for phenylketonuria became universally accepted while the pundits of the time carefully considered the broad criteria on which such a programme could be based. These criteria, summarized by Komrower (1974) are:

(1) The disorder should be treatable;
(2) administratively, the screening programme should be feasible;
(3) methods should be simple, quick, inexpensive and reliable;
(4) the programme should be justified on economic grounds.

Treatability: The only point which needs to be made is that although a carefully controlled study about the effectiveness of the low phenylalanine diet has never been attempted on ethical and legal grounds, time has shown that the early introduction of dietary treatment will prevent mental retardation.

Administration: The aim of a smooth administrative process is that an effective centralized system for rapid laboratory diagnosis, prompt treatment and subsequent follow-up of affected children should be available. Some aspects of administration which relate to screening are considered briefly.

Time of blood collection: In the United Kingdom we owe a great deal to the community based nursing staff in giving flexibility in determining the time of blood collection: this was set at 6–14 days when the national screening programme was introduced in 1969 (H.M. (69) 72). This has not changed. In many countries outside the UK the timing of blood collection is determined by obstetric practice whereby the majority of infants are discharged from the hospital between 6 h to 3 days after birth. In such a case the blood is taken before discharge by the hospital staff.

Tests performed very early in life carry the risk of being false negative. The statistical frequency of missed cases of phenylketonuria on the first day is calculated to be about 16% (Scriver, 1982). Starfield and Holtzman (1975) compared the numbers of missed cases in the Republic of Ireland, the UK and the USA. They concluded that the number of false negative tests were greater in Ireland and the USA where tests were carried out early compared to the UK. The Committee on Genetics of the American Academy of Paediatrics has recommended that infants screened at or before 24 h of age should be re-screened at or by 2 weeks of age (American Academy of Pediatrics, 1982). According to the current trends in discharges, this alone would constitute about 20% of repeat testing (Cunningham *et al.*, 1987). In some states a second test is being done as a routine procedure (Guthrie, 1987).

In an attempt to determine the incidence of missed cases of phenylketonuria by the screening programme, Holtzman and colleagues conducted a structured telephone survey in November and December 1983 (Holtzman, N. A., 1986;

Holtzman, C. *et al.*, 1986). The analysis showed that approximately 1:70 of the affected infants covered by the screening programme had been missed. In 14% of the missed cases, either no specimen arrived in the laboratory or the specimen was inadequate. Half of those missed were attributed to laboratory error, although in two-thirds of these cases, the source of error could not be identified. The authors expressed a note of caution that the survey probably represented an underestimate of the true number.

In the UK, where all screening was done by blood testing from 1975, a review of missed cases during each 5-year period, i.e. 1975–1979 and 1980–1984 showed that the incidence was 1% (I. Smith, personal communication of data from the UK PKU Register). A small number of cases had been missed because either the blood specimen card had been lost in transit or a very small increase in phenylalanine was not followed up by the laboratory. But in the majority, of the order of 80–90%, there was laboratory or human error. Where cards have been available for retesting 3 to 4 years later by the same method, a positive result has been obtained in all. Without exception, all false negative results have occurred by Guthrie testing.

Reporting and filing of the results: The essential point to be made about reporting is that all results, normal, doubtful for repeat testing, and abnormal should be reported to the physicians, health clinics or Health Authorities. This will allow results to be validated and identify those specimens lost in transit. Whatever the method of filing, the object is to keep a laboratory record of the result for future reference.

Economic justification: It has been shown that it is cheaper to screen for and treat phenylketonuria than allow the disease to run its natural course (Komrower *et al.*, 1979) so that it becomes the responsibility of the community to care for the patients for the rest of their lives – not to mention the trauma to the families and loss of productive members to the community.

Screening for congenital hypothyroidism: When simple methods became available, there was total acceptance of its inclusion in the screening programme because it met all the criteria set out for phenylketonuria.

LEGISLATION AND SCREENING

In the USA, testing of infants for several diseases including some inborn errors of metabolism is required by law in many states. The intention of these compulsory screening programmes is the early detection, treatment or prevention of disease. Honourable as the intention may be to test all babies, has the legislation achieved its objective?

For a mandated programme, only one report of a study in New York State to compare the number of live births with the number of specimens tested by a screening laboratory is available. In the four regions, a survey showed that during the 20-year period from 1965 to 1984, between 1–4% of the newborns may not have been tested (Amador and Carter, 1986). However, no indication is given in this paper of the number of missed cases. Compare that with the result in Maryland, where there is no legislation and where parents must be informed of screening and consent taken. A survey showed that the refusal rate was only 0.05% (Faden *et al.*, 1982). In the UK there is no legislation. In the Manchester region the refusal rate is less than 0.02% and in the UK as a whole, at least 99.5% of the infants are screened although it is difficult to determine the exact figure (I. Smith, personal communication of data from the UK PKU Register). Legislation may not have achieved its objective in full in New York State, but it probably has assured resources for the total programme in the USA.

GALACTOSAEMIA

For the mass screening of the newborn, no metabolic disorder has generated so much debate, and aroused such strong emotions, as galactosaemia. The following is an attempt to examine the case in a rational way, for or against mass screening for galactosaemia.

There is little doubt that administratively the screening programme could be enlarged to include galactosaemia with little effort if the dried blood spot method of blood collection for phenylketonuria screening is already in practice. For those centres using other methods of sample collection and analysis, e.g. one-dimensional paper chromatography of plasma obtained from capillary tubes of blood, considerable expense and alteration of working practice would be necessary to accommodate galactosaemia screening. The timing of the sample collection would also be critical.

The incidence of galactosaemia is low and varies from 1:26 000 in Ireland to 1:667 000 or 1:1 000 000 in Japan (Ng *et al.*, 1987; Kawamura, 1987). In the UK, screening for galactosaemia is carried out in Scotland where the incidence is 1:70 000. On the assumption that a similar incidence prevails in England and Wales, one case of galactosaemia would be identified every 16 months in the Manchester region which has a birth rate of about 55 000 a year at an estimated additional cost of a minimum of US$ 25 000 at the current rate of exchange.

On the other hand, the majority if not all of the patients with classical galactosaemia present clinically either with a textbook picture or as sick infants with non-specific symptoms in the first 10 days of life. These features should be sufficient for a clinician to request an urgent test for metabolic investigation including galactosaemia. This is one view.

Those who support the concept of mass screening present different views. The earlier the diagnosis is made the better the ultimate outcome in respect of intellectual development. There is no support for this belief. The present evidence suggests that there is no difference in the outcome between the infants who have been treated from before the age of 2 weeks – amongst them some from birth – and those whose treatment started between 2–6 weeks (Sardharwalla and Wraith, 1987). On the whole the results are disappointing! The other view is that some babies may die from galactosaemia and early detection by screening may prevent death. Most infants can be detected on clinical grounds if a strong index of suspicion is maintained and a test to exclude galactosaemia is considered in all 'sick neonates'. This combined with ease of access to specialized laboratories for urgent metabolic investigation would identify almost all cases of galactosaemia.

It is for these reasons that mass screening for galactosaemia has not been considered in our region. Perhaps for the same reasons screening for galactosaemia has not been universally accepted. In the USA Guthrie (1983) estimated that 40% of infants are not screened, there is no screening programme in England and Wales and in some regions in Australia and in several countries in Europe. The case for mass screening for galactosaemia is not strong; its place lies with the urgent screening of the sick newborn.

CONGENITAL ADRENAL HYPERPLASIA

Several centres have undertaken pilot studies for screening for congenital adrenal hyperplasia (CAH) caused by steroid 21-hydroxylase deficiency. The method entails assaying elevated levels of 17α-hydroxyprogesterone in dried blood spots. The following account discusses the logistics of screening for CAH.

First the incidence. In the most recent review of a world-wide survey of screening for congenital adrenal hyperplasia an overall incidence of 1:14000 was reported (Pang *et al.*, 1988). There were regional variations of 1:11000 to 1:26000. However, the incidence in Alaskan Eskimos and one overseas province of France is much higher.

Taking the average incidence of 1:14000, the screening programme would detect a maximum of four cases with CAH a year in the Manchester region. Two of these would be female who would be expected to present with ambiguous genitalia at birth. Of the two males, one could be a salt-waster although recent information is that the incidence of salt-wasting CAH may be three times higher and the chances are high in this case that the diagnosis would be made on clinical grounds. Therefore the cost of detecting one case of the non-salt-losing variety of CAH who does not carry any long-term financial burden to the community would not be justified.

HAEMOGLOBINOPATHIES

It is worth considering screening for glucose-6-phosphate dehydrogenase deficiency and sickle cell disease because the criteria for mass screening already mentioned are probably not applicable to these disorders, but they introduce a different concept.

Glucose-6-phosphate dehydrogenase deficiency: Although there is no treatment for glucose-6-phosphate dehydrogenase deficiency, environmental avoidance of trigger factors can markedly reduce morbidity in affected individuals. In Greece a newborn screening programme has been in operation since 1977 (Missiou-Tsagarakis, 1987). Out of 1 million infants screened an incidence of 1:21 in males and 1:40 in females who were either homozygotes or heterozygotes with marked reduction in enzyme activity was found. The annual cost of screening was calculated at $29000 for 110000 tests. The benefit of the screening programme was shown in the fourfold reduction in the hospital admission of patients for the treatment of haemolytic crisis. Unfortunately there are no figures for the actual number of patients so treated before and after the screening, nor analysis of costing for the services which needed to be set up or added to the existing health programmes for counselling of the families so that a reliable assessment of cost effectiveness can be made. Nevertheless the screening may be justified on the grounds of a national health problem which requires special consideration in terms of funding.

Sickle cell disease: Screening for sickle cell disease, is undertaken in the USA, Jamaica and two regions in the UK. The experience of the screening programme in the USA gives the best opportunity for discussion.

This programme was based on a concept different from that for phenylketonuria or congenital hypothyroid screening. The element of cost effectiveness was not considered; there was a major health problem which needed attention. The programme was targeted to a high risk population, i.e. Americans of African origin. It was recognised that sickle cell disease carried a high mortality and morbidity in the paediatric population and early detection by screening followed by specialized care would reduce the mortality. New York State which has a black population of about 21% (Pass, 1987), has the largest experience of a sickle cell disease programme. Here, reference is made to that experience to illustrate some points.

Screening must be done on all babies as selection of samples for a defined population could be administratively cumbersome and expensive. Out of a total of about 2.4 million infants screened during the 10-year period from 1975–1984, an incidence of 1:520 of sickle cell disease was obtained in the black population.

Are there any indications that the objective of the screening programme, i.e. reducing the mortality and morbidity, has been achieved? In this respect it is worth referring to the review by Wethers and Grovers (1986) on the subject and examine their data of the effectiveness of an intensive follow-up programme for prevention of infection and counselling in New York City. Of the 736 sickle cell disease infants referred for medical care over 5 years from 1980–1984, 590 (80%) were reported to be under continuous supervision during this period. Out of 590, 11 children, or less than 2%, died. This is significantly lower than the 15–20% reported incidence for the same age in the USA and elsewhere (Warren *et al.*, 1982; Rogers *et al.*, 1978).

This is the good side of the programme. Are there any problems? Feelings of stigmatism, distrust of the health 'establishment' and discovery of non-paternity leading to domestic difficulties are a few we could mention. However, the major problem is concerned with the follow-up of heterozygote infants – about 4000 a year in New York City alone. Detection of sickle cell trait is a by-product which cannot be disregarded. Injection of additional resources will be needed to deal with this problem.

CYSTIC FIBROSIS

Recently cystic fibrosis screening has received considerable attention and needs a brief review. At present it is difficult to allocate an appropriate place for cystic fibrosis in the general concept of newborn screening. Certainly immunoreactive trypsinogen assay has been shown to be sensitive and specific and it costs relatively little. The recently reported 4% false negative result (Wilcken and Brown, 1987) would not be considered serious for cystic fibrosis but would not be acceptable for phenylketonuria screening. Futhermore it will not eliminate the need for sweat testing though it may reduce it.

Evidence has been presented to show that early diagnosis produces short-term benefit in a reduction in hospital admissions in the first year or two of life, thus introducing an element of cost effectiveness (Wilcken and Chalmers, 1985). To know the true cost effectiveness, it is necessary to know the cost of extended treatment if early identification and treatment will further improve the long-term survival (if at all) of these patients. Cystic fibrosis is not treatable in the same sense as phenylketonuria so the emphasis is now being placed on 'quality of life', which modifies the first criterion.

Taking an overall view, it seems clear that screening for cystic fibrosis cannot be considered to be in the same league as phenylketonuria screening, and a different reason will have to be found to justify screening. Knowing the current attitude of the government to health funding in the UK, the proposal for a national screening programme for cystic fibrosis may not receive priority consideration.

FUTURE

Virtually all screening tests, at the present time, are designed to measure accumulating metabolites or enzyme activities but not the primary genetic defect. The development in the area of recombinant DNA could lead to an expansion of screening. If automation of a technique such as the polymerase chain reaction were to become widely available, and fulfilled the criterion of being inexpensive and reliable, this would change the concept of and approach to screening.

The test could be performed on cord blood and this would allow the treatment to be started very early in life. The identification of the mutation at the DNA level should reduce the risk of false negative and false positive. Indeed, the screening would still be limited to those disorders which are treatable.

If technology allowed for mass screening for the carrier state for those disorders which are untreatable, e.g. cystic fibrosis or Duchenne muscular dystrophy, then it is not too difficult to predict that emphasis would be placed on prenatal diagnosis. At the antenatal clinics, carrier detection of mothers for some diseases could become a routine procedure. Introduction of gene therapy could cause a shift in attitude from abortion to early treatment.

A word of caution: countless cards with dried blood spots are stored away and there may be a great temptation to test them for genetic defects. Such enthusiastic action might raise legal questions about the ownership of specimens, consent for testing and disposal of information. One should also consider conditions in which the phenotype manifests much later in life, e.g. Huntington's chorea or Alzheimer's disease. Should infants be screened for these disorders? The burden of knowledge will be considerable for those families and individuals who have the mutant genotype. A great deal of careful thought is required to address these questions if we are to avoid many problems for generations to come.

Resource management: In this day of shrinking resources for health care, each screening laboratory should be prepared to undertake periodically its own assessment of the programmes to ensure that prudent use of available resources is made. Otherwise a time may come (it has already arrived in the UK) when external audit may become unavoidable. Needless to say, if resources were unlimited, then the question as to which genetic disease would qualify for mass screening, does not arise.

Screening of the newborn is here to stay and the anticipated development in DNA technology will offer a very promising future for it. Perhaps a few years from now the Society for the Study of Inborn Errors of Metabolism will review the topic and find that most of what we are doing today has become history.

REFERENCES

Amador, P. S. and Carter, T. P. Historical review of newborn screening in New York State: Twenty years experience. In Carter, T. P. and Wiley, A. M. (Eds.), *Genetic Disease: Screening and Management*, Alan R. Liss, Inc., New York, 1986, 343–357

American Academy of Pedriatics, Committee on Genetics. New issues in newborn screening for phenylketonuria and congenital hypothyroidism. *Pediatrics* 69 (1982) 104–106

Cunningham, G. C., Kan, K. and Mordaunt, V. L. Phenylalanine level of newborns in their first few days of life. In Therrell, Jr. B. L. (Ed.), *Advances in Neonatal Screening*, Elsevier Science Publishers, Amsterdam, 1987, 179–181

Faden, R. R., Chevalow, A. J., Holtzman, N. A. and Horn, S. D. A survey to evaluate parental consent as public policy for neonatal screening. *Am. J. Public Health* 72 (1982) 1347–1352

Guthrie, R. Lawsuits involving missed cases of PKU: lessons learned. In Therrell, Jr. B. L. (Ed.), *Advances in Neonatal Screening*, Elsevier Science Publishers, Amsterdam, 1987, 585–587

Guthrie, R., Bloom, S., Murphey, W. and Susi, A. A comparison of three newborn screening tests for galactosaemia. In Naruse, H. and Irie, M. (Eds.), *Neonatal Screening*, Excerpta Medica, Amsterdam, 1983, 243–251

H. M. (69) 72. *National Health Service. Screening for early detection of phenylketonuria*, Department of Health and Social Security, London, 1969

Holtzman, C., Slazyk, W. E., Cordero, J. F. and Hannon, W. H. Descriptive epidemiology of missed cases of phenylketonuria and congenital hypothyroidism. *Pediatrics* 78 (1986) 553–558

Holtzman, N. A. Genetic screening: criteria and evaluation – a message for the future. In Carter, T. P. and Willey, A. M. (Eds.), *Genetic Disease: screening and management*, Alan R. Liss, Inc., New York, 1986, 3–18

Kawamura, M. Neonatal screening for galactosaemia in Japan. In Therrell, Jr. B. L. (Ed.), *Advances in Neonatal Screening*, Elsevier Science Publishers, Amsterdam, 1987, 227–230

Komrower, G. M., The Philosophy and practice of screening for inherited diseases. *Paediatrics* 53 (1974) 182–188

Komrower, G. M., Sardharwalla, I. B., Fowler, B. and Bridge, C., The Manchester regional screening programme: a 10-year exercise in patient and family care. *Br. Med. J.* 2 (1979) 635–638

Missiou-Tsagarakis, S. Greek neonatal screening program for glucose-6-phosphate dehydrogenase deficiency. In Therrell, Jr. B. L. (Ed.), *Advances in Neonatal Screening*, Elsevier Science Publishers, Amsterdam, 1987, 425–428

Ng, W. G., Kawamura, M. and Donnell, G. N. Galactosaemia screening: methodology and outcome from worldwide data collection. In Therrell, Jr. B. L. (Ed.), *Advances in Neonatal Screening*, Elsevier Science Publishers, Amsterdam, 1987, 243–249

Pang, S., Wallace, M. A., Hofman, L., Thuline, H. C., Dorche, C., Lyon, I. C. T., Dobbins, R. H., Kling, S., Fujieda, K. and Suwa, S. Worldwide experience in newborn screening for classical congenital adrenal hyperplasia due to 21-hydroxylase deficiency. *Pediatrics* 81 (1988) 866–874

Pass, K. A. Newborn screening for sickle cell disease in New York. In Therrell, Jr. B. L. (Ed.), *Advances in Neonatal Screening*, Elsevier Science Publishers, Amsterdam (1987) 409–414

Rogers, D. W., Clarke, J. M. and Cupidore, L. Early deaths in Jamaican children with sickle cell disease. *Br. Med. J.* (1978) 1515–1517

Sardharwalla, I. B. and Wraith, J. E. Galactosaemia. *Nutr. Health* 5 (1987) 175–188

Scriver, C. R. Screening for medical intervention: The PKU experience. In Bonne-Tamir, B. and Cohen, T. (eds.) *Human Genetics, Part B; Medical Aspects*, Alan R. Liss, Inc., New York, 1982, 437–445

Starfield, B. and Holtzman, N. A. A comparison of effectiveness of screening for phenylketonuria in the United States, United Kingdom and Ireland. *N. Engl. J. Med.*, 293 (1975) 118–121

Warren, N. S., Carter, T. P., Humbert, Jr. and Rowley, P. T. Newborn screening for hemoglobinopathies in New York State: experience of physicians and parents of affected children. *J. Pediatr.* 100 (1982) 373

Wethers, D. L. and Grover, R. Screening the newborn for sickle cell disease: is it worth the effort? In Carter T. and Willey, A. M. (Eds.) *Genetic Disease: Screening and Management*, Alan R. Liss, Inc., New York, 1986, 123–136

Wilcken, B. and Brown, A. R. D. Screening for cystic fibrosis in New South Wales, Australia: evaluation of the results of screening 400 000 babies. In Therrell, Jr. B. L. (Ed.), *Advances in Neonatal Screening*, Elsevier Science Publishers, Amsterdam, 1987, 385–390

Wilcken, B. and Chalmers, G. Reduced morbidity in patients with cystic fibrosis detected by newborn screening. *Lancet* 2 (1985) 1319–1321

J. Inher. Metab. Dis. 12 Suppl. 1 (1989) 64–88

A Clinical Biochemist's View of the Investigation of Suspected Inherited Metabolic Disease

W. BLOM, J. G. M. HUIJMANS and G. B. VAN DEN BERG
Department of Pediatrics, Metabolic Laboratory, Sophia Children's Hospital, Erasmus University Rotterdam, Gordelweg 160, 3038 GE Rotterdam, The Netherlands

Summary: The necessity for a multi-disciplinary approach to the study of genetic disease is discussed. The progress of laboratory investigation programmes made it not feasible and inefficient to run a full metabolic investigation programme in every new patient suspected of inherited metabolic disease. An application form for metabolic investigation is described, which can be used to collect clinical information relevant to metabolic disease. On the basis of the patient's clinical information, selection criteria are given to decide which laboratory investigation programme has to be performed in the individual patient. A full metabolic laboratory investigation programme is described and illustrated with some examples of abnormal metabolite patterns. Diagnostic results over a 2-year period are presented.

In the past, a pediatrician confronted with a child suspected of an inborn error of metabolism collaborated with a biochemist or a biochemical laboratory to set up methods for making the laboratory diagnosis and to control therapeutic trials. Depending on the accidental interest of clinicians and biochemists small teams were formed concerned with the diagnostics and therapy of metabolic disease.

During the 1970s more systematic laboratory investigation programmes to detect abnormal metabolite patterns in body fluids were evaluated. Due to technological progress, analytical instrumentation became available to facilitate metabolic investigations. Enzyme assays in blood cells or tissues were developed to confirm a diagnosis. In the middle 1970s cultured skin fibroblasts and amniotic fluid cells extended the possibilities of pre- and postnatal enzyme diagnosis. During the last 5 years chorionic villus biopsies have permitted early prenatal diagnosis and the application of DNA analysis to investigate genetic disease is rapidly increasing.

There is no doubt that the main progress in gaining knowledge of genetic disease is the result of advances in basic research in molecular genetics, biochemistry and cell biology. Working alone or in small groups in the field of genetic disease has been rendered out of date. The work is divided into different highly specialized fields. Centralization of organization and knowledge by the collaboration of different specialist teams is the only guarantee of an up-to-date approach to diagnosis, therapy, genetic counselling and prevention of congenital disease.

In the developed industrialized countries congenital disease has become the major cause of infant mortality, accounting for 25–35% of all infant deaths. There is a growing need for extensive information about the risks of pregnancy and confinement and about the various possibilities of preventing congenital handicaps. The increasing costs of health care have directed the attention of many governments towards programmes that aim at the prevention of disorders which are associated with long-term physical and/or mental handicaps. However, it takes a long time before this macroeconomic view of the problems of congenital disease will be interpreted in microeconomic solutions. In The Netherlands the Institutes or Centres of Clinical Genetics are an example of a national approach.

INSTITUTES OF CLINICAL GENETICS

Since 1979 an Institute or Centre of Clinical Genetics has been established in every university with a medical faculty in The Netherlands. They are non-profit organizations and they are financially independent of the university and the academic hospital, in such a way that the Ministry of Public Health can directly control their financial and economic status. The output and quality of work, however, is the responsibility of the university and the academic hospital. In Figure 1 the organization-scheme of the Institute of Clinical Genetics in Rotterdam is shown. The Institute serves the South-western part of the Netherlands, covering a population of about 3 million people. It is an example of a centralized, multi-disciplinary approach to the investigation and prevention of congenital disease. In this publication we shall concentrate on the working method and the function of the Metabolic Laboratory.

METABOLIC LABORATORY

The activities of the Metabolic Laboratory started in 1971 within the routine Laboratory of Clinical Paediatric Chemistry. At the end of 1975 the Metabolic Laboratory was separated from the Laboratory of Clinical Paediatric Chemistry and became part of the Department of Paediatrics. In 1979 the Metabolic Laboratory was transferred to the Institute of Clinical Genetics.

During the development of the Metabolic Laboratory in the 1970s it became clear that a gap had arisen between the Clinic and the Metabolic Laboratory. Clinicians were not aware of, or did not understand, the advanced possibilities and strengths of the Metabolic Laboratory. The interpretation of laboratory results was difficult if no clinical information on the patient was available. The progress of laboratory investigation programmes made it not feasible nor efficient to run a full investigation programme on every new patient. The need for a selective screening programme, dependent on the clinical symptoms of the patient was forced on us. We therefore formulated two principal questions:

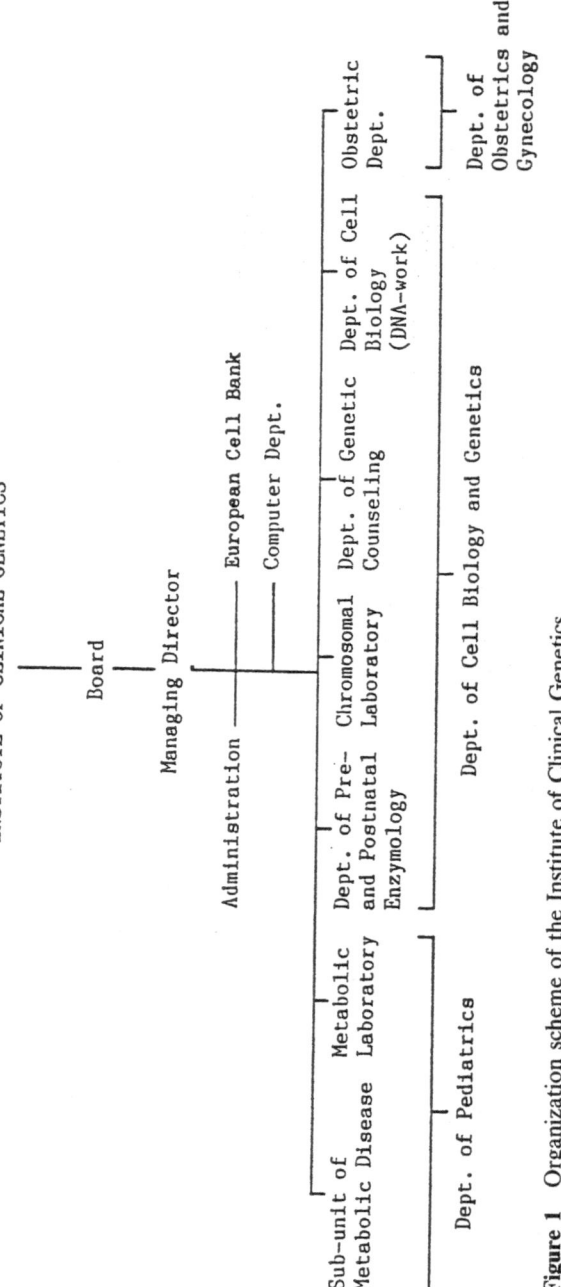

Figure 1 Organization scheme of the Institute of Clinical Genetics

(1) Who decides to do a metabolic screening for a patient and on the basis of which clinical symptoms?

(2) If there is a clinical selection of patients, who decides which laboratory investigations will be performed?

To answer these questions we searched the literature for clinical symptoms related to inborn errors of metabolism. We structured these clinical symptoms and designed a request form for metabolic investigation. On this application form, the pediatrician, neurologist or other clinician marks the patient's clinical abnormalities and sends the application form together with a 24-h urine and/or plasma to the Metabolic Laboratory. On the basis of the given clinical picture a metabolic laboratory investigation programme is made on the Metabolic Laboratory. An English version of the application form is shown in Figure 2.

In addition to the clinical symptoms information is obtained about routine clinical chemistry investigations, nutrition, genetics and medication. Using this approach, a selective laboratory screening programme and reliable interpretation of laboratory results can be made. In addition we discovered remarkable benefits:

(1) the application form has an educative function. The clinician, using the application form, is confronted every time with relevant clinical symptoms of patients with inborn errors of metabolism;

(2) a relationship of confidence was built up between the clinicians and the Metabolic Laboratory;

(3) the yield of diagnoses of inborn errors of metabolism rapidly increased in newly investigated patients.

As far as we know, the request form is already successfully used by various laboratories in several European countries.

METABOLIC LABORATORY INVESTIGATION PROGRAMME

Dividing the diagnostic tasks between the departments of the Institute of Clinical Genetics allows each department to specialize and develop expertise. The Metabolic Laboratory is concerned only with the estimation of abnormal metabolites. The Metabolic Laboratory could develop a broad investigation programme, and large investments in instrumental analysis could be justified. The programme of metabolic investigations is given in Table 1.

Depending on the clinical picture of the patient a selective choice out of the investigation programme is made for every individual patient.

Preliminary examination programme

Every urine is examined for abnormal colour or smell. Some metabolites in organic acidurias give a particular smell to a urine.

A dipstick urine test gives general information about the presence of protein, glucose, ketones, urobilinogen, bilirubin and blood, but is also a check on the

Blom et al.

INSTITUTE OF CLINICAL GENETICS
METABOLIC LABORATORY
SOPHIA CHILDREN'S HOSPITAL
GORDELWEG 160, 3038 GE ROTTERDAM
THE NETHERLANDS
(10) 4656566 - EXT. 2737

APPLICATION FOR
LABORATORY INVESTIGATION
IN HER. METABOLIC DISEASE

PLASMA NUM:
URINE NUM:

PATIENT IDENTIFICATION
NAME   :
DATE OF BIRTH:
ADDRESS   :
POSTCODE   :
CITY   :

SAMPLE DATE:
APPLICANT :
DEPT   :
HOSPITAL :

VOLUME	COLLECTION TIME		
ml	☐ hrs	☐ 12 hrs	☐ 24 hrs

☐ URINE
☐ PLASMA   SAMPLE TIME:
☐ CSF   SAMPLE TIME:
☐ 1th INVESTIGATION ☐ REPETITION
☐ RESEARCH

IN CASE OF REPEATED INVESTIGATION: RESULT(S) PREVIOUS INVESTIGATION(S):

SUMMARY CASE HISTORY + SPECIAL DEMANDS

CLINICAL INFORMATION

I GENERAL PHYSICAL ABNORMALITIES
1 ☐P ☐3 ☐10 ☐50 ☐90 length _ _ _ cm
2 ☐P ☐3 ☐10 ☐50 ☐90 weight f. length
3   weight _ _ _ kg
4 ☐P ☐3 ☐10 ☐50 ☐90 headcir. _ _ cm
5 ☐ abnormal face
6 ☐ hepatomegaly
7 ☐ splenomegaly
8 ☐ ascites
9 ☐ oedema
10 ☐ icterus
11 ☐ tachypnea
12 ☐ hyperventilation
13 ☐ hair + nail abnormalities
14 ☐ skin abnormalities
15 ☐ eye abnormalities
16 ☐ deafness
17 ☐ strange smell

II NEUROLOGICAL ABNORMALITIES
1 ☐ mental retardation
2 ☐ motor retardation
3 ☐ ataxia
4 ☐ spasticity
5 ☐ hypertonia
6 ☐ muscle dystrophia/weakness
7 ☐ nystagmus
8 ☐ chorea-athetosis
9 ☐ convulsions
10 ☐ lethargy/coma
11 ☐ behavioral abnormalities

III GASTROINTESTINAL ABNORMALITIES
1 ☐ vomiting
2 ☐ diarrhea
3 ☐ refusal of nutrition
4 ☐ constipation

IV NEPHROLOGICAL ABNORMALITIES
1 ☐ renal stones
2 ☐ polyuria
3 ☐ strange colour/smell urine
4 ☐ _ _ _ _ _ _ _ _ _ _ _ _ _ _

V X-RAY ABNORMALITIES
1 ☐ bone-age retardation
2 ☐ skeletal abnormalities
3 ☐ osteoporosis
4 ☐ rachitis

VI IMMUNOLOGICAL ABNORMALITIES
1 ☐ recurrent infections
2 ☐ _ _ _ _ _ _ _ _ _ _ _ _ _ _

VII HEMATOLOGICAL ABNORMALITIES
1 ☐ anemia
2 ☐ neutropenia
3 ☐ thrombopenia
4 ☐ thrombo-embolic abnormalities
5 ☐ bleeding tendency
6 ☐ lymphocyte vacuoles
7 ☐ leucocyte granula
8 ☐ abnormal bonemarrow

VIII LABORATORY ABNORMALITIES
1 ☐ acidosis
2 ☐ hypoglycemia
3 ☐ hyperglycemia
4 ☐ ketosis
5 ☐ hyperammonemia
6 ☐ _ _ _ _ _ _ _ _ _ _ _
7 ☐ _ _ _ _ _ _ _ _ _ _ _

IX NUTRITION
1 ☐ oral
2 ☐ parenteral
3 ☐1 ☐2 ☐3 ☐4 ☐5 g/kg protein int.
4 ☐ formula _ _ _ _ _ _ _ _ _ _ _

X GENETICS
1 ☐ consanguinity
2 ☐ metabolic disease in family
3   _ _ _ _ _ _ _ _ _ _ _ _ _ _

XI MEDICATION

Figure 2   Request form for the laboratory investigation of metabolic disease

Table 1   Metabolic laboratory investigation programme

1. *Preliminary examination urine*
   Colour/smell
   Urine dipstick analysis for nitrite, pH,
      protein, glucose, ketones, urobilinogen,
      bilirubin, blood
   Clinitest (Benedict's reaction)
   (Sulphite reaction)

2. *Group screening tests*

Group	Method[a]	Specimen[b]
Amino acids	HVE, amino acid analyser	ser, pla, u, csf, af
Organic acids	Capillary GC/MS	ser, pla, u, csf, af
Very long-chain fatty acids	Capillary GC/MS	pla
Acyl-carnitines	FAB/MS	u
Mono- and disaccharides	TLC	u
Oligosaccharides	TLC	u
Imidazoles	2d TLC	u
Purines/pyrimidines	2d TLC	u
Tryptophan+indoles	2d TLC+HPLC, capillary GC/MS	u
Kynurenine+metabolites	2d TLC+HPLC, capillary GC/MS	u
Cerebrosides/sulphatides	TLC	u
Mucopolysaccharides	Spot test + CPC p-test	u
	Q. as hexuronic acid	u, af
	2d electrophoresis	
Porphyrins	Chemical test, TLC	u

3. *Specific metabolite assays*

Metabolite	Method	Specimen
Methylmalonic acid	Spectrophotometric	ser, pla, u
Orotic acid	Spectrophotometric	u
Uric acid	Spectrophotometric	ser, u
Phytanic acid	Capillary GC/MS	ser, u
Tryptophan (free and total)	HPLC	pla
Serotonin	HPLC	wb, csf
Oxalic acid + glycollic acid	Capillary GC/MS	u
Oxalic acid	Enzymatic	pla
Sialic acid	Spectrophotometric	u

[a] HVE = high voltage electrophoresis; GC/MS = gas chromatography–mass spectrometry; FAB/MS = fast atom bombardment mass spectrometry; TLC = thin-layer chromatography; 2d = two dimensional; HPLC = high performance liquid chromatography; CPC p-test = cetyl pyridinium chloride precipitation test; Q. = quantitative.
[b] Ser = serum; pla = plasma; u = urine; csf = cerebrospinal fluid; af = amniotic fluid; wb = whole blood

quality of the urine. If the nitrite concentration is positive and/or the pH is increased, the urine might be contaminated by bacteria due to an urinary tract infection or the urine may not have been collected, stored or transported correctly. A high urinary pH may also suggest renal bicarbonate loss.

On every urine we perform a Clinitest (Benedict's reaction) to detect reducing substances. Antibiotics may interfere with the Clinitest. If a patient is suspected of sulphite oxidase deficiency, we perform a test for sulphite in a fresh portion of urine.

Group screening tests

Amino acids: Screening of amino acids by high-voltage electrophoresis (HVE) is performed in the urine of every new patient. In the case of an abnormal pattern, quantitative amino acid analysis will be done, using an amino acid analyser. See Figures 3 and 4. A summary of amino acid metabolic abnormalities is given in Table 2.

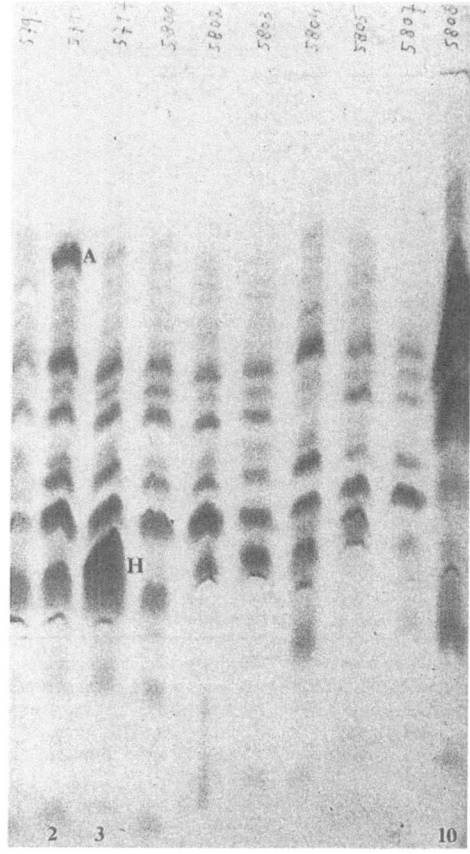

Figure 3 High-voltage electrophoretogram of amino acids in urine. Abnormalities: lane 2, A = antibiotics; lane 3, H = histidine due to histidinaemia; lane 10, pattern of argininosuccinic aciduria

Quantitative amino acid analysis can be used to a limited degree for prenatal diagnosis. In Table 3 the result of amino acid analysis is given for a pregnancy at risk for argininosuccinic aciduria. In the maternal urine, and in amniotic fluid, increased levels of argininosuccinic acid and the related cyclic anhydrides could be detected. The diagnosis of citrullinaemia can also easily be made by amino acid

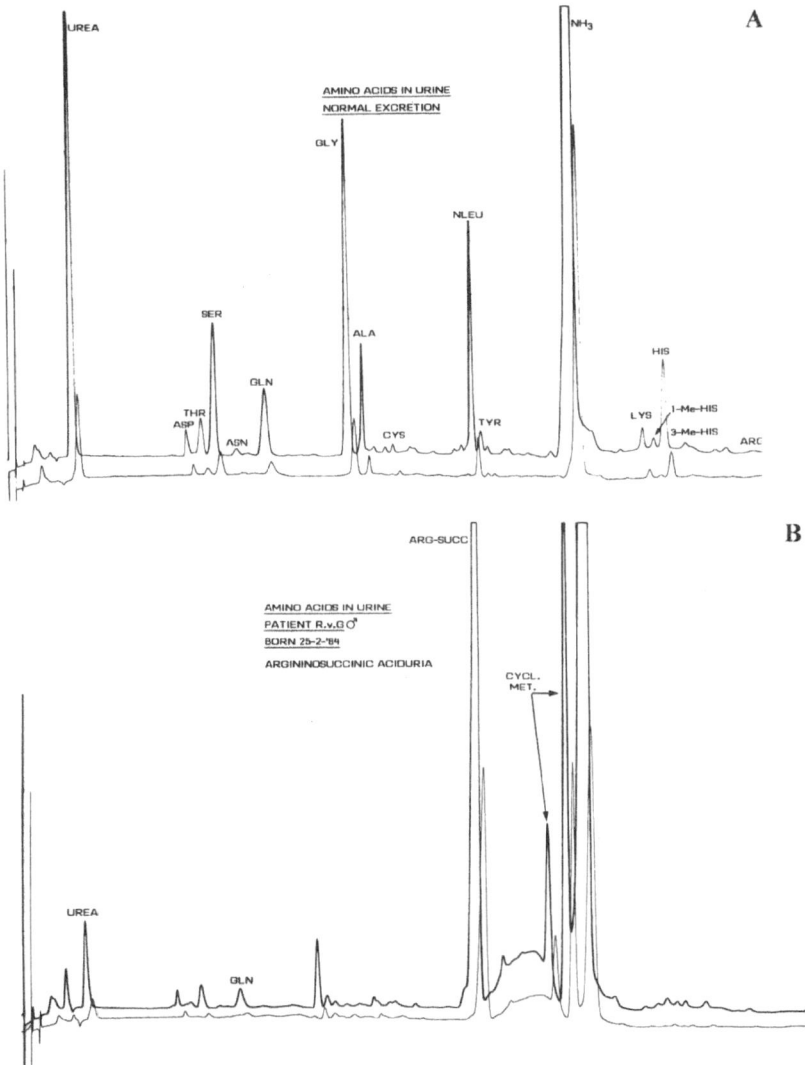

Figure 4 (A) Normal amino acid chromatogram of urine; (B) amino acid chromatogram of a 10 times diluted urine of a patient with argininosuccinic aciduria

analysis in amniotic fluid (Kleijer *et al.*, 1984a). Table 4 shows that citrulline is markedly increased in amniotic fluid if the fetus is affected by citrullinaemia.

Organic acids: Organic acids are analysed in the urine of every new patient by gas chromatography. In our routine method the organic acids are methylated and keto-groups are converted into ethoximes. In special cases we also silylate the

Table 2 Primary and secondary aminoacidopathies observed in urine

Amino acid	Primary metabolic disorder	Secondarily increased (decreased) in:
Taurine	Not described	Catabolic state; high protein intake; acute liver failure; sulphite-oxidase deficiency
Phosphoethanolamine	Hypophosphatasia (bone alkaline-phosphatase deficiency)	Some endocrine disorders; hypertension; bone diseases
Aspartylglucosamine	Aspartylglucosaminuria (lysosomal aspartylglycosylaminase deficiency)	Not described
Aspartic acid	Dicarboxylic aminoaciduria (transport disorder in combination with glutamic acid and proline)	Decomposition of asparagine
4-Hydroxyproline	Hydroxyprolinaemia (hydroxyproline oxidase deficiency)	Newborn infants; chronic uraemia; bone disease
Threonine	Not described	Vitamin B6 deficiency; liver cirrhosis
Serine	Not described	Vitamin B6 deficiency; (Decreased in folic acid deficiency, and bacterial decomposition of the urine)
Asparagine	Not described	Not described
Glutamic acid	1. Dicarboxylic aminoaciduria (transport disorder together with aspartic acid and proline) 2. Glutamic acidaemia	Decomposition of glutamine
Glutamine	Not described	All conditions with hyperammonaemia together with alanine; acute sick newborn infants
Sarcosine	Hypersarcosinaemia (sarcosine dehydrogenase deficiency)	Glutaric aciduria Type 2; folic acid deficiency
2-Aminoadipic acid	2-Aminoadipic aciduria (no enzyme defect detected)	2-Ketoadipic aciduria; severe convulsive conditions
Proline	1. Hyperprolinaemia Type 1 (proline oxidase deficiency) 2. Hyperprolinaemia Type 2 (Δ^1-pyrroline-5-carboxylic acid dehydrogenase deficiency) 3. Iminoglycinuria (transport defect for proline, OH-proline and glycine)	Iminodipeptiduria (prolidase deficiency); newborn infants
Glycine	Nonketotic hyperglycinaemia (deficiency of the cleavage enzyme)	1. Ketotic hyperglycinaemia due to (a) propionic acidaemia, (b) methylmalonic acidaemia, (c) isovaleric acidaemia, or (d) 2-methylacetoacetic aciduria 2. D-Glyceric aciduria 3. Hyperprolinaemia Type 1, or iminoglycinuria 4. Hypersarcosinaemia 5. Infants up to 6 months of age 6. Starvation 7. Bacterial decomposition of hippuric acid 8. Valproic acid therapy (Decreased in folic acid deficiency)

Table 2 (continued) Primary and secondary aminoacidopathies observed in urine

Amino acid	Primary metabolic disorder	Secondarily increased (decreased) in:
Alanine	Not described	All conditions with lactic acidaemia; together with glutamine in hyperammonaemia; bacterial contamination of the urine; (Decreased in ketotic hypoglycaemia)
Citrulline	Citrullinaemia (argininosuccinate synthetase deficiency)	Argininosuccinic aciduria; saccharopinuria; renal insufficiency; hyperargininaemia
2-Aminobutyric acid	Not described	Hyperaminoaciduria
Valine	1. Hypervalinaemia (transaminase defect) 2. Maple syrup urine disease	Not described
Cystine	1. Isolated cystinuria (transport defect) 2. Dibasic aminoaciduria together with ornithine, lysine and arginine (transport defect) 3. (Increased in leukocytes and cultured fibroblasts in cystinosis)	Conditions of homocystinuria due to a remethylation defect; infants during the first months of life; renal defects; (Decreased in homocystinuria and cystathioninuria)
Homocitrulline	Not described	Young infants; various hyperammonaemia syndromes
Cystathionine	Cystathioninuria (β-cystathioninase deficiency)	Vitamin B_6 deficiency; neuroblastoma and hepatoblastoma; liver cirrhosis
Methionine	1. Hypermethioninaemia (methionine-adenylotransferase deficiency) 2. Methionine malabsorption syndrome	Homocystinuria; tyrosinosis; (Decreased in homocystinuria due to remethylation defects)
Alloisoleucine	Not described	Maple syrup urine disease
Isoleucine	Maple syrup urine disease	Not described
Leucine	Maple syrup urine disease	Not described
Argininosuccinic acid	Argininosuccinic aciduria (argininosuccinate lyase deficiency)	Detectable in hyperornithinaemia
Tyrosine	1. Tyrosinosis Type 1 (fumarylacetoacetase deficiency) 2. Tyrosinosis Type 2 (cytosolic tyrosine-aminotransferase deficiency)	Transient tyrosinosis in newborns; high protein intake; galactosaemia; fructose intolerance; liver disease (hepatitis, Wilson's disease)
β-Alanine	Hyper-β-alaninaemia (β-alanine-2-oxo-glutarate-amino-transferase deficiency)	After kidney transplantation, when the kidney is rejected; carnosinuria
Phenylalanine	1. Phenylketonuria (phenylalanine hydroxylase deficiency) 2. Hyperphenylalaninaemia (dihydropteridine reductase deficiency) 3. Hyperphenylalaninaemia (various disorders of dihydropteridine biosynthesis)	Newborns (especially in maternal PKU); high protein intake; tyrosinosis

Table 2 (continued)   Primary and secondary aminoacidopathies observed in urine

Amino acid	Primary metabolic disorder	Secondarily increased (decreased) in:
β-Aminoisobutyric acid	β-Aminoisobutyric aciduria – occurs in 6–10% of the normal population in N.W. Europe (not considered as a disease)	Various types of neoplastic disease; excessive tissue break-down
Homocystine	1. Homocystinuria (cystathionine-β-synthase deficiency) 2. Homocystinuria (N^5,N^{10}-methylene-THF-reductase deficiency) 3. Homocystinuria (N^5-methyl-THF-methyl-transferase deficiency)	Vitamin B_{12} malabsorption or deficiency together with methylmalonic acid; vitamin B_6 deficiency
γ-Aminobutyric acid	Not described with an expression in urine	β-Alaninaemia; intestinal dysbacteriosis
Tryptophan	Tryptophan pyrrolase deficiency (?)	Hartnup disease; hypoalbuminaemia; (Decreased in intestinal tryptophan malabsorption; chronic diarrhoea or constipation)
Ethanolamine	Ethanolaminosis (hepatic ethanolamine kinase deficiency)	Liver cirrhosis; hyperlysinaemia; hypersarcosinaemia; newborns
Ornithine	1. Hyperornithinaemia (ornithine-2-oxo-acid-amino-transferase deficiency) 2. Dibasic aminoaciduria (transport defect)	Not described
Lysine	1. Hyperlysinaemia (lysine-2-oxoglutarate reductase deficiency) 2. Dibasic aminoaciduria (transport defect) 3. Lysinuric protein intolerance (transport defect)	Newborns together with cystine; hyperammonaemia (sometimes together with homocitrulline and arginine); saccharopinuria
1-Methylhistidine	Not described	Renal insufficiency; by alimentary cause (chicken)
Histidine	Histidinaemia	Newborns; folic acid deficiency
3-Methylhistidine	Not described	Malnutrition; starvation
Carnosine	Carnosinaemia (carnosinase deficiency)	High meat diet (especially chicken, turkey, etc.); infants up to 2 years of age
Anserine	Carnosinaemia (carnosinase deficiency)	High intake of meat, especially poultry
Arginine	1. Hyperargininaemia (arginase deficiency) 2. Dibasic aminoaciduria (transport defect) 3. Lysinuric protein intolerance (transport defect)	Lysinaemia; ornithinaemia

Table 3   Amino acid analysis for a pregnancy at risk of argininosuccinic aciduria

Specimen	Date	Arginosuccinic acid (mmol L^{-1})	Cyclic anhydride I (mmol L^{-1})	Cyclic anhydride II (mmol L^{-1})
Mother's urine	13.8.79	2.14	0.21	0.40
Amniotic fluid	27.8.79	0.73	0.06	0.08
Cord blood plasma:	27.8.79			
arterial		0.29	trace	0.09
venous		0.27	trace	trace
Patient H.N. born 27.8.79:				
plasma	28.8.79	1.42	0.16	0.31
CSF	28.8.79	0.65	0.13	0.08

Table 4   Citrulline concentrations in amniotic fluid of three pregnancies at risk for citrullinaemia

Amniotic fluid	Citrulline (μmol L^{-1})
At risk A$_1$	170
At risk A$_2$	130
At risk B	160
Control range ($n = 5$)	9–12
Literature range ($n = 58$)	6–23

organic acids, e.g. to detect oxalic acid or (poly)hydroxy acids. An FID and an NPFID detector are simultaneously used in our gas chromatographs. The NPFID detector indicates the presence of nitrogen in the metabolite. In this manner we can easily detect the ethoximes, e.g. (glycine-) conjugates and drugs or drug metabolites. For example see Figure 5. If abnormal peaks appear in the gas chromatogram, the identity is established or confirmed by gas chromatography–mass spectrometry.

Many organic acidaemias can give acute peri- or neonatal problems. Although metabolic acidosis is an important symptom, one persistent misunderstanding is that organic acid analysis is *only* indicated in the case of metabolic acidosis. Many of our diagnosed patients with organic acidaemias had a very mild or no metabolic acidosis.

Prenatal diagnosis of organic acidaemias by means of stable isotope dilution mass spectroscopy analysis is of increasing importance (Jacobs, 1989). Organic acid analysis is not only important in the diagnosis of an organic acidaemia but also gives much information about nutritional status, abnormal bacterial metabolism in the intestine, other gastrointestinal abnormalities, vitamin deficiencies, liver function disorders, (drug) intoxications, etc. Because the Metabolic Laboratory is informed about the clinical picture of the patient, we were able to correlate many organic acid abnormalities with general paediatric problems. For general information and references to organic acidaemias we refer to two handbooks: Goodman and Markey (1981) and Chalmers and Lawson (1982).

J. Inher. Metab. Dis. 12 Suppl. 1 (1989)

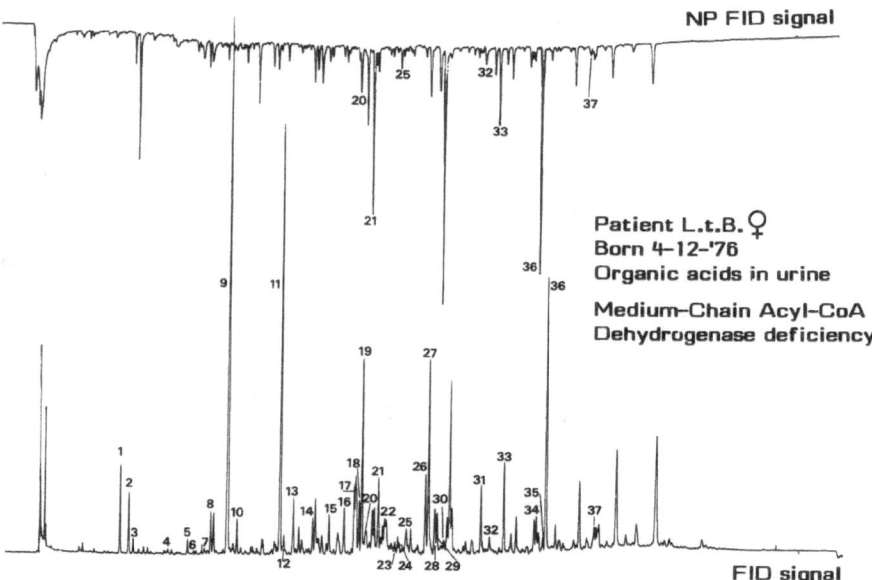

Figure 5 Gas chromatogram of organic acids in the urine of a patient with medium-chain acyl-CoA dehydrogenase deficiency. All the numbered peaks are from metabolites related to the disease. Peaks detected by the FID as well as the NPFID detector: 20 = hexanoyl-glycine, 21 = octanoyl-glycine, 25 = decanoyl-glycine, 32 = adipyl-glycine, 33 = phenyl-propionyl-glycine, 36 = suberyl-glycine and 37 = sebacyl-glycine

In consultation with the Departments of Neonatology and of Intensive Care we made two agreements:

(1) In all acute patients the first portion of urine at admission is collected and sent to the Metabolic Laboratory. Then a 24-h urine is collected.

(2) In all neonates with a sepsis-like picture urine is collected immediately. If a bacterial culture is negative and/or the patient does not respond to antibiotics, the urine is sent to the Metabolic Laboratory.

The first sample of urine is important because this urine is a reflection of the acute metabolic state of the patient. If an inborn error is diagnosed a 24-h urine is directly available for further investigations. Many acutely ill neonates with an inborn error of amino acid or organic acid metabolism have a sepsis-like picture. During admission symptomatic therapy can mask the metabolic picture or the patient can suddenly die. In those cases there is always an early urine taken at the time of admission. If it turns out that a patient has no metabolic problem, the urine can be thrown away. This procedure is very important in, for example, urea cycle disorders, tyrosinosis or organic acidaemias.

Very long-chain fatty acids: Very long-chain fatty acids in plasma are estimated in patients suspected of a peroxisomal disorder. For example Zellweger syndrome or neonatal adrenoleukodystrophy (Poll-The, 1988).

Acyl-carnitines: Acyl-carnitines are analysed by means of fast atom bombardment mass spectrometry, according to Millington and co-workers (1984) and Roe and co-workers (1985). Abnormal carnitine esters are excreted in urine in many organic acidaemias, in disorders of fatty acid β-oxidation and in valproic acid therapy. However, most patients with these abnormal metabolic conditions are carnitine deficient, resulting in a reduction of the excretion of abnormal carnitine esters. The effect of carnitine therapy, in the metabolic disorders mentioned and in valproic acid therapy, can be controlled by the estimation of acyl-carnitines.

Mono- and disaccharides: Indications of mono- and disaccharide (sugar) analysis are given in Table 5. In the newborn, sugar analysis is a simple screening method to diagnose galactosaemia or other disorders of galactose metabolism. However, when a urine of a patient suspected of galactosaemia is analysed, one has to confirm that the patient received lactose in the nutrition and/or that the patient did not

Table 5 Indications for sugar analysis

Poor growth
Nutritional problems
Hepatomegaly
Bowel distension
Ascites, oedema
Cataract
Lethargy, coma
Anaemia, bleeding tendency
Hyperbilirubinaemia
Positive Benedict's test

recently have a blood exchange transfusion. The non-specific symptoms in the acute galactosaemic patient are usually treated by glucose infusions, in which case galactose rapidly disappears from the urine. After exchange transfusion galactose-1-phosphate uridyltransferase activity is introduced into the blood of the patient. This can mask the enzyme deficiency, at least in the enzymatic assay. Hereditary fructose intolerance can also be diagnosed by means of sugar analysis. In this case one has to be certain that the patient has had sucrose in feeds before a negative result excludes the diagnosis. In liver insufficiency, different mono- and disaccharides can frequently be detected in urine, e.g. in hepatitis or Wilson's disease.

Oligosaccharides: Indications for oligosaccharide analysis are given in Table 6. Humbel and Collart (1975) described a thin-layer chromatographic method for detection of oligosaccharides in urine. However, the oligosaccharides often appear as diffuse bands in the chromatogram and this method does not take into account concentration variabilities of different urines. Interpretation of oligosaccharide patterns is then difficult. Blom and co-workers (1983) published an improved TLC method with a desalting procedure for the urine; the amount of urine spotted on the thin-layer plate is dependent on the creatinine concentration and an age-

78

Blom et al.

Table 6 Indications for oligosaccharide analysis

The same as for mucopolysaccharidosis (Table 8)
Cherry-red spot in fundus
Hyperplasia of the gingiva
Muscle weakness, hypotonia, hypertonia
Muscle dystrophy
Convulsions
Skin abnormalities (keratosis)
Positive sweat-test without cystic fibrosis

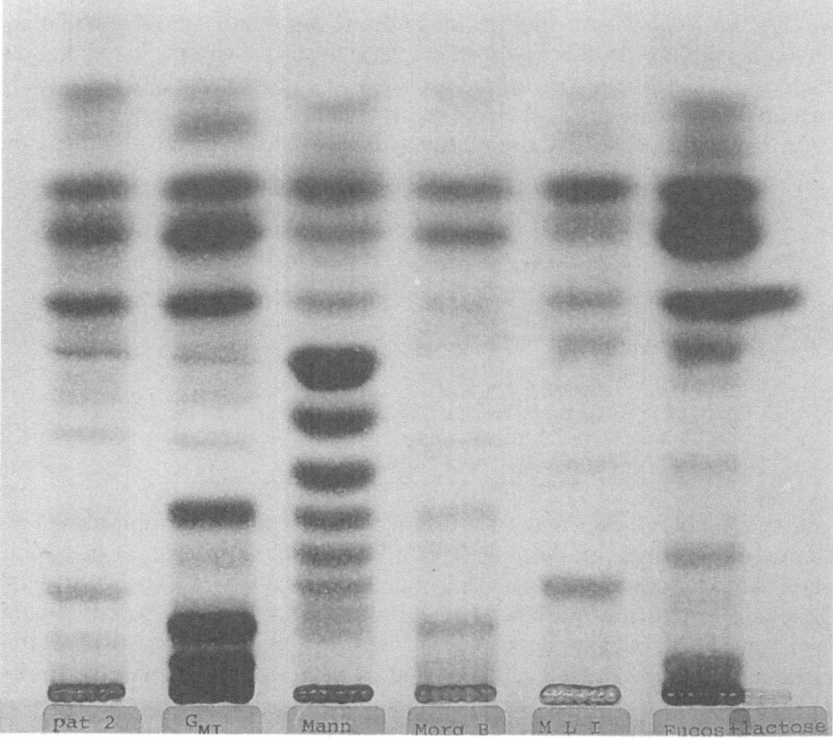

Figure 6 Thin-layer chromatogram of oligosaccharides in urine of patients with the diagnosis: lane 1, α-N-acetylgalactosaminidase deficiency; lane 2, G_{M1}-gangliosidosis; lane 3, α-mannosidosis; lane 4, Morquio B syndrome; lane 5, mucolipidosis type I; lane 6, α-fucosidosis (+ overlapping lactose as a standard)

dependent factor. Some examples of abnormal oligosaccharide patterns are presented in Figure 6. In lane 1 of the figure the abnormal oligosaccharide pattern of a patient with N-acetylgalactosaminidase deficiency is shown. This new lysosomal storage disease was recently described in detail (Van Diggelen *et al.*, 1988). The desalting procedure with ion-exchange resins does not work in aspartylglycosylaminase deficiency because the accumulating aspartylglucosamine is bound to the cation-exchange resin but the aspartylglucosamine can easily be detected with amino acid analysis. In breast-fed newborns an abnormal oligosaccharide excretion pattern is observed. The pattern on first examination resembles the pattern seen in α-mannosidosis. Developing the TLC plate twice with the same solvents gives a characteristic difference between α-mannosidosis and a breast-fed newborn oligo-

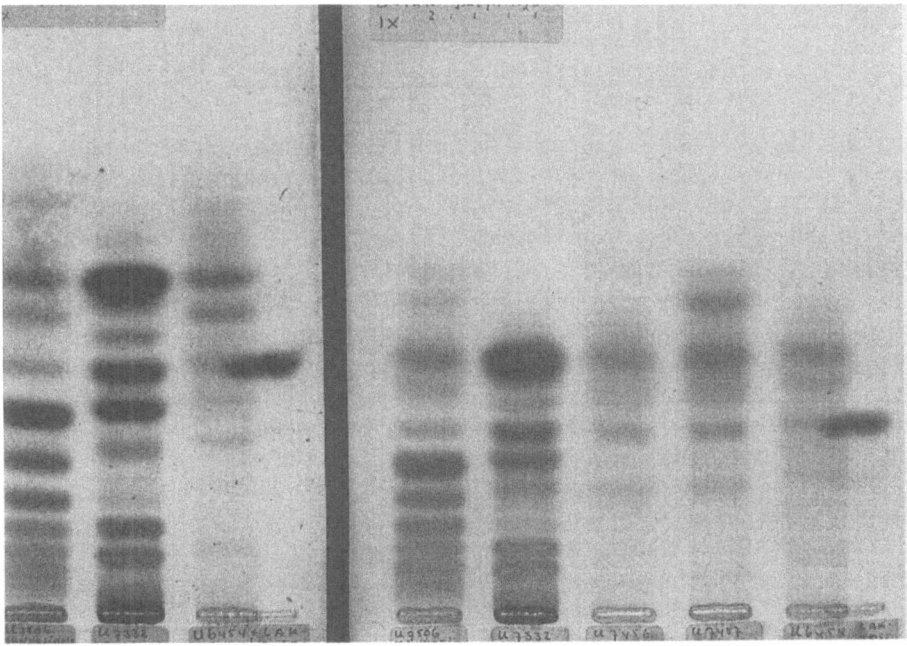

Figure 7   Thin-layer chromatogram of oligosaccharides in urine. The left plate with lanes 1–3 is developed twice with the same organic solvent mixture; the right plate with lanes 4–8 is developed once. Lanes 1 and 4 present the pattern of α-mannosidosis; lanes 2 and 5 present the pattern in the urine of a breast-fed patient. All the other oligosaccharide patterns are normal. Overlapping with the urine lactose is spotted in lanes 3 and 8

saccharide pattern (Figure 7). Performing oligosaccharide analysis in the mother's milk, we detected the same oligosaccharides as we observed in the urine of breast-fed newborns.

Imidazoles, purines and pyrimidines: Imidazoles are histidine metabolites. Indications for imidazole analysis are given in Table 7. By two-dimensional thin-layer chromatography abnormal pictures can be obtained in histidinaemia but also in other diseases like coeliac disease, xanthinuria or adenylosuccinase deficiency. In coeliac disease spots of *N*-acetyl and *N*-propionylhistamine, imidazolonpropionic acid, 4-amino-imidazole-5-carboxyamide (AICA) and 4-amino-imidazole-5-carboxyamide riboside (AICAR) can be observed, as a result of intestinal dysbacteriosis and folic acid deficiency. In xanthinuria a characteristic elongated spot of

Table 7   Indications for imidazole analysis

Anorexia with poor growth
Vomiting, diarrhoea
Distended abdomen, abnormal stools
Osteoporosis
Muscle dystrophy
Renal stones
Histidinaemia
Microcephaly, mental retardation
Spasticity, epilepsy

xanthine appears. On the same place on the TLC chromatogram an antibiotic spot may be visible, but this spot is not elongated. To confirm the presence of xanthine, the same TLC development can be used, but using the staining procedure for purines and pyrimidines. Xanthine and hypoxanthine will colour blue, while the antibiotic spots remain orange. In adenylosuccinase deficiency a clear spot of succinyl-4-amino-imidazole-5-carboxyamide riboside (SAICAR) can be detected.

Tryptophan and metabolites: At the end of the 1950s and in the early 1960s amino acids were analysed by means of paper chromatography by which tryptophan could be detected. With the introduction of automated amino acid analysers publications on abnormal tryptophan excretion in urine (e.g. Hartnup disease) declined remarkably because tryptophan is destroyed to a large extent in the amino-acid analyser and thus is not detected. Therefore we developed a two-dimensional TLC method for indole analysis at the end of the 1970s.

Table 8   Indications for indole analysis

Skin abnormalities:
    dry, scaly skin, erythematous rash
    photosensitivity, pellagra
Neurological abnormalities:
    cerebellar ataxia, hypertonia
    (intentional) tremor
    abnormal reflexes
    abnormal EEG, convulsions
    diplopia, nystagmus
Diarrhoea, constipation
Psychiatric abnormalities:
    depression, anxiety
    obsession–compulsion
    hyperactivity, chaotic behaviour
    irritability, aggression
    automutilation, sleep problems

In Table 8 the indications for indole analysis are shown. Using this TLC method we can detect intestinal tryptophan malabsorption syndromes like Hartnup disease and blue diaper syndrome. But we also discovered abnormal indole excretion in urine of patients with various psychiatric disorders (e.g. Blom *et al.*, 1985, 1986). After a tryptophan loading test increased excretion in urine of metabolites of the kynurenine pathway can be detected. Using our gas chromatograph method of organic acid analysis many indolic metabolites can be detected after a tryptophan loading test. Quantitation of indolic compounds can be performed by HPLC (Figures 8 and 9).

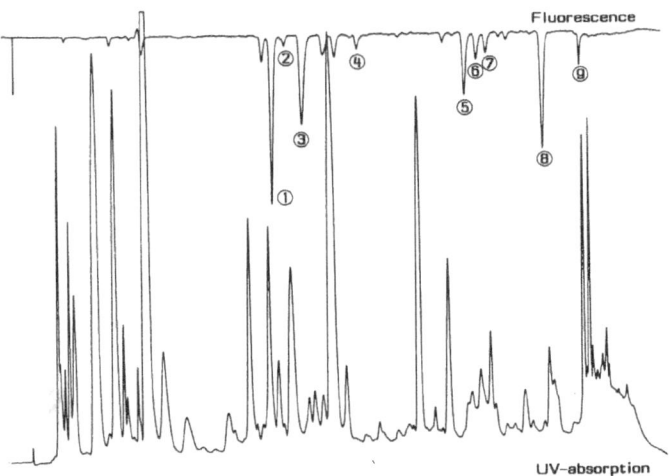

Figure 8 HPLC chromatogram of indoles in the first 12-h urine after a tryptophan loading (110 mg kg^{-1}) test. Identification of the peaks: 1 = tryptophan; 2 = 5-OH-indole; 3 = indican; 4 = 5-OH-indoleacetic acid; 5 = unknown; 6 = indolelactic acid; 7 = *N*-acetyltryptophan; 8 = indoleacetic acid; 9 = indolepyruvic acid

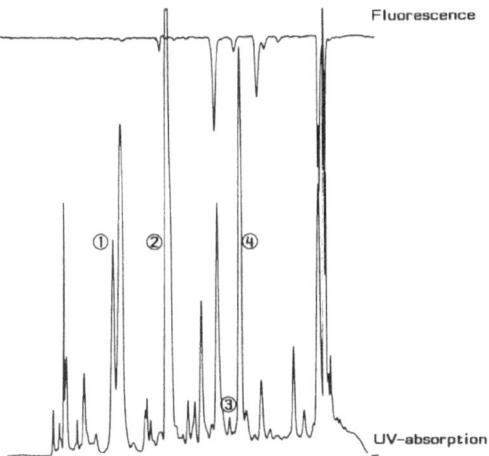

Figure 9 HPLC chromatogram of kynurenine+metabolites in the first 12-h urine after a tryptophan loading (110 mg kg^{-1}) test. Identification of the peaks: 1 = 3-OH-kynurenine; 2 = kynurenine; 3 = xanthurenic acid; 4 = kynurenic acid

J. Inher. Metab. Dis. 12 Suppl. 1 (1989)

Cerebrosides and sulphatides: After filtration of the sediment of a 24-h urine, cerebrosides and sulphatides can be extracted and purified from the filtered sediment. The extract is evaporated to dryness and resolved. The final solution can be investigated for cerebrosides and sulphatides by TLC.

In most lysosomal storage diseases in which cerebrosides accumulate in the lysosomes no abnormalities can be detected in urine. Only in Fabry disease (α-galactosidase deficiency) can characteristic abnormal cerebrosides (digalactosylceramide and ceramide trihexoside) be observed with this TLC method. In metachromatic leukodystrophy (aryl-sulphatase A deficiency) abnormal sulphatide bands appear in the thin-layer chromatogram (Figure 10).

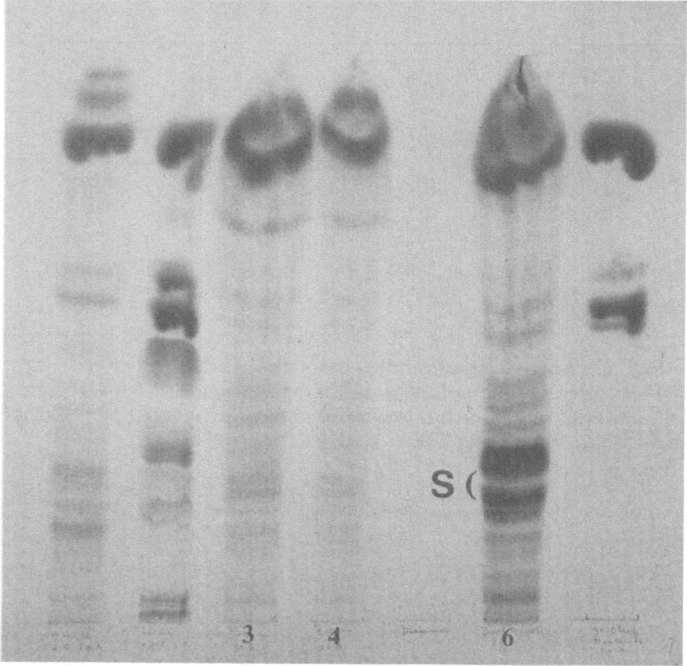

Figure 10   Thin-layer chromatogram of cerebrosides and sulphatides. Lanes 3 and 4, pattern of a normal urine; lane 6, pattern in the urine of a patient with metachromatic leukodystrophy (arylsulphatase A deficiency): S = sulphatides

This method for cerebroside and sulphatide analysis can be useful to confirm the diagnosis of Fabry disease or metachromatic leukodystrophy, if enzyme analysis does not discriminate between homo- and heterozygosity. This problem can occur, if the enzyme assay is performed in leukocytes.

Mucopolysaccharides: A number of simple screening tests are available for the demonstration of increased amounts of mucopolysaccharides in the urine. These tests may give false negative or false positive results. For this reason we always perform two screening tests (*o*-toluidine blue test and the cetyl-pyridinium chloride precipitation test). The precipitation test can often be false positive in concentrated urines. In Morquio disease, with an increased excretion of keratan sulphate in the urine, both these screening tests are negative because keratan sulphate does not react. Table 9 gives the indications for mucopolysaccharide analysis.

Table 9   Indications for mucopolysaccharide analysis

Abnormal face (gargoylism)
Cornea clouding
Deafness
Hepatosplenomegaly
(Disproportional) growth retardation
Skeletal abnormalities
Mental retardation
Abnormal behaviour (aggression, hyperactivity)

If one or both of the screening tests are positive, or if the patient is suspected of Morquio disease, two-dimensional electrophoresis of the mucopolysaccharides is performed. By two-dimensional electrophoresis various types of mucopolysaccharidosis can be diagnosed. The method does not discriminate between different types of Sanfilippo syndromes, or, for example, between Hunter, Hurler and Scheie syndromes.

The combination of mucopolysaccharide electrophoresis and TLC of oligosaccharides can be used to distinguish Morquio A syndrome (*N*-acetyl-galactosamine-6-sulphate sulphatase deficiency) from Morquio B syndrome (β-galactosidase deficiency) (Van der Horst *et al.*, 1983). In both Morquio syndromes keratan sulphate excretion in urine is increased, but only in the Morquio B syndrome can an abnormal oligosaccharide pattern, resembling the pattern seen in G_{M1}-gangliosidosis, be detected (see also Figure 6).

With slight modifications, the two-dimensional electrophoresis can be used for prenatal diagnosis of mucopolysaccharidosis, which we described in 1984 (Kleijer *et al.*, 1984b). Figures 11 and 12 are examples of abnormal electrophoretic pictures in amniotic fluid.

Porphyrins: A screening test on porphyrins is performed in 10 mL of fresh urine, acidified with 0.1 mL acetic acid and stored in the dark. The urine is extracted, centrifuged and the organic layer is observed under UV light (366 nm). The test is positive if the organic phase fluoresces orange-red. We use another qualitative test for the detection of urobilinogen and porphobilinogen. If the screening tests are positive, we perform a thin-layer method to detect different porphyrins in order to discriminate between the various porphyrias.

Specific metabolite assays

Methylmalonic acid is quantitated, if it is increased in the gas chromatogram of organic acids in urine, or to control therapy in methylmalonic acidemia.

Orotic acid is quantitatively estimated, if the patient is suspected of orotic aciduria or of a hyperammonaemia syndrome. Carbamylphosphate synthetase and *N*-acetyl-

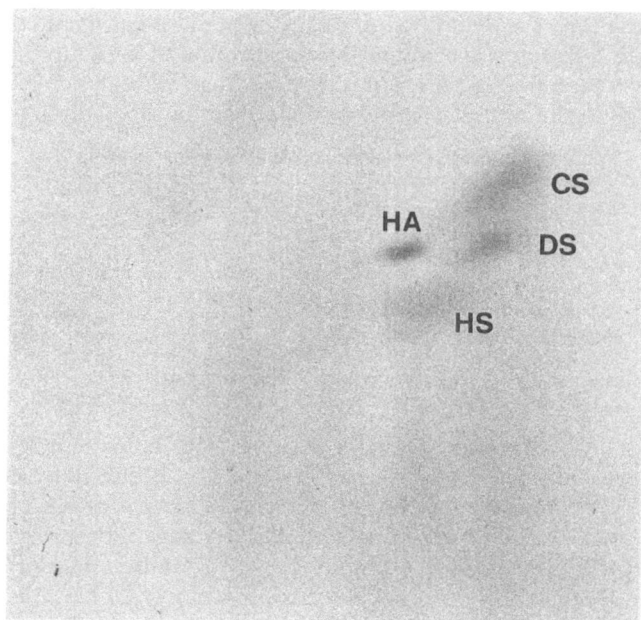

Figure 11 Two-dimensional electrophoretogram of mucopolysaccharides in amniotic fluid of a pregnancy at risk for Hurler syndrome: DS = dermatansulphate and HS = heparansulphate (both increased); HA = hyaluronic acid and CS = chondroitin-4-sulphate (both normal)

glutamate synthetase deficiency can be distinguished from ornithine transcarbamylase deficiency by orotic acid quantitation. In carbamylphosphate synthetase and *N*-acetylglutamate synthetase deficiency orotic acid excretion in the urine is low or normal, whereas in ornithine transcarbamylase deficiency orotic acid is found in large quantities in the urine. Therapeutic control in hyperammonaemic syndromes using urinary orotic acid quantitation is very useful.

Uric acid estimation can be used as a screening test for disorders of purine metabolism, e.g. in Lesch–Nyhan syndrome, or to detect an increase of urinary uric acid in urolithiasis.

Phytanic acid is looked for if the patient is suspected of a peroxisomal disorder, e.g. Refsum disease.

Tryptophan and serotonin are estimated in tryptophan metabolism or transport disorders and in specific (child) psychiatric abnormalities.

Oxalic acid and glycollic acid or glyceric acid are determined in oxalate urolithiasis due, respectively to oxalosis type 1 or type 2, and to control therapy in these disorders.

Free and total sialic acid is estimated in the urine of patients suspected of sialuria, Salla disease, generalized *N*-acetylneuraminic acid storage disease or mucolipidosis type 1 and 2.

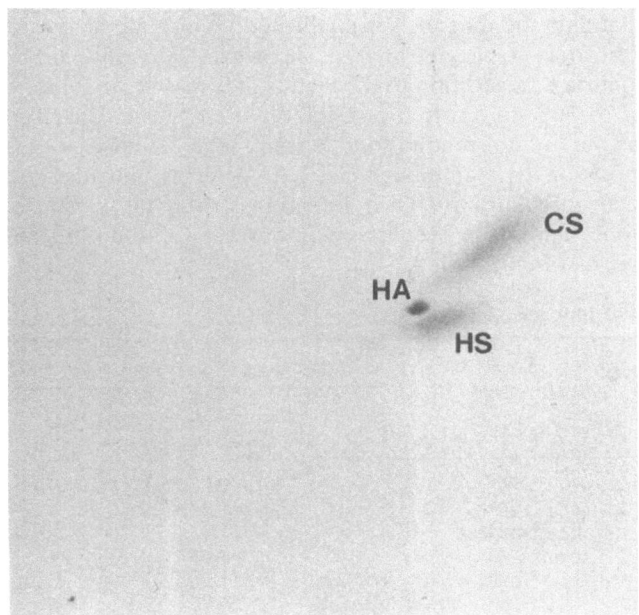

Figure 12 Two-dimensional electrophoretogram of mucopolysaccharides in amniotic fluid of a pregnancy at risk for Sanfilippo A syndrome: HS = heparansulphate (increased); HA = hyaluronic acid and CS = chrondroitin-4-sulphate (both normal)

Table 10   Diagnoses in 1985 and 1986

		1985		1986	
		Types	*Total*	*Types*	*Total*
Aminoacidopathies		9	38	9	33
Organic acidaemias		9	12	8	10
Carbohydrate metabolic disorders		2	3	2	2
Lysosomal storage diseases		2	4	6	8
Peroxisomal disorder		—	—	1	1
	Total	22	57	26	54
Number of new patients			876		850
Yield in %			6.5		6.4

DIAGNOSTIC RESULTS

Many metabolic laboratories present diagnostic results in absolute number of diagnoses per year or per investigation period, but yields of diagnostic results are rarely published. In Table 10 we present our complete diagnostic results for the years 1985 and 1986. A yield of approximately 6.5% is very acceptable. It is obvious that aminoacidopathies and organic acidaemias are the major metabolic diseases.

J. Inher. Metab. Dis. 12 Suppl. 1 (1989)

In most of the patients the diagnosis is confirmed by enzyme analysis. In some of the amino acid disorders no enzyme analysis is performed because it is not necessary (e.g. phenylketonuria). In addition to the results of Table 10, we observe metabolic abnormalities in 20–30% of newly investigated patients which (partly) explain the clinical problems but are not related to inherited metabolic diseases, e.g. transient neonatal tyrosinosis or hyperammonaemia, keto-acidosis, nutritional deficiencies, intestinal dysbacteriosis, urinary tract infections, drug intoxications, etc. Also negative metabolic laboratory results are important for the clinician because a metabolic disease can be excluded.

Table 11   Origin of patients

	1985		1986	
	SCH	*Other hospital*	*SCH*	*Other hospital*
Aminoacidopathies	7	31	10	23
Organic acidaemias	4	8	4	6
Carbohydrate metabolic disorders	3	—	1	1
Lysosomal storage disorders	—	4	1	7
Peroxisomal disorder	—	—	—	1
Total	14	43	16	38
Number of new patients	233	643	250	600
Yield in %	6.0	6.7	6.4	6.3

SCH = Sophia Children's Hospital.

Table 11 shows that there is no difference between the yield of diagnostic results in the Sophia Children's Hospital and other hospitals served by our laboratory which we consider remarkable. This indicates that in general there is a good clinical selection of patients, which may be as a result of the use of our request form.

DISCUSSION

We have tried to emphasize that the process of diagnosis, therapy, genetic counselling and prevention of congenital disease is complex. Differentiation of tasks, specialization and collaboration are essential. Institutes of Clinical Genetics in The Netherlands are an example of a national approach.

Within the setting of the Institute of Clinical Genetics our Metabolic Laboratory is a highly specialized, dedicated diagnostic centre, concerned with (abnormal) metabolite screening, identification and quantitation. The philosophy of work and the working methods are completely different from those of routine clinical chemistry laboratories. Every individual patient with clinical symptoms suspected of a metabolic disease has to be a challenge for a metabolic laboratory. Every metabolic abnormality, known or unknown, has to be interpreted biochemically and clinically.

The efficiency and cost–benefit ratio of the metabolic diagnostic work require not an at-random laboratory screening, but a selective approach based on clinical indications. With the request form for metabolic investigation we made an attempt to bridge the gap between the Clinic and the Metabolic Laboratory and to improve the quality of work, the concept of biochemical and clinical coherence, and the diagnostic yield.

In the metabolic field a steady state will never be reached. We have to be alert and to anticipate new developments in diagnostic methods, interpretation of laboratory results, analytical instrumentation, computerization, etc. We have to stress the timely replacement or extension of analytical laboratory instruments and the requirement for sufficient laboratory staff. We have to realize that diagnosing many patients means additional investigations in the patient and/or his family and above all longitudinal control of therapy in treatable metabolic disorders. The amount of work to control treatment is growing year after year and takes up a substantial part of our laboratory activities. And, of course, we have to study new relevant literature and to publish!

REFERENCES

Blom, W., Luteyn, J. C., Kelholt-Dijkman, H. H., Huijmans, J. G. M. and Loonen, M. C. B. Thin-layer chromatography of oligosaccharides in urine as a rapid indication for the diagnosis of lysosomal acid maltase deficiency (Pompe's disease). *Clin. Chim. Acta* 134 (1983) 221–227

Blom, W., van den Berg, G. B., Huijmans, J. G. M. and Sanders-Woudstra, J. A. R. Successful nicotinamide treatment in a autosomal dominant behavioral and psychiatric disorder. *J. Inher. Metab. Dis.* 8 Suppl. 2 (1985) 107–108

Blom, W., van den Berg, G. B., Huijmans, J. G. M., Przyrembel, H., Fernandes, J., Scholte, H. R. and Sanders-Woudstra, J. A. R. Neurologic action of megadosis of vitamins. *Bibliothec. Nutr. Dieta* 38 (1986) 120–135

Chalmers, C. A. and Lawson, A. M. *Organic Acids in Man. The analytical chemistry, biochemistry and diagnosis of the organic acidurias*, Chapman and Hall Ltd, London and New York, 1982

Goodman, S. I. and Markey, S. P. Diagnosis of organic acidemias by gas chromatography-mass spectrometry. *Laboratory and Research Methods in Biology and Medicine*, Vol. 6, Alan R. Liss, Inc., New York, 1981

Humbel, R. and Collart, M. Oligosaccharides in urine of patients with glycoprotein storage diseases. I. Rapid detection by thin-layer chromatography. *Clin. Chim. Acta* 60 (1975) 143–145

Jacobs, C. A. J. M. Prenatal diagnosis of inherited metabolic disorders by stable isotope dilution GC–MS of amniotic fluid: review of four year experience. *J. Inher. Metab. Dis* (1989) In press.

Kleijer, W. J., Blom, W., Huijmans, J. G. M., Mooyman, M. C. T., Berger, R. and Niermeijer, M. F. Prenatal diagnosis of citrullinemia: elevated levels of citrulline in the amniotic fluid of three affected pregnancies. *Prenat. Diagn.* 4 (1984a) 113–118

Kleijer, W. J., Huijmans, J. G. M., Blom, W., Gorska, D., Kubalska, J., Wasalek, M. and Zaremba, J. Prenatal diagnosis of Sanfilippo disease type B. *Hum. Genet.* 66 (1984b) 287–288

Millington, D. S., Roe, C. R. and Maltby, D. A. Application of high resolution fast atom bombardment and constant B/E ratio linked scanning to the identification and analysis of acylcarnitines in metabolic disease. *Biomed. Mass Spectr.* 11 (1984) 236–241

Poll-The, B. T. Genetic peroxisomal disorders. Thesis, University of Amsterdam, 1988

Roe, C. R., Millington, D. S., Maltby, D. A., Bohan, T. P., Kahler, S. G. and Chalmers, R. A. Diagnostic and therapeutic implications of medium-chain acylcarnitines in medium-chain acyl-CoA dehydrogenase deficiency. *Pediatr. Res.* 19 (1985) 459–466

Van der Horst, G. T. J., Kleijer, W. J., Hoogeveen, A. T., Huijmans, J. G. M., Blom, W. and van Diggelen, O. P. Morquio B syndrome: a primary defect in β-galactosidase. *Am. J. Hum. Genet.* 16 (1983) 261–275

Van Diggelen, O. P., Schindler, D., Willemsen, R., Boer, M., Kleijer, W. J., Huijmans, J. G. M., Blom, W. and Galjaard, H. α-N-acetylgalactosaminidase deficiency, a new lysosomal storage disorder. *J. Inher. Metab. Dis.* 11 (1988) 349–357

J. Inher. Metab. Dis. 12 Suppl. 1 (1989) 89–96

Genetic Aspects of Prenatal Diagnosis

J. M. CONNOR

Duncan Guthrie Institute of Medical Genetics, Yorkhill, Glasgow, G3 8SJ, UK

Summary: With improved control of environmental agents, genetic conditions are now a major cause of residual handicap and mortality in all age groups. Primary prevention of this diverse group of over 5000 distinct disorders is not yet possible and effective therapy is, as yet, available for very few. Hence, the present emphasis on prevention is directed towards the identification and testing of pregnancies at risk in order to allow the option of early selective termination of pregnancy. Although over 400 distinct conditions have already been successfully prenatally diagnosed, the identification of at-risk pregnancies on the basis of a positive family history alone can identify only a minority of affected pregnancies. In contrast, genetic screening during (or before) pregnancy offers a real prospect for detection of a majority of affected pregnancies and hence for reducing the birth frequency of serious genetic conditions. This is exemplified by the impact of the maternal serum α-fetoprotein screening programme for neural tube defects and is under active development for autosomal aneuploidies and certain other major congenital malformations. These screening programmes will result in a reduced frequency of mental and physical handicap in the community but their implementation will require a comprehensive team approach with supraregional (or national) funding and co-ordination.

SIZE OF THE PROBLEM

Genetic diseases affect all populations and have been apparent since prehistory. They have, however, grown rapidly in importance with the improved control of infections and other environmental agents and now constitute a major cause of residual handicap and mortality in all age groups. This is exemplified by the infant mortality rate for England and Wales which was 154/1000 in 1900 with 4.5/1000 of the total due to genetic disease. By 1980 the infant mortality rate had fallen to 12/1000 but the number due to genetic disease was unaltered: hence the genetic contribution to the infant mortality rate has risen from 3 to 40%. Between 0.3 and 0.4% of school-age children are severely mentally retarded and a further 1% have a significant physical handicap. Nowadays most of this handicap is genetic and, furthermore, chronic diseases with a significant genetic component affect at least 10–20% of the adult population.

Genetic diseases may be subdivided into chromosomal disorders (with a microscopically visible abnormality), single gene disorders, and multifactorial conditions

Journal of Inherited Metabolic Disease. ISSN 0141–8955. Copyright © SSIEM and Kluwer Academic Publishers, PO Box 55, Lancaster, UK.

(where one or more genes interact with one or more factors in the environment). Chromosomal disorders affect 0.6% of live births and multifactorial conditions are nowadays the most commonly identified cause of major congenital malformations (2% of live births) and chronic disorders of adulthood (see above). Diagnosis of chromosomal and multifactorial disorders is usually straightforward and counselling utilizes empiric (observed rather than calculated) recurrence risks and either fetal karyotyping or detailed ultrasound scanning for prenatal diagnosis in pregnancies at risk (Harper, 1988; Whittle and Connor, 1989). Collectively the single gene disorders affect just over 1% of Caucasian live births but their diagnosis and management is complicated by their diversity with 4344 distinct recognized conditions (2557 autosomal dominant, 1477 autosomal recessive and 310 X-linked traits; McKusick, 1988). Clinically many of these are difficult to distinguish and this genetic heterogeneity is a major potential pitfall for meaningful genetic counselling and prenatal diagnosis. Even this large number of single gene disorders is only a fraction of the true total (estimated at over 50 000) with, because of the limited symptomatic repertoire of each organ, many conditions yet to be delineated. The problem is further compounded by rapid developments in both laboratory and obstetric aspects of prenatal diagnosis with over 500 publications *per annum* on this subject. These difficulties have led to the development of the speciality of medical genetics and to the creation of regional genetics centres to assist in the provision of sophisticated genetic risk assessment and counselling.

IDENTIFICATION OF AT-RISK PREGNANCIES

Table 1 shows the factors which are identifiable either prior to or during a pregnancy which can alert the clinician to an increased risk for a chromosomal disorder, single gene disorder or multifactorial malformation. A positive family history can be a vital clue but the customary enquiry 'Is there a family history of diabetes, tuberculosis or epilepsy?' is completely inadequate if a serious attempt is to be made to prevent genetic disease. Conversely, in a busy clinic it is impractical to construct a full pedigree for every patient and a compromise is to document previous outcomes of pregnancy, to record the maternal age, to enquire if the couple are blood relatives and to ask if there is any family history of note and specifically any history of malformed or handicapped children. A positive response to any of these questions will necessitate further evaluation and possibly referral to a genetic counselling centre.

GENETIC ASSESSMENT AND COUNSELLING

Within a region, genetic assessment and counselling clinics are usually held on a centre–satellite basis. Adequate time in an appropriate setting is essential and in general we allocate 30–45 min for a new family to allow time to take a history, construct a pedigree and examine key family members. Precision of diagnosis is the cornerstone of medical genetics and hence counselling should be deferred until all data from specialized investigations and/or evaluation of medical records of

Table 1   Identifiable risk factors for genetic conditions

I. *Chromosomal disorders* (0.6% of live births)
Factors identifiable prior to a pregnancy:
   Increased maternal age
   Positive family history
   Previous obstetric history

Factors identifiable during a pregnancy
   Abnormal ultrasound appearance
   Elevated or low maternal serum α-fetoprotein

II. *Single gene disorders* (1% of live births)
Factors identifiable prior to a pregnancy:
   Parental consanguinity
   Ethnic origin
   Positive family history
   Previous obstetric history

Factors identifiable during a pregnancy
   Abnormal ultrasound appearance
   Elevated maternal serum α-fetoprotein assay (congenital nephrosis, Meckel syndrome)

III. *Congenital malformations* (2% of live births)
Factors identifiable prior to a pregnancy:
   Parental consanguinity
   Ethnic origin
   Positive family history
   Previous obstetric history
   Maternal illness or medication

Factors identifiable during a pregnancy:
   Abnormal ultrasound appearance
   Elevated maternal α-fetoprotein
   Polyhydramnios
   Oligohydramnios
   Maternal infection
   Maternal exposure to teratogens/drugs

other family members are available. Both parents should be counselled and neither the corner of a hospital ward nor a crowded clinic room is adequate. Further, it is inappropriate to counsel too soon (usually within 3 months) after recent bereavement or after the initial shock of a serious diagnosis.

Counselling needs to consider all aspects of the condition and the depth of explanation should be matched to the educational background of the couple. Generally geneticists consider a risk of more than 1 in 10 as high, and less than 1 in 20 as low, but the risks have to be considered in relation to the degree of disability. Couples often feel very guilty or stigmatized and it is important to recognize and allay this and other common misconceptions about heredity (Table 2).

Counselling must be non-directive. The aim is to provide a balanced version of the facts which will allow the couple to reach their decision with regard to their

Table 2   Common misconceptions about heredity

Absence of other affected individuals means that a disorder is not genetic and *vice versa*
Any condition present at birth must be inherited
Upsets, mental and physical, of the mother in pregnancy cause malformations
Genetic diseases are untreatable
If only males of females are affected in the family this indicates sex linkage
A 1 in 4 risk means that the next three children will be unaffected

reproductive future. Where the couple have a high recurrence risk for a serious untreatable abnormality the possibility of prenatal diagnosis needs to be covered, with practical details about the tests available and their diagnostic limitations. Often assessment and counselling can be accomplished in one sitting and it is our policy to follow this session with a letter which summarizes the situation and invites the couple to return if new questions arise. We also ask the couple for their assistance in contacting other family members at risk and for their permission to enter their pedigree number on a genetic register so that they may be readily recalled when relevant research developments occur.

UPTAKE OF PRENATAL DIAGNOSTIC SERVICES

Most couples who seek genetic counselling make an appropriate decision with respect to the information and the majority of couples faced with a high recurrence risk for a serious untreatable disorder will forego further pregnancies in the absence of a test for prenatal reassurance. The growth in uptake of prenatal diagnosis and the shifting choice of test can be seen in Table 3 which compares invasive diagnostic procedures for the years 1969–1977, inclusive, with a single year ending 31 March 1988 for couples from the West of Scotland.

The marked rise in the annual number of tests reflects increased awareness and acceptance of these procedures by patients and their clinicians and the growing list of conditions which can now be diagnosed in the fetus (Whittle and Connor, 1989). In detailed analyses of reasons for non-uptake of prenatal diagnosis, 8% of pregnant women are opposed to all prenatal tests on moral grounds, some present too late in pregnancy, and the remainder are not offered a test. This last group is potentially of very serious concern since in the UK every doctor has medico-legal responsibility to identify patients in their care whose illness is genetic and to provide access for all family members at risk to sophisticated genetic counselling and, if appropriate, prenatal diagnosis. Failure to do this, whether from religious objections or ignorance, does not constitute a defence.

By conventional biochemical analysis, 96 autosomal recessive inborn errors of metabolism have now been successfully prenatally diagnosed and this represents 15.3% of the 626 validated total. Within this group nearly half (46) have also been successfully prenatally diagnosed on the basis of chorionic villus samples. Further, over 30 single gene disorders have been prenatally diagnosed by either direct DNA

Table 3 Indications for routine invasive prenatal diagnostic tests in the West of Scotland

Indication	*Nine-year period 1969–1977 inclusive*		*Year ending 31 March 1988*	
	Amnio	*CVS*	*Amnio*	*CVS*
Chromosomal				
Maternal age 35–39 yrs	18% (405)	—	47% (654)	62% (125)
Maternal age 40+ yrs	20% (432)	—	9% (129)	10% (20)
Low maternal serum α-fetoprotein assay	—	—	6% (86)	—
Previous chromosome abnormality	9% (210)	—	2% (29)	13% (26)
Family history of chromosome abnormality	4% (83)	—	3% (45)	—
Parental translocation	1.5% (32)	—	0.5% (7)	2.5% (5)
Maternal anxiety	4% (94)	—	4% (55)	1% (2)
Sexing	1% (26)	—	—	4% (8)
Single gene disorders				
DNA analysis	—	—	—	3% (6)
Biochemical analysis	1% (28)	—	0.5% (6)	2.5% (5)
Multifactorial disorders				
Raised maternal serum α-fetoprotein	7% (156)	—	18% (243)	—
Previous neural tube defect	31% (707)	—	6% (83)	—
Family history of neural tube defect	2% (52)	—	1% (13)	—
Other	1.5% (37)	—	3% (38)	2% (4)
Total	100% (2262)	—	100% (1388)	100% (201)

Amnio = amniocentesis; CVS = chorionic villus sampling

analysis or by indirect gene tracking with linked markers. Although this number is small in comparison to the total of 4344 recognized single gene defects (2208 fully validated and 2136 not yet fully validated) it includes most of the more frequent of these conditions (e.g. cystic fibrosis, familial hypercholesterolaemia, adult polycystic kidney disease, Duchenne muscular dystrophy and the haemophilias) and it is estimated that DNA diagnosis is now possible for two-thirds of the potential demand for prenatal diagnosis generated by the single gene disorders.

GENETIC SCREENING IN PREGNANCY

Overall less than 20% of pregnancies at risk of important single gene disorders can be predicted on the basis of a positive family history; for multifactorial malformations the figure is only 10% and for chromosomal disorders under 5% could be predicted on the basis of an affected individual in the family. Hence selective testing of pregnancies on the basis of a positive family history, whilst of direct benefit to the families concerned, can never have a major impact on the birth frequency of these genetic conditions.

The idea of screening the entire population at risk originated with the neonatal screening for inborn errors of metabolism and this approach has already produced an important impact for neural tube defects and is currently being developed for chromosomal disorders and certain other major congenital malformations. Screening for neural tube defects by maternal serum α-fetoprotein assay is at present confined to 16–20 weeks and a result is defined as elevated if it is greater than two multiples of the median value (2MOM) for the appropriate gestation. If elevated (5% of all pregnancies) the gestation needs to be confirmed (by ultrasound), pregnancy complications such as twins or threatened/missed abortion excluded and the maternal serum α-fetoprotein assay repeated. If the second value is under 2MOM no further action is necessary but if also elevated (3.5% of all pregnancies) detailed ultrasound scanning and an amniocentesis need to be considered as within this group with two elevated maternal serum α-fetoprotein assay values 1 in 20 will have a neural tube defect (as compared with a 1 in 30 risk with only a single elevated assay value). In the West of Scotland experience to 31 May 1988, 290 000 pregnancies have been screened in this manner with 851 neural tube defects detected and 127 open spina bifida pregnancies missed. Thus in our experience the sensitivity of this screening programme for neural tube defect detection is 87% and selective termination of affected pregnancies has reduced the birth frequency of this defect by over 70% (Table 4; Ferguson-Smith, 1983).

Table 4   Screening programme for neural tube defects (NTD) in the West of Scotland

	Expected year of confinement									
	1977	1978	1979	1980	1981	1982	1983	1984	1985	1986
Total pregnancies	33 984	35 081	37 714	37 651	38 201	35 784	34 714	35 070	37 974	35 530
Proportion screened (%)	34.1	49.1	60.8	69.9	73	79.4	79.2	75.3	74	80
NTD terminations	40	62	95	77	99	92	74	71	61	78
NTD births	111	117	102	80	79	59	37	34	29	30
NTD birth frequency/1000	3.3	3.3	2.7	2.1	2.1	1.6	1.1	1.0	0.8	0.8

Spina bifida occulta, syndromes and neural tube defects secondary to chromosomal causes are excluded

Maternal serum α-fetoprotein assay levels are reduced (to about 70% of expected) in pregnancies with trisomy 21, 18 or 13. This reduction can be combined with the known maternal age-related risk for these major chromosomal abnormalities in order to make amniocentesis more selective. Using a cut off of 1 in 280, which is equivalent to the mid-trimester risk for a 35 year old, it is predicted that 37% of trisomies 21, 18 and 13 could be detected by offering amniocentesis to 6.6% of pregnant women (Cuckle *et al.*, 1987). In contrast, if amniocentesis is offered to women 35 years and over (irrespective of maternal serum α-fetoprotein assay) then only 30% of trisomies will be detected for an amniocentesis rate of 6.7%. Prospective studies are in progress to evaluate these claims, but our own detection rate for autosomal trisomies has risen from 1 abnormality per 124 amnioceteses (on the basis of maternal age alone) to 1 abnormality per 100 amniocenteses (combined risk from maternal serum α-fetoprotein assay and maternal age). More recently retrospective studies have indicated that this selectivity can be further enhanced by the simultaneous measurement of maternal serum unconjugated oestriols and HCG and it is predicted that with such a combination over 60% of Down's syndrome pregnancies could be detected for an amniocentesis rate of 5% (Wald *et al.*, 1988a and b).

In addition to this current interest in biochemical screening for chromosomal disorders, there is also interest in utilizing detailed ultrasound anomaly scans to screen for chromosomal disorders (Benacerraf *et al.*, 1988; Lockwood *et al.*, 1987), neural tube defects (Nicolaides *et al.*, 1986) and other major malformations especially congenital heart defects (Allan *et al.*, 1986; Benacerraf *et al.*, 1987). These programmes will need careful evaluation to determine their sensitivity, specificity, and predictive values in clinical practice (Connor, 1989) but public opinion both in Europe and the USA would appear to favour an increase of screening during pregnancy. The principal justification for such screening relates to the currently unquantified effects on the consumer, including the provision of authoritative information, the relief from uncertainty, support during a period of crisis and the expansion of an individual's scope for exercising choice. The King's Fund forum (1987) concluded that these advantages outweighed the potential harm of introduction of worrying delay whilst confirmatory tests are conducted, the distress which may result from false positive tests and the illusory reassurance given by false negative tests. All current prenatal screening programmes have been developed in a climate of fierce competition for scarce resources and this has led to an undue emphasis on tangible benefits (i.e. resources saved *versus* the actual cost of each programme). Sophisticated calculations clearly show the cost-efficacy of such programmes but these benefits, as indicated above, are of secondary importance to those enjoyed by the pregnant mother. They do, however, help to counter the financial arguments against the introduction and development of screening programmes with a view to reducing the burden of genetic disease and handicap in the community.

REFERENCES

Allan, L. D., Crawford, D. C., Chita, S. K. and Tynan, M. J. Prenatal screening for congenital heart disease. *Br. Med. J.* 292 (1986) 1717–1719
Benacerraf, B. R., Miller, W. A. and Frigoletto, F. D. Sonographic detection of fetuses with trisomy 13 and 18: accuracy and limitations. *Am. J. Obstet. Gynecol.* 158 (1988) 404–409
Benacerraf, B. R., Pober, B. R. and Sanders, S. P. Accuracy of fetal echocardiography. *Radiology* 165 (1987) 4847–4849
Connor, J. M. Screening for genetic abnormality. *Fetal Med. Rev.* 1 (1989) 13–25
Cuckle, H. S., Wald, N. J. and Thompson, S. G. Estimating a woman's risk of having a pregnancy associated with Down's syndrome using her age and serum α-fetoprotein level. *Br. J. Obstet. Gynecol.* 94 (1987) 387–402
Ferguson-Smith, M. A. The reduction of anencephalic and spina bifida births by maternal serum alpha fetoprotein screening. *Br. Med. Bull.* 39 (1983) 365–372
Harper, P. S. *Practical Genetic Counselling*, 3rd edn., Wright, Bristol, 1988

King's Fund forum. Consensus statement: screening for fetal and genetic abnormality. *Br. Med. J.* 295 (1987) 1551–1553

Lockwood, C., Benacerraf, B., Krinsky, A., Blakemore, K., Belanger, K., Mahoney, M. and Hobbins, J. A sonographic screening method for Down's syndrome. *Am. J. Obstet. Gynecol.* 157 (1987) 803–808

McKusick, V. A. *Mendelian Inheritance in Man*, 8th edn., Johns Hopkins University Press, Baltimore and London, 1988

Nicholaides, K. H., Campbell, S., Gabbe, S. G. and Guidetti, R. Ultrasound screening for spina bifida: cranial and cerebellar signs. *Lancet* 2 (1986) 72–74

Wald, N. J., Cuckle, H. S., Densem, J. W., Nanchahal, K., Canick, J. A., Haddow, J. E., Knight, G. and Palomaki, G. E. Maternal serum unconjugated estriol as an antenatal screening test for Down's syndrome. *Br. J. Obstet. Gynecol.* 95 (1988a) 334–341

Wald, N. J., Cuckle, H. S., Densem, J. W., Nanchahal, K., Royston, P., Chard, T., Haddow, J. E., Knight, G. J., Palomaki, G. E. and Canick, J. A. Maternal serum screening for Down's syndrome in early pregnancy. *Br. Med. J.* 297 (1988b) 883–887

Whittle, M. J. and Connor, J. M. (Eds.). *Prenatal Diagnosis in Obstetric Practice*, Blackwell Scientific Publications, Oxford and Edinburgh, 1989

J. Inher. Metab. Dis. 12 Suppl. 1 (1989) 97–104

Obstetric Aspects of Prenatal Diagnostic Methods

M. J. Whittle, D. H. Gilmore and M. B. McNay
The Department of Midwifery, The Queen Mother's Hospital, Yorkhill, Glasgow, G3 8SH, Scotland

Summary: The vast improvements in ultrasound technology have proved to be an important starting point for invasive investigative procedures in obstetrics. These methods not only allow a more precise diagnosis to be made but also offer considerable scope for *in utero* therapy.

The fetus is being considered increasingly as a patient in its own right so that when an anomaly is found or suspected it is becoming mandatory to establish a diagnosis with the same degree of precision as would be acceptable in adult medicine. Since the ability to undertake these investigations tends to be limited to a few specialized centres it may be necessary to arrange the transfer of the patient some distance but nevertheless it is believed that this is a worthwhile undertaking. Of course the diagnosis is often obvious, for example in anencephaly or gross body stalk anomalies, and under these circumstances termination of pregnancy can be offered without further investigation. Other cases are, however, less clear so that, for example, the fetus with renal anomalies or an anterior abdominal wall defect may need detailed study to establish viability.

The purpose of this review is to describe the various techniques available for confirming fetal diagnosis which allow the obstetrician to plan management using the scheme shown in Figure 1.

Prenatal detection of fetal anomaly concerns both screening and diagnostic programmes. Screening methods are not fully discussed here but it is vital that those involved in prenatal care are aware of the factors that place any individual pregnancy in an at-risk category for fetal anomaly. Thus the common indications for detailed ultrasound evaluation include a positive past obstetric history, raised maternal serum α-fetoprotein concentration, a family history of anomaly or a suspicious screening ultrasound scan (Table 1).

The diagnostic methods to be discussed here include detailed ultrasound scanning, amniocentesis, chorionic villus sampling and fetal blood sampling.

ULTRASOUND SCANNING

Ian Donald, who was Professor of Midwifery at the University of Glasgow, is considered by most to be the founder of obstetric ultrasound, appreciating at an

97

Journal of Inherited Metabolic Disease. ISSN 0141-8955. Copyright © SSIEM and Kluwer Academic Publishers, PO Box 55, Lancaster, UK.

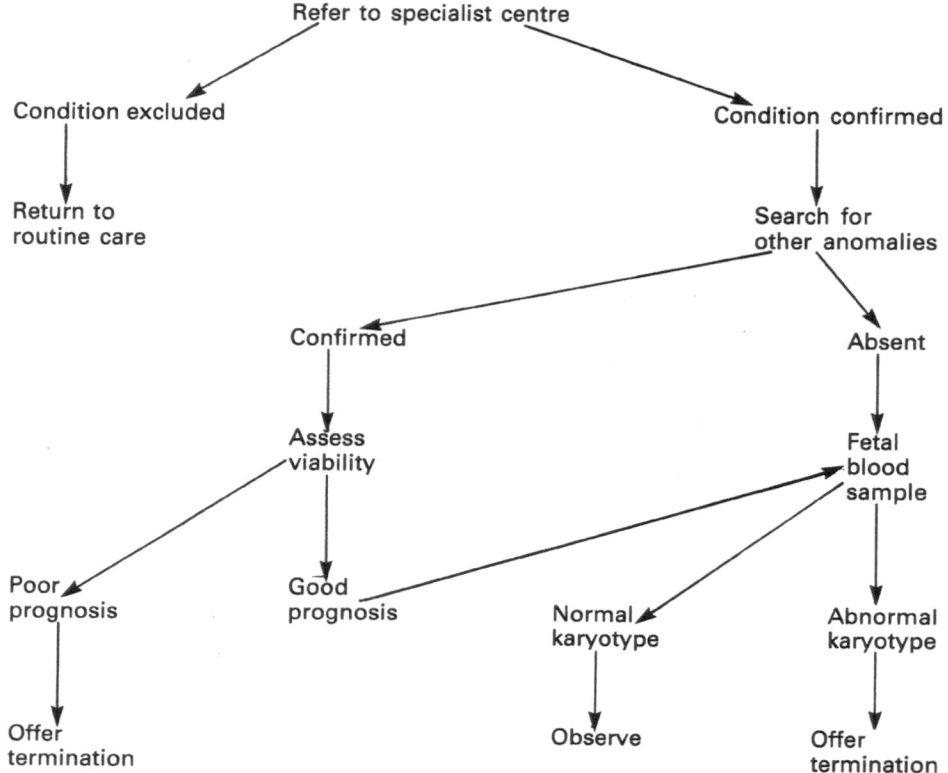

Figure 1   The management of a pregnancy with a suspected fetal abnormality

Table 1   Indications for detailed anomaly scans[a]

Past history of anomaly	35.0%
Raised α-fetoprotein	35.0%
Family history of anomaly	10.0%
Clinical suspicion	7.0%
Ultrasound suspicion	7.0%
Complex	6.0%

[a] The Queen Mother's Hospital, Glasgow, 1987

early stage the significance of the technique in pregnancy evaluation. Since 1954, when the pioneering work commenced, enormous improvements have transformed ultrasound from a useful method of fetal measurement to a technique which, through the production of superb images, allows the accurate evaluation not only of fetal anatomy but also fetal behavioural characteristics. As shown in Table 2, the majority of important structures are identifiable by about 20 weeks (Zador *et al.*, 1988) and it is on this basis that ultrasound screening for anomalies is arranged to be undertaken at a gestational age of between 18 and 20 weeks.

Table 2 Proportion of fetal organs clearly visualized by 20 weeks[a]

Cerebral ventricles	85.0%
Stomach	95.0%
Bladder	89.0%
Spine	76.0%
Extremities	97.0%
Kidneys: left	23.0%
right	31.0%
Diaphragm	43.0%
Heart	15.0%

[a] From Zador *et al.*, 1988

The reliable identification of normal fetal anatomy requires rigorous discipline to ensure that all structures are properly evaluated. Failure to identify a particular item should not be assumed to be due to adverse scanning conditions but might, in fact, be the first indication that a fetal anomaly exists. It is, therefore, imperative that the mother is recalled until all the relative structures have been seen.

Although the advantages of detailed ultrasound evaluation undertaken in mid-pregnancy may seem obvious, there are no supportive substantive data although prospective studies are in progress. In our own practice the maternal serum α-fetoprotein concentration is used as the primary screening test with ultrasound being used as a second line of evaluation. The introduction of the maternal serum α-fetoprotein screening programme has led to a marked reduction in the incidence of babies born at term with neural tube defects (Ferguson-Smith, 1983). However, without the use of detailed ultrasound to exclude the 29 out of 30 babies whose mothers have raised serum α-fetoprotein concentration but are perfectly normal, the screening programme would result in many unnecessary amniocenteses. The programme also helps to identify other anomalies, such as anterior abdominal wall defects, chromosomal disorders and other potential obstetric problems such as twins. In the absence of a maternal serum α-fetoprotein screening programme, a detailed fetal anomaly scan would seem desirable not only for the detection of neural tube defects but also other common anomalies such as those which may be found in the renal tract and cardiovascular system.

When patients are referred for detailed scans a number of important markers of fetal condition need to be noted and perhaps the most striking of these relates to the volume of amniotic fluid present. Polyhydramnios may suggest that the fetus is having deglutition problems as in oesophageal atresia, diaphragmatic hernia or even facial abnormalities such as micrognathia; alternatively there may be a bowel obstruction as in duodenal or jejunal atresia or complex mechanisms such as those seen in babies with neural tube defects. Oligohydramnios, conversely, is more likely to be the result of renal tract anomalies and great care must be taken in evaluating this system, which can be difficult when fluid volumes are reduced.

Other markers of fetal anomaly include polydactyly, absent radii and non-immune hydrops. One important rule in ultrasound diagnosis is that if one anomaly is found then another should be assumed to be present and positively searched for; this includes eliminating the possibility of chromosomal anomalies.

Although the value of ultrasound may appear obvious, the debate about its usefulness in practice continues. Concern about the safety of ultrasound has led to the production of a number of publications: some support ultrasound as a harmless investigation but others suggest potential danger. Following a detailed analysis of the literature, The Royal College of Obstetricians and Gynaecologists concluded that there were no substantive data to support the view that ultrasound, properly used by adequately trained personnel, was harmful and indeed that it was likely to be beneficial (RCOG, 1984).

AMNIOCENTESIS

The indications for amniocentesis are shown in Table 3. It is undoubtedly the most commonly performed invasive prenatal diagnostic test and because of this there is a great deal of information concerning its safety and limitations. However, it seems likely that in the majority of cases the amniocentesis is performed blind or at least only after placental localization by ultrasound.

Table 3   Indications for amniocentesis[a]

Maternal age	181 (67.5%)
Raised α-fetoprotein	46 (17.0%)
Past history	26 (10.0%)
Other	15 (5.5%)
Total	268

[a] The Queen Mother's Hospital, Glasgow, 1985

These methods are unsatisfactory and may lead to a failure to obtain a sample of fluid, require multiple attempts or cause placental or fetal damage. It has been shown that 'discolouration' of the fluid (not necessarily blood-staining) indicates an approximately ten-fold increased risk of fetal loss (Tabor *et al.*, 1986) and the same study suggested that transplacental amniocentesis should be avoided if possible since it may carry about a 2.6-fold increase in risk of fetal loss. Particular care to avoid the placenta during amniocentesis is required when the woman is rhesus negative so that the risks of rhesus sensitization can be minimized – all should, of course, receive anti-D following the procedure.

These problems can be avoided by performing amniocentesis under direct ultrasound control by use of either a needle guide system attached to the ultrasound transducer or a freehand technique. Using these methods it is possible precisely to identify a clear space and to watch the passage of the needle into a pocket of amniotic fluid.

The risk of pregnancy loss following amniocentesis varies not only from centre to centre but also with the indications for the test. In our own practice the risk of loss is about 1% and this has been consistent for a number of years. A large randomized study of amniocentesis (Tabor *et al.*, 1986) found a spontaneous abortion rate of 1.7% following the procedure which was undertaken in a low-risk population using an 18-gauge needle under ultrasound control. The spontaneous loss rate in the control population was 0.7%, giving a relative risk of abortion for the procedure of 2.3. However, the outcome does seem to be related to the indication: when amniocentesis has been performed because of a raised serum α-fetoprotein, loss rates rise about eight-fold.

Long-term complications are difficult to assess, but there does appear to be a slight increase in prematurity. The association of limb abnormalities, apparent from earlier studies (MRC, 1978), does not seem to have been confirmed (Tabor *et al.*, 1986), although there was still an increased incidence of respiratory problems in those babies from the amniocentesis group.

CHORIONIC VILLUS SAMPLING

Although amniocentesis has proved to be a useful practical method for the prenatal detection of chromosomal anomalies, metabolic disease and even DNA diagnoses of gene-linked disorders, its most serious disadvantage is the lateness of the definitive diagnosis. This arises because the procedure is not routinely performed prior to about 15 weeks and the cells in the amniotic fluid must first be cultured – a process which may take from between 2 and 3 weeks. In the presence of a confirmed abnormality, therefore, the mother will be faced with a late termination which can be an unpleasant and harrowing experience for the parents and attendants alike.

The development of chorionic villus sampling in the late 1970s provided the potential for obtaining material which would represent the fetal karyotype. It also became clear that direct preparation of the actively dividing surface cells of the trophoblast would enable a chromosomal diagnosis to be made within about 48 h of sampling. This, taken together with the fact that the procedure itself could be performed prior to 12 weeks of pregnancy, meant that in those cases with an adverse result the pregnancy could be terminated by suction curettage under general anaesthesia.

A further benefit of chorionic villus sampling was that the material obtained was a good source of DNA, allowing such studies to be undertaken immediately without the need for prior culture; the same advantage applied to biochemical assays.

The initial attempts at chorionic villus sampling involved the passage of a small endoscope through the cervix to enable the direct visualization of the trophoblast which was then biopsied. Performance of this technique required considerable skill and the most frequent complication was perforation of the fetal membranes. Later techniques included the passage of a fine catheter into the trophoblastic tissue via the cervix under ultrasound control; some variety of this approach is the one used most frequently today.

The transabdominal approach offers an alternative technique and is performed in a similar way to an amniocentesis. This is the method adopted in The Queen Mother's Hospital and to the end of June 1988 some 190 procedures have been performed. A 20-gauge needle is passed through the abdominal wall under ultrasound guidance and into the trophoblastic tissue. A 10 mL syringe is attached to the needle and suction applied. The aspirated material is examined under a microscope to ensure that sufficient material has been obtained: at least 10 mg being required for a karyotypic diagnosis and about 30 mg for a DNA assessment. Although this single-needle technique is relatively simple, the volume of tissue removed is sometimes small so several insertions may be required. To overcome this problem, some groups are using a double-needle technique in which the outer needle is inserted to the myometrium and the inner needle is used to make multiple aspirations of the trophoblastic tissue.

The main indication for chorionic villus sampling at The Queen Mother's Hospital is maternal age (75%), with X-linked disorders (7%) and previous abnormality (7%) being the next most common indications. Only 3% had the procedure for a DNA diagnosis.

The safety of these techniques is difficult to evaluate and the results of a multicentre randomized study will not be available for a while. One problem in evaluating the risk of spontaneous abortion after chorionic villus sampling is the difficulty in determining the background loss rate early in pregnancy. It has been suggested that when a fetal pole and heart beat have been identified the background risk of subsequent abortion is around 2% overall, with a level of about 10% by the time the mother has reached the age of 40 years (Gilmore and McNay, 1985). Against this the Chorionic Villus Sampling Fetal Loss Registry would indicate an overall loss rate following chorionic villus sampling of around 3.5% (Table 4); the rates for the various methods are also shown. It would seem, therefore, that chorionic villus sampling may not contribute to any greater loss than amniocentesis.

Table 4 **Comparison of loss rates for transabdominal and transcervical chorionic villus samples**[a]

	Number of centres	Number of patients	Losses
Transabdominal	25	3977	2.3%
Transcervical (portex)	43	21895	2.8%
All methods	153	41521	3.5%

[a] Chorionic Villus Sampling Fetal Loss Registry, March, 1988

A more recent concern with chorionic villus sampling is, however, its diagnostic reliability. Several reports have now suggested that it has not been possible to confirm in the fetus certain anomalous karyotypes detected in the trophoblast (Callen *et al.*, 1988). In most cases these were mosaic forms identified in the direct preparations, and thus involving the surface trophoblast cells, and the fact that the fetus was actually normal was only confirmed once the trophoblastic core had been cultured. The chance of this form of discordance is probably about 1% and although similar problems can arise in amniotic fluid culture the risks are about 20-fold less. Perhaps of greater concern are the cases in which direct testing suggests a normal fetus although in fact it has a karyotypic abnormality. Long-term culture helps to exclude this extremely rare event.

Experience with chorionic villus sampling is still relatively limited and in our own practice the role of the technique is still emerging, particularly for karyotypic diagnosis in low-risk (<37 years old) mothers. However, the technique clearly has major advantages for early diagnosis in pregnancies at high risk of chromosome disorders, when a metabolic problem is anticipated, and when a DNA diagnosis is required.

FETAL BLOOD SAMPLING

Attempts at fetal blood sampling, which were first made in the mid-1950s, required some method for visualizing the fetal vessels. Scrimgeour, in the late 1960s, used a fetoscope introduced into the uterus via a small hysterotomy incision under general anaesthesia and, although reasonable views of the uterine contents were achieved, and indeed several fetuses with spina bifida identified, the procedure was clearly unacceptable.

The development of fibre-optic systems enabled a small fetoscope to be produced which could be introduced into the uterus under local anaesthesia alone. Both Rodeck in the UK and Hobbins in the USA have described the use of this instrument not only to visualize the fetus but also to identify the fetal vessels in the cord as a prelude to blood sampling.

Initially blood sampling was performed as a method of diagnosing haemoglobino-pathies, the fetal blood obtained being examined by electrophoresis. However, the indications for sampling have gradually changed over the years so that now the common indications are for rapid karyotype in the presence of an ultrasonically identified anomaly and the evaluation of potential erythroblastosis fetalis. In other countries, such as France, the most common indication includes the investigation of fetal infection by *Toxoplasmosis*.

Although the early work on blood sampling was by use of the fetoscope the enormous improvements in ultrasound technology have allowed the development of ultrasound guided procedures. The advantage of this approach is that it is less traumatic since only a 20- or 22-gauge needle is employed and the procedure is conducted in a similar way to an amniocentesis.

The first descriptions of the procedure appeared in 1983, when Daffos, working in Paris, discussed its potential. Since then there have been a number of reports from various groups around the world, although the individual experience is still small. The risks of the procedure are difficult to judge because outcome relates strongly to the indication for the procedure. Obviously the baby undergoing investigation because of fetal anomaly or non-immune hydrops will not have a good prognosis with or without sampling. The most useful figures, because they relate largely to normal fetuses merely at risk of infection, are probably from the group in Paris (Daffos *et al.*, 1986) in which the fetal loss rate was about 1.7%. When the results from accumulated figures are considered the risk of fetal loss is seen to be about 7% (Table 5), but, as previously mentioned, this will include many cases in which poor outcome might be anticipated. Interestingly these data also demonstrated that in experienced hands fetoscopy may be associated with fewer losses than cordocentesis. However, the likely explanation for the difference is the indication for the procedure which, for the fetoscopy group, was mainly the investigation of haemoglobinopathies.

Table 5   Fetal blood sampling: world experience August 1986–July 1987[a]

	Cordocentesis	Fetoscopy
Patients	1570	926
Procedures	1709	944
Elective abortions	246 (15.0%)	202 (28.0%)
Losses <28 weeks	46 (3.4%)	29 (4.0%)
Losses >28 weeks	48 (3.6%)	6 (0.8%)

[a] Data presented at International Fetoscopy Working Group, Boston, Massachusetts, 1987

The ability to gain access to the fetal circulation either by fetoscopy or by ultrasound guided procedures has widened the horizons for fetal therapy. Already the use of the intravascular approach to the treatment of rhesus disease is becoming accepted as a useful and potentially lifesaving procedure and the treatment of inborn errors of metabolism by correction of the enzyme defect using the intravascular route, while futuristic, remains an exciting possibility.

REFERENCES

Callen, D. F., Korban, G., Dawson, G., Gugasyan, L., Krumins, E. J. M., Eichenbaum, S., Petrass, J., Purvis-Smith, S., Smith, A., Den Dulk, G. and Martin, N. Extra embryonic/fetal karyotypic discordance during CVS. *Prenat. Diagn.* 8 (1988) 453–460

Daffos, F., Capella-Pavlosky, M. and Forestier, F. Fetal blood sampling during pregnancy with the use of a needle guided by ultrasound: a study of 606 consecutive cases. *Am. J. Obstet. Gynecol.* 153 (1986) 655–660

Ferguson-Smith, M. A. The reduction of anencephalic and spina bifida births by MSAFP screening. *Br. Med. Bull.* 39 (1983) 365–372

Gilmore, D. H. and McNay, M. B. Spontaneous fetal loss rate in early pregnancy. *Lancet* 1 (1985) 107

MRC. The assessment of the hazards of amniocentesis. *Br. J. Obstet. Gynecol.* 85 Suppl. 2 (1978)

Royal College of Obstetricians and Gynaecologists. Report of the RCOG working party on routine ultrasound examination in pregnancy, 1984

Tabor, A., Madsen, M., Obel, E. B., Philip, J., Bang, J. and Norgaard-Pedersen, B. Randomized controlled trial of genetic amniocentesis in 4606 low risk women. *Lancet* 1 (1986) 1287–1293

Zador, I. E., Buttons, S. F., Tse, G. M., Brindley, B. A. and Sokol, R. J. Normograms for ultrasound visualization of fetal organs. *J. Ultrasound Med.* 7 (1988) 197-201

J. Inher. Metab. Dis. 12 Suppl. 1 (1989) 105–117

Chorionic Villus Sampling: Diagnostic Uses and Limitations of Enzyme Assays

B. FOWLER, L. GILES, A. COOPER and I. B. SARDHARWALLA
Willink Biochemical Genetics Unit, Royal Manchester Children's Hospital, Pendlebury, Manchester, M27 1HA, UK

Summary: Control ranges for enzymes in uncultured chorionic villi were established, based on: (1) 21 of 22 enzymes (mainly lysosomal) in villi had similar properties to the enzyme in cultured fibroblasts; (2) isoenzyme patterns in villi were similar to those in fibroblasts for five lysosomal enzymes but different for aryl sulphatases; (3) control ranges were determined for 12 enzymes in abortion villi and for 21 enzymes in biopsy villi, values tending to be higher in the latter for those enzymes studied in both types of sample; (4) storage of samples under various conditions revealed no major changes in activity of seven lysosomal enzymes.

A number of potential pitfalls in the use of chorionic villus samples for diagnosis of metabolic disorders by enzyme assay are described: (1) the presence of aryl sulphatase C in chorionic villi, an isoenzyme which may interfere in assays of aryl sulphatase A; (2) the presence of maternal enzyme in chorionic villus material illustrated by the detection of the A isoenzyme of B-hexosaminidase in chorionic villus from a pregnancy affected with Sandhoff's disease; (3) the finding of falsely normal levels of α-iduronidase in chorionic villus samples from a pregnancy affected with Hurler's disease, probably due to contamination with maternal tissue which has relatively high levels of this enzyme compared with fetal chorionic material: (4) the inadequacy of indirect assays of incorporation of radiolabel into macromolecules using chorionic villi, for example [14C]propionate incorporation for prenatal diagnosis of methylmalonic aciduria.

Provided that such pitfalls are recognized and great care is taken in selection of villus samples and interpretation of results, chorionic villus sampling allows reliable prenatal diagnosis of a large number of disorders using enzyme asays.

This paper describes detailed control studies of several enzymes (mostly lysosomal) in samples of chorionic villi obtained both from abortion material and by biopsy as a basis for this approach to prenatal diagnosis. Emphasis was given to assays performed directly on uncultured samples, which we believe to be the best approach, although assays on cultured villi have a role to play for some disorders which are difficult to diagnose on uncultured villi and for confirmation of initial results. Two disadvantages of using cultured chorionic villi are the risk of over-

Journal of Inherited Metabolic Disease. ISSN 0141–8955. Copyright © SSIEM and Kluwer Academic Publishers, PO Box 55, Lancaster, UK.

growth by maternal cells which has been documented (Besley and Broadhead, 1989) and the 3 to 4 week delay in obtaining the result. Specific activities and a number of properties of a large number of enzymes were determined in chorionic villi from abortion material. Control ranges were then established for 21 enzymes in up to 56 control biopsy chorionic villus samples. Conditions of transport and storage of samples were investigated by studying several enzyme activities in samples kept in different media at different temperatures for various times.

Based on previous reports, and considering the nature of chorionic villus samples, we recognized a number of potential pitfalls in using this approach for prenatal diagnosis of inherited metabolic disorders. First, the presence of unusual isoenzymes, for example of aryl sulphatases which could explain the finding of normal aryl sulphatase A activity in chorionic villi from a fetus shown subsequently to be affected with metachromatic leucodystrophy (Sanguinetti *et al.*, 1986). Second, the presence of maternal tissue, which is possible even with meticulous selection of villi from biopsies and is especially important when the particular enzyme activity is higher in maternal than fetal tissue. Third, the possibility of cross-over of enzyme from the maternal to the fetal side of the placenta, which could explain the higher residual enzyme activity seen in fetal placenta compared with fetal cultured fibroblasts in a case of methylmalonic aciduria (Fowler *et al.*, 1988) and a case of Hunter's syndrome (Kleijer *et al.*, 1984). Fourth, the unusual results obtained in chorionic villi with indirect assays based on incorporation of radiolabelled substrate into macromolecules. For example Vimal and coworkers (1984) reported normal incorporation of label from citrulline into protein in uncultured chorionic villi but reduced levels in cultured villus cells in a pregnancy affected with argininosuccinic aciduria. To illustrate these pitfalls and the potential influence on the reliability of prenatal diagnosis by enzyme assay on chorionic villi we describe our detailed studies on four enzymes:

(1) aryl sulphatases in control chorionic villi revealing the presence of an extra isoenzyme;

(2) β-hexosaminidases in controls and two cases at risk for Sandhoff's disease illustrating the isoenzyme patterns and the presence of maternal enzyme;

(3) α-iduronidase in two cases at risk for Hurler's disease and comparison of control fetal and maternal chorionic tissue;

(4) methylmalonyl-CoA mutase activity and incorporation of [^{14}C]propionic acid into protein in a pregnancy affected with methylmalonic aciduria.

METHODS

Methods for the biopsy technique and selection of chorionic villus samples have been reported elsewhere (Giles *et al.*, 1987). Lysosomal enzymes were assayed in cell-free extracts prepared with 0.1% Triton X-100 as previously described (Giles *et al.*, 1987). Acid neuraminidase (EC 3.2.1.18), β-mannosidase (EC 3.2.1.25), β-hexosaminidase (EC 3.2.1.30), acid phosphatase (EC 3.1.3.2), α-fucosidase (EC

3.2.1.51), β-galactosidase (EC 3.2.1.23), acid esterase (EC 3.1.1.3), α-glucosidase (EC 3.2.1.20), β-glucosidase (EC 3.2.1.45), α-mannosidase (EC 3.2.1.24), α-galactosidase (EC 3.2.1.22), α-iduronidase (EC 3.2.1.76), α-hexosaminidase (EC 3.2.1.50) and β-glucuronidase (EC 3.2.1.31) were assayed fluorimetrically; aryl sulphatase A (EC 3.1.6.1), β-galactocerebrosidase (EC 3.2.1.46) and sphingomyelinase (EC 3.1.4.12) were assayed colorimetrically; sulphamidase (EC 3.10.1.1), *N*-acetylgalactosamine-6-sulphate sulphatase (EC 3.1.6.4) and acetyl-CoA:2-amino-2-deoxy-α-glucoside *N*-acetyltransferase were assayed with radiolabelled substrates, all as previously described (Cooper *et al.*, 1988). Iduronate sulphate sulphatase was assayed radioisotopically as described by DiNatale and Ronsisvalle (1981). Methylmalonyl-CoA mutase (EC 5.4.99.2) and cystathionine β-synthase (EC 4.2.1.22) were assayed as previously described in cell-free extracts prepared in the buffer used in the respective enzyme assays (Fowler *et al.*, 1978, 1988).

RESULTS AND DISCUSSION

Control studies

Conditions of enzyme assay: Studies of the effect of varying protein content and time of assay, the pH optimum and Michaelis constant, carried out using control chorionic villus tissue from abortion material, revealed no important differences when compared with our fibroblast data for each of 22 lysosomal enzymes studied (A. Cooper and L. Giles, unpublished observations) except for aryl sulphatase A (see Giles *et al.*, 1987). This suggested that for these enzymes there were no major differences between activities in chorionic villi and cultured skin fibroblasts and allowed selection of optimum conditions of assay. The only modifications made to the assays referred to above for chorionic villus samples were increases of the incubation time of assay for α-iduronidase (increased to 90 min), β-galactosidase (increased to 15 min), sphingomyelinase (increased to 6 h), sulphamidase, *N*-acetylgalactosamine-6-sulphate sulphatase and acetyl-CoA:amino-2 deoxy-α-glucoside *N*-acetyltransferase each increased to 18 h.

Control ranges in abortion and biopsy chorionic villi: The levels of enzyme activities in chorionic villi, stored at $-70°C$ prior to assay, from controls, both abortion and biopsy samples are shown in Figures 1–5 and compared with our control values for fibroblasts for reference.

In 22 samples from abortion material satisfactory ranges were found for total β-hexosaminidase, acid phosphatase and acid esterase (Figure 1) and for α-glucosidase, β-glucosidase, α-mannosidase and α-galactosidase (Figure 2) which were similar to the ranges for cultured fibroblasts. α-Fucosidase activities (Figure 1) were clearly higher whilst β-galactosidase (Figure 1), sphingomyelinase (Figure 2) and aryl sulphatase A (Figure 3) activities were clearly lower than in cultured fibroblasts. Also in abortion villi, the range of methylmalonyl-CoA mutase activity was satisfactory (Fowler *et al.*, 1988) whereas cystathionine synthase activity ($n = 8$) was very low (Figure 3) precluding prenatal diagnosis of homocystinuria due to deficiency of this enzyme by assays on uncultured villus samples.

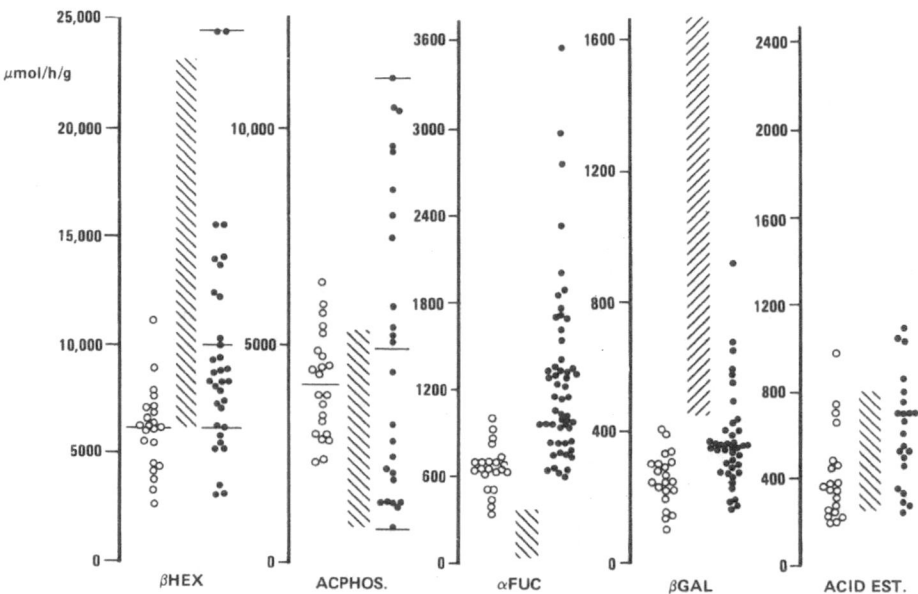

Figure 1 Lysosomal enzyme activities in μmol (g protein)$^{-1}$h^{-1}, for control uncultured chorionic villi obtained from (O) abortion material and (●) biopsies: βHEX = β-hexosaminidase; ACPHOS = acid phosphatase; αFUC = α-fucosidase; βGAL = β-galactosidase; ACID EST = Acid esterase. The hatched areas represent our control ranges for cultured skin fibroblasts

In samples obtained by biopsy, except for sphingomyelinase ($n = 25$) the ranges tended to be higher than those in abortion villi for total β-hexosaminidase ($n = 35$), acid phosphatase ($n = 25$), β-galactosidase ($n = 41$), acid esterase ($n = 24$), β-glucosidase ($n = 25$) and α-galactosidase ($n = 27$) (Figures 1 and 2). This difference was more marked for α-fucosidase ($n = 56$) (Figure 1), α-glucosidase ($n = 25$) and α-mannosidase ($n = 25$) (Figure 2). These differences indicate the value of establishing control values in biopsy material rather than abortion material for this approach to prenatal diagnosis. Control ranges for further enzymes were established in biopsy samples only. The values of β-hexosaminidase A ranged from 33 to 68% of the total activity ($n = 14$, mean = 49.5%) determined by DEAE cellulose chromatography (see later). Satisfactory ranges of β-mannosidase and β-galactocerebrosidase were found whilst the levels of neuraminidase (Figure 4) were relatively low, indicating the need for great care in performing prenatal diagnosis of sialidosis using uncultured chorionic villi. The ranges of activity of seven enzymes deficient in several types of mucopolysaccharidosis are shown in Figure 5. The values of α-iduronidase in 53 control biopsy samples were appreciably lower than in fibroblasts, indicating possible difficulties in prenatal diagnosis of Hurler's disease (see later). The ranges of iduronate sulphate sulphatase, α-hexosaminidase, acetyl-CoA:amino α-glucoside *N*-acetyltransferase, β-glucuronidase, *N*-acetylgalactosamine-6-sul-

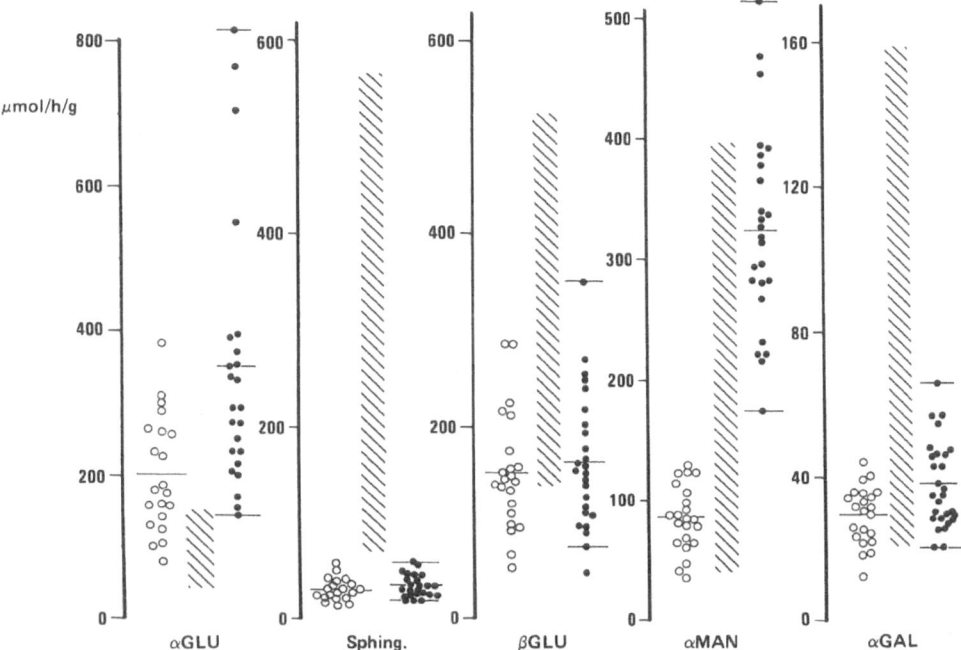

Figure 2 Lysosomal enzyme activities, in μmol (g protein)$^{-1}$h^{-1}, for control uncultured chorionic villi obtained from (O) abortion material and (●) biopsies: αGLU = α-glucosidase; Sphing = sphingomyelinase; βGLU = β-glucosidase; αMAN = α-mannosidase; αGAL = α-galactosidase

phate sulphatase and sulphamidase were satisfactory although relatively low for the last of these.

The range of activities of many of these enzymes in control samples appear to be rather wide, probably reflecting the heterogenous nature of chorionic villus tissue. Similar wide ranges have been reported by three other groups, Poenaru and coworkers (1984) who measured 13 enzymes in 20 samples, Gatti and coworkers (1985), 15 enzymes in 7–41 samples and Evans and coworkers (1986), nine enzymes in 11 samples.

Storage and transport conditions: Previous studies had revealed no differences in activity of 13 lysosomal enzymes in fresh, unstored chorionic villi compared with samples frozen at −70°C prior to assay (A. Cooper and B. Fowler, unpublished observations). Similar observations were also reported by Evans and coworkers (1986). To study further the effect of storage conditions on enzyme activity in chorionic villi, seven representative lysosomal enzymes were assayed in control villus material stored in various ways. Samples of villi from control abortions were placed in either saline (0.9% w/v, sterile) or tissue culture medium (Eagles MEM with 10% fetal calf serum) and cell-free extracts prepared for assay: (1) within 2 h; (2) after storage at room temperature for 24, 48 and 72 h; (3) after storage at 4°C for 24, 48 and 72 h; (4) after storage at −70°C for 8 weeks.

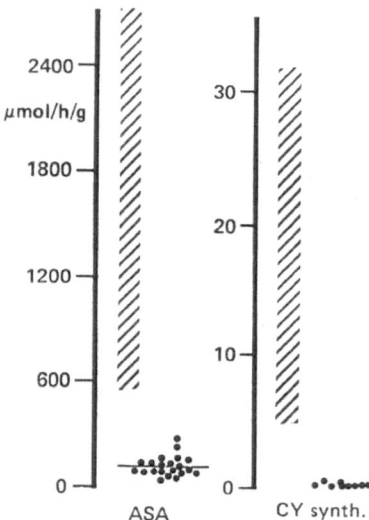

Figure 3 Enzyme activities in μmol (g protein)$^{-1}$h^{-1}, for control uncultured chorionic villi obtained from abortion material: ASA = aryl sulphatase A; CY synth = cystathionine synthase. The hatched areas represent our control ranges for cultured skin fibroblasts

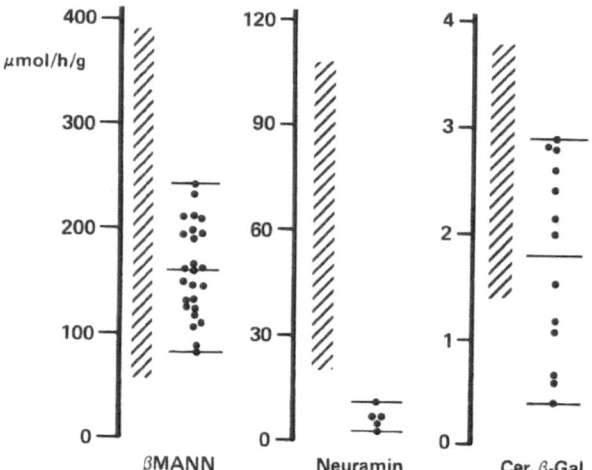

Figure 4 Lysosomal enzyme activities in μmol (g protein)$^{-1}$h^{-1}, for control uncultured chorionic villi obtained from biopsies: βMANN = β-mannosidase; Neuramin = neuraminidase; Cer-β-Gal = β-galactocerebrosidase. The hatched areas represent our control ranges for cultured skin fibroblasts

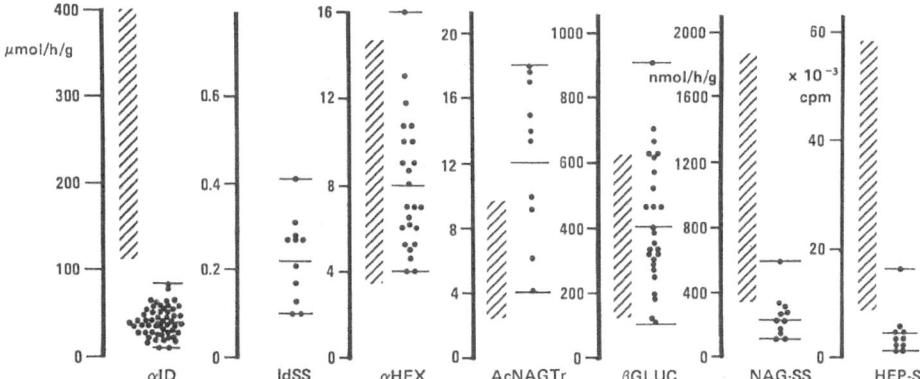

Figure 5 Activities of enzymes deficient in mucopolysaccharide disorders, in μmol(g protein)$^{-1}$h^{-1}, for control uncultured chorionic villi from biopsies: αID = α-iduronidase; IdSS = iduronate sulphate sulphatase; αHEX = α-hexosaminidase; AcNAGTr = acetyl-CoA: 2-amino-2-deoxyglucoside *N*-acetyltransferase; HEP-S = sulphamidase. The hatched areas represent our control ranges for cultured skin fibroblasts

The activities of α-fucosidase, β-galactosidase, β-glucuronidase, α-mannosidase, β-glucosidase, α-glucosidase and β-hexosaminidase varied no more under each of these storage conditions than in different samples from the same abortus. No major losses of enzyme activity were seen and values in samples stored in each of these ways remained within our control range. There were no differences between samples stored in sterile saline or culture medium. These studies suggest that chorionic villus biopsies for assay of at least those lysosomal enzymes studied here can be transported in saline or culture medium for up to 48 h at room temperature after which they should be assayed or stored frozen at −70°C.

Potential pitfalls in the use of chorionic villus samples

Detailed studies of four enzymes in control or at-risk chorionic villus samples are described which highlight several problems in the use of chorionic villi for prenatal diagnosis of metabolic disorders:

(1) aryl sulphatases revealing an extra isoenzyme in chorionic villi which could interfere in assays of aryl sulphatase A;

(2) β-hexosaminidases in samples from controls and two cases at risk for Sand-hoff's disease illustrating the isoenzyme patterns and the presence of maternal enzyme;

(3) α-iduronidase in two cases at risk for Hurler's disease and in control fetal and maternal tissue indicating problems associated with maternal contamination;

(4) methylmalonyl-CoA mutase activity and incorporation of [^{14}C]propionate into protein in a pregnancy affected with methylmalonic aciduria revealing conflicting results with these two assays. This study also indicated difficulties

with diagnosis of vitamin responsive forms of this condition using chorionic villi.

Aryl sulphatases in chorionic villi: As shown in Figure 3, the activity of aryl sulphatase A, assayed by the standard colorimetric assay, is much lower in villi than in fibroblasts. Furthermore our detailed studies of aryl sulphatases in chorionic villi (Giles *et al.*, 1987) showed different properties of aryl sulphatase A with respect to pH optimum, K_m and linearity with time of incubation. Further studies using DEAE cellulose chromatography with continuous fluorimetric assay revealed a large quantity of an extra isoenzyme in villi compared with fibroblasts. This isoenzyme was shown to have similar properties to aryl sulphatase C. These findings were supported by electrophoretic studies and we concluded that this extra isoenzyme in villi has some activity in the standard colorimetric assay used for diagnosis of metachromatic leukodystrophy using leukocytes or cultured fibroblasts. The presence of this extra isoenzyme explains the false normal result in chorionic villus in a fetus affected with metachromatic leukodystrophy reported by Sanguinetti and colleagues (1986) who presented additional evidence for the presence of aryl sulphatase C in chorionic villi.

It is clear that the colorimetric assay for aryl sulphatase A activity used on other tissues is not suitable for chorionic villus samples although modification of the conditions for extraction of enzyme may minimize interference by aryl sulphatase C (Sanguinetti *et al.*, 1986). The most reliable alternative methods are based on separation of sulphatases. For example by DEAE cellulose chromatography or electrophoresis (Giles *et al.*, 1987) or by immunoprecipitation and electrophoresis as described by Poenaru *et al.* (1988).

β-Hexosaminidases in Sandhoff's disease: We have reported detailed studies of β-hexosaminidase isoenzymes in chorionic villi from controls and in two pregnancies at risk for Sandhoff's disease (Giles *et al.*, 1988). In the first case total β-hexosaminidase activity was normal, $6365 \, \mu mol \, (g \, protein)^{-1} h^{-1}$ controls 3227–$24\,495 \, \mu mol \, (g \, protein)^{-1} h^{-1}$, in contrast to clearly reduced activity in case 2, $672 \, \mu mol \, (g \, protein)^{-1} h^{-1}$, although the value was somewhat higher than that usually found in samples from patients with Sandhoff's disease. The level of total β-hexosaminidase activity in cultured amniotic fluid cells from case 1, $(3360 \, \mu mol \, (g \, protein)^{-1} h^{-1}$, controls 6016–$20\,622 \, \mu mol \, (g \, protein)^{-1} h^{-1}$, and in fetal tissue of case 2, $73 \, \mu mol \, (g \, protein)^{-1} h^{-1}$, controls 4796–$5799 \, \mu mol \, (g \, protein)^{-1} h^{-1}$, confirmed the diagnosis of an unaffected and affected pregnancy, respectively.

More detailed investigation of the β-hexosaminidase isoenzymes in the chorionic villus samples was performed by DEAE cellulose chromatography with continuous enzyme assay using the fluorogenic substrate. In case 1, which had normal total activity, the pattern of β-hexosaminidases was normal with major peaks of 'B' and 'A' isoenzymes and smaller amounts of the so-called intermediate isoenzymes 'I_1' and 'I_2'. Incidentally we have observed that these intermediate isoenzymes tend to be considerably higher in chorionic villi than in other cells and tissues. In case 2, which had low total activity, the pattern was very different with the presence of two extra isoenzymes, the so-called 'S' isoenzymes which are characteristic of

Sandhoff's disease. However there was a clearly detectable quantity of the normal 'A' isoenzyme which would be expected to be completely absent in Sandhoff's disease. In contrast, β-hexosaminidase isoenzymes in fetal tissue were the same as in Sandhoff's disease with no detectable 'A' isoenzyme. Therefore the small quantity of the 'A' isoenzyme in chorionic villi of this affected fetus is most likely of maternal origin. It is emphasized that the chorionic villus sample was a good one and rigorously selected using the accepted criteria for identification of fetal villus material.

We conclude that the identification of β-hexosaminidase isoenzymes in chorionic villi by DEAE cellulose chromatography allows reliable first-trimester diagnosis of both Tay–Sachs and Sandhoff's disease. In Sandhoff's disease the presence of the unusual 'S' isoenzyme provides a qualitative difference between affected and unaffected cases, allowing reliable diagnosis even if maternal contamination is present or if the total β-hexosaminidase activity is on the borderline of the control range. The presence of the 'A' isoenzyme in what appeared to be 'pure' villi from our case affected with Sandhoff's disease must reflect either a small degree of maternal contamination which cannot be recognized visually or placental cross-over of maternal enzyme. Poenaru and colleagues (1984) also reported the presence of β-hexosaminidase A in chorionic villi from a fetus affected with Sandhoff's disease but suggested this could be due to contamination with maternal enzyme during conservation of the sample at $-70°C$ for 3 months, not an explanation for our observations found in fresh tissue.

Other isoenzymes studied in control chorionic villi: We have studied isoenzymes of five other lysosomal enzymes in control chorionic villi from abortion material, namely α-glucosidase, β-glucosidase, α-mannosidase, acid esterase and α-fucosidase. The methods used and the isoenzymes identified are listed in Table 1. We conclude that for these five enzymes there are no unusual isoenzymes in chorionic villi that would interfere in diagnostic studies and that the patterns are similar to those seen in cultured fibroblasts.

α-Iduronidase in control and at-risk chorionic villi: maternal decidua vs *fetal activities*: α-Iduronidase activities found in chorionic villi from two cases at risk

Table 1 Isoenzymes in chorionic villi

Enzyme	Method of identification	Isoenzymes
α-Glucosidase	Thermostability at 50°C	Acidic, neutral – similar to skin fibroblasts
β-Glucosidase	Thermostability at 45°C	Mainly acidic, some neutral – similar to skin fibroblasts
α-Mannosidase	DEAE cellulose chromatography at pH 6.0, gradient 0–0.3 mol L⁻¹ NaCl	Acidic A+B, neutral – similar to skin fibroblasts
Acid esterase	Electrophoresis (Coates *et al.*, 1978)	Two bands (acidic, neutral) – similar to skin fibroblasts
α-Fucosidase	DEAE cellulose chromatography at pH 6.0. Gradient 0–0.3 mol L⁻¹ NaCl	Similar to liver (Chester *et al.*, 1977)

for Hurler's disease are shown in Figure 6. The values in two separate samples from case 1, which were obtained when there was very little experience of the technique, were well within the control range. These were rather poor samples and maternal contamination was suspected. Follow-up studies on amniotic fluid indicated an affected fetus which was confirmed following termination of the pregnancy. In contrast there was a marked deficiency of α-iduronidase in chorionic villi from case 2, $0.27\,\mu\text{mol}\,(\text{g protein})^{-1}\text{h}^{-1}$, controls $10\text{--}83\,\mu\text{mol}\,(\text{g protein})^{-1}\text{h}^{-1}$, and an affected fetus was confirmed following termination.

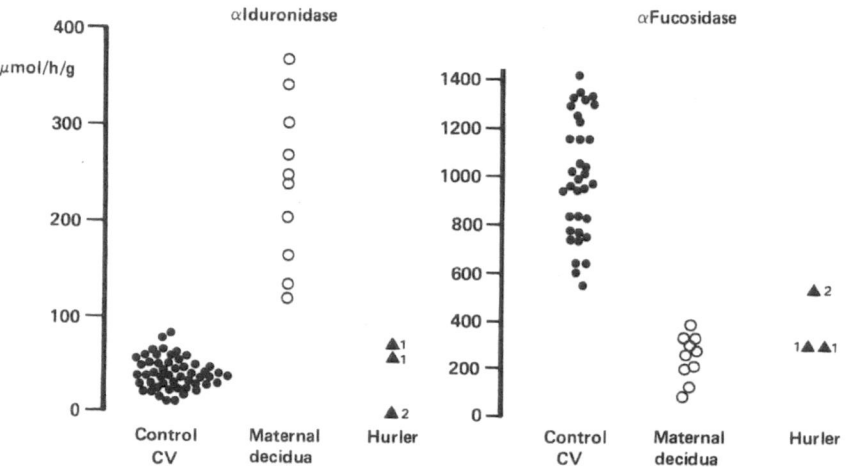

Figure 6 α-Iduronidase and α-fucosidase activities, in $\mu\text{mol}\,(\text{g protein})^{-1}\text{h}^{-1}$, for chorionic villi and maternal decidua: (●) control chorionic villi from biopsies; (○) control maternal decidua; (▲) chorionic villi from biopsies in two cases 'at risk' for Hurlers disease. Note that only the lower part of the control range for α-fucosidase is shown

We studied levels of α-iduronidase, α-fucosidase (Figure 6) and β-galactosidase in ten samples ·of maternal decidua, a potential source of contamination. α-Iduronidase activity (Figure 6) was considerably higher in this maternal tissue than in chorionic villi whereas β-galactosidase was similar in both types of sample: control chorionic villi, $167\text{--}920\,\mu\text{mol}\,(\text{g protein})^{-1}\text{h}^{-1}$; maternal decidua, $227\text{--}915$.

This supports the idea that contamination of chorionic villi with maternal tissue can give a falsely normal value of α-iduronidase in chorionic villus samples. It is of interest that the levels of α-fucosidase activity were considerably lower in maternal tissue than in control chorionic villi (Figure 6). The activity of this enzyme was also low in the samples from case 1, suspected of maternal contamination and well within the range for maternal decidua. In contrast we have found α-fucosidase activity to be within the control chorionic villi range in samples of each of 12 pregnancies in which the result obtained in villi was confirmed either on fetal material or postnatally. These observations suggest that measurement of α-fucosidase activity is useful and when low may indicate maternal contamination of chorionic villi samples.

J. Inher. Metab. Dis. 12 Suppl. 1 (1989)

Methylmalonyl-CoA mutase: methylmalonic aciduria: We have reported the measurement of methylmalonyl-CoA mutase activity in uncultured chorionic villi from controls and pregnancies at risk for methylmalonic aciduria (Fowler *et al.*, 1988). In controls, appreciable levels of mutase activity were found when assayed in the presence of added coenzyme, i.e. total (apo+holo-) mutase and this was deficient in one pregnancy confirmed to be affected with methylmalonic aciduria. Therefore diagnosis of the apo-mutase deficient form of this condition is possible on chorionic villi. However, this assay is unreliable for detection of the coenzyme synthesis defective form of this condition using uncultured chorionic villi, due to the relatively low activity found in the absence of added coenzyme (holo-mutase) and the possibility that coenzyme from the mother could accumulate in fetal tissues.

The measurement of [^{14}C]propionate incorporation into cell proteins has been profitably used in studies on fibroblasts of patients and is low in all forms of methylmalonic aciduria. However this assay gave conflicting results in chorionic villi of the fetus with mutase deficiency described above. Two different portions of the same biopsy gave different values of propionate incorporation. One was clearly low, the other was 40% of the mean control value and approached the lower limit of the normal range. Further analysis of cell proteins by hydrolysis and chromatographic analysis of amino acids clearly indicated that the higher value was due to incorporation of label into aspartic acid and glutamic acid. This confirms that the higher value reflects true activity of the propionate to succinate pathway rather than non-specific binding of radioactivity. In villi obtained from the placenta at termination and cultured fetal fibroblasts from this pregnancy, the values in this assay were clearly abnormal ruling out the possibility of alternate pathways of propionate metabolism in placental tissue as an explanation for the ambiguous result.

Also Sachs and coworkers (1988) reported normal propionate incorporation in villi of two cases affected with methylmalonic aciduria; similar findings have been reported with the assay of incorporation of citrulline into protein in a pregnancy affected with argininosuccinic aciduria (Vimal *et al.*, 1984).

Experience of enzyme assays on chorionic villi

There have been many detailed reports of individual positive cases diagnosed on chorionic villi. Many disorders of amino acid, lysosomal storage, organic acid and carbohydrate disorders have been diagnosed accurately in the first trimester by enzyme assay. Two large series of prenatal diagnosis of metabolic disorders using chorionic villi have been reported. Poenaru (1987) described 258 cases, 56 of which were affected. A second series totalling 98 cases (when diagnosis by DNA studies are excluded) with 26 positive, has been reported by Sachs and colleagues (1988). The total numbers of cases included in these studies are large but the numbers of individual metabolic disorders included are also large so that the numbers of pregnancies at risk for each disorder is often small. For example the first series included 38 disorders, for nine of which only one unaffected pregnancy was studied. In the second there were 25 disorders, for seven of which only only pregnancy was examined. Experience, however, is growing rapidly and other series have been presented (Young *et al.*, 1988; Besley and Broadhead, 1989).

Because of the potential problems with some enzymes, and distinct differences between chorionic villi and cultured cells, it is important to establish the technique for each individual disorder by experience of adequate numbers of both positive and negative cases.

CONCLUSIONS

Enzyme assays on uncultured chorionic villus biopsies allow reliable, rapid, first-trimester diagnosis of many metabolic disorders. It is emphasized that great care is needed in selection of chorionic villi and interpretation of results. Some disorders are difficult to diagnose using chorionic villi, although these difficulties can some-times be overcome by modifying or increasing the specificity of the assay. Cultured chorionic villi can be useful for those disorders which are difficult to diagnose in uncultured samples and for back-up of results obtained. The validity of indirect assays of isotope incorporation into macromolecules using uncultured chorionic villus samples must be questioned. Finally for those individual metabolic disorders for which there is not adequate experience we recommend that all normal results in chorionic villi be backed up by cultured villi or amniocentesis.

REFERENCES

Besley, G. T. N. and Broadhead, D. M. Prenatal diagnosis of inherited metabolic disease by chorionic villus analysis: The Edinburgh experience. *J. Inher. Metab. Dis.* 12 Suppl. 2 (1989) 263–266

Chester, M. A., Hultberg, B. and Sjoblad, S. A comparison of the α-fucosidase activities of human liver and serum. *Biochim. Biophys. Acta* 485 (1977) 147–155

Coates, P. M., Cornter, J. A., Mennuti, M. T. and Wheeler, J. E. Prenatal diagnosis of Wolman's disease. *Am. J. Med. Genet.* 2 (1978) 397–407

Cooper, A., Hatton, C., Thornley, M. and Sardharwalla, I. B. Human β-mannosidase deficiency: Biochemical findings in plasma, fibroblasts, white cells and urine. *J. Inher. Metab. Dis.* 11 (1988) 17–29

DiNatale, P. and Ronsisvalle, L. Identification and partial characterisation of two enzyme forms of iduronate sulfatase from human placenta. *Biochim. Biophys. Acta* 661 (1981) 106–111

Evans, M. I., Moore, C., Kolodny, E. H., Casassa, M., Schulman, J. D., Landsberger, E. J., Karson, E. M., Dorfman, A. D., Larsen Jr., J. W. and Barranger, J. A. Lysosomal enzymes in chorionic villi, cultured amniocytes, and cultured skin fibroblasts. *Clin. Chim. Acta* 157 (1986) 109–114

Fowler, B., Kraus, J., Packman, S. and Rosenberg, L. E. Homocystinuria: Evidence for three distinct classes of cystathionine β-synthase mutants in cultured fibroblasts. *J. Clin. Invest.* 61 (1978) 645–653

Fowler, B., Giles, L., Sardharwalla, I. B., Donnai, P. and Clayton, J. K. First trimester diagnosis of methylmalonic aciduria. *Prenat. Diagn.* 87 (1988) 207–213

Gatti, R., Lombardo, C., Filcamo, F., Borrone, C. and Porro, E. Comparative study of 15 lysosomal enzymes in chorionic villi and cultured amniotic fluid cells. Early prenatal diagnosis in seven pregnancies at risk for lysosomal storage diseases. *Prenat. Diagn.* 5 (1985) 329–336

Giles, L., Cooper, A., Fowler, B., Sardharwalla, I. B. and Donnai, P. Aryl Sulphatase isoenzymes of chorionic villi: Implications for prenatal diagnosis. *Prenat. Diagn.* 7 (1987) 245–252

Giles, L., Cooper, A., Fowler, B., Sandharwalla, I. B. and Donnai, P. First trimester prenatal diagnosis of Sandhoff's disease. *Prenat. Diagn.* 8 (1988) 199–205

Kleijer, W. J., Van Diggelen, O. P., Janse, H. C., Galjaard, H., Dumez, Y., Boue, J. First trimester diagnosis of Hunter syndrome on chorionic villi. *Lancet* 2 (1984) 472

Poenaru, L. First trimester prenatal diagnosis of metabolic diseases: A survey in countries from the European Community. *Prenat. Diagn.* 7 (1987) 333–341

Poenaru, L., Castelnau, L., Besancon, A-M., Nicolesco, H., Akli, S. and Theophil, D. First trimester prenatal diagnosis of metachromatic leukodystrophy in chorionic villi by 'immunoprecipitation-electrophoresis'. *J. Inher. Metab. Dis.* 11 (1988) 123–130

Poenaru, L., Kaplan, L., Dumez, J. and Dreyfus, J. C. Evaluation of possible first trimester prenatal diagnosis in lysosomal diseases by trophoblast biopsy. *Pediatr. Res.* 18 (1984) 1032–1034

Sachs, E. S., Jahoda, M. G. J., Kleijer, W. J., Pijpers, L. and Galjaard, H. Impact of first-trimester chromosome, DNA and metabolic studies on pregnancies at high genetic risk: Experience with 1000 cases. *Am. J. Med. Genet.* 29 (1988) 293–303

Sanguinetti, N., Marsh, J., Jackson, M., Fensom, A. H., Warren, R. C. and Rodeck, C. H. The aryl sulphatases of chorionic villi: potential problems in the first-trimester diagnosis of metachromatic leucodystrophy and Maroteaux–Lamy disease. *Clin. Genet.* 30 (1986) 302–308

Vimal, C. M., Fensom, A. H., Heaton, D., Ward, R. H. T., Garrod, P., Penketh, R. J. A. Prenatal diagnosis of argininosuccinic aciduria by analysis of cultured chorionic villi. *Lancet* 2 (1984) 521–522

Young, E. P., Whitfield, A. E. and Patrick, A. D. Experience of prenatal diagnosis of chorionic villi in approximately 100 pregnancies at risk for an inherited metabolic disorder. Abstracts of the 26th Annual Symposium of the Society for the Study of Inborn Errors of Metabolism, Glasgow, 1988, Abstract No. 04

J. Inher. Metab. Dis. 12 Suppl. 1 (1989) 118–134

Prenatal and Perinatal Diagnosis of Peroxisomal Disorders

R. B. H. Schutgens[1], G. Schrakamp[2], R. J. A. Wanders[1],
H. S. A. Heymans[1]*, J. M. Tager[3] and H. van den Bosch[2]

[1]*Department of Pediatrics, University Hospital Amsterdam, AMC, Meibergdreef
9, 1105 AZ Amsterdam, The Netherlands;* [2]*Laboratory of Biochemistry, State
University of Utrecht, Padualaan 8, 3584 CK Utrecht, The Netherlands; and*
[3]*Laboratory of Biochemistry, University of Amsterdam, AMC, Meibergdreef 15,
1105 AZ Amsterdam, The Netherlands*

Summary: Peroxisomes play an essential role in human cellular metabolism.
Peroxisomal disorders, a group of genetic diseases caused by peroxisomal
dysfunction, can be classified into three groups: (1) disorders of peroxisome
biogenesis with a generalized loss of peroxisomal functions (Zellweger syndrome, neonatal adrenoleukodystrophy, infantile Refsum disease, hyperpipecolic acidaemia); (2) disorders with a loss of multiple peroxisomal functions
(rhizomelic chondrodysplasia punctata and Zellweger-like syndrome; (3)
disorders with loss of a single peroxisomal function (X-linked adrenoleukodystrophy, peroxisomal thiolase deficiency, bifunctional protein deficiency, acyl-
CoA oxidase deficiency, classic Refsum disease, hyperoxaluria type I and
acatalasaemia). Prenatal diagnosis is indicated in all these genetic disorders
with the exception of classic Refsum disease, most types of hyperoxaluria
type I and acatalasaemia.

A variety of techniques is available now for the prenatal diagnosis of
peroxisomal disorders in the first or second trimester of gestation. Prenatal
diagnosis was performed by us in 70 pregnancies at risk for a disorder of
peroxisome biogenesis, three for rhizomelic chondrodysplasia punctata, four
for X-linked adrenoleukodystrophy and two for a defect in peroxisomal β-
oxidation. Fourteen affected fetuses were identified; no false negative cases
were obtained.

INTRODUCTION

Peroxisomes

In mammals each type of subcellular organelle (endoplasmic reticulum, mitochon-
drion, lysosome, peroxisome) plays a distinct and essential role in cellular metabolism. As a consequence each organelle in principle catalyses a characteristic set

---

* Present address: Department of Pediatrics, University of Groningen, Groningen, The
Netherlands.

Journal of Inherited Metabolic Disease. ISSN 0141–8955. Copyright © SSIEM and Kluwer Academic
Publishers, PO Box 55, Lancaster, UK.

of enzyme reactions and houses a specific set of enzyme proteins. However, some overlap in function between peroxisomes and other organelles, including mitochondria and the endoplasmic reticulum, has been found, e.g. in the β-oxidation of fatty acids.

Peroxisomes (microbodies) are apparently ubiquitous in mammalian cells, with the exception of mature erythrocytes, but their size and abundance varies considerably (Novikoff *et al.*, 1973).

Peroxisomal proteins are encoded by nuclear genes and synthesized on free polyribosomes in the cytosol (for review see Lazarow, 1987). Studies in rat liver have shown that this includes not only all the matrix enzyme proteins studied so far, but also the core protein urate oxidase and the integral membrane proteins (Suzuki *et al.*, 1987). Subsequently the newly synthesized peroxisomal proteins are imported post-translationally, generally at their final sizes into pre-existing peroxisomes. This leads to the progressive enlargement of the peroxisomes followed by division and the formation of new peroxisomes. At present, much work is being done by different groups to unravel the details of the mechanisms involved in the biogenesis of peroxisomes.

Essential metabolic processes in which peroxisomes are involved are summarized in Table 1. These include the metabolism of hydrogen peroxide (de Duve and Baudhuin, 1966), biosynthesis of ether-phospholipids (Hajra, 1984), the β-oxidation of (very) long-chain fatty acids (Lazarow and de Duve, 1976; Singh, I. *et al.*, 1984; Singh, H. *et al.*, 1987; Wanders *et al.*, 1987a), the β-oxidation of dicarboxylic acids (Kolvraa and Gregersen, 1986), polyunsaturated fatty acids (Hiltunen *et al.*, 1986; Hovik and Osmundsen, 1987), prostaglandins (Diczfalusy *et al.*, 1987; Schepers *et al.*, 1988) and xenobiotics (Yamada *et al.*, 1986), and side-chain cleavage during the conversion of tri- and dihydroxycholestanoic acid to bile acids (see review by Pedersen *et al.*, 1987). Moreover, peroxisomes play a role in glyoxylate catabolism since alanine glyoxylate aminotransferase, a pyridoxal phosphate dependent enzyme, is exclusively a peroxisomal enzyme in man (Noguchi, 1987). Peroxisomes are also involved in polyamine catabolism (Höltta, 1977; Beard *et al.*, 1985) and in cholesterol and in dolichol synthesis (Appelkvist and Dallner, 1987; Thompson *et al.*, 1987).

Recently we found that in humans the first step in L-pipecolic acid degradation is catalysed by the enzyme L-pipecolic acid oxidase, present in peroxisomes (Wan-

Table 1   Established functions of peroxisomes in mammalian cells

Hydrogen peroxide metabolism
Ether-phospholipid biosynthesis
β-Oxidation of (very) long-chain fatty acids, dicarboxylic acids, poly-unsaturated fatty acids, prostaglandins and zenobiotics
β-Oxidation of tri- and dihydroxycholestanoic acid
Glyoxylate catabolism (in man)
Polyamine catabolism
Cholesterol and dolichol synthesis
Pipecolic acid degradation (in man)

ders *et al.*, 1988b). In agreement with these findings is the report that in man the conversion of [³H]-L-pipecolic acid to [³H]-α-aminoadipic acid takes place in peroxisomes (Mihalik and Rhead, 1988). Finally, in contrast to the rat in which phytanic acid oxidation unequivocally occurs in liver mitochondria (Skjeldahl *et al.*, 1987), at least one step in this metabolic process must take place in peroxisomes in man since phytanic acid accumulates in patients deficient in peroxisomes (Poulos *et al.*, 1984).

Peroxisomal disorders

In recent years it has become clear that in man an impairment of one or more peroxisomal functions often results in serious disease. No animal model has been described so far. A growing number of genetic diseases originating from a deficiency of one or more peroxisomal enzymes is being recognised (Schutgens *et al.*, 1986a; Wanders *et al.*, 1988e; Lazarow and Moser, 1989). Peroxisomal disorders can tentatively be classified into three groups (Table 2).

Table 2   Classification of peroxisomal disorders

A.	*Disorders of peroxisome biogenesis with general loss of peroxisomal functions:* Cerebro-hepato-renal (Zellweger) syndrome Neonatal adrenoleukodystrophy Infantile Refsum disease Hyperpipecolic acidaemia
B.	*Disorders with loss of limited number of peroxisomal functions:* Rhizomelic chondrodysplasia punctata Zellweger-like syndrome
C.	*Disorders with loss of a single peroxisomal function:* Adrenoleukodystrophy (X-linked) Thiolase deficiency (pseudo-Zellweger syndrome) Bifunctional protein deficiency Acyl-CoA oxidase deficiency (pseudo-neonatal adrenoleukodystrophy) Hyperoxaluria type I Acatalasaemia

Group A: consists of disorders of peroxisome biogenesis with a generalized loss of peroxisomal functions. The clinical characteristics of the different disorders of this group (Zellweger syndrome; neonatal adrenoleukodystrophy; infantile Refsum disease; hyperpipecolic acidaemia) have been described in detail (Goldfischer and Reddy, 1984; Schutgens *et al.*, 1986a; Lazarow and Moser, 1989). In addition to the classic form of Zellweger syndrome milder variants have been described (Barth *et al.*, 1985; Bleeker-Wagemakers *et al.*, 1986). The genetic relationship between the different disorders in this group has been studied by complementation analysis after somatic cell fusion (Roscher *et al.*, 1986; Brul *et al.*, 1988; Poll-Thé, 1989). We have identified four different complementation groups within group A, demonstrating that there is not only genetic heterogeneity within the group of peroxisome deficiency disorders but also within the Zellweger syndrome. The basic biochemical defect in this group appears to involve the formation or maintenance of the peroxisomal structure. Already in 1973, Goldfischer and coworkers reported that patients affected by the cerebro-hepato-renal (Zellweger) syndrome lacked demonstrable peroxisomes in liver and kidney. This finding has been confirmed by many others. Subsequently, biochemical evidence was presented for a deficiency of peroxisomes in these disorders (Wanders *et al.*, 1984). It was shown that several peroxisomal proteins are synthesized normally in cultured fibroblasts from patients with Zellweger syndrome but that the newly synthesized enzyme proteins are subsequently degraded rapidly in these cells due to the deficiency of peroxisomes (Schram *et al.*, 1986). This accounts for the multiple enzyme defects found in Zellweger syndrome. However, some of the newly synthesized peroxisomal enzymes in Zellweger cells, like catalase, D-amino acid oxidase, L-α-hydroxyacid oxidase and alanine glyoxylate aminotransferase, escape rapid degradation and are metabolically active in the cytoplasm (Wanders *et al.*, 1984, 1987b; Goldfischer *et al.*, 1985).

The generalized loss of peroxisomal functions results in a variety of biochemical abnormalities, including an impaired ability to synthesize plasmalogens and bile acids, defective peroxisomal β-oxidation and the deficient catabolism of phytanic acid and pipecolic acid.

Group B: comprises disorders characterized by a loss of multiple peroxisomal functions and presumably normal peroxisomes and at present consists of two genetic disorders, namely rhizomelic chondrodysplasia punctata and Zellweger-like syndrome.

In rhizomelic chondrodysplasia punctata deficiencies have been found both of the two peroxisomal enzymes involved in phospholipid synthesis, acyl-CoA:dihydroxyacetone phosphate acyltransferase and alkyl dihydroxyacetone phosphate synthase, and there is an impairment of phytanic acid oxidation (Heymans *et al.*, 1986; Schutgens *et al.*, 1988). Moreover, in liver and in fibroblasts from patients with rhizomelic chondrodysplasia punctata the peroxisomal 3-oxoacyl-CoA thiolase protein is present only in the unprocessed form (Hoefler *et al.*, 1988). Other peroxisomal functions are normal in this disorder. Clinical characteristics of rhizomelic chondrodysplasia punctata have been described earlier (Spranger *et al.*, 1971).

Zellweger-like syndrome resembles classical Zellweger syndrome in its clinical presentation. However, it differs biochemically from the Zellweger syndrome since the biogenesis of peroxisomes is not impaired. Multiple defects of the enzymes of peroxisomal β-oxidation and dihydroxyacetone phosphate acyltransferase are found (Paturneau-Jouas *et al.*, 1987; Suzuki *et al.*, 1988). Biosynthesis of ether-phospholipids and catabolism of phytanic acid and pipecolic acids seem normal.

Group C: consists of genetic disorders characterized by the loss of only a single peroxisomal function.

In *X-linked adrenoleukodystrophy* and its variant adrenomyeloneuropathy, the deficient enzyme activity is the peroxisomal very-long-chain acylcoenzyme A synthetase, which normally activates the very-long-chain fatty acids to their CoA-esters before they enter the β-oxidation process (Wanders *et al.*, 1988a). All other peroxisomal functions are normal in adrenoleukodystrophy. The clinical features of the different adrenoleukodystrophy types have been described in detail elsewhere (Moser *et al.*, 1987b).

In *peroxisomal 3-oxoacyl-CoA thiolase deficiency* (pseudo-Zellweger syndrome) the biochemical defect is a deficiency of the peroxisomal 3-oxoacyl-CoA thiolase enzyme protein as shown by immunoblotting (Schram *et al.*, 1987). Other peroxisomal functions are normal. The only patient described with this disorder so far presented with clinical abnormalities very similar to classic Zellweger syndrome (Goldfischer *et al.*, 1986).

Bifunctional protein deficiency has been found in one child (Watkins *et al.*, 1989).

Acyl-CoA oxidase deficiency (pseudo-neonatal adrenoleukodystrophy) has been found in two siblings (Poll-Thé *et al.*, 1988). Clinical manifestations were very similar to those observed in patients suffering from neonatal adrenoleukodystrophy. Hepatic peroxisomes were increased in number and of enlarged size. Biochemical studies revealed a deficiency of acyl-CoA oxidase, the first enzyme in peroxisomal β-oxidation. Other peroxisomal functions were found to be normal.

Finally, in performing biochemical studies in patients suspected of a peroxisomal disorder, we have recently identified a growing number of patients with a defect in peroxisomal β-oxidation; immunoblotting and other detailed biochemical studies still have to be done in order to identify the deficient peroxisomal β-oxidation enzyme in these patients.

Hyperoxaluria type I can be classified in group C of the peroxisomal disorders; the peroxisomal enzyme alanine glyoxylate aminotransferase (AGT) is deficient in this disorder (Danpure and Jennings, 1986; Wanders *et al.*, 1987b, 1988c).

METHODS

Very-long-chain fatty acids in chorionic villus cells, in chorionic villus fibroblasts and in cultured amniotic fluid cells have been fractionated and quantitated essentially as described by Moser and coworkers (1984), with minor modifications as reported earlier (Wanders *et al.*, 1987c). Acyl-CoA dihydroxyacetone phosphate acyltransferase (DHAPAT) activity in chorionic villus cells, chorionic villus fibroblasts and amniotic fluid cells was measured as described (Schutgens *et al.*, 1986b).

De novo plasmalogen biosynthesis in chorionic villus fibroblasts and amniotic fluid cells was analysed as described by Schrakamp *et al.* (1988).

Particle-bound catalase was quantitated essentially as reported by Wanders *et al.* (1984). For direct analyses of chorionic villus cells, the fetal cells, taken by biopsies at 8–10 weeks of gestation, were transported in a frozen condition to the University Hospital, Amsterdam. For culturing of fibroblasts from the chorionic villus cells the biopsy material was placed in a plastic culture flask and fibroblasts were cultured according to standard procedures (Wanders *et al.*, 1987c). Amniotic fluid cells were obtained after amniocentesis at about the 16th week of gestation and cultured in F10 medium supplemented with 25% (v/v) fetal calf serum.

PRENATAL DIAGNOSIS

In our opinion prenatal diagnosis is indicated in classic Zellweger syndrome, neonatal adrenoleukodystrophy, infantile Refsum disease and hyperpipecolic acidaemia (Group A in Table 2), in rhizomelic chondrodysplasia punctata and Zellweger-like syndrome (Group B in Table 2), and in X-linked adrenoleukodystrophy, peroxisomal thiolase deficiency, bifunctional protein deficiency, acyl-CoA oxidase deficiency and the infantile type of hyperoxaluria type I. All of these disorders are characterized by severe clinical abnormalities and usually result in early death since there is currently no effective postnatal treatment.

Treatment of Zellweger syndrome has been tried by supplementation of the diet with precursors of ether-phospholipids (Wilson *et al.*, 1986) with only marginal clinical effects. Administration of clofibrate has failed to induce liver peroxisomes in Zellweger syndrome patients (Lazarow *et al.*, 1985; Björkhem *et al.*, 1985). The potential of postnatal treatment in Zellweger syndrome, Zellweger-like syndrome and thiolase deficiency is *a priori* limited by the multiple malformations and defects that originate in fetal life.

In X-linked adrenoleukodystrophy patients, plasma very-long-chain fatty acids can be normalized at least in part by a dietary regimen based on restriction of the intake of very-long-chain fatty acids and supplementation with trioleate (Rizzo *et al.*, 1986; Moser *et al.*, 1987a) or *trioleate* plus erucate (C26:1) (Rizzo, 1989) to inhibit endogenous chain elongation of long-chain fatty acids. However, it is still uncertain whether this approach results in any long-term positive effect on the clinical condition of the patients.

Techniques

A variety of techniques are available for the prenatal diagnosis of the peroxisomal disorders either in the first or the second trimester of gestation. A summary of these techniques is given in Table 3.

They include the direct analysis of chorionic villus samples by cytochemical staining for plasmalogens, which would be expected to be absent in disorders of peroxisome biogenesis and in rhizomelic chondrodysplasia punctata (Roels *et al.*, 1987) or by indirect immunofluorescence using anti-catalase antiserum in order to distinguish between cells containing peroxisomes (punctate fluorescence due to the fact that catalase is concentrated in peroxisomes) and those deficient in peroxisomes (diffuse fluorescence) (Wanders *et al.*, 1988d). Other procedures for prenatal diagnosis of disorders of peroxisome biogenesis are based on the demonstration of increased very-long-chain fatty acid levels or their impaired oxidation (Moser *et al.*, 1984; Solish *et al.*, 1985; Rocchiccioli *et al.*, 1987; Wanders *et al.*, 1987c), deficient plasmalogen synthesis (Hajra *et al.*, 1985; Schutgens *et al.*, 1985), lowered levels of particle-bound catalase (Wanders *et al.*, 1986), deficient phytanic acid oxidase activity (Poll-Thé *et al.*, 1985; Poulos *et al.*, 1986) or elevated levels of intermediates of bile acids biosynthesis (Stellaard *et al.*, 1988). For the prenatal diagnosis of X-linked adrenoleukodystrophy, 3-oxoacyl-CoA thiolase deficiency, bifunctional protein deficiency or acyl-CoA oxidase deficiency, respectively, re-

Table 3 Methods for prenatal diagnosis in peroxisomal disorders

Peroxisomal disorder	Material[a]	Parameter analysed[b]
Disorders of peroxisome biogenesis	CV	VLCFA, DHAPAT, peroxisomes, plasmalogens
	CVF, AFC	VLCFA, DHAPAT, plasmalogen biosynthesis, particle-bound catalase, phytanic acid oxidase, C26:0 β-oxidation
	AF	bile acids
Rhizomelic chondrodysplasia punctata	CV	DHAPAT, plasmalogens
	CVF, AFC	DHAPAT, plasmalogen biosynthesis, phytanic acid oxidase
Zellweger-like syndrome	CV	VLCFA, DHAPAT
	CVF, AFC, DHAPAT	VLCFA, DHAPAT, plasmalogen biosynthesis
Adrenoleukodystrophy (X-linked)	CV	VLCFA, DNA-RFLP
	CVF, AFC	VLCFA, DNA-RFLP, C26:0 β-oxidation
Thiolase deficiency	CV	VLCFA
	CVF, AFC	VLCFA, C26:0 β-oxidation, thiolase protein
	AF	bile acids
Acyl-CoA oxidase deficiency	CV	VLCFA
	CVF, AFC	VLCFA, C26:0 β-oxidation, acyl-CoA oxidase protein
Hyperoxaluria type I	fetal liver	Alanine glyoxylate aminotransferase

[a]CV = chorionic villus biopsy; CVF = cultured chorionic villus fibroblasts, AFC = cultured amniotic fluid cells; AF = amniotic fluid.
[b]DHAPAT = acyl-CoA:dihydroxyacetone phosphate acyltransferase; VLCFA = very-long-chain fatty acids; RFLP = restriction length fragment polymorphism

liance must be placed on very-long-chain fatty acid studies, since plasmalogen synthesis or peroxisome biogenesis is not affected. In X-linked adrenoleukodystrophy linkage analysis of DNA, using a highly polymorphic probe (ST14), has also been used (Boué *et al.*, 1985). Prenatal detection of rhizomelic chondrodysplasia punctata depends upon measurement of plasmalogen synthesis and phytanic oxidation activities as very-long-chain fatty acid metabolism is not affected in this condition.

Finally, in families in which a child has died in infancy because of primary hyperoxaluria type I in its acute neonatal form with rapid progression, prenatal diagnosis is indicated in subsequent pregnancies. However, this can only be done by measuring the alanine glyoxylate aminotransferase activity in fetal liver obtained by biopsy, as the enzyme activity is not expressed in fibroblasts or amniocytes (Wanders, 1988c). Prenatal diagnosis has been reported recently in two pregnancies at risk for this type of hyperoxaluria (Danpure *et al.*, 1988).

Heterozygote detection

Heterozygotes for X-linked ALD can be detected using very-long-chain fatty acid analysis (Moser *et al.*, 1981; Tönshoff *et al.*, 1982) or restriction fragment length polymorphism using the DNA probe ST14 (Aubourg *et al.*, 1987). In Zellweger syndrome and the other peroxisome deficiency disorders, no heterozygote detection is possible at present since the abnormalities observed in the patients are secondary effects resulting from a primary lesion the nature of which is not yet known. In the peroxisomal β-oxidation enzyme deficiencies it should in principle be possible to detect heterozygotes by measuring the activity of the enzyme involved.

Experience at the University Hospital, Amsterdam

Since 1983, we have monitored 70 pregnancies at risk for disorders of peroxisome biogenesis, three at risk for rhizomelic chondrodysplasia punctata, five at risk for X-linked adrenoleukodystrophy and two at risk for a defect in peroxisomal β-oxidation. We have identified 14 affected fetuses (Table 4). We had one false positive case in which the prenatal diagnosis of a defect in peroxisomal β-oxidation

Table 4 Prenatal diagnosis of peroxisomal disorders at the University Hospital, Amsterdam, from January 1983 to September 1988

At-risk pregnancy for:	*Type of sample*[a] *(number of analyses)*			*Outcome*	
	CV	*CVF*	*AFC*	*Affected*	*Not affected*
Zellweger syndrome	12	26	35	10	53
Infantile Refsum disease	3	1	4	2	3
Neonatal adrenoleukodystrophy	1	1	1	0	2
Rhizomelic chondrodysplasia punctata	2	2	2	0	3
Adrenoleukodystrophy (X-linked)	0	1	4	1	4
Defects of peroxisomal β-oxidation	0	2	0	1	1

[a]CV = chorionic villus biopsy material; CVF = cultured chorionic villus cells; AFC = amniotic fluid cells

could not be confirmed by postmortem examination of the fetus (see discussion). There have been no false negative tests. Only in 23 cases biochemical studies in the index patient were done before prenatal studies; in all other cases no material from the index patient was available for biochemical studies. Initially, we only utilized cultured amniotic fluid cells (Schutgens *et al.*, 1985); since 1986 we have also carried out direct analyses of chorionic villus cells and/or analyses of cultured chorionic villus fibroblasts (Table 4). The detailed results of the analyses in these three cell types are presented in Table 5.

Direct analysis of disorders of peroxisome biogenesis in chorionic villus cells was based on measurement of the dihydroxyacetone phosphate acyltransferase activity. In chorionic villus cells from 10 controls an enzyme activity of 6.3 ± 2.0 nmol (mg protein)$^{-1}$ (2h)$^{-1}$ was found. As a control enzyme we also measured the activity of

Table 5 Results of analyses of chorionic villus (CV), cultured chorionic villus fibroblasts (CVF) or cultured amniotic fluid cells (AFC) from pregnancies at risk for a disorder of peroxisome biogenesis

	CV		CVF		AFC	
	Not affected[a]	Affected[b]	Not affected[a]	Affected[b]	Not affected[a]	Affected[b]
DHAPAT activity (nmoles/2 h/mg protein)	6.7±2.3 (12)	0.08–0.46 (5)	6.8±2.5 (12)	0.04–0.35 (6)	6.4±2.3 (31)	0.04–0.51 (3)
Fatty acids ratio:						
C26:0/C22:0	n.m.	n.m.	0.12±0.05 (12)	0.30–1.36 (4)	0.10±0.06 (8)	0.53–0.94 (3)
C24:0/C22:0	n.m.	n.m.	1.42±0.45 (12)	2.37–3.48 (4)	1.50±0.32 (8)	2.76–3.23 (3)
De novo plasmalogen biosynthesis[c]						
pPE in PE	n.m.	n.m.	84.7±4.7 (20)	5.0–18.6 (5)	89.8±6.8 (21)	11.9–16.3 (3)
pPC in PC	n.m.	n.m.	10.8±3.9 (20)	0.6–1.2 (5)	19.8±8.8 (21)	1.2–2.6 (3)
$[^3H]/[^{14}C]$ ratio in						
alkenyl PE	n.m.	n.m.	1.2±0.5 (17)	21.0–105 (5)	1.0±0.3 (16)	n.m.
alkenyl PC	n.m.	n.m.	0.6±0.3 (17)	3.8–10.3 (5)	0.6±0.3 (16)	n.m.
Catalase latency[d]	n.m.	n.m.	+ (18)	– (6)	+ (32)	– (3)

Values are [a] means ±SD. [b] ranges; number of pregnancies in parentheses; n.m. = not measured.
[c] PE = total phosphatidylethanolamine; pPE = plasmalogen phosphatidylethanolamine; PC = total phosphatidyl choline; pPC = plasmalogen phosphatidylcholine; alkenyl PE = alkenyl chains of pPE; alkenyl PC = alkenyl chains of pPC.
[d] For catalase latency, + and – indicate that >65% and <5%, respectively, of total cellular catalase activity is particle-bound.

glutamate dehydrogenase. In five of the 16 pregnancies in which direct analysis of chorionic villus cells was performed a deficient dihydroxyacetone phosphate acyltransferase activity was found; two pregnancies were terminated immediately, whereas in the other three the results of the analyses of chorionic villus fibroblasts were awaited before termination. Subsequent studies, in fibroblasts from fetal skin obtained postmortem, confirmed the results of the prenatal diagnosis in all five cases. Direct analysis of chorionic villus cells in two pregnancies at risk for rhizomelic chondrodysplasia punctata indicated that dihydroxyacetone phosphate acyltransferase activities were normal. Healthy children were born subsequently.

Chorionic villus fibroblasts were studied in 28 pregnancies at risk for a disorder of peroxisome biogenesis. In most cases at least two different assays were performed in order to have a valuable cross-check. The results obtained from these studies both of affected fetuses and unaffected fetuses, respectively, are given in Table 5. Data obtained earlier, in studies with cultured skin fibroblasts from controls and from patients with a disorder of peroxisome biogenesis (Schutgens *et al.*, 1985, 1987b), were used for evaluation of the results. In seven of the 28 at-risk pregnancies analysed using chorionic villus fibroblasts, including three pregnancies in which a deficient dihydroxyacetone phosphate acyltransferase activity was found earlier in direct chorionic villus analysis, abnormal values were found, subsequently resulting in termination of the pregnancies in all cases. Confirmation of the diagnosis was obtained in six cases; in one case no fetal material became available for biochemical studies.

Chorionic villus fibroblasts were also analysed in two pregnancies at risk for rhizomelic chondrodysplasia punctata by measuring both dihydroxyacetone phosphate acyltransferase activity and *de novo* plasmalogen biosynthesis. No indication for rhizomelic chondrodysplasia punctata was found in the fetal cells.

One pregnancy at risk for X-linked adrenoleukodystrophy was evaluated by measuring very-long-chain fatty acid levels in chorionic villus fibroblasts; normal values were found in this case. We also analysed peroxisomal parameters in chorionic villus fibroblasts from one pregnancy in which earlier studies in fibroblasts from the index patients had indicated that the pregnancy was at risk for a defect in peroxisomal β-oxidation. Normal values were found and a healthy child born. However, in another pregnancy in which the index patient had died and the diagnosis of Zellweger syndrome had been based on clinical parameters only, chorionic villus fibroblast analysis revealed increased very-long-chain fatty acid levels (C26:0/C22:0 ratio = 0.51), but normal *de novo* plasmalogen biosynthesis excluding Zellweger syndrome but indicating a defect in peroxisomal β-oxidation. Subsequent biochemical analysis of fetal skin fibroblasts confirmed this diagnosis. Our findings stress the importance of biochemical studies on material from index patients.

Amniotic fluid cells were analysed in 40 pregnancies at risk for a disorder of peroxisome biogenesis; in two of them normal peroxisomal parameters had been found earlier in chorionic villus fibroblast analyses; in one an affected fetus had already been identified by chorionic villus fibroblast studies. The results of the amniotic fluid cell studies are presented in Table 5. In four cases, including the one in which chorionic villus fibroblast studies had already revealed abnormalities, values were obtained indicative of a disorder of peroxisome biogenesis. In all four cases the diagnosis was confirmed subsequently in postmorten examination of the fetus.

Plasmalogen synthesis was measured in amniotic fluid cells from two pregnancies at risk for rhizomelic chondrodysplasia punctata; normal values were found. Finally, the very-long-chain fatty acid levels were measured in amniotic fluid cells in four pregnancies at risk for X-linked adrenoleukodystrophy in which fetal sexing had indicated a male fetus. Increased values were found in one case (C26:0/C22:0 ratio = 0.94) indicating the fetus was affected. No material became available for confirmation studies in this positive case.

PERINATAL DIAGNOSIS

Several recent reviews have summarized the clinical characteristics and a variety of biochemical assays that can be used for the postnatal and perinatal diagnosis of the different peroxisomal disorders (see Kelly, 1983; Schutgens *et al.*, 1986, 1987; Wilson *et al.*, 1986; Lazarow and Moser, 1989). In classic Zellweger syndrome, Zellweger-like syndrome and peroxisomal thiolase deficiency, clinical characteristics of central diagnostic importance at birth are the typical face (high forehead, upslanting palpebral fissures, hypoplastic supraorbital ridges, epicanthal folds), severe weakness and hypotonia. Infants with these disorders rarely survive for more than a few months due to severe hypotonia, feeding difficulty, seizures and liver involvement, often combined with cardiac defects. No biochemical studies in cord blood from Zellweger patients have been reported so far, but assays of blood samples from patients taken after a few days of life revealed increased concentrations of very-long-chain fatty acids, bile acid intermediates, and a deficiency of plasmalogens. However, blood phytanic acid levels in patients are initially normal in very early life presumably because phytanic acid originates from dietary sources. Depending upon the diet, elevated blood phytanic acid levels can be found in patients at 2 to 6 months of life. Increased levels of plasma and urinary pipecolic acid may not be demonstrable in infants with Zellweger syndrome less than 4 weeks old (for review see Lazarow and Moser, 1989). Absence or deficiency of liver peroxisomes can be demonstrated directly in patients with Zellweger syndrome by liver biopsy, provided catalase cytochemistry and appropriate controls are included (Roels *et al.*, 1987). The selection of a test for diagnosis of disorders of peroxisome biogenesis is influenced by the availability of laboratory resources. In our experience assay of dihydroxyacetone phosphate acyltransferase activity in platelets and of plasma very-long-chain fatty acids represent the least invasive and most informative procedures as these assays will also differentiate between disorders of peroxisome biogenesis and disorders such as Zellweger-like syndrome, peroxisomal thiolase deficiency and acyl-CoA oxidase deficiency. More detailed analyses can subsequently be performed in cultured skin fibroblasts.

In X-linked adrenoleukodystrophy, increased very-long-chain fatty acids levels can probably already be found in very early life. However, no data for cord blood are available in the literature. Diagnosis can also be based on the finding of an impairment of *in vitro* C26:O β-oxidation in leukocytes of patients.

Patients suffering from the acute neonatal form of hyperoxaluria type I can be diagnosed in early life on the basis of grossly increased urinary excretion of oxalate and glycollate (Williams and Smith, 1983).

DISCUSSION

Substantial experience has been gained in recent years in the prenatal diagnosis of peroxisomal disorders. Most information is available for the disorders of peroxisome biogenesis, Zellweger syndrome, neonatal adrenoleukodystrophy, infantile Refsum disease and hyperpipecolic acidaemia. Lazarow and Moser (1989) recently reported that at the Kennedy Institute, Baltimore, USA, 72 pregnancies at risk for this group of peroxisomal disorders were monitored, identifying 13 affected fetuses. They also monitored four pregnancies at risk for rhizomelic chondrodysplasia punctata and identified one affected fetus (Hoefler *et al.*, 1988). No false negative cases were found. Moser and coworkers also monitored a substantial number of pregnancies at risk for X-linked adrenoleukodystrophy.

In this paper we report the outcome of prenatal diagnosis in 80 pregnancies: 70 pregnancies at risk for a disorder of peroxisome biogenesis, three for rhizomelic chondrodysplasia punctata, five for X-linked adrenoleukodystrophy and two for a defect in peroxisomal β-oxidation. Fourteen affected fetuses were identified. No false negative cases were found. However, one false positive diagnosis was obtained. In this case the clinical diagnosis in the index patient had been Zellweger syndrome. Unfortunately no biochemical studies of the index patient had been done before monitoring the at-risk pregnancy as no material was available. Analysis of the limited amount of cultured amniotic fluid cells available in this pregnancy revealed a normal dihydroxyacetone phosphate acyltransferase activity and normal catalase latency, excluding Zellweger syndrome. However, we judged the very-long-chain fatty acid profile as pathological with C26:0/C22:0 and C24:0/C22:0 fatty acids ratios of 0.23 and 2.15, respectively. As we could not fully exclude pseudo-Zellweger syndrome or pseudo-neonatal adrenoleukodystrophy the pregnancy was terminated. No confirmation of an affected fetus could be obtained in analyses of fetal fibroblasts since very-long-chain fatty acid levels and C26:0 β-oxidation were found to be normal in these cells.

Both Lazarow and Moser (1989) and we have found that direct analysis of very-long-chain fatty acids in samples of chorionic villi fails to provide sufficiently reliable differentiation and can result in false positive cases. We have therefore abandoned this procedure. However, recent results by Rocchiccioli *et al.* (1987) suggest that this procedure can be feasible. In our experience, measurement of the dihydroxyacetone phosphate acyltransferase activity is a far better discriminating parameter in analysing chorionic villus samples both in disorders of peroxisome biogenesis and in rhizomelic chondrodysplasia punctata. We always recommend that one proceeds to analyse chorionic villus fibroblasts in cases in which a normal dihydroxyacetone phosphate acyltransferase activity is found in the direct analysis of chorionic villus samples; the finding of a deficient dihydroxyacetone phosphate acyltransferase activity (but normal activity of glutamate dehydrogenase) is considered to be sufficient for the prenatal diagnosis of an affected fetus. Nevertheless, in these cases also our policy at present is to await the results of chorionic villus fibroblast studies before deciding whether or not to advise termination of the pregnancy. When chorionic villus fibroblast samples are used, the possibility of a false negative result due to maternal overgrowth must be kept in mind (Carey *et al.*, 1986).

We conclude that ample experience has been gained in recent years in the prenatal and perinatal diagnosis of peroxisomal disorders and that reliable techniques are now available for genetic counselling.

ACKNOWLEDGEMENTS

We thank many colleagues for sending us material from their patients. Some of the chorionic villus biopsy material from controls was provided by Dr W. Kleijer, Rotterdam.

The research reported in this paper was supported by a grant from the Princess Beatrix Fund (The Hague, The Netherlands). The authors gratefully acknowledge the expert help of Corrie van den Berg and Paula Zwaal in preparation of the manuscript.

REFERENCES

Appelkvist, E. L. and Dallner, G. Dolichol metabolism and peroxisomes. In: Fahimi, H. D. and Sies, H. (Eds.), *Peroxisomes in Biology and Medicine*, Springer-Verlag, Berlin, 1987, pp. 53–66
Aubourg, P. R., Sack, G. H., Meyers, D. A., Lease, J. J. and Moser, H. W. Linkage of adrenoleukodystrophy to a polymorphic DNA probe. *Ann. Neurol.* 21 (1987) 349–352
Barth, P. G., Schutgens, R. B. H., Bakkeren, J. A. J. M., Dingemans, K. P., Heymans, H. S. A., Douwes, A. C. and van der Kley-van Moorsel, J. J. A milder variant of Zellweger syndrome. *Eur. J. Pediatr.* 144 (1985) 338–342
Beard. M. E., Baker, R., Conomos, P., Pugatch, D. and Holzman, E. Oxidation of oxalate and polyamines by rat liver peroxisomes. *J. Histochem. Cytochem.* 33 (1985) 460–464
Björkhem, I., Blomstrand, S., Glaumann, H. and Strandvik, B. Unsuccessful attempts to induce peroxisomes in two cases of Zellweger disease by treatment with clofibrate. *Pediatr. Res.* 19 (1985) 590–593
Bleeker-Wagemakers, E. M., Oorthuys, J. W. E., Wanders, R. J. A. and Schutgens, R. B. H. Long term survival of a patient with the cerebro-hepato-renal (Zellweger) syndrome. *Clin. Genet.* 29 (1986) 160–164
Boué, J., Oberle, I., Heilig, R., Mandel, J. L., Moser, H. W., Larsen, J. W. Jr., Dumez, Y. and Boué, A. First trimester prenatal diagnosis of adrenoleukodystrophy by determination of very long chain fatty acid levels and by linkage analysis to a DNA probe. *Hum. Genet.* 69 (1985) 272–274
Brul, S., Westerveld, A., Strijland, A., Wanders, R. J. A., Schram, A. W., Heymans, H. S. A., Schutgens, R. B. H., van den Bosch, H. and Tager, J. M. Genetic heterogeneity in the cerebro-hepato-renal (Zellweger) syndrome and other inherited disorders with a generalized impairment of peroxisomal functions: a study using complementation analysis. *J. Clin. Invest.* 81 (1988) 1710–1715
Carey, W. F., Robertson, E. F., van Crugten, C., Poulos, A. and Nelson, P. N. Prenatal diagnosis of Zellweger's syndrome by chorionic villus sampling – and a caveat. *Prenat. Diagn.* 6 (1986) 227–229

Danpure, C. J., and Jennings, P. R. Peroxisomal alanine: glyoxylate aminotransferase deficiency in primary hyperoxaluria type I. *FEBS Lett.*, 201 (1986) 20–24

Danpure, C. J., Cooper, P. J., Jennings, P. R., Wise P. J., Penketh, R. J. and Rodeck, C. H. Enzymatic prenatal diagnosis of primary hyperoxaluria type 1: successes and potential problems. *26th SSIEM Annual Symposium*, 1988, Abstract 012

de Duve, C. and Baudhuin, P. Peroxisomes (microbodies and related particles). *Physiol. Rev.*, 46 (1966) 323–357

Diczfalusy, U., Alexson, S. E. H. and Pedersen, J. I. Chain shortening of prostaglandin PGF$_{2\alpha}$. *Biochem. Biophys. Res. Commun.* 144 (1987) 1206–1213

Goldfischer, S., Moore, C. L., Johnson, A. B., Spiro, A. J., Valsamis, M. P., Wisniewski, H. K., Ritch, R. H., Norton, W. T., Rapin, I. and Gartner, L. M. Peroxisomal and mitochondrial defects in the cerebro-hepato-renal syndrome, *Science* 182 (1973) 62–64

Goldfischer, S. and Reddy, J. K. Peroxisomes (microbodies) in cell pathology. *Int. Rev. Exp. Pathol.* 26 (1984) 45–84

Goldfischer, S., Collins, J., Rapin, I., Coltoff-Schiller, B., Chang, C. H., Nigro, M., Black, V. H., Javitt, N. B., Moser, H. W. and Lazarow, P. B. Peroxisomal defects in neonatal-onset and X-linked adrenoleukodystrophies. *Science* 227 (1985) 69–71

Goldfischer, S., Collins, J., Rapin, I., Neumann, P., Neglia, W., Spiro, A. J., Ishii, T., Roels, F., Vamecq, J. and van Hoof, F. Pseudo-Zellweger syndrome: deficiencies in several peroxisomal oxidative activities. *J. Pediatr.* 108 (1986) 25–32

Hajra, A. K. Biosynthesis of O-alkylglycerol ether lipids. In: Mangold, J. K. and Paltauf, F. (Eds.), *Ether Lipids: Biochemical and biomedical aspects*, Academic Press, Orlando, 1984, 85–106

Hajra, A. K., Datta, N. S., Jackson, L. B., Moser, A. B., Moser, H. W., Larsen, J. W. Jr. and Powers, J. Prenatal diagnosis of Zellweger cerebro-hepato-renal syndrome. *N. Engl. J. Med.* 312 (1985) 445–446

Heymans, H. S. A., Oorthuys, J. W. E., Nelck, G., Wanders, R. J. A., Dingemans, K. P. and Schutgens, R. B. H. Peroxisomal abnormalities in rhizomelic chondrodysplasia punctata. *J. Inher. Metab. Dis.* 9 Suppl. 2 (1986) 329–331

Hiltunen, J. K., Karki, T., Hassinen, I. E. and Osmundsen, H. β-oxidation of polyunsaturated fatty acids by rat liver peroxisomes. A role for 2,4-dienoyl-Coenzyme A reductase in peroxisomal β-oxidation. *J. Biol. Chem.* 261 (1986) 16484–16493

Hoefler, G., Hoefler, S., Watkins, P. A., Chen, W. W., Moser, A., Baldwin, V., McGillivary, B., Charrow, J., Friedman, J. M., Rutledge, L., Hashimoto, T. and Moser, H. W. Biochemical abnormalities in rhizomelic chondrodysplasia punctata. *J. Pediatr.* 112 (1988) 726–733

Höltta, E. Oxidation of spermine and spermidine in rat liver: purification and properties of polyamine oxidase. *Biochemistry* 16 (1977) 91–100

Hovik, R. and Osmundsen, H. Peroxisomal β-oxidation of long-chain fatty acids possessing different extents of unsaturation. *Biochem. J.* 247 (1987) 531–535

Kelley, R. I. The cerebro-hepato-renal syndrome of Zellweger. Morphological and metabolic aspect. *Am. J. Med. Genet.* 16 (1983) 502–517

Kolvraa, S. and Gregersen, N. *In vitro* studies on the oxidation of medium-chain dicarboxylic acids in rat liver. *Biochim. Biophys. Acta* 876 (1986) 515–525

Lazarow, P. B. Biogenesis of peroxisomes: Implications for Zellweger syndrome. In Vogel, F., Sperling, K. (Eds.), *Human Genetics*, Springer Verlag, Berlin, 1987, 369–376

Lazarow, P. B. and de Duve, C. A fatty acyl-CoA oxidizing system in rat liver peroxisomes: enhancement by clofibrate, a hypolipidemic drug. *Proc. Natl. Acad. Sci. USA*, 73 (1976) 2043–2046

Lazarow, P. B. and Moser, H. W. Disorders of Peroxisome biogenesis. In Scriver, C. R., Beaudet, A. L., Sly, W. S., Valle, D. (Eds.), *The Metabolic Basis of Inherited Disease*, 6th edn., McGraw-Hill, New York, 1989, in press

Lazarow, P. B., Black, V., Shio, H., Fujiki, Y., Hajra, A. K., Datta, N. S., Bangaru, B. S. and Dancis, J. Zellweger syndrome: biochemical and morphological studies on two patients treated with clofibrate. *Pediatr. Res.* 19 (1985) 1356–1364

Mihalik, S. J. and Rhead, W. J. L-pipecolic acid catabolism in mammals. *Trans. Am. Soc. Neurochem.* 19 (1988) 72 (Abstract)

Moser, H. W., Moser, A. B., Frayer, K. K., Chen, W., Schulman, J. D., O'Neill, B. P. and Kishimoto, Y. Adrenoleukodystrophy: Increased plasma content of saturated very long chain fatty acids. *Neurology* 31 (1981) 1241–1249

Moser, A. E., Singh, I., Brown, F. R. III, Solish, G. I., Kelley, R. I., Benke, P. J. and Moser, H. W. The cerebro-hepato-renal (Zellweger) syndrome: increased levels and impaired degradation of very long fatty acids and prenatal diagnosis. *N. Engl. J. Med.* 310 (1984) 1141-1146

Moser, H. W., Naidu, S., Kumar, A. J. and Rosenbaum, A. E. The adrenoleukodystrophies. *Crit. Rev. Neurobiol.*, 5 (1987b) 29–88

Moser, A. E., Borel, J., Odone, A., Naidu, S., Cornblath, D., Sanders, D. B. and Moser, H. W. A new dietary therapy for adrenoleukodystrophy: biochemical and preliminary clinical results in 36 patients. *Ann. Neurol.* 21 (1987a) 240–249

Noguchi, T. Amino acid metabolism in animal peroxisomes. In Fahimi, H. D. and Sies, H. (Eds.), *Peroxisomes in Biology and Medicine*, Springer-Verlag, Berlin, 1987, 234–243

Novikoff, A. B., Novikoff, P. M., Davis, C. and Quintana, N. Studies on microperoxisomes. V. Are microperoxisomes ubiquitous in mammalian cells? *J. Histochem. Cytochem.* 21 (1973) 737–755

Paturneau-Jouas, E., Taillard, A., Gansmuller, J. Mikol, J. Aigrot, M. S. and Sereni, C. Clinical, biochemical and pathological aspects of a 'Zellweger-like' peroxisomal disorder. In Salvayre, R. (Ed.), *Lipid Storage Disorders*, Nato-Inserm, Toulouse (1987) 133–134 (Abstract)

Pedersen, J. J., Kase, B. F., Prydz, K. and Björkhem, I. Liver peroxisomes and bile acid formation. In Fahimi, H. D. and Sies, H. (Eds.), *Peroxisomes in Biology and Medicine*, Springer-Verlag, Berlin, 1987, 67–77

Poll-Thé, B. T., Poulos, A., Sharp, P., Boué, J., Ogier, H., Odievre, M. and Saudubray, J. M. Antenatal diagnosis of infantile Refsum's disease. *Clin. Genet.*, 27 (1985) 524–526

Poll-Thé, B. T., Skjeldal, O. H., Stokke, O., Poulos, A., Demaugre, F. and Saudubray, J. M. Phytanic acid alpha-oxidation and complementation analysis of classical Refsum and peroxisomal disorders. *Hum. Genet.* 81 (1989) 175–181

Poll-Thé, B. T., Roels, F., Ogier, H., Scotto, J., Vamecq, J., Schutgens, R. B. H., van Roermund, C. W. T., van Wijland, M. J. A., Schram, A. W., Tager, J. M. and Saudubray, J. M. A new peroxisomal disorder with enlarged peroxisomes and a specific deficiency of acyl-CoA oxidase (pseudo neonatal adrenoleukodystrophy). *Am. J. Hum. Genet.* 42 (1988) 422–434

Poulos, A., Sharp, P. and Whiting, M. Infantile Refsum's disease (phytanic acid storage disease): a variant of Zellweger's syndrome? *Clin. Genet.* 25 (1984) 579–586

Poulos, A., van Crugten, C., Sharp, P., Carey, W. F., Robertson, E., Becroft, B. M. D., Saudubray, J. M., Poll-Thé, B. T., Christensen, E. and Brandt, N. Prenatal diagnosis of Zellweger syndrome and related disorders: impaired degradation of phytanic acid. *Eur. J. Pediatr.* 145 (1986) 507–510

Rizzo, W. B. Personal communication

Rizzo, W. B., Watkins, P. A., Phillips, M. W., Cranin, D., Campbell, B. and Avigan, J. Adrenoleukodystrophy: Oleic acid lowers fibroblast saturated C22–C26 fatty acids. *Neurology* 26 (1986) 357–361

Rocchiccioli, F., Aubourg, P. and Choiset, A. Immediate prenatal diagnosis of Zellweger syndrome by direct measurement of very long chain fatty acids in chorionic villus cells. *Prenat. Diagn.* 7 (1987) 349–354

Roels, F., Verdonck, V., Pauwels, M., Lissens, W. and Liebaers, I. Visualization of peroxisomes and plasmalogens in first trimester chorionic villus. *J. Inher. Metab. Dis.* 10 Suppl. 2 (1987) 349–354

Roscher, A., Hoefler, S., Hoefler, G., Paschke, E. and Paltauf, F. Neonatal adrenoleuko-dystrophy and cerebro-hepato-renal syndrome: genetic complementation analysis of impaired peroxisomal plasmalogen biosynthesis. In *Inborn Errors of Cellular Organelles*, 24th SSIEM Symposium, Amersfoort, 1986, 03 (Abstract)

Schepers, L., Casteels, M., Vamecq, J., Parmentier, G., van Veldhoven, P. P. and Manna-erts, G. P. β-Oxidation of the carboxyl side chain of prostaglandin E_2 in rat liver peroxisomes and mitochondria. *J. Biol. Chem.* 263 (1988) 2724–2731

Schrakamp, G., Schalkwijk, C. G., Schutgens, R. B. H., Wanders, R. J. A., Tager, J. M. and van den Bosch, H. Plasmalogen biosynthesis in peroxisomal disorders. *J. Lipid Res.* 29 (1988) 325–334

Schram, A. W., Strijland, A., Hashimoto, T., Wanders, R. J. A., Schutgens, R. B. H., van den Bosch, H. and Tager, J. M. Biosynthesis and maturation of peroxisomal β-oxidation enzymes in fibroblasts in relation to the Zellweger syndrome and infantile Refsum disease. *Proc. Natl. Acad. Sci. USA* 83 (1986) 6156–6158

Schram, A. W., Goldfischer, S., van Roermund, C. W. T., Brouwer-Kelder, E. M., Collins, J., Hashimoto, T., Heymans, H. S. A., van den Bosch, H., Schutgens, R. B. H., Tager, J. M. and Wanders, R. J. A. Human peroxisomal 3-oxoacyl-coenzyme A thiolase deficiency. *Proc. Natl. Acad. Sci. USA* 84 (1987) 2494–2496

Schutgens, R. B. H., Schrakamp, G., Wanders, R. J. A., Heymans, H. S. A., Moser, H. W., Moser, A. E., Tager, J. M., van den Bosch, H. and Aubourg, P. The cerebro-hepato-renal (Zellweger) syndrome: prenatal detection based on impaired biosynthesis of plasmalogens. *Prenat. Diagn.* 5 (1985) 337–344

Schutgens, R. B. H., Heymans, H. S. A., Wanders, R. J. A., van den Bosch, H. and Tager, J. M. Peroxisomal disorders: A newly recognised group of genetic diseases. *Eur. J. Pediatr.* 144 (1986a) 430–440

Schutgens, R. B. H., Romeyn, G-J., Ofman, R., van den Bosch, H., Tager, J. M. and Wanders, R. J. A. Acyl-CoA: dihydroxyacetone phosphate acyltransferase in human skin fibroblasts: study of the properties using a new assay method. *Biochim. Biophys. Acta* 879 (1986b) 286–291

Schutgens, R. B. H., Wanders, R. J. A., Heymans, H. S. A., Schram, A. W., Tager, J. M., Schrakamp, G. and van den Bosch, H. Zellweger syndrome: biochemical procedures in diagnosis, prevention and treatment. *J. Inher. Metab. Dis.* 10 Suppl. 1 (1987) 33–45

Schutgens, R. B. H., Heymans, H. S. A., Wanders, R. J. A., Oorthuys, J. W. E., Tager, J. M., Schrakamp, G., van den Bosch, H. and Beemer, F. A. Multiple peroxisomal enzyme deficiencies in rhizomelic chondrodysplasia punctata: comparison with Zellweger syndrome, Conradi–Hunermann syndrome and the X-linked dominant type of chondrodysplasia punctata. In Moss, D. W., Schmidt, E., Schmidt, F. W. (Eds.) *Advances in Clinical Enzymology*, Karger, Basel, 6 1988, 57–65

Singh, I., Moser, A. B., Goldfischer, S. and Moser, H. W. Lignoceric acid is oxidized in the peroxisome: implications for the Zellweger cerebro-hepato-renal syndrome and adrenoleukodystrophy. *Proc. Natl. Acad. Sci. USA* 81 (1984) 4203–4207

Singh, H., Derwas, N. and Poulos, A. Very long chain fatty acid β-oxidation by rat liver mitochondria and peroxisomes. *Arch. Biochem. Biophys.* 259 (1987) 382–390

Skjeldal, O. H., Stokke, O., Refsum, S., Norseth, J. and Petit, H. Clinical and biochemical heterogeneity in conditions with phytanic acid accumulation. *J. Neurol. Sci.* 77 (1987) 87–96

Solish, G. I., Moser, H. W., Ringer, L. D., Moser, A. E., Tiffany, C. and Schutta, E. The prenatal diagnosis of the cerebro-hepato-renal syndrome of Zellweger. *Prenat. Diagn.* 5 (1985) 27–34

Spranger, J. W., Opitz, J. M. and Bidder, U. Heterogeneity of chondrodysplasia punctata. *Hum. Genet.* 11 (1971) 190–212

Stellaard, F., Langelaar, S. A., Kok, R. M., Kleijer, W. J., Schutgens, R. B. H. and Jakobs, C. Prenatal diagnosis of Zellweger syndrome by determination of trihydroxycoprostanoic acid in amniotic fluid. *26th SSIEM Annual Symposium*, Glasgow, P129 (Abstr.)

Suzuki, Y., Orii, T., Takiguchi, M., Mori, M., Hijikata, M. and Hashimoto, T. Biosynthesis of membrane polypeptides of rat liver peroxisomes. *J. Biochem.* 101 (1987) 491–496

Suzuki, Y., Shimozawa, N., Orii, T., Igarashi, N., Kono, N., Matsui, A., Inoue, Y., Yokata, S. and Hashimoto, T. Zellweger-like syndrome with detectable hepatic peroxisomes: A variant form of peroxisomal disorder. *J. Pediatr.* 113 (1988) 841–845

Thompson, S. L., Burrow, R., Laub, R. J. and Krisans, S. K. Cholesterol synthesis in rat liver peroxisomes. *J. Biol. Chem.* 262 (1987) 17420–17425

Tönshoff, B., Lehnert, W. and Ropers, H. H. Adrenoleukodystrophy: diagnosis and carrier detection by determination of very long chain fatty acids in cultured fibroblasts. *Clin. Genet.* 22 (1982) 25–29

Wanders, R. J. A., Kos, M., Roest, B., Meijer, A. J., Schrakamp, G., Heymans, H. S. A., Tegelaers, W. H. H., van den Bosch, H., Schutgens, R. B. H. and Tager, J. M. Activity of peroxisomal enzymes and intracellular distribution of catalase in Zellweger syndrome. *Biochem. Biophys. Res. Commun.* 123 (1984) 1054–1061

Wanders, R. J. A., Schrakamp, G., van den Bosch, H., Tager, J. M. and Schutgens, R. B. H. A prenatal test for the cerebro-hepato-renal (Zellweger) syndrome by demonstration of the absence of catalase-containing particles (peroxisomes) in cultured amniotic fluid cells. *Eur. J. Pediatr.* 145 (1986) 136–138

Wanders, R. J. A., van Roermund, C. W. T., van Wijland, M. J. A., Heikoop, J., Schutgens, R. B. H., Schram, A. W., van den Bosch, H., Poll-Thé, B. T., Saudubray, J. M., Moser,

H. W. and Moser, A. B. Peroxisomal very long chain fatty acid β-oxidation in human skin fibroblasts: activity in Zellweger syndrome and other peroxisomal disorders. *Clin. Chim. Acta* 166 (1987a) 255–263

Wanders, R. J. A., van Roermund, C. W. T., Westra, R., Schutgens, R. B. H., van de Ende, M. A., Tager, J. M., Monnens, L. A. H., Baadenhuysen, H., Govaerts, L., Przyrembel, H., Wolff, E. D., Blom, W., Huymans, J. G. M. and Laerhoven, F. G. M. Alanine glyoxylate aminotransferase and the urinary excretion of oxalate and glycollate in hyperoxaluria type I and the Zellweger syndrome. *Clin. Chim. Acta* 165 (1987b) 311–319

Wanders, R. J. A., van Wijland, M. J. A., van Roermund, C. W. T., Schutgens, R. B. H., van den Bosch, H., Tager, J. M., Nijenhuis, A. and Tromp, A. Prenatal diagnosis of Zellweger syndrome by measurement of very long chain fatty acid ($C26:0$) β-oxidation in cultured chorionic villus fibroblasts: implications for early diagnosis of other peroxisomal disorders. *Clin. Chim. Acta* 165 (1987c) 303–310

Wanders, R. J. A., van Roermund, C. W. T., van Wijland, M. J. A., Schutgens, R. B. H., van den Bosch. H. and Tager, J. M. Direct demonstration that the deficient oxidation of very long chain fatty acids in X-linked adrenoleukodystrophy is due to an impaired ability of peroxisomes to activate very long chain fatty acids. *Biochem. Biophys. Res. Commun.* 153 (1988a) 618–624

Wanders, R. J. A., Romeyn, G. J., van Roermund, C. W. T., Schutgens, R. B. H., van den Bosch, H. and Tager, J. M. Identification of L-pipecolic oxidase in human liver and its deficiency in the Zellweger syndrome. *Biochem. Biophys. Res. Commun.* 154 (1988b) 33–38

Wanders, R. J. A., van Roermund, C. W. T., Jurriaans, S. Schutgens, R. B. H., Tager, J. M., van den Bosch, H., Wolff, E. D., Przyrembel, H., Berger, H., Schaaphok, F. G., Reitsman, W. and van Luyk, W. H. J. Diversity in residual alanine glyoxylate aminotransferase activity in hyperoxaluria type I: Correlation with pyridoxine responsiveness. *J. Inher. Metab. Dis.* 11 Suppl. 2 (1988c) 208–211

Wanders, R. J. A., Wiemer, E. A. C., Brul, S., Schutgens, R. B. H., van den Bosch, H. and Tager, J. M. Prenatal diagnosis of Zellweger syndrome via a method directly visualizing peroxisomes in chorionic villus fibroblasts and amniocytes. *26th SSIEM Annual Symposium*, 1988d, Abstract, p.163

Wanders, R. J. A., Heymans, H. S. A., Schutgens, R. B. H., Barth, P. G., van den Bosch, H. and Tager, J. M. Peroxisomal disorders in neurology. *J. Neurol. Sci.* 88 (1988e) 1–39

Watkins, P. A., Chen, W. W., Harris, C. J., Hoefler, G., Hoefler, S., Blake, Jr., D. S., Balfe, A., Kelley, R. I., Moser, A. B., Beard, M. E. and Moser, H. W. Peroxisomal bifunctional enzyme deficiency. *J. Clin. Invest.* 83 (1989) 771–777

Williams, H. E. and Smith, L. H. Primary hyperoxaluria. In Stanbury, J. B., Wijngaarden, J. B., Fredrickson, D. S., Goldstein, J. L. and Brown, M. S. (Eds.), *The Metabolic Basis of Inherited Disease*, 5th edn. McGraw-Hill, New York, 1983, 204-228

Wilson, G. N., Holmes, R. G., Custer, J., Lipkowitz, J. L., Stover, J., Datta, N. and Hajra, A. Zellweger syndrome: Diagnostic assays, syndrome delineation and potential therapy. *Am. J. Med. Genet.* 24 (1986) 69–82

Yamada, J., Itoh, S., Horie, S., Watanabe, T. and Suga, T. Chain-shortening of a xenobiotic acyl compound by the peroxisomal β-oxidation system in rat liver. *Biochem. Pharmacol.* 35 (1986) 4363–4368

Note added in proof: Recently we also have identified a fetus affected by rhizomelic chondrodysplasia punctata in an at-risk pregnancy. In chorionic villus fibroblasts we found a deficient DHAPAT activity and an impaired *de novo* plasmalogen biosynthesis.

J. Inher. Metab. Dis. 12 Suppl. 1 (1989) 135–173

Prenatal Diagnosis and Prevention of Inherited Abnormalities of Collagen

F. M. Pope, S. C. M. Daw, P. Narcisi, A. R. Richards and
A. C. Nicholls
*Dermatology Research Group, Clinical Research Centre and Northwick Park
Hospital, Watford Road, Harrow, Middlesex, UK*

Summary: There is now strong evidence for the implication of collagen $\alpha1(I)$, $\alpha2(I)$ and $\alpha1(III)$ mutations in many forms of osteogenesis imperfecta and inherited arterial aneurysms (Ehlers Danlos syndrome type IV). A sizeable proportion of these disorders have detectable abnormalities by conventional protein chemistry, immunofluorescence, or more sophisticated DNA analysis. Everyone of them with specific defects or with linkage to appropriate gene markers is therefore amenable to prevention using conventional prenatal diagnosis by chorionic villus biopsy (with fibroblast culture), fetoscopic biopsy (with fibroblast culture), ultrasound diagnosis of the severely deformed fetus, or gene linkage studies by chorionic villus biopsy or amniocentesis.

Already many collagen $\alpha1(I)$, $\alpha2(I)$ and $\alpha1(III)$ mutations have been characterized including point mutations, small and large deletions and regulatory mutations. Many others are likely to be rapidly studied by exploiting recent advances in DNA technology, and other strong candidate genes include collagen II (some chondrodystrophies), collagen VI (certain arterial and cardiovascular diseases) and collagen VII (dystrophic epidermolysis bullosa). Other important common diseases are likely to include osteoporosis, osteoarthritis and cerebral aneurysms.

A detailed review is provided of collagen interstitial genes and proteins, together with a description of the various forms of osteogenesis imperfecta and Ehlers Danlos syndrome in which either collagen $\alpha1(I)$, $\alpha2(I)$ or $\alpha1(III)$ mutations have been identified. Appropriate restriction length polymorphisms (RFLPs) useful in identifying carriers of these mutant genes are also described.

One of the most practical and important advances in human genetic disease has been the development of reliable methods of genetic disease prevention. These include population screening, retrospective and family counselling and antenatal diagnosis. It is with this latter element that we are concerned in this Symposium. Current methods of antenatal diagnosis for human genetic diseases include first and second trimester fetal sampling by methods including chorionic villus sampling (first trimester), amniocentesis, direct inspection of the fetus, fetal blood sampling and fetal skin biopsy. Some or all of these methods are certainly directly applicable

135

Journal of Inherited Metabolic Disease. ISSN 0141–8955. Copyright © SSIEM and Kluwer Academic Publishers, PO Box 55, Lancaster, UK.

to the prevention of inherited defects of connective tissue. So far very little has been attempted for this important group of diseases. Here we review the background information for collagen genes and proteins, indicating those with identified abnormalities. Children with some specific defects could already be prenatally diagnosed and other closely related disorders with similar mechanisms are also candidates for this approach. Techniques likely to be utilized include the ultrasound diagnosis of severely crippled fetuses, the immunofluorescent detection of abnormal collagen protein, the detailed characterization of collagen proteins produced from cultured fetal or chorionic fibroblasts and the detection of faulty mutated collagen gene sequences using standard methods of DNA analysis and amplification, both for direct point mutations, gene deletions and insertions and also by indirect analysis with the candidate gene using standard RFLP analysis.

COLLAGEN GENES AND PROTEINS

Collagen proteins are a family of structural elements serving a mechanical and scaffolding role in a variety of connective tissues. These include arteries, bone, cartilage, tendons, skin, heart valves, pleuroperitoneum and gastrointestinal stroma. Collagens also form basement membranes and associated elements in skin, lung, intestine, glomeruli and various epithelia and very probably play a crucial directing role in embryogenesis and morphology. Absent or faulty components produce fetal blighting and death *in utero*. Difficulties in conception or premature rupture of fetal membranes are commonplace. Although initially described over 30 years ago as a single protein type, a wide variety of collagen genes and proteins has rapidly been discovered, presently including at least 12 collagen types coded by a minimum of 20 genes (Tsipouras and Ramirez, 1987). More genes and proteins are also possible at least two of which have been identified indirectly by gene cloning techniques, resulting in gene sequences currently without a protein product.

Gene defects of collagen I ($\alpha 1(I)$ and $\alpha 2(I)$ proteins coded by genes on chromosomes 17 and 7) (Pope *et al.*, 1985b) and collagen III on chromosome 2 (Pope *et al.*, 1986; Pope *et al.*, 1987) are well characterized and will form the main subject of this paper. Defects for collagen II are just beginning to be described in association with various cartilage defects (Francomano *et al.*, 1988). Other important collagens awaiting diseases include collagen VII (Bentz *et al.*, 1983), which forms anchoring fibrils attaching epidermal to underlying dermal components, collagens VI and VIII (Sage *et al.*, 1985) which are widely dispersed in arteries and endothelia, and collagens IX, X and XI which are cartilage-associated. Several types of collagen IV occur in basement membranes. Rapidly advancing evidence indicates important associations between various collagen components so that types I and III, types II and IX and types VI and III collagens associate specifically with one another and other non-collagenous components of connective tissue. Very probably specific molecular regions of various connective tissue components combine in an ordered way with several others and incorrect associations will produce specific structural abnormalities and disease. Thus type III collagen binds to minority collagens IX and X and type I collagen associates with type III and type VI collagens.

DEFECTS OF TYPES I AND III COLLAGENS

These diseases are clinically diverse and present to many specialities including paediatrics, general medicine, clinical genetics, dermatology, rheumatology, vascular surgery, neurosurgery, neurology and orthopaedic surgery (Pope *et al.*, 1985a; Tsipouras and Ramirez, 1987). They cause both rare and common diseases and, for example, type I collagen abnormalities of $\alpha 1(I)$ and $\alpha 2(I)$ chains cause hereditary brittle bone disease (McKusick 16620–26) and some common forms of osteoporosis (McKusick 25940–25942). Type III collagen mutations cause rare inherited aneurysms (lethal Ehlers Danlos syndrome type IV) (McKusick 13005, 22535) but can also cause subarachnoid haemorrhage from common berry aneurysms. Some types of osteoporosis affect up to 50% of women by the age of 75 years (Lewis, 1981; Jensen *et al.*, 1982), osteoarthritis occurs in 10% of radiological surveys (Dieppe, 1987) and berry aneurysms of the Circle of Willis cause 4000 deaths per annum in the United Kingdom (Mortality Statistics, 1977). Overall therefore, inherited abnormalities of collagen produce a significant burden of disease, at least some of which could justifiably be prevented by prenatal diagnosis.

Recent advances in recombinant DNA analysis theoretically allow the detailed examination of any human (or other) gene. If the gene itself is unidentified then its localization to particular chromosomal sites using random population variations in gene sequence (restriction fragment length polymorphisms) allows the identification of the mutant gene by so-called reverse genetics. Collagen gene analysis is amenable to both these approaches. In the case of the type I and III collagen defects abnormalities have been specifically recognized by histology, protein chemistry and DNA analysis combined with detailed examination of the clinical patterns of disease (phenotype). Thus, for example, osteogenesis imperfecta specifically produces congenitally thin collagen-depleted bones which fracture easily (Williams *et al.*, 1988) (Figure 1) and type III collagen-deficient Ehlers Danlos syndrome (EDS IV) is characterized by a specific clinical phenotype with collagen-depleted elastin-rich skin and arteries (Pope *et al.*, 1988b) (Figure 2). Collagen protein analysis in the majority of cases shows reduction or alteration of type III collagen proteins. Generally those individuals affected by type I and III collagen mutations have clinical phenotypes linked to the candidate $\alpha 1(I)$, $\alpha 2(III)$ genes even when no abnormality of the mutant protein is detectable.

GENERAL PROPERTIES OF INTERSTITIAL COLLAGEN GENES

The interstitial collagen genes (collagens I, II, III and V but also XI) are the best studied and collagens, I, II and III have been cloned in animals (Chu *et al.*, 1984; Weiss *et al.*, 1982; Myers *et al.*, 1983) and humans and share a very similar structure and organization. At the protein level, all of them are proteins of 120 kDa with globular N and C terminal extensions, the latter having extensive interchain disulphide bonds. (Prockop and Kivirriko, 1984). There is also a regular central α helix which self-assembles to form hetero- or homotrimers, as in type I and III collagens, respectively. Glycine occurs in every third position within the helix to form a heteropolymer of general formula (Gly XY). Frequently X and Y residues

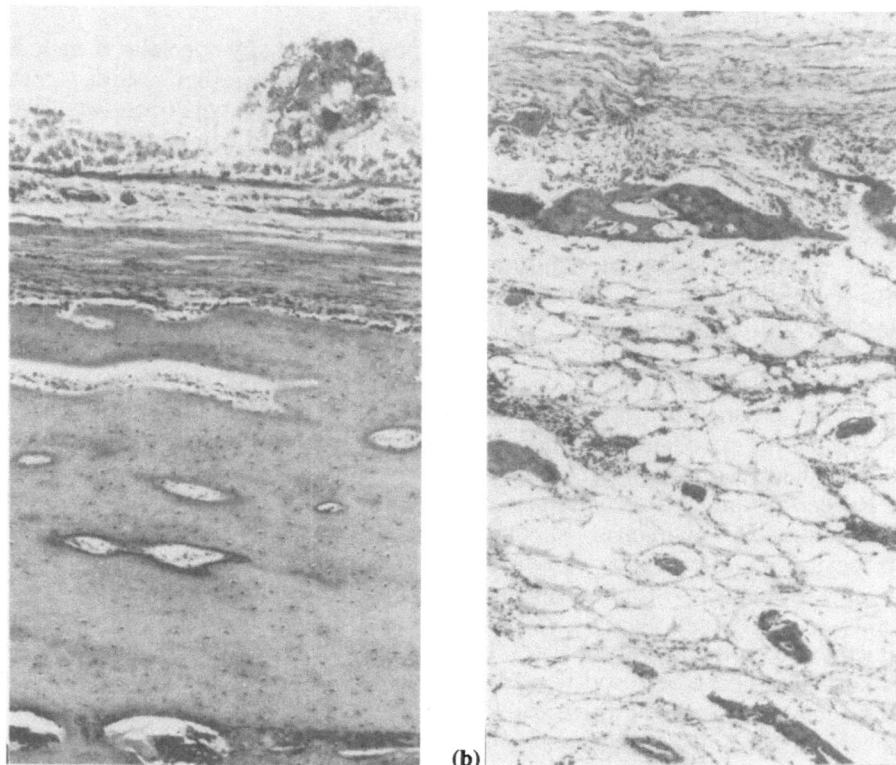

(a) (b)

Figure 1 Comparison of haematoxylin and eosin stained femoral shafts from (a) normal control and (b) severe osteogenesis imperfecta lethal cortical bone. Whilst both bones clearly have a normal periosteum there is a dearth of bone matrix material in the osteogenesis imperfecta bone (×157)

are either proline 10% or lysine 4% and the regular glycine repeat is biophysically crucial for helix stability and coherence. As we will see later, the replacement of helical glycines by other residues seriously disturbs collagen stability and strength, producing (in the main) catastrophic disease and seriously weakened connective tissues. Other crucial properties of the collagen triple helix include the important function of the C propeptides in aligning collagen triple helix prior to fibril formation, and stability of even small alterations within one component of the triple helix to seriously affect its normal companions within the helix (called suicide mutations by Prockop) (Figure 3a,b). One of the striking analogies discovered by gene cloning and sequencing interstitial collagen genes is the heavy conservation of intron sizes for all domains of the collagen molecules. Thus exons coding for helical sequences, in which the protein structure is $(GlyXY)_n$ and therefore coded by a basic 9 base pair (3 amino acid motif), are all 9 base pair multiples with 45, 54, 72, 107 and 162 base pair elements forming the so-called cassette model for

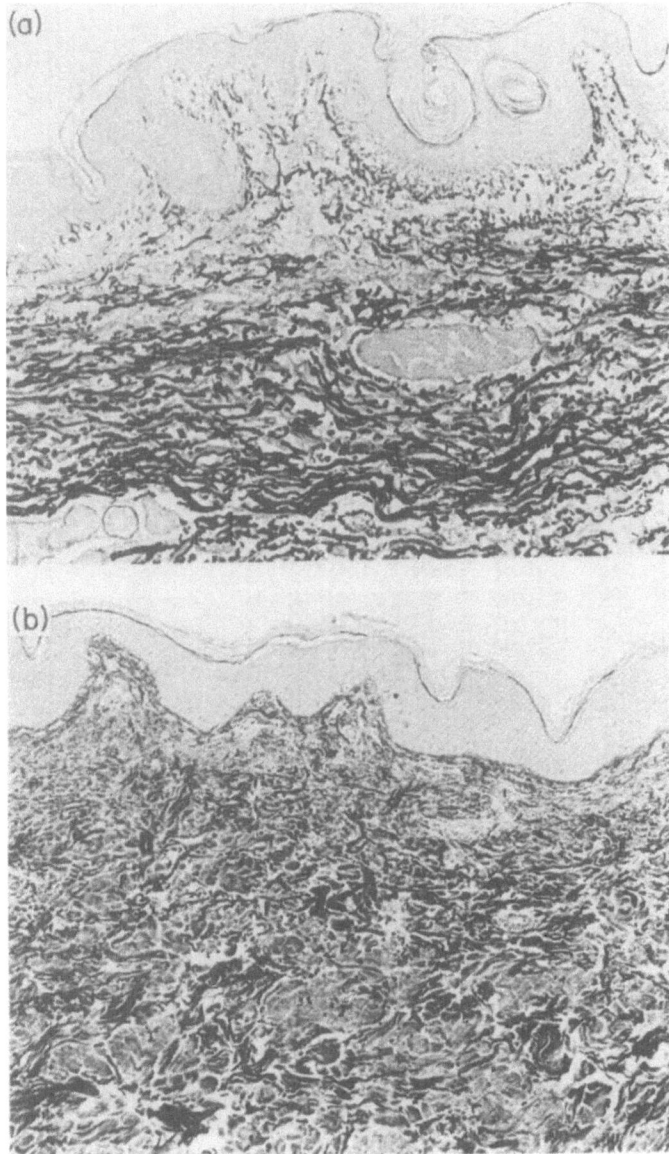

Figure 2 Histological features of skin biopsy from (a) Ehlers Danlos syndrome type IV patient compared with (b) normal control, stained for collagen and elastic fibres. Note relative increase in elastic fibres and collagen depletion in Ehlers Danlos syndrome type IV sample compared with control (×157)

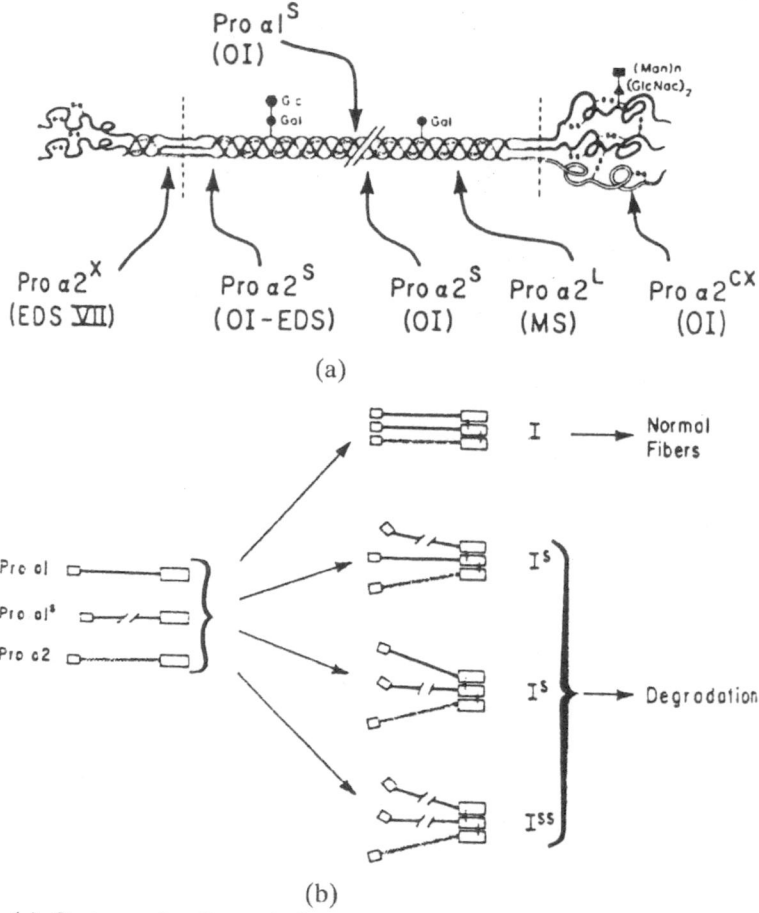

Figure 3 (a) Cartoon of collagen helix showing globular N and C extension and triple helical core; (b) Diagrammatical representation of altered triple helical assembly in the presence of one or two mutated chains

interstitial collagens (Frischauf *et al.*, 1978; Boyd *et al.*, 1980; Wozney *et al.*, 1981; Myers *et al.*, 1983).

Similarly, there is tight conservation of exons coding for the 3' (C terminal) and 5' N terminal propeptide sequences. For example, exons coding for the 3' sequence of α1(I), α2(I), α1(II) and α1(III) genes code for important junctional regions including specific lysine cross-linking and carbohydrate attachment regions (Myers *et al.*, 1983, 1985; Chu *et al.*, 1985b). There is similarly tight conservation of the N terminal coding sequences which contain, amongst others, specific lysine cross-linkage and pepsin cleavage sequences. Quite clearly (see later) mutations of these essential regions produce specific disorders of collagen fibril size and assembly (producing Ehlers Danlos syndrome type VII in the case of N terminal sequences and various forms of osteogenesis imperfecta (α1(I) and α2(I) sequences). On the other hand, intron sizes are not conserved and vary widely between interstitial collagen types (Ramirez *et al.*, 1985). Nevertheless, in common with all intron sequences which require excision and splicing, there is tight conservation of 5' and 3' intron splice acceptor and donation sites, mutation of which results in exon skipping and deletion (see later) (D'Alessio *et al.*, 1988).

The precise reason for such rigid conservation of interstitial collagen exon order and arrangement is not entirely clear, but probably is connected with the very specific constraints upon ordered fibril structure and assembly dictated by physical constraints and requirements for bone rigidity and strength, arterial pulsation and elasticity and the cushioning properties of articular cartilage. Certainly, specific mutations (see below) of these substances seriously interfere with the mechanical stability, strength and coherence of all these structures. In marked contrast, non-interstitial collagen genes have diverged significantly from this structural pattern. Type IV collagen is an excellent example and consists of at least two collagen chains forming amorphous (non-fibrillar elements) of the lamina densa of basement membrane (Timpl *et al.*, 1985; Poschl *et al.*, 1988). At the protein and rotary shadowing level there are obvious interruptions to the regular fibrillar (GlyXY regions); these non-collagenous (NC) regions induce kinks and bends into the molecule, presumably required for its non-rigid fibrillar structure and crucial for the supportive and filtration functions of basement membranes in regions such as lung, kidneys, placenta and blood vessels. The type IV genes are remarkable as they have a common promotor region situated centrally, whilst the genes are transcribed in opposite orientations in the 5' and 3' directions. Type VII collagen has very large C and N terminal extensions with a central helical interruption whilst the gene for type X collagen has no intervening sequences. Collagen VIII is secreted by endothelial cells and collagens IX, X (Olsen *et al.*, 1985; Ninomiya *et al.*, 1986), and XI together with II and VI form significant elements of cartilage components.

MUTATIONS OF COLLAGEN GENES AND PROTEINS

Mutations of the interstitial collagen type I and III molecules (and genes) resemble those causing various haemoglobinopathies. They include amino acid substitutions, gene deletions and insertions, nonsense mutations and regulatory mutations with absent, greatly diminished or physically faulty proteins. Unlike the haemoglobino-pathies which show clustering, genetic drift and selective advantage in affected heterozygotes, collagen type I mutations are private abnormalities quite different in each family. This in turn implies an absence of selective pressure generated by the heterozygote advantages in the defects of globin. From this point of view, collagen mutations resemble more closely those causing phenylketonuria or Duchenne muscular dystrophy. Type III collagen mutations, in contrast, are more uniform both clinically as they frequently have a 'family' resemblance to each other, but also at the biochemical level as they either retain a very poorly secreted protein intracellularly (in small amounts) or secrete reduced quantities of the protein without retention. Whether the intracellular retainers have clusters of mutations in certain regions of the mutant type III collagen awaits clarification. Structural mutations are rarer in the type III collagen mutations, although several workers have now found apparent alterations in cyanogen bromide peptide α1(III) CB5 or α1(III) CB9, both of which are at the 3' end of the gene (Stolle *et al.*, 1985; Cole, personal communication, 1988; Narcisi *et al.*, 1989). Other abnormalities include mutations of the procollagen peptidase cleavage site at the N terminal end of both pro α1(I) and pro α2(I) collagens (Eyre *et al.*, 1985; Cole *et al.*, 1986; Weil *et al.*, 1988). Both these defects cause Ehlers Danlos syndrome type VII (McKusick 13006, 22541), characterized by extreme joint laxity and short stature, with thin easily torn and fragile skin. Bones and blood vessels are normal, however.

So far, convincing abnormalities have been identified only for α1(I), α2(I) and α1(III) genes or proteins (Pope *et al.*, 1987; Tsipouras and Ramirez, 1987), although the type II gene is strongly suspected in certain rare inherited defects of cartilage such as the Stickler syndrome and spondyloepiphyseal dysplasia congenita (Francomano *et al.*, 1988; Lumadue *et al.*, 1988). Similarly, type VII collagen is absent from the basement membrane zone in some forms of dystrophic epidermolysis bullosa (McKusick 13170, 22645) (Eady, 1987). No doubt considerable genetic heterogeneity in these diseases awaits clarification and, as similar mutations can be expected in some or all of the other collagen genes, many other defects await characterization and detailed analysis. Compound heterozygosity from combinations of mutations is also likely, as well as phenocopies of different mutants caused by interacting elements amongst various collagen and other connective tissue components.

TYPE I COLLAGEN MUTATIONS

Collagen type I is widely distributed in skin, ligaments, bones, tendons and blood vessels and the major clinical effects of mutations in these substances predominantly affect bones and ligaments. Diseases caused by inherited abnormalities of type I collagen α1(I) and α2(I) chains include hereditary brittle bone disease (osteogenesis imperfecta) and Ehlers Danlos syndrome type VII in which fragile skin and joint laxity predominate. Intermediate (overlap) syndromes produce loose-jointed patients with fragile bones (which can occur either early or in adolescence or adulthood). The latter include various common types of osteoporosis. Other physical features of this disease group include blue sclerae (whose thinness has a light scattering effect upon the underlying retinal pigment), deafness, dentinogenesis imperfecta, high palatal arching, kyphoscoliosis and mitral valve prolapse (Pope *et al.*, 1985b). Occasionally premature aortic rupture and cerebral aneurysms have also been described. There is partial correlation with the biochemical situation of the mutation within the collagen protein helix, so that C terminal or central helical mutations cause severe or catastrophic osteogenesis imperfecta. N terminal mutations, on the other hand, produce milder osteogenesis imperfecta, inherited osteoporosis with Ehlers Danlos-like features or variants of Ehlers Danlos syndrome type VII (Prockop *et al.*, 1985). Mutations outside the main collagen helix and the C terminal propeptide produce very mild osteogenesis imperfecta. A single patient with the Marfan syndrome has been described in detail by Byers and colleagues (1981), but its significance is unclear as linkage studies have so far excluded the α2(I) gene as a candidate in other typical Marfan families. In the main, collagen type I mutations most often cause various forms of osteogenesis imperfecta.

CLINICAL FEATURES OF OSTEOGENESIS IMPERFECTA

The clinical and pathological features are those of an inherited osteoporosis. The pathology in the more severe forms shows severe bone matrix deficiency (Williams *et al.*, 1988). Under these circumstances (Figure 1) the periosteum persists and the cartilage chondrocyte columns of the epiphyseal plates may be slightly atypical (Pope *et al.*, 1985b). Radiologically the disease ranges from a mild osteoporosis with occasional fractures to a widespread skeletal abnormality with absence of skull calcification, multiple rib fractures, platyspondyly with spinal collapse and multiply fractured modelled or unmodelled long bones. These changes are reflected in the clinical severity of disease which ranges from a normal-looking child with occasional fractures to a lethal crippling short-limbed dwarfism (fatal either *in utero* or perinatally) (Figure 4a–d). This variability is recognized by a number of clinical classifications, of which the best and most practicable is that devised by Sillence and colleagues (1979, 1984). Two of these groups are mild and autosomal dominant, whilst two are lethal or very severely crippling and can be either autosomal recessive or lethal new dominant mutations. Type I Sillence osteogenesis imperfecta is a mild disease usually presenting in infancy or childhood, although it can occur at birth with perinatal fractures. Notable features include autosomal dominant inheritance (multiple generations with transmission to and through either sex), blue sclerae, variable short stature, childhood fractures which improve at adolescence and recur in menopausal women. Deafness and dentinogenesis imperfecta may also be common (and the presence or absence of dentinogenesis imperfecta breeds true within affected families). The dentinogenesis imperfecta can present in either or both the first and second dentitions and is caused by thin, poorly canalized dentine to which enamel is not well attached, producing easily worn, discoloured and opalescent teeth (Figure 5a–c). Type IV resembles type I osteogenesis imperfecta except that the sclerae are white or blueish grey in contrast to the bright blue sclerae of Sillence type I disease. There also seems to be more overlap between Sillence type IV (white-eyed) osteogenesis imperfecta and more severe disease – presumably because some white-eyed type II or III mutants are mistakenly included in this subgroup. I prefer to restrict the type IV classification to milder disease.

Sillence type II osteogenesis imperfecta is a severely crippling and often lethal disease. There are three main types originally subclassified by Sillence as IIa, IIb and IIc (Figure 6). Sillence type IIa is an invariably lethal disease in which every bone is multiply fractured, osteoporotic and distorted in shape with little sign of modelling (into diaphysis and metaphyses) (Figure 6a). The skull is poorly calcified and the disease is usually fatal *in utero* or from bronchopneumonia in infancy. The

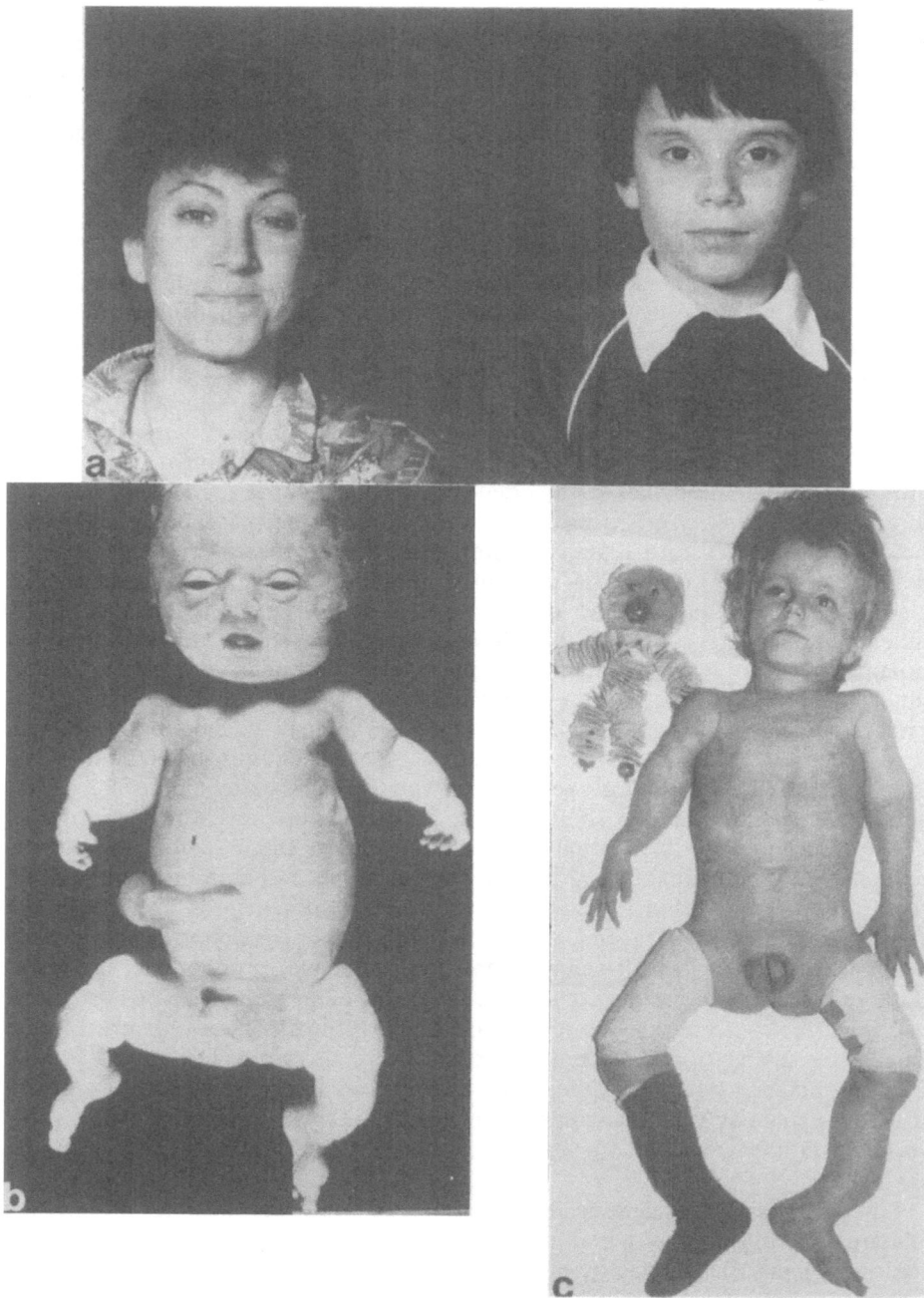

Figure 4 Clinical spectrum of osteogenesis imperfecta phenotypes showing (a) normal facial appearance of affected mother and son with Sillence type I osteogenesis imperfecta; (b) typical short-limbed dwarfism of lethally affected fetus with Sillence type IIa osteogenesis imperfecta; and (c) severely deformed limbs of patient with Sillence type III osteogenesis imperfecta

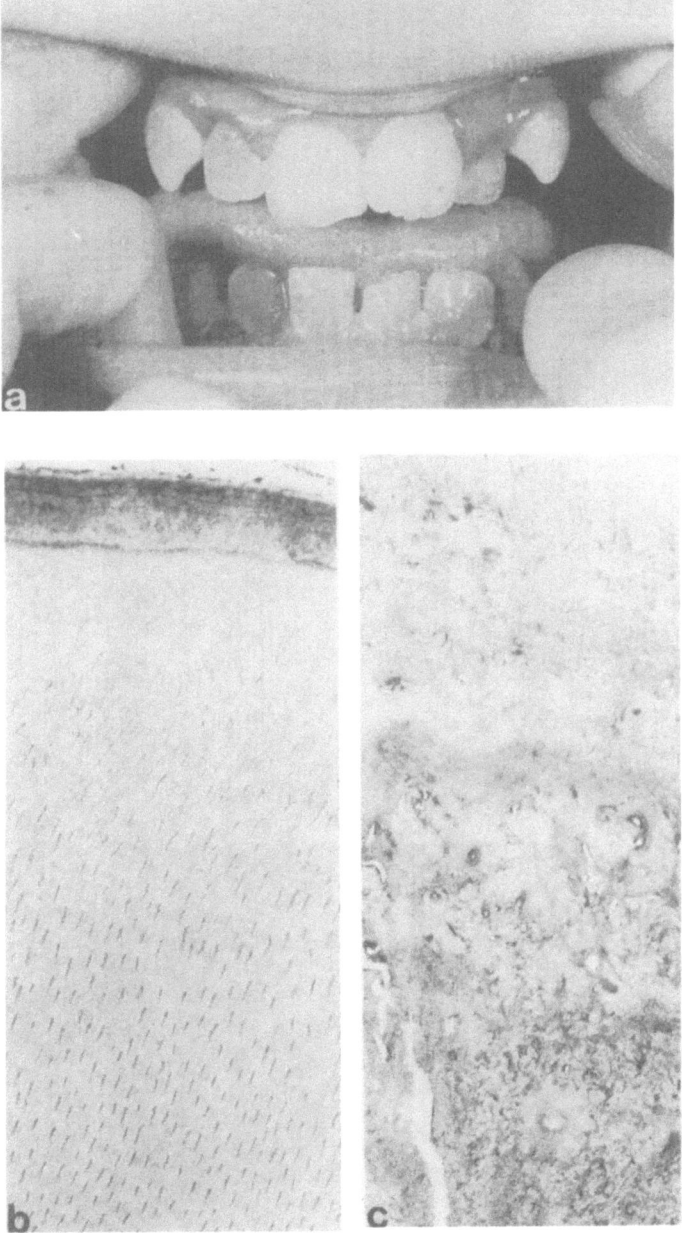

Figure 5 (a) Clinical dental appearance of child with dentinogenesis imperfecta showing patchy involvement of secondary teeth; (b) Histological appearance of normal tubular root dentine compared with (c) pattern from osteogenesis imperfecta teeth (×62.5)

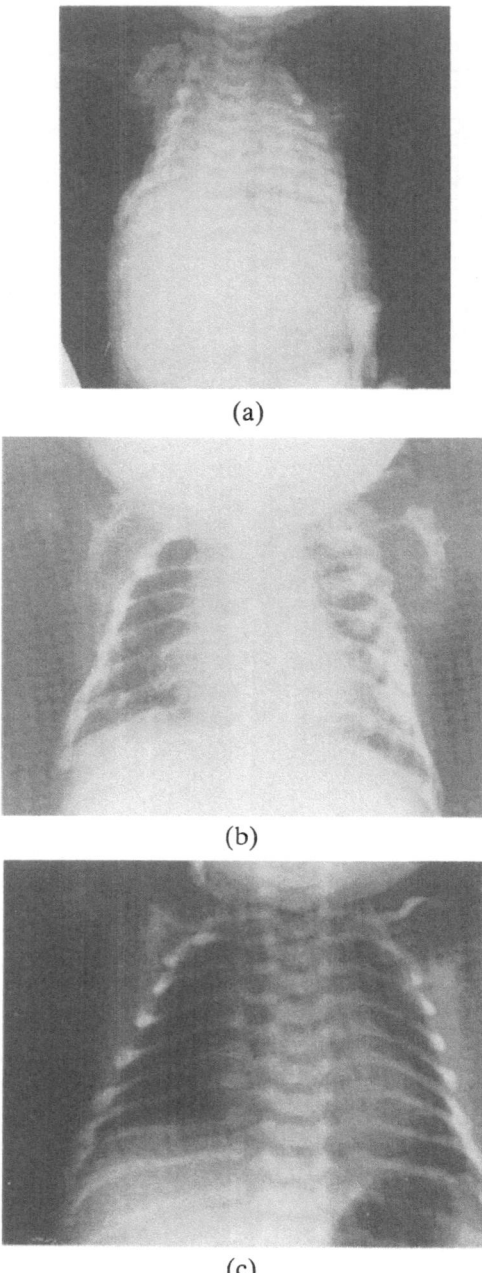

(a)

(b)

(c)

Figure 6 Typical chest X-ray appearances of lethal affected Sillence type II fetuses. (a) with generalized bone involvement, (b) similar to (a) except with nodular ribs, and (c) with the thin-ribbed variant. These correspond respectively with Sillence types IIa, IIc and IIb/III osteogenesis imperfecta

disease is easy to diagnose by ultrasound near the 18th week of pregnancy. Although Sillence originally considered the inheritance to be autosomal recessive, most currently available evidence suggests new dominant lethal mutations (Thompson *et al.*, 1987). There is good evidence to show that rare families with several affected siblings have been examples of gonadal mosaicism, although there is still a distinct possibility of either compound heterozygosity or occasional autosomal recessive inheritance within this group. Thompson has modified Sillence's classification and regards those children with IIa-like limbs and skull but with nodular ribs to have type IIb osteogenesis imperfecta (Figure 6b). She calls the thin-ribbed, thin-limbed variant infantile type III osteogenesis imperfecta and reserves the classification of IIc to thin-ribbed variants with particularly distorted limbs. To some extent this alters Sillence's original classification in which the thin-boned type was called IIb and the type with nodular ribs, IIc (Figure 6c). Thompson's classification is more logical and orderly and progresses from completely broadened fractured unmodelled ribs and limbs to narrowed well modelled limbs and ribs. Byers and colleagues (1988b) have described five type II subgroups of which 1 and 2 correspond to IIa, 3 corresponds to IIb and 4 and 5 are the equivalents of IIc and infantile type III osteogenesis imperfecta. These subgroups should be regarded as good clinical guides to severity but are not foolproof or comprehensive. Generally, both Thompson/Sillence type IIb and IIc variants are usually autosomal recessive or genetic compounds and carry a 1 in 4 recurrence risk. Autosomal dominant lethal forms of type IIb are also likely, whilst type IIa is usually from new dominant mutations. Type IIc/infantile type II osteogenesis imperfecta is either a childhood lethal or produces very severely crippling disease and the distinction between infantile IIc and III osteogenesis imperfecta is by no means as clear cut as Thompson suggests. We also have excellent evidence that at least one form of type IIc/III infantile osteogenesis imperfecta is inherited as an autosomal recessive, produces a severe deficiency of bone matrix, has abnormalities of collagen type I proteins, but does not appear to be genetically linked to either the $\alpha 1(I)$ or $\alpha 2(I)$ genes of type I collagen. This strongly suggests that molecules other than type I collagen cause some forms of inherited osteogenesis imperfecta (Williams *et al.*, 1988).

EXAMPLES OF TYPE I COLLAGEN MUTATIONS IN OSTEOGENESIS IMPERFECTA

Almost all the molecular defects so far identified in osteogenesis imperfecta have affected either $\alpha 1(I)$ or $\alpha 2(I)$ proteins or genes (Pope *et al.*, 1985; Prockop *et al.*, 1985). This is not surprising since bone matrix protein consists largely of type I collagen with traces of types III and V collagens (Pope *et al.*, 1980a). Generally, there is a variety of recognized mutations which does not consistently correlate with the clinical picture, although, as will become clear in the case of various cysteine mutations, apparently very similar mutations can have drastically different effects depending upon their precise localization with the collagen type I molecule (Byers *et al.*, 1988). Equally, some mutations are very much more likely to cause lethal diseases than others. Thus cysteine mutations in the C terminal $\alpha 1(I)$ peptide α1(I) CB6 can cause both lethal Sillence type II osteogenesis imperfecta and mild autosomal dominant osteogenesis imperfecta tarda (Steinemann *et al.*, 1984, 1986). In the lethal form a glycine to cysteine mutation due to a single amino acid/base change at position 988 produces lethal Sillence type II disease, with generalized bone matrix depletion and altered melting characteristics of the collagen helix, which becomes pepsin-susceptible 3°C lower than usual. Model building experiments show a disturbance of the collagen helix at this point and a severely impaired helix structure. A Gly–Cys mutation at position 748 introduces a physical kink into the abnormal chain and subsequently interferes by slippage with cross-linkage at the N terminal end of the chain (Vogel *et al.*, 1988).

In contrast, the mild Sillence type I mutant that we have studied also lies in CB6 (Nicholls *et al.*, 1984a) but does not affect the melting properties of the triple helix, which is normally susceptible to pepsin digestion at 41°C (Steinemann *et al.*, 1986) (Figure 7). We speculated initially that this might have been explained by a second or third position mutation of arginine or serine to cysteine. In fact, there is a glycine to cysteine mutation but occurring in the first 3′ glycine residue of the collagen α helix within the non-helical telopeptide sequence (Cohn *et al.*, 1988). Obviously this causes less disruption than more helical defects, which is reflected in the normal biochemical melting profiles and the very mild clinical changes.

A number of glycine to cysteine mutations have now been identified, as have some glycine to arginine mutations (Steinmann *et al.*, 1984; Cohn *et al.*, 1986; De Vries and de Wet, 1986; Bateman *et al.*, 1987, 1988; Vogel *et al.*, 1987; Constantinou *et al.*, 1988). These show a range of clinical osteogenesis imperfecta syndromes but invariably C terminal or central helical lesions cause lethal disease whereas non-helical or defects at the 5′ end of the gene (N terminal-protein) cause much milder disorders (Byers *et al.*, 1984). Detection of these defects is difficult unless a charge or cross-linking mutation such as arginine or cysteine occurs. No doubt, other lethal glycine mutations are also localized in the helical region.

Byers and colleagues have been mainly responsible for locating kinked or other faults within the collagen helix by virtue of the fact that defects impairing the C to N terminal winding of the collagen triple helix cause overhydroxylation of the mutant protein (Bonadio and Byers, 1985). This is because of tardiness of ribosomal release of the mutant partially unwound protein. Such overmodification occurs at the N terminal from the faulty product and can be detected by a combination of one- and two-dimensional protein electrophoresis. Knowing the order of type I collagen cyanogen bromide peptides allows deduction of the peptide within which the fault lies. A combination of protein and gene sequencing of the mutant peptide can then identify the precise gene location. Byers and colleagues have also devised cosmid vectors which specifically accept large 23–27 kb gene inserts covering the majority of α1(I) and α2(I) gene defects, leading directly to gene amplification of mutant regions using the polymerase chain reaction to multiply gene sequences homologous to specific oligonucleotide primers (Cohn *et al.*, 1986, 1988; Byers *et al.*, 1988).

A number of other mutations have also been discovered including small and large gene deletions which can be in or out of phase, gene insertions and increased

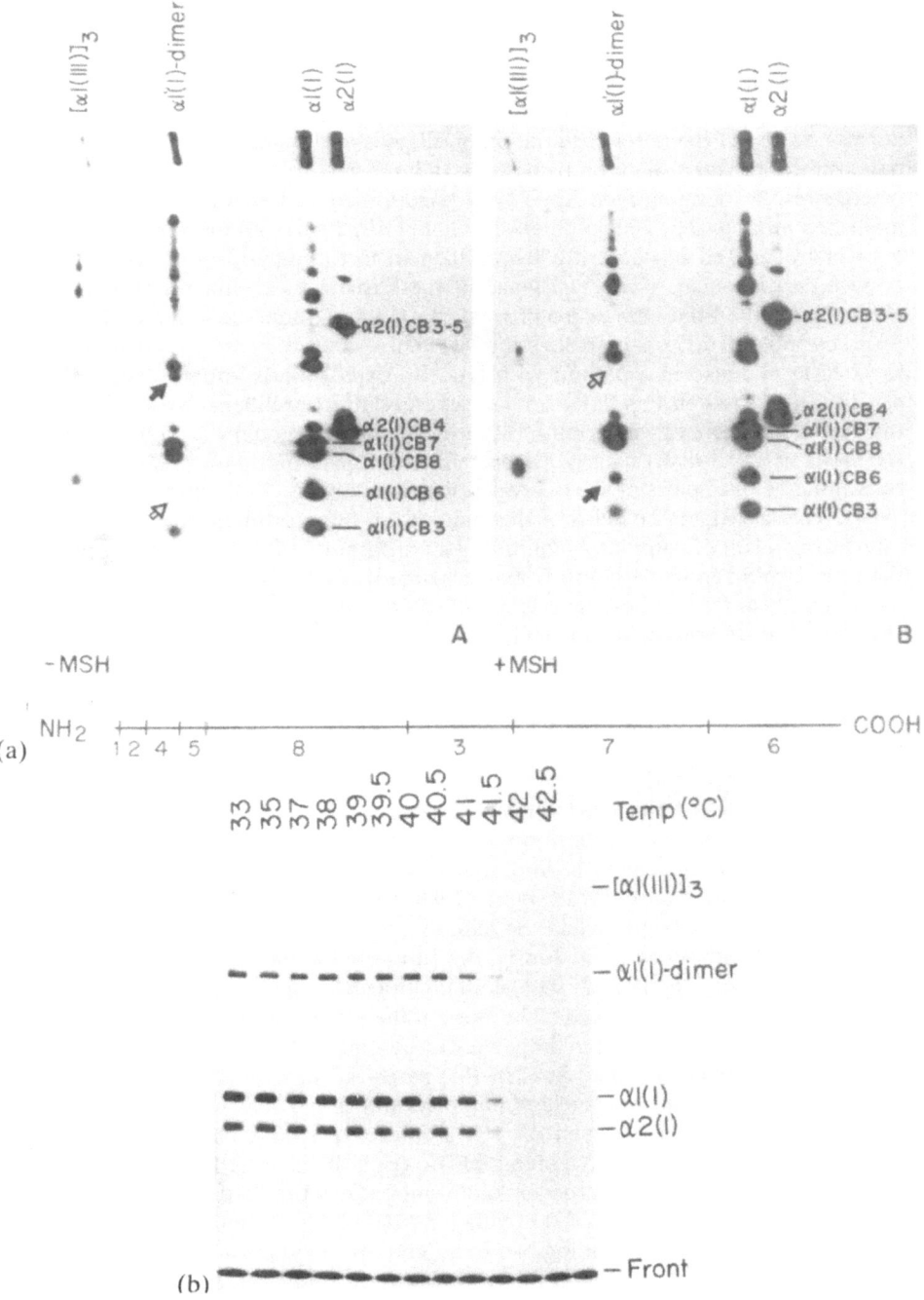

Figure 7 Composite autofluorogram showing (a) localization of the mutant cystein dimer to collagen peptide α1(I) CB6 (b) showing the normal melting profiles of the mutant and normal α(I) chains. Both substances melt as expected at 40°C

J. Inher. Metab. Dis. 12 Suppl. 1 (1989)

III/I collagen ratios with apparent reductions in collagen type I mRNA (Barsh *et al.*, 1981, 1982). Some of these mutations are mild and autosomal dominant Sillence Type I mutants, whilst others produce catastrophic lethal type II osteogenesis imperfecta. Presumably, in the former case the remaining allele is relatively normal, whilst in the latter case the other allele is also mutant. The first large gene deletion to be identified in osteogenesis imperfecta was a 500 bp deletion in osteogenesis imperfecta type IIa. This was examined both by Prockop's group who identified an apparent 500 bp deletion (Chu *et al.*, 1985) and by Byers' group who later characterized in detail a 650 bp intron to intron deletion removing residues between amino acids 327–411 (84aa) in the triple helical domain (Barsh *et al.*, 1985). Since then they have also characterized a 179 amino acid deletion between residues 586 and 765 of the collagen α2(I) chain, caused by a 4.5 kb deletion from the α2(I) gene also in a patient with type IIa osteogenesis imperfecta (Willing *et al.*, 1988). A smaller 4 bp deletion in a severely affected Sillence type III child (of third cousin heterozygote parents) (Figure 8a–d homozygous) with α2(I) deficiency (Nicholls *et al.*, 1984b) causes a frameshift nonsense mutation (Figure 9) in the remaining 96 base pairs of the C propeptide (Deak *et al.*, 1983; Pihlajaniemi *et al.*, 1984). The last 32 amino acids of this mutant are therefore nonsense. This has the interesting result of completely inhibiting incorporation of the mutant α2 chain into the type I collagen triple helix. Collagen trimers of α1(I) chains form instead and α2 chains are intracellularly degraded and do not leave the cytoplasm of fibroblast cultures. Presumably collagen α1(I)$_3$ is inadequate as a bone matrix framework and, although collagen fibril diameters *in vivo* looked relatively normal (Figure 8a), the clinical result is of poorly mineralized osteopenic bones with severe deformity and popcorn expansion of distal femur and proximal tibial metaphyses (Figure 8d). The heterozygous normal-looking parents of the affected child have premature osteoporosis.

Another defect of the procollagen C propeptide has also been discovered in which excessive mannosylation occurs (Peltonen *et al.*, 1980), causing severe Sillence type III osteogenesis imperfecta. Gene insertions are very much less common than other mutations. Byers (1988a) have identified 50–70 extra amino acid residues in the triple helical domain of type I collagen between amino acids 123 and 212, although anomalously the abnormal molecules produced by this mutation are not lengthened. The mutant molecules have an abnormal melting temperature and are asymmetrical because of the extra residues, and probably have alterations of structure within important cross-linked regions of the triple helix nearer the N terminus than usual in this case. All other rearrangements so far recognized have been between the amino terminus and residue 402, marking the junction (methionine) between α1 (CB3) and α1(I) CB8 peptides. These also produce out-of-register arrangements of the triple helix. The functional elements here include intermolecular cross-linked lysines at position 9 of the amino terminal telopeptide and position 87 of the collagen helix. This domain is also crucial for interactions with mineral binding proteins. The proteolytic conversion of procollagen to collagen also requires in-phase registration of all three peptides which, if defective, would affect collagen processing and secondary fibrillogenesis.

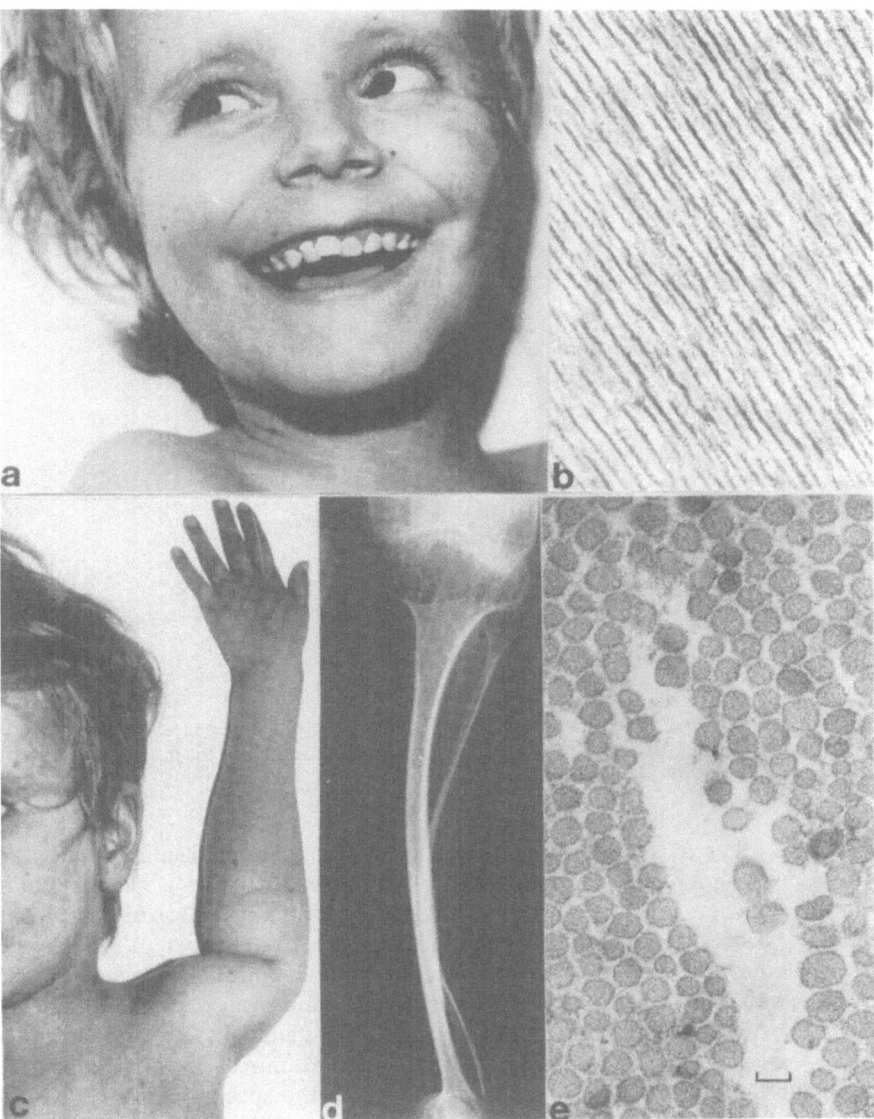

Figure 8 Clinical, radiological and histological features of homozygously affected child with Sillence type III osteogenesis imperfecta and α2 chain deletion. (a) Facial appearance showing clinically normal teeth; (b) light microscopy of dentine showing normal pattern (stained with picrothionine ×102); (c) abnormally twisted left upper arm caused by a persistent humoral pseudoarthrosis; (d) radiological appearance of lower limbs with pop-corned expansion of lower femur, upper and lower tibia; and (e) electron microscopical appearance of dermal collagen fibrils in formaldehyde-fixed skin sample. The bar represents 100 nm

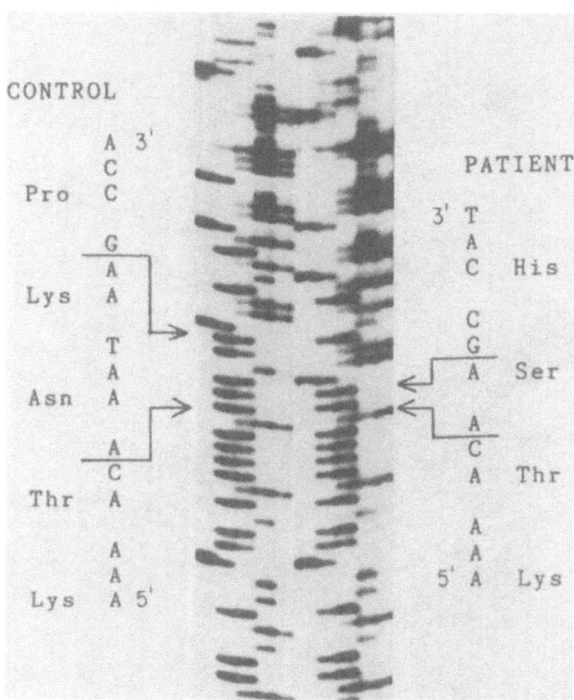

Figure 9 Sequenced 3' end of mutant and wild type α2(I) genes showing 4 base pair mutations deleting AATA from the normal (expected) sequence. This makes the subsequent downstream sequences out of phase

Various other α2(I) mutations include an N terminal deletion in Sillence type I osteogenesis imperfecta (Sippola *et al.*, 1984), probably due to a splicing mutation and a similar defect in patients with premature familial osteoporosis that we have studied (Nicholls, Heath, Pope, unpublished data). A number of α2(I) cysteine mutations have also been described in mild white-eyed Sillence type IV patients (Cohn *et al.*, 1988a). Furthermore, gene linkage studies suggest that all autosomal dominant Sillence type IV mutants have α2(I) gene linkage and presumably mutations (Tsipouras *et al.*, 1983; Tsipouras and Ramirez, 1987). Sillence type I osteogenesis imperfecta on the other hand (as in the specific examples described above) is linked either with α1(I) or α2(I) mutations (Sykes *et al.*, 1988).

Possibly genes other than α1(I) or α2(I) may also be defective. We have recently made a detailed clinical biochemical and genetic study of an unique Irish traveller family with Sillence type IIb/III osteogenesis imperfecta (Williams *et al.*, 1988). Here three consecutively affected children with severe Sillence type II osteogenesis imperfecta were born to first cousin parents (Figure 10a). One of them died shortly after birth, the next survived with the clinical phenotype of Sillence type III osteogenesis imperfecta (Figure 11) and the third affected pregnancy was terminated

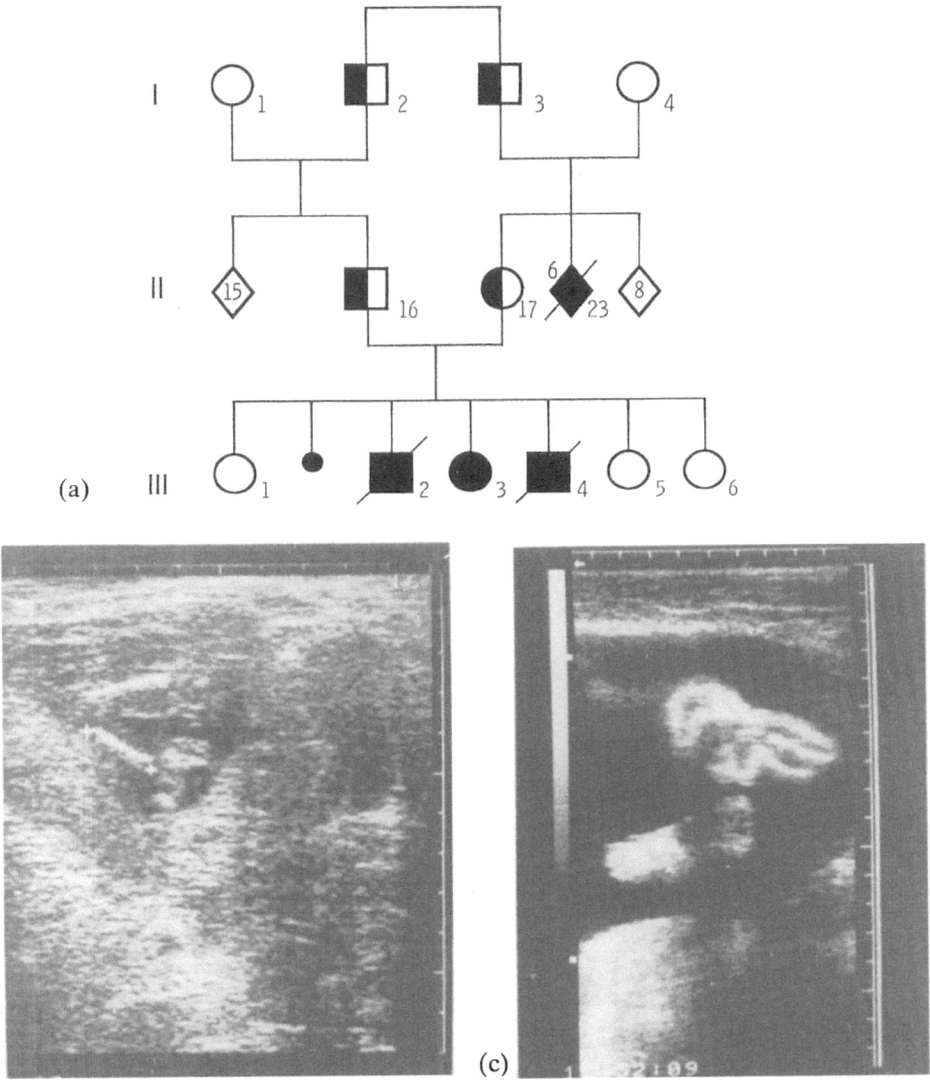

Figure 10 (a) Pedigree of affected Irish traveller family showing heterozygous first cousin parents and three consecutively affected children. III.3 survives currently aged 7 years, III.2 died perinatally of a respiratory infection whilst III.4 was terminated at the 30th week of pregnancy; (b) real-time ultrasound scan of lower limb of normal fetus compared with (c) the ultrasound appearance of the distorted upper and lower leg of an affected fetus

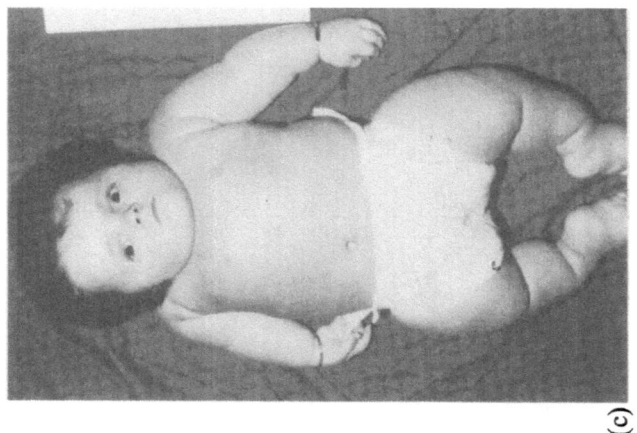

(c)

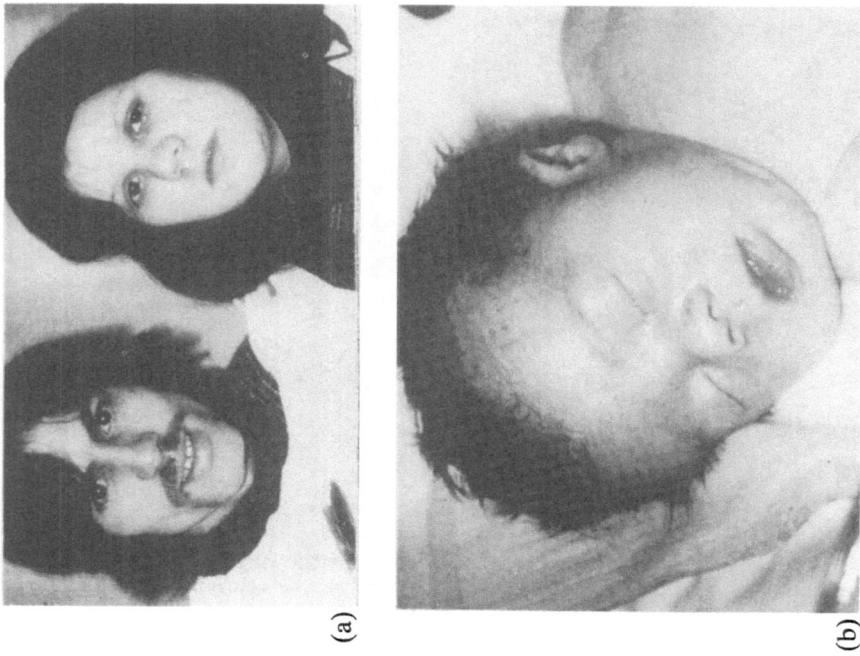

(a)

(b)

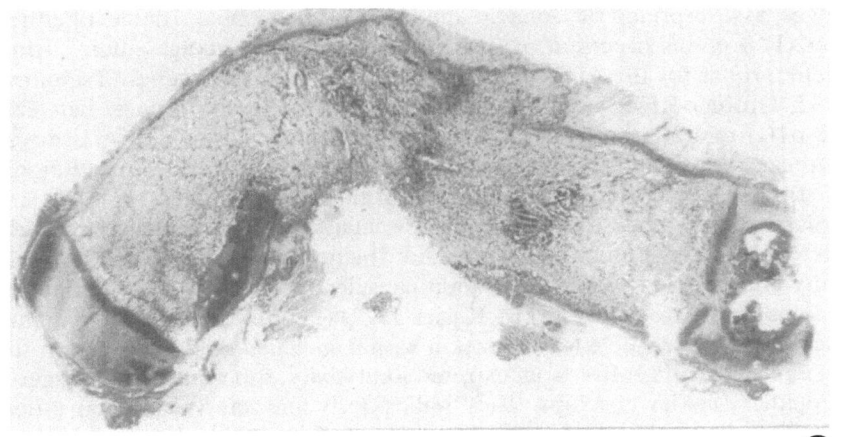

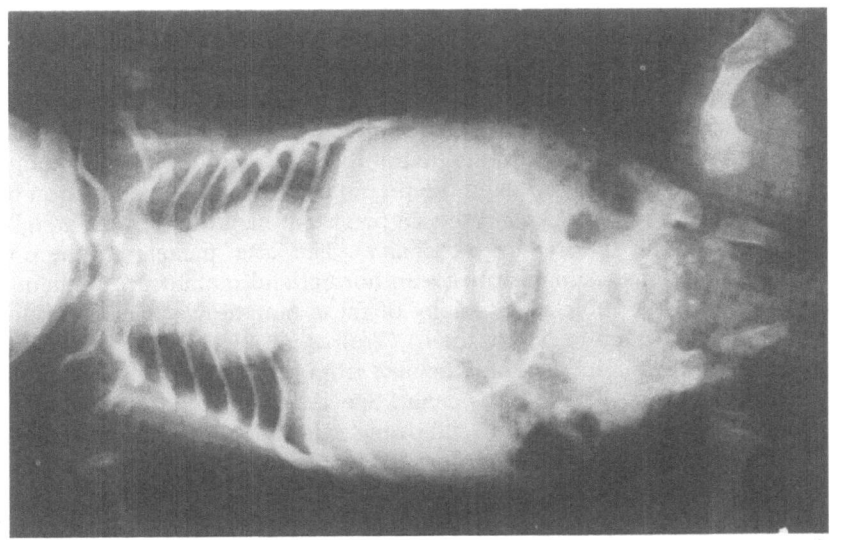

Figure 11 Clinical appearance of (a) normal parents II.16 and II.17, (b) lethally affected child III.2, and (c) surviving child. (d) Shows the typical radiological phenotype of an affected child, and (e) shows the distorted matrix-depleted femur in longitudinal section

at the 28th week of gestation (Figure 10b). The bone pathology clearly shows collagen-depleted bone matrix (Figures 1 and 11e) and the biochemistry shows overmodified α1(I) and α2(I) chains along the length of the chain, as judged by cyanogen bromide peptide mapping (Daw *et al.*, 1988). The clear implication of such changes, as interpreted by Bonadio and Byers (1985), is that a defect of either α1(I) or α2(I) proteins occurs at or near the C terminus. Linkage studies using various gene probes for the α1(I) (Sykes *et al.*, 1986) and α2(I) genes (Tsipouras *et al.*, 1982; Grobler-Rabie *et al.*, 1985) do not show common linkage between either the α1(I) or α2(I) genes. This strongly implies the occurrence of a novel mechanism causing secondary alteration in collagen type I molecules, resulting in a specific structural deficiency of bone matrix in this affected family.

A completely different non-osteogenesis imperfecta phenotype can also be caused by certain type I collagen mutations. Instead of fractured bones, the main physical abnormality affects skin ligaments and joint capsules, producing the syndrome of Ehlers Danlos syndrome type VIII (McKusick 1972) (Figure 12). Affected patients have hyperextensible fragile easily torn skin with a so-called criss-cross pattern to the palms and soles, and suffer from extreme joint laxity, especially of the fingers, wrists, shoulders, ankles and hips. They walk poorly and late (as infants), often have congenital dislocation of the hips and may be diagnosed as having inherited muscle disease (Pope and Nicholls, 1986). Three distinct causes of this phenotype have been recognized. One closely resembles so-called dermatosporaxis of sheep and cattle (Lenears *et al.*, 1971), where the peptidases which cleave the N and C terminal propeptides are deficient or defective (Lichtenstein *et al.*, 1974). Collagen fibril assembly is disturbed and, instead of regular cylindrical fibrils, affected . animals have misassembled hieroglyphic fibrils (in cross-section). Since then two human variants of Ehlers Danlos syndrome VII have been described, one affecting the α1(I) and the other α2(I) N terminal propeptide area (Eyre *et al.*, 1985; Cole *et al.*, 1986). Both mutations affect that region of the N propeptide which contains an important lysine cross-link region and the pepsin cleavage site. Examination of pepsinized procollagens in both cases detects a persistent higher molecular weight form (which runs along with normal pro α chains). The latter means that there is insufficient peptide loss to distinguish between normal and mutant pro α chains. Preliminary studies of the molecular biology of these mutations suggests exon 6 deletions in all cases (proven in one of them) (Weil *et al.*, 1987; D'Alessio *et al.*, 1988). In one instance 24 amino acids are deleted from pro α1(I) chains and in the other 18 amino acids from the pro α2(I) chain. Specific splice mutations of the 5′ splice donor site GT have mutated to GC allowing exon skipping with an in-phase deletion. Possibly all Ehlers Danlos syndrome VII structural mutations have similar abnormalities in this region of the gene or at least will have abnormalities of the lysine cross-link site.

Presumably the various type I collagen mutations, resulting in osteogenesis imperfecta on the one hand and Ehlers Danlos type VII syndrome on the other result from the specific biophysical effects of the mutations upon particular physical properties and interactions of type I collagen with other matrix components. Certainly, overlap syndromes with features both of Ehlers Danlos syndrome and

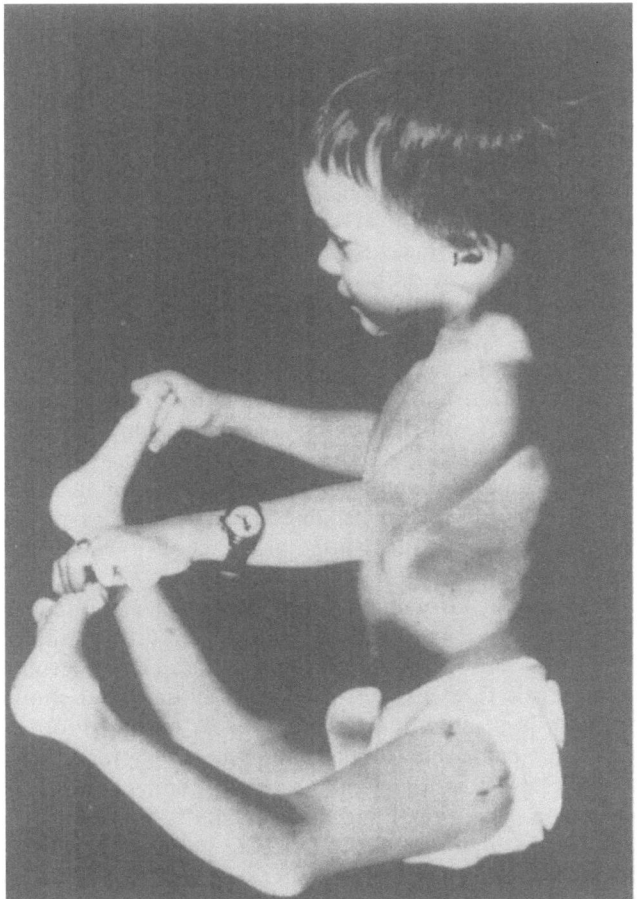

Figure 12 Clinical features of patient affected with Ehlers Danlos syndrome type VII. Note extreme joint laxity of the hips which has caused the knees to rotate 180° (i.e. they are back to front)

osteogenesis imperfecta occur especially with mutations of the N terminus. Prockop has elegantly explained the disastrous effects of single autosomal mutations upon a triple helical molecule with two α1 and α2 chains (Prockop *et al.*, 1985). The stoichiometry of assembly is such that 3 out of 4 of such chains will contain a mutant product, which, if shortened, lengthened or distorted results in the 'suicide' of that trimer by disturbance of the correct winding, assembly and melting profile of the fibre, followed subsequently by degradation of the faulty product.

TYPE III COLLAGEN MUTATIONS

Defects of type III collagen chiefly affect blood vessels, skin, pleuroperitoneal linings and gastrointestinal tract (Pope and Nicholls, 1986). These are all regions in which type III collagen is abundant, although it forms only 35% of the collagenous components of skin but 70% of arterial collagen (Epstein, 1973). The most dramatic physical signs of disease are produced in the cardiovascular system with dangerous or lethal arterial rupture of small and medium-sized vessels. Internal and external carotid aneurysms including abnormalities of the cavernous sinus and the Circle of Willis (Fox *et al.*, 1988) are commonplace as are aneurysms of the ascending, descending and abdominal aorta, renal, splenic, iliac, femoral, popliteal and axillary vessels. Venous problems also occur but in the main are confined to varicose veins (sometimes very prematurely). Easy bruising is common especially in childhood (Roberts *et al.*, 1984), but there is a disease spectrum ranging from a lethal premature ageing syndrome (Ehlers Danlos syndrome type IV – acrogeric type) to virtually normal-looking individuals with the benign hypermobile syndrome (Ehlers Danlos syndrome type III). This latter group is heterogeneous but we have studied several families forming a distinct subgroup with superadded lumbosacral striae, mitral valve prolapse and aortic rupture. Because they sometimes are tall (but frequently slightly built) there are resemblances to the Marfan syndrome. They are clearly distinguishable by the normal arm span and equal upper segment/lower segment ratios (Pope and Nicholls, 1986). They also do not dislocate lenses.

Typical Ehlers Danlos syndrome type IV patients, however, have a very characteristic phenotype and share the common clinical features of thin easily bruised skin with easily visible veins, prematurely aged hands and feet (from the thin skin) and a very characteristic face (Figure 13). Typically the latter shows a madonna-like appearance with large slightly protruding eyes, thin lips, lobeless ears and a pinched nose. In some cases this can be reminiscent of systemic sclerosis but is in fact quite distinct. These features combine with a tendency to short stature and slim build (with some exceptions) and affected patients are easily recognized in infancy and childhood (Pope and Nicholls, 1986; Pope *et al.*, 1988).

Type III collagen secretion is usually drastically diminished and in our experience can range from 10 to 80% of the expected normal values (Figure 14a). In other cases a 50% reduction in normally secreted proteins occurs (Figure 14b). Type III collagen levels are technically difficult to measure accurately on polyacrylamide gels and there are advantages and disadvantages to all commonly used methods. These include measurement as an unreduced disulphide-linked trimer, interrupted reduction (for various times) and non-reduction. For accurate measurement and peptide mapping of the mutant protein (when present in sufficient quantities) immunoprecipitation by specific type III antibodies is useful.

In our hands most affected patients are poor secretors and retain a moderate amount of mutant protein intracellularly (Pope *et al.*, 1988a,b). Occasionally, we see this as a temperature-sensitive mutation correctable at lower than normal culture temperatures (Narcisi, unpublished data). We have also noted that the degree of overmodification of the mutant protein varies (when co-electrophoresed) and we strongly suspect that this indicates different mutation sites (similar to those of osteogenesis imperfecta) (Figure 15).

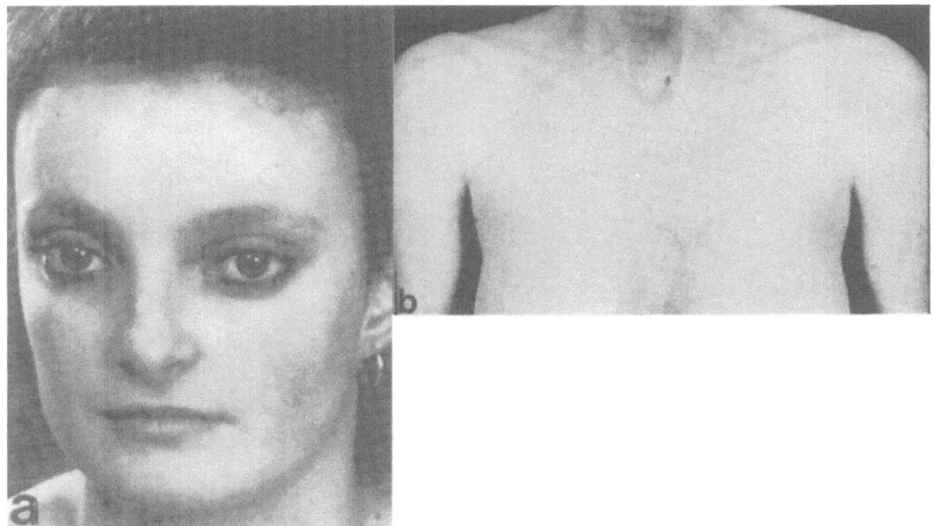

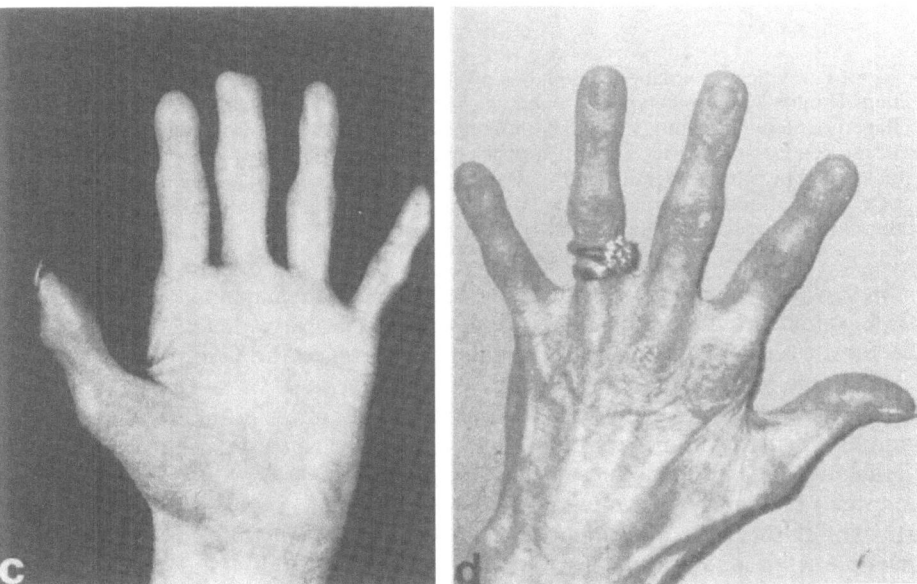

Figure 13 Characteristic clinical phenotype of Ehlers Danlos syndrome type IV patients showing (a) typical large-eyed, thin-nosed face, (b) characteristic thin skin with easily visible veins, (c) and (d) palmar and dorsal appearance of prematurely aged hands

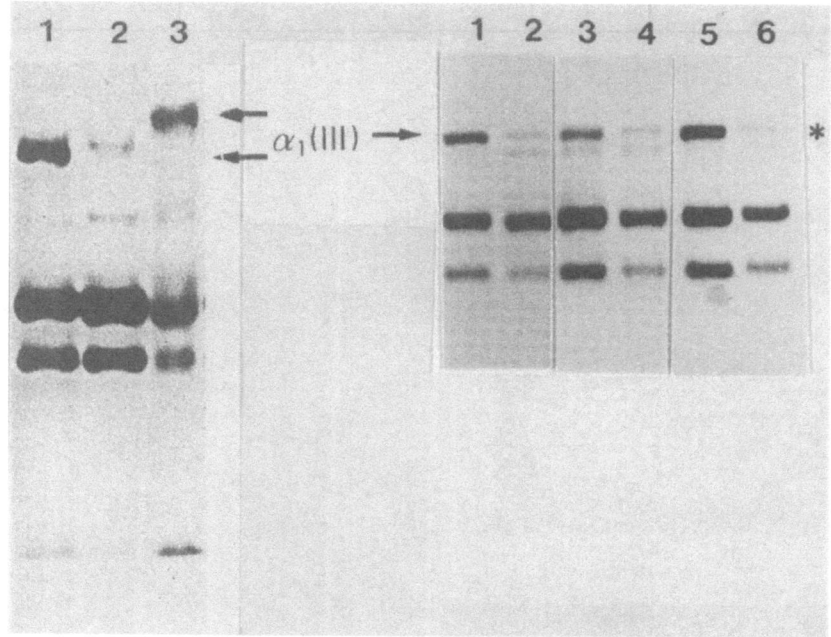

Figure 14 Typical radiolabelled collagen profiles from (a) acrogeric, and (b) non-acrogeric Ehlers Danlos syndrome type IV patients. The acrogeric pattern characteristically shows collagen-depleted medium (track 2) compared with the normal control (track 1). The mutant cell line retains substantial quantities of an overmodified mutant protein in the cell layer (track 3). The non-acrogeric Ehlers Danlos syndrome type IV patients (b) sometimes produce diminished quantities of type III collagen (tracks 1 and 3) without much intracellular retention compared with the normal control tracks 5 and 6

Most workers in the field have not found peptide mapping of overmodified proteins to be as useful as in osteogenesis imperfecta. Nevertheless, we expect that the most overmodified chains have mutations closer to the C terminal end of the protein than less overmodified protein. When the type III collagen occurs in easily detectable quantities it is theoretically possible to peptide map them using cyanogen bromide, hydroxylamine, trypsin, V8 proteinase, collagenase and other enzymes. Mutant type III proteins have been difficult to detect although they have been described previously by Stolle and colleagues (1985) (a possible gene insertion in $\alpha 1$(III) CB5 near the C terminus). We have also recently detected either a gene deletion or an amino acid substitution in the same peptide (Narcisi *et al.*, 1989). Superti-Furga and his colleagues have found a large protein and gene deletion which appears to be intron to intron and in phase at the end of the gene (N terminal end of the protein) (Superti-Furga *et al.*, 1987, 1988). Very probably similar defects to the osteogenesis imperfecta mutants await detection and are likely to produce amino acid substitutions, gene deletions, splicing abnormalities and gene insertions similar to those of osteogenesis imperfecta.

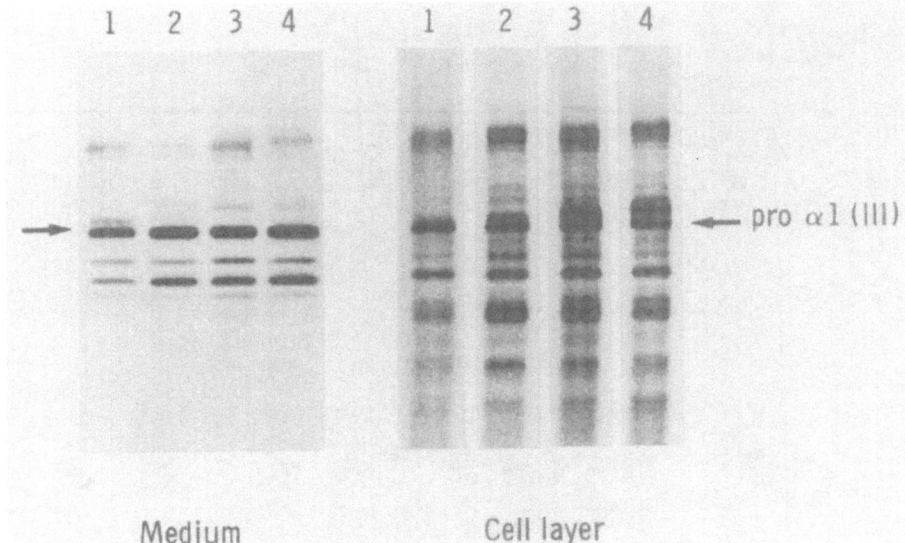

Figure 15 Radiolabelled medium and cell layer procollagens from normal control track 1 compared with three affected Ehlers Danlos syndrome type IV patients tracks 2, 3 and 4. The patients secrete little or no type III procollagen into the medium but retain substantial quantities in the cell layer (medium tracks 2–4 and cell layer tracks 2–4). Importantly, the migration distances of the retained pro type III increase progressively from track 2 to 4, suggesting different degrees of overhydroxylation implying differing mutation sites. By analogy with various osteogenesis imperfecta mutants, we expect the most delayed proα1(III) to be nearest the C terminus relative to the least delayed

In our experience phenocopies of acrogeric Ehlers Danlos syndrome type IV with apparently normal or slightly lowered type III collagen profiles are common. Mutations within the apparently normally migrating protein are very likely and our family mentioned above with the CB5 mutation is a good example. We were encouraged by the clinical phenotype to carry out a linkage study to the type III gene which proved to be positive (Nicholls *et al.*, 1988) (Figure 16). Analysis of the purified protein then allowed accurate genetic mapping.

Analysis of defects in the common intracellular retention mutants is difficult, probably because the mutations are small (and must therefore be undetectable with conventional Southern and Northern blotting). The most profitable approach to these types of mutations will come from the rapid analysis of small point mutations or deletions using appropriate cDNA or genomic markers for the cloned type III gene to carry out S1 nuclease (Kuivaniemi *et al.*, 1988), or RNAse A mapping (Grange *et al.*, 1988). This, combined with oligonucleotide primed polymerase chain reaction amplified DNA, theoretically leads to the rapid automated sequencing of amplified DNA (Prockop, 1988, personal communication). Mutants previously analysed over months or years will probably be characterized in days or weeks.

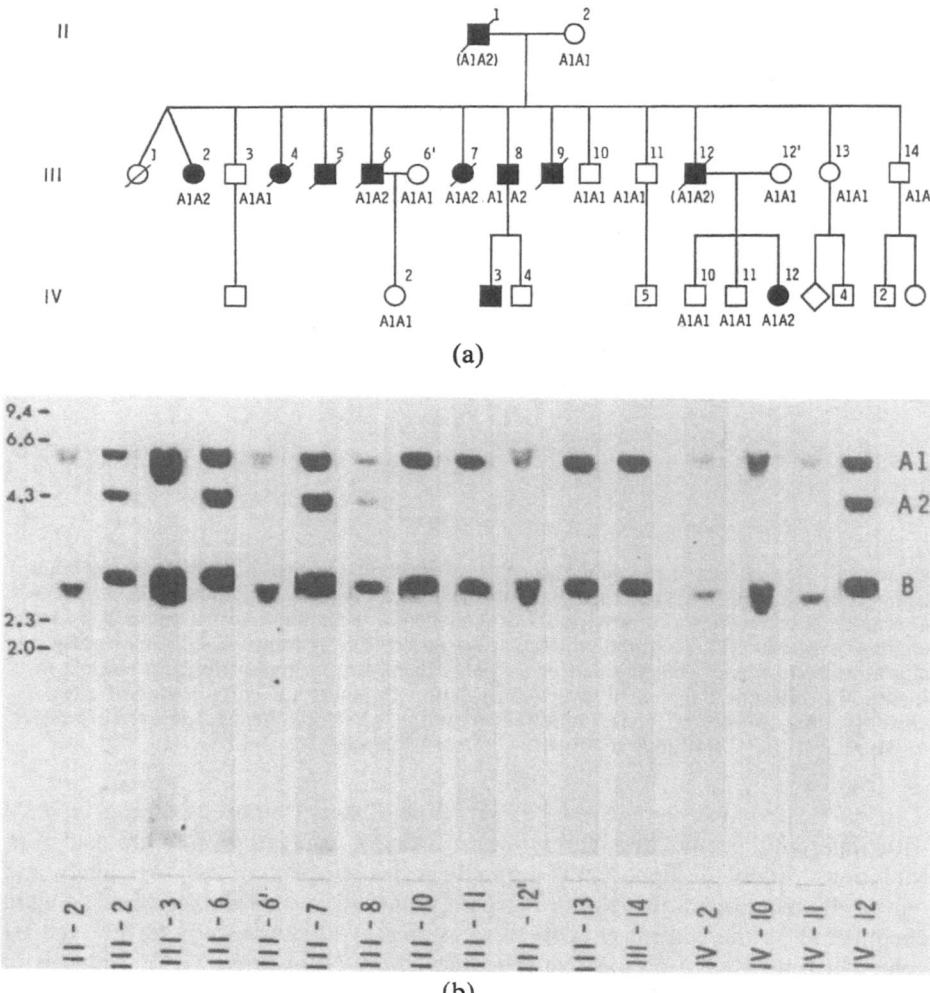

Figure 16 (a) Pedigree of affected three generation family with Ehlers Danlos syndrome type IV and arterial aneurysms; (b) Southern blotting experiments show segregation of the α2 allele with the disease

Similar considerations will equally well apply to other type III mutations other than Ehlers Danlos syndrome type IV. These include annular aortic ectasia, type III deficient Ehlers Danlos syndrome type III, some patients with Ehlers Danlos syndrome type I and substantial numbers of sporadic cerebral aneurysms of the Circle of Willis. The latter cause 4000 deaths per annum in young or middle-aged adults in the UK and occur in 2% of postmortem examinations.

DEFECTS OF OTHER COLLAGENS

Type II collagen is the main collageneous component of cartilage which also contains collagens VI, IX and X depending upon its precise anatomical site and function. Type II collagen has been cloned and partially sequenced (Weiss *et al.*, 1982) and a number of gene probes and RFLPs have been identified and characterized (Pope *et al.*, 1984; Stoker *et al.*, 1985; Sykes *et al.*, 1985, 1988b). Evidence for gene linkage of the α1(II) gene to various relevant inherited chondrodysplasias has produced somewhat contradictory evidence. Wordsworth and colleagues (1988) have summarized the British position and have observed discordant segregation between the α1(II) gene (COL2A1) and the following diseases: achondroplasia, pseudo-achondroplasia (McKusick 17115, 17117, 26415, 26416), hypochondroplasia (McKusick 14600), multiple epiphyseal dysplasia (McKusick 13243), autosomal recessive spondyloepiphyseal dysplasia tarda (McKusick 27160, 27163), diaphyseal aclasis (McKusick 13370) and the trichorhinophalangeal syndrome (McKusick 19035, 27550). He did not have informative pedigrees with autosomal dominant spondyloepiphyseal dysplasia tarda (McKusick 18410) or metaphyseal chondrodysplasia (McKusick 25040, 25022–5) but concluded that collagen type II gene defects were uncommon in the heritable chondrodysplasias. American groups examining similar patients with comparable gene probes have had somewhat different experiences in several diseases. Francamono and her colleagues (1988) have studied in detail eight families with the Stickler syndrome (McKusick 10830). They found definite linkage to the cartilage α1(II) gene RFLPs in four of them and excluded linkage in two families, two others being uninformative. The same authors have also found abnormalities of α1(II) gene markers in Kniest disease (McKusick 24519) and very recently have reported a 3 kb unique deletion localized to exon 19 of the α1(II) gene in a patient with spondyloepiphyseal dysplasia congenita (McKusick 18390) (Lumadue *et al.*, 1988). This latter observation is interesting especially in view of the observation of Wordsworth and his colleagues of weakly positive lod scores in spondyloepiphyseal dysplasia congenita, spondylometaphyseal dysplasia and diastrophic dysplasia and does quite strongly hint that certain inherited chondrodysplasias with significant cartilage pathology have actual structural abnormalities of their α1(II) gene structure.

No doubt such abnormalities are heterogeneous but significant cartilage gene involvement is likely in at least some of them. Of course, the several other cartilage gene components will also need exclusion as relevant or irrelevant to disease causation. There are also hints that type II collagen defects occur more commonly than expected in patients with osteoarthritis. Clear linkage was detected in a large Finnish family with inherited osteoarthritis and RFLPs for the α1(II) gene (Vaisanen *et al.*, 1986). One major impediment to better understanding of the various chondrodysplasias and also osteoarthritis has been the difficulties in characterizing cartilage chondrocytes by culturing chondrocytes which unfortunately revert to a fibroblastic phenotype after relatively few passages. To some extent this has now been overcome, by culturing chrondrocytes in agar suspension (Horton *et al.*, 1988). Under these circumstances they retain their cartilaginous phenotype so allowing the potential for detailed protein analysis, as has proved so successful in inherited diseases of arteries and bones. Although cartilaginous proteins can certainly be successfully extracted and characterized in tissues, this approach has the drawback that intracellular non-exported mutants would not be identified by this technique, which would detect only alterations of secreted protein (probably due to point mutations, deletions or insertions).

Basement membrane specific and associated collagens such as types IV and VII are likely to be very important in disorders of epithelial stromal interactions; particularly the dermo-epidermal type VII collagen, which is closely associated with the physical adhesion of the epidermis to the dermis, as it connects the lamina lucida of basement membrane to underlying interstitial collagen fibrils (Briggaman *et al.*, 1971; Lunstrum *et al.*, 1986). Similarly type IV collagen is localized to the lamina lucida of basement membrane. The type VII collagen protein is concentrated in distinctive cross-striated anchoring fibrils which are easily detectable by electron microscopical examination of stratified squamous epithelium (Figure 17). Type VII collagen antibodies brightly fluoresce in normal skin but such staining is missing from sections of autosomal recessive dystrophic epidermolysis bullosa skin (Eady, 1987). Some patients with autosomal recessive epidermolysis bullosa also have elevated human collagenase levels whereas other do not. In those that do the disappearance of anchoring fibrils might be a secondary effect.

So far no obvious diseases have been recognized with abnormalities of collagens VI, VIII, IX and X, although they form substantial components of skin, arterial walls and cartilage. Certainly, previously unexplained abnormalities affecting skin, tendons and cartilage could sometimes be explained by type VI collagen abnormalities (some forms of spondyloepiphyseal dysplasias are good examples). Similarly, other more cartilage-localized dysplasias could be associated with collagens VI, IX and X and vascular abnormalities in which type III defects have been excluded are candidates for type VI and VIII abnormalities. There are also strong possibilities of interactions between various collagen types so that theoretically similar phenotypes may be caused by abnormalities of very different collageneous (and non-collageneous) components. The clinical variabilities of inherited defects of connective tissue are so diverse that such interactions and phenocopies are likely to be the rule rather than the exception.

RESTRICTION FRAGMENT LENGTH POLYMORPHISMS (RFLPs)

Common, random variations in DNA sequence which lie close to particular genes (or even within them) are very useful markers for gene linkage studies. They are usually sufficiently close to candidate genes of interest to segregate with them (usually) and therefore minimize meiotic cross-overs. The *HpaI* variable site which detects 75% of black Americans with the sickle cell mutation 1423, 4800 was the first to be detected and is an excellent example. It was very quickly realized that as few as 200 gene markers might be sufficient to map most important human genes and also it was quickly apparent that RFLPs dispersed sufficiently widely could be used to map the genes for specific human (and animal) diseases. This technique is

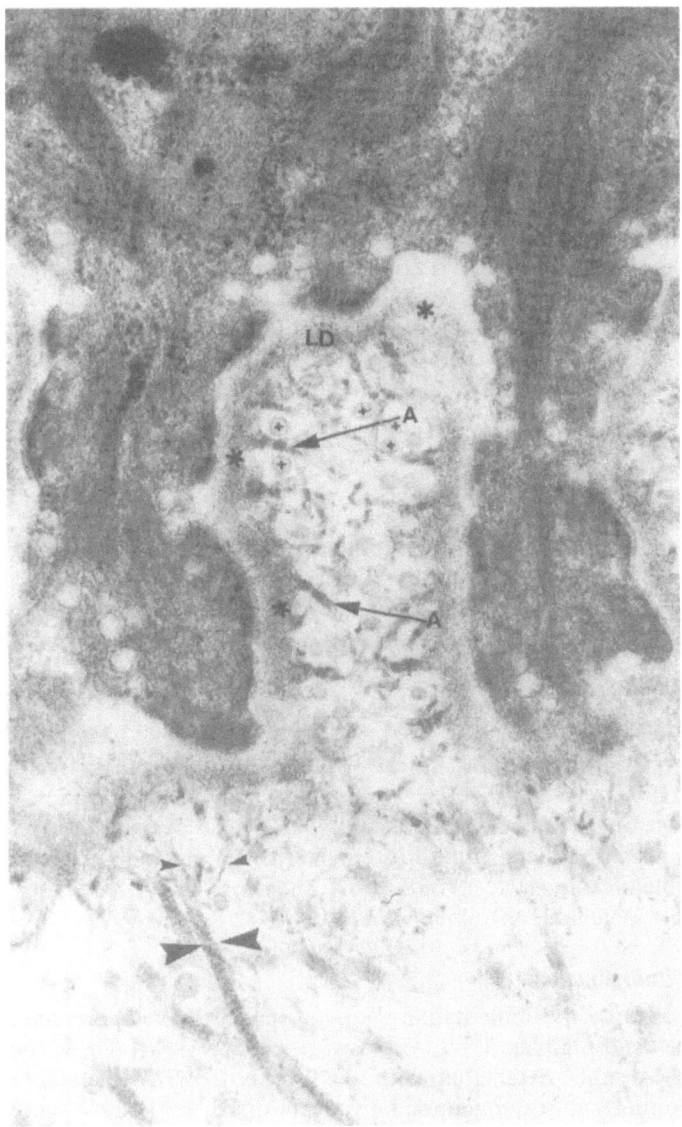

Figure 17 Electron micrograph of junctional zone of single epidermal cell and underlying basal stroma. This clearly shows the lamina densa of basement membrane (starred and labelled LD), associated with anchoring fibrils (arrowed A). These are closely associated with reticular dermal interstitial collagen fibrils (seen here in transverse section and indicated with crosses). Dermally, extensions of the anchoring fibrils (small arrowheads) are in close association with underlying interstitial fibrils (large arrowheads) (×36000). With kind permission of Dr Pat Fryer

called reverse genetics – find a gene marker closely linked with a disease then move ('walk') from the marker to the responsible gene.

Collagen-related RFLPs are used to map inherited defects of collagen in a similar fashion to the haemoglobinopathies (i.e. as markers in families with diseases for which the mutant gene has already been identified). They can also be used in the reverse genetics way to identify the chromosomal location for which the candidate gene or protein is so far unidentified but in which a connective tissue abnormality is very likely. Good examples would be the Marfan syndrome (McKusick 15470), pseudo-xanthoma elasticum (McKusick 17785, 17786, 26480, 26481), inherited aneurysms not linked to type III collagen mutations and those chondrodystrophies in which type II cartilage gene linkage has been excluded. Prenatal diagnosis using RFLPs would be possible in any autosomal dominant or recessive disorder of type I or III collagen and has already been successfully achieved in certain families with osteogenesis imperfecta and Ehlers Danlos syndrome type VI.

TYPE I COLLAGEN GENES

α1(I) polymorphisms

Although these have been difficult to identify, Sykes and his colleagues have now characterized an *MspI* RFLP 30 kb 5' of the gene and an intragenic *RsaI* variable site 10 kb 3' of the gene. So far these markers have been associated with classical autosomal dominant Sillence types I and IV osteogenesis imperfecta (Sykes *et al.*, 1988b).

α2(I) polymorphisms

These were identified earlier, more easily and in greater numbers than the α1(I) markers. *EcoR1* and *Msp1* RFLPs are well known at the 5' end of this gene and have been strongly linked with Sillence type IV osteogenesis imperfecta but also some patients with Sillence type I osteogenesis imperfecta (Tsipouras Myers *et al.*, 1983; Grobler-Rabie *et al.*, 1985). *BglII* and *EcoR1* RFLPs at the 3' end of the gene are also available (Brebner *et al.*, 1985).

α1(II) polymorphisms

Several intragenic and some flanking polymorphisms have been recognized for this gene (Sykes and Ogilvie, 1965; Wordsworth *et al.*, 1988). These include *HindIII* and *PvuII* variants detectable with the 9.2 kb *EcoR1* subclone which do not segregate either with osteogenesis imperfecta or Ehlers Danlos syndrome type II. The *HindIII* RFLP has been tightly linked to familial osteoarthritis (McKusick 16570) in a large autosomal dominant Finnish pedigree (Vaisanen *et al.*, 1986). There is a *BamH1* intragenic RFLP which appears twice as commonly in Caucasian patients with early osteoarthrosis as in a control population (24% compared with 10%) (Hull *et al.*, 1985). Furthermore there is definite linkage of the *HindIII* and *PvuII* RFLPs to some families with Stickler syndrome in which there is abnormal epiphyseal development, loose jointedness, retinal detachment and myopia (Francamono *et al.*, 1988). Other families were unlinked to the gene. Gene linkage has also been observed in the Kniest syndrome where myopia, retinal detachment and large epiphyses occur. Also a gene deletion has been detected in a single patient with spondyloepiphyseal dysplasia congenita (see earlier) (Lumadue *et al.*, 1980). This evidence therefore strongly suggests a pathological role for the cartilage collagen α1(II) gene in the mechanism of at least some forms of degenerative joint disease.

A very variable *EcoR1/BamH1* polymorphic deletion detectable with the 4.3 kb *EcoR1* subclone which includes 3′ flanking regions of the gene shows an unique satellite hypervariable deletion in a unusual repetitive region close hypervariable deletion in an unusual repetitive region close to the gene. This produces deletions and duplications in mutiples of 30 bp and population frequencies varying at least to some extent with racial origin (Stoker *et al.*, 1986).

α1(III) markers

An *EcoRl* RFLP in a 2.1 kb *EcoRl* fragment close to the 3′ end of the gene produces a two allele polymorphism with a variant 1.6 kb band (Byers *et al.*, 1986). An *AvaII* RFLP maps to the flanking region of this gene and is detectable with a cDNA probe for this region (Dalgleish *et al.*, 1985). The *EcoRl* RFLP successfully detected linkage to the gene in two American families with Ehlers Danlos syndrome type IV. We have used the *AvaII* RFLP to establish linkage of the disease to the type III gene in a large Belgian pedigree with familial aneurysmal Ehlers Danlos syndrome type IV but a relatively normal protein profile. This both identifies and confirms the type III gene as the mutant locus and provides a prenatal marker for the diseased gene (Nicholls *et al.*, 1988).

Type VI RFLPs

Genes for the α1, α2 and α3 type VI collagens have been cloned and partially sequenced. The α1 and α2 chains are located on chromosome 2 and the α3 chain on chromosome 2. Well away from type III and type V collagens RFLPs have just been identified (Weaver *et al.*, 1988) and are not linked to the Marfan syndrome (Cutting *et al.*, 1988). Other important candidate diseases have already been mentioned on page 164.

CONCLUSION

Human genes with collagen sequences have been identified on chromosomes 1 and 6 but so far have not been further characterized in detail. Still others such as human α1(V), α1(VII), α1(IX) and α1(X) await cloning and chromosome assignment. The prenatal diagnosis and prevention of all those particular molecular defects described above is already feasible although not yet a reality. We can expect steady progress in the prenatal diagnosis, prevention and genetic counselling of common and rare collagen mutations. These include osteogenesis imperfecta, some osteoporoses, the arterial form of Ehlers Danlos syndrome, berry and aortic aneurysms, Stickler syndrome, Kniest disease, spondyloepiphyseal dysplasia congenita and some forms of familial common osteoarthritis. Other disorders of connective tissue in which specific defects have not yet been recognized include Ehlers Danlos syndrome other than types IV, VI and VII, the Marfan syndrome, some forms of osteogenesis imperfecta, various chondrodystrophies other than those mentioned above, Cutis laxa of various types and common forms of joint hypermobility. We can confidently expect identifiable defects in many of them to become recognized and delineated within the near future.

REFERENCES

Barsh, G. S. and Byers, P. H. Abnormal secretion of type I procollagen in a variety of osteogenesis imperfecta. *Proc. Natl. Acad. Sci. USA* 8 (1981) 5142–5146

Barsh, G. S., David, K. and Byers, P. H. Type 1 osteogenesis imperfecta; a non-functional allele for pro α1(I) chains of type I procollagen. *Proc. Natl. Acad. Sci. USA* 79 (1982) 3838–3842

Barsh, G. S., Roush, C., Bonadio, J. *et al.* Intron mediated recombination may cause a deletion in an α1(I) collagen chain in a lethal form of osteogenesis imperfecta. *Proc. Natl. Acad. Sci. USA* 82 (1985) 2870–2874

Bateman, J. F., Chan, D., Walker, I. D. *et al.* Lethal perinatal osteogenesis imperfecta due to a substitution of arginine for glycine at residue 391 of the α1(I) chain of type I collagen. *J. Biol. Chem.* 262 (1987) 7021–7027

Bateman, J. F., Lamande, S. R., Dahl, H-H. M. *et al.* Substitution of arginine for glycine 664 in the collagen α1 chain in lethal perinatal OI. *J. Biol. Chem.* 263 (1988) 11625–11630

Bentz, H., Morris, N. P., Murray, L. W. *et al.* Isolation and partial characterization of a new human collagen with an extended triple-helical structural domain. *Proc. Natl. Acad. Sci. USA* 80 (1983) 3168–3172

Bonadio, J. F. and Byers, P. H. Subtle structural alterations in the chains of type I procollagen produce osteogenesis imperfecta type II. *Nature (London)* 316 (1985) 363–366

Boyd, C. C., Tolstoshev, P., Schafer, M. P. *et al.* Isolation and characterisation of a 15 kilobase genomic sequence coding for part of the pro α2 chain of sheep type I collagen. *J. Biol. Chem.* 225 (1980) 3212–3220

Brebner, D. K. and Rabie, A. F. Two new polymorphic markers in the human pro α2(I) collagen gene. *Human Genet.* 70 (1985) 25–27

Briggaman, R. A., Daldorf, F. G. and Wheeler, C. E. Formation and origin of basal lamina and anchoring fibrils in adult human skin. *J. Cell Biol.* 51 (1971) 384–395

Byers, P. H., Siegel, R. C., Peterson, K. E. *et al.* Marfan syndrome: abnormal α2 chain in type I collagen. *Proc. Natl. Acad. Sci. USA* 78 (1981) 7745–7749

Byers, P. H., Starman, B. J., Cohn, D. J. and Horwitz, A. L. A novel mutation causes a perinatal lethal form of osteogenesis imperfecta. *J. Biol. Chem.* 263 (1988a) 7855–7861

Byers, P. H., Tsipouras, P., Bonadio, J. F., Starman, B. J. and Schwartz, R. C. Perinatal lethal osteogenesis imperfecta (OI type II): a biochemically heterogeneous disorder usually due to new mutations in the genes for type I collagen. *Am. J. Hum. Genet.* 42 (1988b) 237–248

Chu, M-L., Williams, C. J., Pepe, G. *et al.* Internal deletion in a collagen gene in a perinatal lethal form of osteogenesis imperfecta. *Nature (London)* 304 (1983) 78–80

Chu, M-L., de Wet, W., Bernard, M. *et al.* Human pro α1(I) collagen gene structure reveals evolutionary conversion of a pattern of introns and exons. *Nature (London)* 310 (1984) 337–340

Chu, M-L., Garguilo, V., Williams, D. J. *et al.* Multiexon deletion in an osteogenesis imperfecta variant with increased type III collagen mRNA. *J. Biol. Chem.* 260 (1985a) 691–694

Chu, M-L., Weil, D., de Wet, W. *et al.* Isolation of cDNA and genomic clones encoding human pro α1(III) collagen. *J. Biol. Chem.* 260 (1985b) 4357–4363

Cohn, D. H., Byers, P. H., Steinmann, B. *et al.* Lethal osteogenesis imperfecta resulting from a single nucleotide change in one human pro α1(I) collagen allele. *Proc. Natl. Acad. Sci. USA* 83 (1986) 6045–6047

Cohn, D. H., Apone, S., Eyre, D. R., Starman, B. J., Andreassen, P., Charbonneau, H., Nicholls, A. C., Pope, F. M. and Byers, P. H. Substitution of cysteine for glycine within the carboxyl terminal telopeptide of the α1 chain of type I collagen produces mild osteogenesis imperfecta. *J. Biol. Chem.* 263 (1988a) 14605–14607

Cohn, D. H., Wenstrup, R. J., Willing, M. C. *et al.* General strategies for isolating the genes encoding type I collagen and for characterising mutations which produce osteogenesis imperfecta. *IIIrd International Conference on osteogenesis imperfecta*, Pavia, Italy, September 1987 (in press). *Ann. NY Acad. Sci.* (1988b)

Cole, W. G., Chan, D., Chamber, G. W. *et al.* Deletion of 24 aminoacids from the pro α1(I) chain of type I procollagen in a patient with the Ehlers Danlos syndrome type VII. *J. Biol. Chem.* 261 (1986) 5496–5503

Constantinou, G. D., Nielsen, K. B. and Prockop, D. J. A lethal variant of osteogenesis imperfecta has a single base mutation that substitutes cysteine for glycine 904 of the α1(I) chain of type I procollagen. The asymptomatic mother has an unidentified mutation producing an over-modified and unstable type I procollagen. *J. Clin. Invest.* (1988) (in press)

Cutting, G., Francomano, C. A., Chu, M. L., Timpl, M. K., McCormick, A. C., Warren, A. C., Hong, H. K., Pyeritz, R. E. and Antonarakis, S. E. Genetic linkage analysis and macrorestriction mapping of COL6A1 and COL 6A2 structural genes of type VI collagen. *Am. J. Hum. Genet.* 43 (1988) Suppl. pA141

D'Alessio, M., Weil, D., Prince, J., Bateman, J., Cole, W., Hollister, D. and Ramirez, F. Differential expression of splicing mutations in the two type I procollagen genes. *Am. J. Hum. Genet.* 43 (1988) Suppl. p A141

Dalgleish, R., Woodhouse, M. and Reeders, S. An RFLP associated with the human type III collagen gene. *Nucleic Acids Res.* 13 (1985) 4609

Daw, S., Nicholls, A. C., Williams, E. M. *et al.* Autosomal recessive osteogenesis imperfecta. Excess post transitional modification of collagen but linked to either CollA1 or CollA2. *J. Med. Genet.* 25 (1988) 275

Deak, S. B., Nicholls, A. C., Pope, F. M. *et al.* The molecular defect in a non lethal variant of osteogenesis imperfecta. *J. Biol. Chem.* 258 (1983) 15192–15197

Dieppe, P. Osteoarthritis and related disorders. *Oxford Textbook of Medicine*, Oxford University Press, Oxford, Melbourne and New York, 1987, 2nd edn., Vol. II, p. 76

De Vries, W. N. and De Wet, W. J. The molecular defect in an autosomal dominant form of osteogenesis imperfecta: synthesis of type I procollagen containing cysteine in the triple helical domain of pro-α1(I) chains. *J. Biol. Chem.* 261 (1986) 9056–9064

Eady, R. A. J. Rashes, blisters and basement membranes. *Clin. Exp. Dermatol.* 12 (1987) 159–170

Eyre, D. R., Shapiro, F. D. and Aldridge, J. F. A heterozygous collagen defect in a variant of the Ehlers Danlos syndrome type VII. *J. Biol. Chem.* 260 (1985) 11322–11329

Epstein, E. H. Jr. α1(III)$_3$ human skin collagen: release by pepsin digestion and preponderance in fetal life. *J. Biol. Chem.* 249 (1974) 3225–3229

Fox, R., Pope, F. M., Narcisi, P., Nicholls, A. C., Kendall, B. E., Hourihan, M. D. and Compston, D. A. S. Spontaneous carotid cavernous fistula in Ehlers–Danlos syndrome. *J. Neurol. Neurosurg. Psychiatr.* 51 (1988) 984–986

Frischauf, A. M., Lehrach, H., Rosner, C. *et al.* Procollagen complementary DNA: a probe for messenger RNA purification and the number of type I collagen genes. *Biochemistry* 17 (1978) 3243–3249

Francomano, C. A., Rowan, B. G., Liberfarb, R. M., Hirose, T., Maumenee, C. H., Stoll, H. U. and Pyeritz, R. E. The Stickler and Wagner syndromes: evidence for genetic heterogeneity. *Am. J. Hum. Genet.* 43 (1988) Suppl. p A83

Grange, D. K., Gottesman, G. S. and Marini, J. C. Detection of point mutations in type I collagen mRNA: application of an RNA/RNA hybrid system in osteogenesis imperfecta. *Am. J. Hum. Genet.* 43 (1988) Suppl. p. A85

Grobler-Rabie, A. F., Brebner, D. K., Vandenplas, S. *et al.* Polymorphism of DNA sequence in the pro α2(I) collagen gene. *J. Med. Genet.* 22 (1985) 182–186

Horton, W. A., Aulthouse, A. L., Marchado, M. A. *et al. In vitro* studies of chondrocyte differentiation in the human chondrodysplasia (Abst.) *J. Med. Genet.* 25 (1988) 276

Hull, R. G., McPheat, J., Cheetham, J. E. *et al.* An apparent collagen type II gene polymorphism in some patients with osteoarthrosis. *J. Rheumatol.* 25 (1986) 120

Jensen, G. F., Christiansen, C., Boesen, J. *et al.* Epidemiology of post menopausal spinal and long bone fractures: a unifying approach to post menopausal osteoporosis. *Clin. Orthopaedics Related Res.* 166 (1982) 75–81

Kuivaniemi, H., Sabol, C., Tromp, G., Sippola-Thiele, M. and Prockop, D. J. A 19-base pair deletion in the pro-α2(I) gene of type I procollagen that causes in-frame RNA splicing from exon 10 to exon 12 in a proband with atypical osteogenesis imperfecta and in his asymptomatic mother. *J. Biol. Chem.* 263 (1988) 11407–11413

Lenaers, A., Ansay, M., Nusgens, B. V. *et al.* Collagen made of extended α chain procollagens in genetically defective dermatosparactic calves. *Eur. J. Biochem.* 23 (1971) 533–543

Lewis, A. F. Fracture of neck of femur: changes in incidence. *Br. Med. J.* 283 (1981) 1217–1220

Lichtenstein, J. R., Martin, G. R., Kohn, L. D. *et al.* Defect in conversion of procollagen in a form of Ehlers Danlos syndrome. *Science* 182 (1974) 298–300

Lumadue, J., Rowan, B. G. and Francomano, C. A. Structural alteration of the type II collagen gene in an individual with spondyloepiphyseal dysplasia congenita. *Am. J. Hum. Genet.* 43 (1988) Suppl. p. A193

Lunstrum, G. P., Sakai, L. Y., Keene, D. B. *et al.* Large complex globular domains of type VII procollagen contribute to the structure of anchoring fibrils. *J. Biol. Chem.* 261 (1986) 9042–9048

McKusick, V. A. *Heritable Disorders of Connective Tissue*, CV Mosby, St. Louis, 1972, pp. 740–856

McKusick, V. A. *Mendelian Inheritance in Man. Catalogs of Autosomal Dominant, Autosomal Recessive and X-linked Phenotypes*, Johns Hopkins University Press Ltd., Baltimore and London, 1988, 8th edn.

Mortality Statistics. Review of Registrar General on Deaths in England and Wales, HMSO, London, 1977, Table 6, p. 29

Myers, J. C., Dickson, L. A., de Wet, W. J. *et al.* Analysis of the 3′ end of the human pro α2(I) collagen gene. *J. Biol. Chem.* 258 (1983) 10128–10135

Myers, J. C., Loidl, H. R., Seyers, J. M. *et al.* Complete primary structure of the human α2 type (V) procollagen COOH-terminal propeptide. *J. Biol. Chem.* 260 (1985) 11216–11222

Narcisi, P., Nicholls, A. C., De Paepe, A. and Pope, F. M. An α1(III) CB5 mutation in Ehlers Danlos syndrome type IV. *J. Med. Genet.* 26 (1989) (in press)

Nicholls, A. C., Craig, D. and Pope, F. M. An abnormal collagen α chain containing cysteine in autosomal dominant osteogenesis imperfecta. *Br. Med. J.* 288 (1984a) 112–113

Nicholls, A. C., Osse, G., Schloon, H. G. *et al.* The clinical features of homozygous α2(I) collagen deficient osteogenesis imperfecta. *J. Med. Genet.* 21 (1984b) 257–262

Nicholls, A. C., De Paepe, A., Narcisi, P. *et al.* Linkage of a polymorphic marker for the type III collagen gene (COL3A1) to atypical autosomal dominant Ehlers Danlos syndrome type IV in a large Belgian pedigree. *Human Genet.* 78 (1988) 276–281

Ninomiya, Y., Gordon, M., van der Rest, M. *et al.* The developmentally regulated type X collagen gene contains a long open reading frame without introns. *J. Biol. Chem.* 261 (1986) 5041–5050

Ogilvie, D. J., Aitchison, K. and Sykes, B. C. An RFLP close to the human collagen I gene COL1A1. *Nucl. Acids Res.* 15 (1987) 4699

Olsen, B. R., Ninomiya, Y., Lozano, G. *et al.* Short chain collagen genes and their expression in cartilage. In Fleischmajer, R., Olsen, B. R. and Kuhn, K. (eds.) *Chemistry and Pathology of Collagen*. Annals of the New York Academy of Sciences, 460, 1985, pp. 141–153

Peltonen, L., Palotie, A. and Prockop, D. J. A defect in the structure of the I procollagen in a patient who had osteogenesis imperfecta: excess mannose in the COOH-terminal propeptide. *Proc. Natl. Acad. Sci. USA* 77 (1980) 6197–6283

Pihlajaneimi, T., Dickson, L. A., Pope, F. M. *et al.* Osteogenesis imperfecta: cloning of a pro-α2(I) collagen gene with a frameshift mutation. *J. Biol. Chem.* 259 (1984) 12941–12944

Pope, F. M., Nicholls, A. D., Eggleton, C. *et al.* Osteogenesis imperfecta: lethal bones contain types III and V collagens. *J. Clin. Pathol.* 33 (1980a) 534–538

Pope, F. M., Nicholls, A. C., Jones, P. *et al.* EDS IV (acrogeria) is heterogeneous. New autosomal dominant and recessive types. *J. R. Soc. Med.* 73 (1980b) 180–186

Pope, F. M., Nicholls, A. C., Narcisi, P. *et al.* Some patients with cerebral aneurysms are deficient in type III collagen. *Lancet* 1 (1981) 973–974

Pope, F. M., Cheah, K. S. E., Nicholls, A. C. *et al.* Lethal osteogenesis imperfecta congenita and a 300 base pair deletion for an α1(I)-like collagen. *Br. Med. J.* 288 (1984) 431–434

Pope, F. M., Martin, G. R., Lichtenstein, J. R. *et al.* Patients with Ehlers Danlos syndrome type IV lack type III collagen. *Proc. Natl. Acad. Sci. USA* 72 (1985a) 1314–1316

Pope, F. M., Nicholls, A. C., McPheat, J. *et al.* Collagen genes and proteins in osteogenesis imperfecta. *J. Med. Genet.* 22 (1985b) 466–478

Pope, F. M. and Nicholls, A. C. Collagen genes and proteins in human diseases. In Champion, R. H. (ed.) *Recent Advances in Dermatology*, Churchill Livingstone, London, 1986, Vol. 7, pp. 23–52

Pope, F. M., Nicholls, A. C., Lewkonia, R. M. *et al.* Clinical and genetic heterogeneity of the Marfan syndrome. In Wuepper, K. D. and Gedde-Duhl, T. Jr. (eds.) *Current Problems in Dermatology*, Karger, Basel, 1987, Vol. 17, pp. 95–110

Pope, F. M., Narcisi, P., Nicholls, A. C., Liberman, M. and Oorthuys, J. W. E. Clinical presentations of Ehlers Danlos syndrome type IV. *Arch. Dis. Child.* 63 (1988a) 1016–1025

Pope, F. M., Nicholls, A. C., Narcisi, P., Temple, A., Chia, Y., Fryer, P., De Paepe, A., de Groote, W. P., McEwan, J. R., Compston, D. A., Oorthuys, H., Davies, J. and Dinwoodie, D. I. Type III collagen mutations in Ehlers Danlos syndrome type IV and other related disorders. *Clin. Exp. Dermatol.* 13 (1988b) 285–302

Poschl, E., Pollner, R. and Kuhn, K. The genes for the α1(IV) and α2(IV) chains of human basement membrane collagen type IV are arranged head-to-head and separated by a bidirectional promoter of unique structure. *EMBO J.* 7 (1988) 2687–2695

Prockop, D. J. and Kivirikko, K. I. Heritable disorders of collagen. *N. Eng. J. Med.* 311 (1984) 376–386

Prockop, D. J., Chu, M-L., de Wet, W. *et al.* Mutations in osteogenesis imperfecta leading to the synthesis of abnormal type I procollagens. In Fleischmajer, R., Olsen, B. R. and Kuhn, K. (eds.) *Biology, Chemistry and Pathology of Collagen*, Annals of the New York Academy of Sciences, 460, 1985, pp. 289–297

Ramirez, F. Bernard, M., Chu, M-L. *et al.* Isolation and characterisation of the human fibrillar collagen genes. In Fleischmeyer, R. M., Olsen, B. R. and Kuhn, K. (eds.) *Biology, Chemistry and Pathology of Collagen*, Annals of New York Academy of Sciences, 460, 1985, pp. 117–129

Roberts, D. L. L., Pope, F. M., Nicholls, A. C. and Narcisi, P. Ehlers Danlos syndrome type IV mimicking non-accidental injury in a child. *Br. J. Dermatol.* 111 (1984) 341–345

Sage, H., Trueb, B., Bornstein, P. *et al.* Biosynthetic and structural properties of endothelial cell type VIII collagen. *J. Biol. Chem.* 258 (1985) 13391–13401

Sillence, D. O., Senn, A. and Danks, D. M. Genetic heterogeneity in osteogenesis imperfecta. *J. Med. Genet.* 16 (1979) 101–116

Sillence, D. O., Barlow, K. K., Garber, A. P. *et al.* Osteogenesis imperfecta type II. Delineation of the phenotype with reference to genetic heterogeneity. *Am. J. Med. Genet.* 17 (1984) 407–423

Sippola, M., Kaffe, S. and Prockop, D. J. A heterozygous defect for structurally altered PNα2 chain of type I procollagen: a mild variant of osteogenesis imperfecta. *J. Biol. Chem.* 259 (1984) 14094–14200

Stacey, A., Bateman, J., Choi, T. *et al.* Perinatal lethal osteogenesis imperfecta in transgenic mice bearing an engineered mutant pro-α1(I) collagen gene. *Nature (London)* 332 (1988) 131–136

Steinmann, B., Rao, V. H., Vogel, A. *et al.* Cysteine in the triple-helical domain of one allelic product of the α1(I) gene of type I collagen produces a lethal form of osteogenesis imperfecta. *J. Biol. Chem.* 289 (1984) 11129–11138

Steinmann, B., Nicholls, A. and Pope, F. M. Clinical variability of osteogenesis imperfecta reflecting molecular heterogeneity: cysteine substitutions in the α1(I) collagen chain producing lethal and mild forms. *J. Biol. Chem.* 261 (1986) 8958–8964

Stewart, R. E., Hollister, D. W. and Rimoin, D. L. A new variant of Ehlers Danlos syndrome: an autosomal dominant disorder of fragile skin, abnormal scarring and generalised periodontitis. *Birth Defects Original Article Series XIII*, 1977, 3B, pp. 85–93, The National Foundation

Stoker, N. G., Cheah, K. S. E., Griffin, J. R. *et al.* A highly polymorphic region 3' to the human type II collagen gene. *Nucl. Acids Res.* 13 (1985) 4613–4622

Stolle, C. A., Pyeritz, R. E., Myers, J. C. *et al.* Synthesis of an altered type III procollagen in a patient with Type IV Ehlers Danlos syndrome. *J. Biol. Chem.* 260 (1985) 1937–1944

Superti-Furga, A., Gitzelmann, R. and Steinmann, B. Dominant Ehlers-Danlos syndrome type IV caused by a shortened mRNA for type III collagen. *J. Med. Genet.* 24 (1987) 636

Superti-Furga, A., Gugler, E., Gitzelmann, R. and Steinmann, B. Ehlers-Danlos syndrome type IV: a multi-exon deletion in one of the two COLA31 alleles affecting structure, stability, and processing of Type III procollagen. *J. Biol. Chem.* 263 (1988) 6226–6232

Sykes, B. and Ogilvie, D. Lethal osteogenesis imperfecta. Is the collagen gene deletion a normal variant rather than a causal mutation? *J. Med. Genet.* 22 (1985) 138

Sykes, B., Ogilvie, D., Wordsworth, P. *et al.* Osteogenesis imperfecta is linked to both type I collagen structural genes. *Lancet* 2 (1986) 69–72

Sykes, B. C., Ogilvie, D. J., Wordsworth, D. P. *et al.* Evidence against the structural gene encoding type II collagen (COL2A1) as the mutant locus in achondroplasia. *J. Med. Genet.* 22 (1988a) 394

Sykes, B., Smith, R., Vipond, S. *et al.* Exclusion of the α1(II) cartilage collagen gene as the mutant locus in type 1a osteogenesis imperfecta. *J. Med. Genet.* 22 (1988b) 187–197

Thompson, E. M., Young, I. D., Hal, C. M. *et al.* Osteogenesis imperfecta. *J. Med. Genet.* 16 (1987) 101–111

Tidman, M. J. and Eady, R. A. J. Evaluation of anchoring fibrils and other components of the dermal–epidermal junction in dystrophic epidermolysis bullosa by a quantitative ultrastructural technique. *J. Invest. Dermatol.* 84 (1988) 374–377

Timpl, R., Oberbaumer, I., Von der Mark, H. *et al.* Structure and biology of the globular domain of basement membrane type IV collagen. In Fleischmajer, R., Olsen, B. R. and Kuhn, K. (eds.) *Biology, Chemistry and Pathology of Collagen*, Annals of New York Academy of Science, 460, 1985, pp. 58–73

Tsipouras, P., Myers, J. C., Ramirez, F. *et al.* Restriction fragment length polymorphism ascribed with the proα1(I) gene of human type I procollagen. Application to a family with an autosomal dominant form of osteogenesis imperfecta. *J. Clin. Invest.* 72 (1982) 1262–1267

Tsipouras, P., Byers, P. H. and Schwartz, R. C. Elhers Danlos syndrome type IV: cosegregation of the phenotype to a COL3A1 allele of type III procollagen. *Human Genet.* 74 (1986) 41–46

Tsipouras, P. and Ramirez, F. Genetic disorders of collagen. *J. Med. Genet.* 24 (1987) 2–8

Vaisanen, P., Elima, K., Palotie, A. *et al.* Studies on RFLPs related to type II collagen gene in Finnish population. Abstract SII.4, *7th International Congress in Human Genetics*, Berlin, 1986

Vogel, B. E., Minor, R. R., Freund, M. *et al.* A point mutation in a type I procollagen gene converts glycine 748 of the α1 chain to cysteine and destabilises the triple helix in a lethal variant of osteogenesis imperfecta. *J. Biol. Chem.* 262 (1987) 14737–14744

Vogel, B. E., Doelz, R., Kadler, K. E., Hojima, Y., Engel, J. and Prockop D. J. A substitution of cysteine for glycine 748 of the α1 chain produces a kink at this site in the procollagen I molecule and an altered *N*-proteinase cleavage site over 225 nm away. *J. Biol. Chem.* 263 (1988) 19249–19255

Weaver, E. J., Chu, M-L. and Knowlton, R. G. Bgl I polymorphism in the type VI (α3) procollagen gene [Cr1 6A3]. *Nucl. Acids Res.* 16 (1988) 11386

Weil, D., Bernard, M., Combates, N., Wirtz, M. K., Hollister, D. W., Steinmann, B. and Ramirez, F. Identification of a mutation that causes exon skipping during collagen pre-mRNA splicing in an Ehlers Danlos syndrome variant. *J. Biol. Chem.* 263 (1988) 8561–8564

Weiss, E. H., Cheah, K. S. U., Grosveld, F. G. *et al.* Isolation and characterisation of a human collagen α1(I)-like gene from a cosmid library. *Nucl. Acids Res.* 10 (1982) 1981–1994

Williams, E. M., Nicholls, A. C., Daw, S. C. M., Mitchell, N., Levin, L. S., Green, B., MacKenzie, J., Evans, D. R., Chudleigh, P. A. and Pope, F. M. Phenotypical features of a unique Irish family with severe autosomal recessive osteogenesis imperfecta. *Clin. Genet.* 35 (1989) 181–190

Willing, M. C., Cohn, D. H., Starman, B. J. *et al.* Heterozygosity for a large deletion in the α2(I) collagen gene has a dramatic effect on type in collagen secretion and produces perinatal lethal osteogenesis imperfecta. *J. Biol. Chem.* 263 (1988) 8398–8404

Wordsworth, P., Ogilvie, D., Priestly, L., Smith, R., Wynne-Davies, R. and Sykes, B. Structural and segregation analysis of the type II collagen gene (COL2A1) in some heritable chondrodysplasias. *J. Med. Genet.* 25 (1988) 521–527

Wozney, J., Hanahan, D., Tate, V. *et al.* Structure of the pro α2(I) collagen gene. *Nature (London)* 294 (1981) 129–135

J. Inher. Metab. Dis. 12 Suppl. 1 (1989) 174–190

Prenatal Diagnosis of Duchenne Muscular Dystrophy: A Three-year Experience in a Rapidly Evolving Field

E. Bakker, E. J. Bonten, H. Veenema, J. T. den Dunnen,
P. M. Grootscholten, G. J. B. van Ommen and P. L. Pearson
*Department of Human Genetics, Sylvius Laboratories, Wassenaarseweg 72,
2333 AL Leiden, The Netherlands*

Summary: Application of molecular genetic techniques has greatly increased diagnostic possibilities of hereditary disorders. In 1983 the first linkage of Duchenne muscular dystrophy with flanking DNA probes was described, which made carrier detection possible in a limited number of cases. The first published prenatal diagnosis for Duchenne muscular dystrophy dates from 1985. DNA-analysis for Duchenne muscular dystrophy and Becker muscular dystrophy has become increasingly informative, firstly by the development of more flanking markers, followed by intragenic probes detecting deletions and, more recently, by the use of cDNA probes detecting a deletion or duplication mutation in over 60% of the Duchenne and Becker muscular dystrophy patients. Although these developments allow a highly reliable (>99%) carrier detection and prenatal diagnosis in over 90% of cases, the continuing introduction of new probes and/or technologies has necessitated constant reappraisal of many families to derive maximum information. During the past 3 years we applied prenatal diagnosis for Duchenne and Becker muscular dystrophies with DNA-analysis on 53 male fetuses in 47 families. Twenty-two healthy male babies were born, after being diagnosed to have a low Duchenne muscular dystrophy risk. Two pregnancies also diagnosed as low risk have not yet come to term. In the other cases a high risk for Duchenne muscular dystrophy was found and the parents chose abortion. Our studies also revealed a number of important diagnostic pitfalls, such as non-paternity, karyotypic anomalies and gonadal mosaicism.

DUCHENNE AND BECKER MUSCULAR DYSTROPHIES

Duchenne muscular dystrophy (McKusick 31020) is a lethal, recessive, X-linked neuromuscular disorder. In affected boys the first symptoms are usually observed in early childhood (2–4 years). Pseudohypertrophy of the calves is typically combined with a waddling gait, tendency to fall and a positive Gowers' sign (climbing up their legs) while getting up from a seated position. At the end of the first decade the patients lose the ability to walk and most of them will die before the age of 20

174

Journal of Inherited Metabolic Disease. ISSN 0141–8955. Copyright © SSIEM and Kluwer Academic Publishers, PO Box 55, Lancaster, UK.

(for review see Emery, 1987). The population frequency of Duchenne muscular dystrophy is one in approximately 3–4000 boys. Assuming that the male and female mutation rate for recessive X-linked lethal disorders is equal and that the reproductive viability of the patients is virtually zero, one third of all patients should result from a new mutation (Haldane's rule). This is in agreement with the observed high mutation rate for the Duchenne muscular dystrophy gene which is about 1 in 10^4 in all Western countries.

Becker muscular dystrophy (McKusick 31010) which is about five- to eight-fold less frequent than Duchenne's form, has a later age of onset. It was first thought to be non-allelic with Duchenne muscular dystrophy, but, as we now know, it is also caused by the same defective gene (Kingston *et al.*, 1983, Kunkel *et al.*, 1986; Monaco *et al.*, 1988). An indirect marker for Duchenne muscular dystrophy is the strongly-elevated creatine kinase concentration in the patient's blood. Two-thirds of the obligate carriers of Duchenne muscular dystrophy have an elevated creatine kinase concentration as well. Carrier detection based on repeatedly elevated creatine kinase concentration has until the DNA-analysis was introduced in 1985, been the only possible carrier detection test but it results in approximately 40% false negative results (Bullock *et al.*, 1979).

DNA RESEARCH IN AN EVOLVING FIELD

Reversed genetics, or the cloning of a gene with unknown function, can be applied to all those monogenic hereditary disorders for which the chromosomal localization is found by linkage analysis or the close association of a specific chromosome rearrangement in disease patients. For example the gene for Duchenne muscular dystrophy was shown to be located on the middle of the short arm of the X-chromosome by cytogenetic studies of various X/autosome translocations observed in female Duchenne muscular dystrophy patients (for review see Boyd *et al.*, 1986). In 1983, linked DNA polymorphisms were found on either side of the Duchenne muscular dystrophy mutation (Davies *et al.*, 1983), see Figure 1A. Shortly thereafter, more restriction fragment length polymorphisms (RFLPs) detected by cloned DNA became available. This resulted in a >98% reliable carrier detection and first trimester prenatal diagnosis in approximately 75% of the cases (Bakker *et al.*, 1985, 1986; see Figure 1B and C).

Two independent selective cloning approaches, followed respectively by Kunkel and coworkers (1985) and by Ray and coworkers (1985) eventually gave access to the coding sequences (for review see Kedes, 1985). Kunkel used the Phenol Enhanced Reassociation Technique (PERT) starting with DNA from a patient (patient B.B. first described by Francke *et al.* (1985)) carrying a sub-microscopic deletion causing a compound syndrome of Duchenne muscular dystrophy, chronic granulomatous disease, retinitis pigmentosa and McLeod syndrome. Ray and coworkers (1985) cloned a translocation breakpoint in a female Duchenne muscular dystrophy patient (X/21 translocation, first described by Verellen-Dumoulin *et al.* (1984). The first probes isolated by these techniques were respectively pERT87 and XJ1.1 (see Figure 1C) both detecting deletions in about 8% of Duchenne

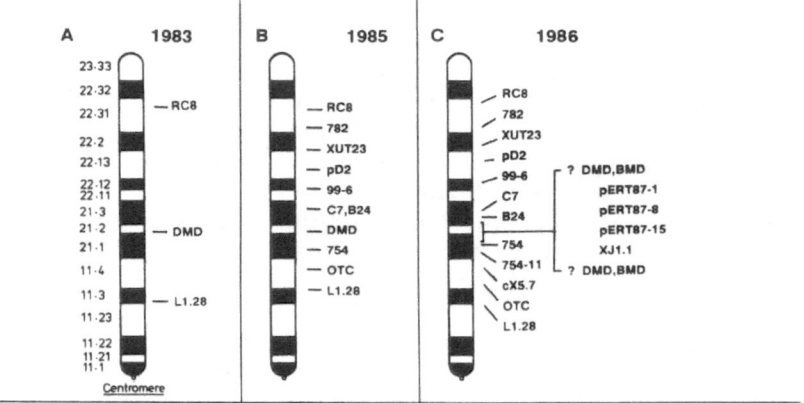

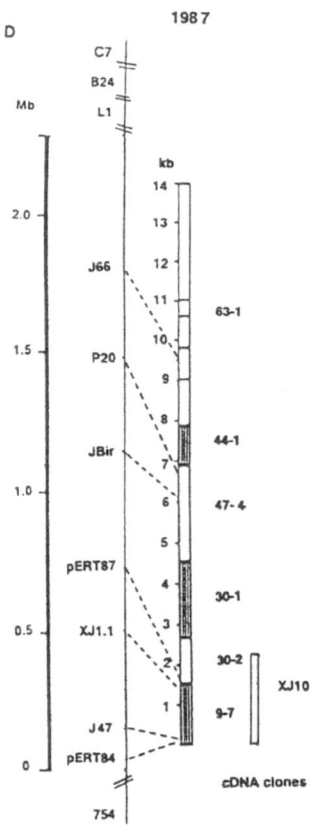

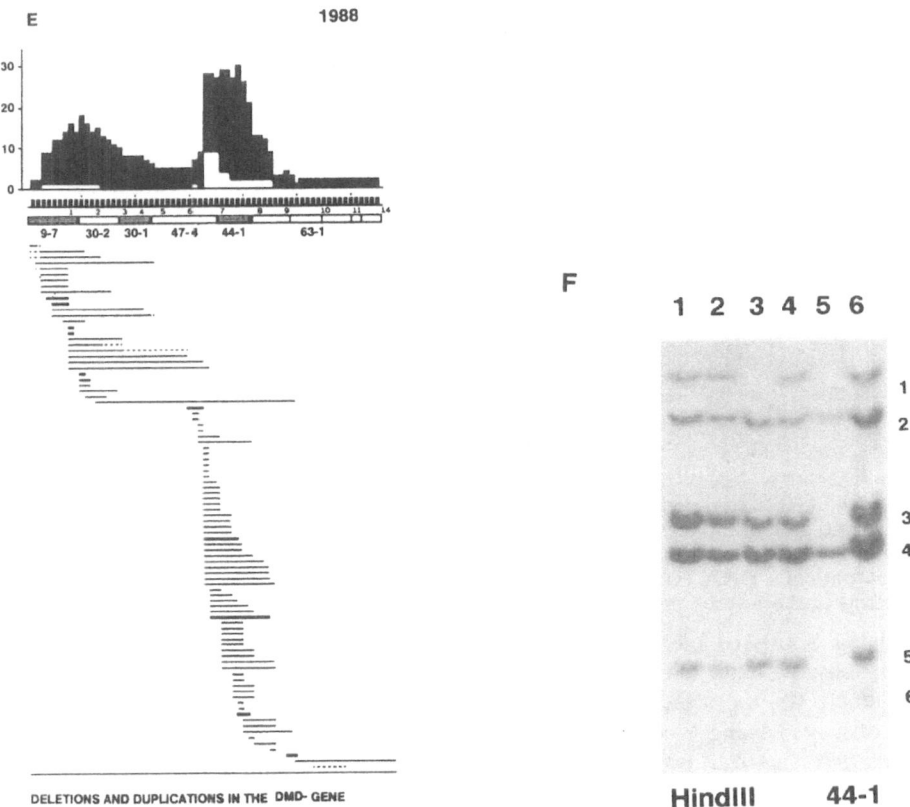

Figure 1 (A) In 1983 the first flanking markers for Duchenne muscular dystrophy (DMD) were available. (B) In 1985 many Xp RFLP-markers were localized and were applied for diagnostic purposes. (C) In 1986, intragenic genomic probes detecting many RFLPs and deletions in approximately 10% of the patients, a standard approach of the diagnosis was necessary. (D) In 1987 the genomic map constructed by use of FIGE analysis showed the huge size of the Duchenne muscular dystrophy gene and the genomic distribution of the cDNA clones. (E) In 1988 the non-random distribution of start and end points of deletions and/or duplication was demonstrated. Results of 92 mutations detected in Leiden by use of the cDNA-probes. (F) Example of a typical Southern blot; *Hind*III digest hybridized with probe 44-1, revealing six *Hind*III fragments containing an exon. In two of these random Duchenne muscular dystrophy patients a deletion was detected. In lane 3 a deletion of bands 1 and 6 is shown, in lane 5 a deletion of bands, 1, 3, 5 and 6 is shown

muscular dystrophy patients (Monaco *et al.*, 1985; Ray *et al.*, 1985; Kunkel *et al.*, 1986).

The coding sequence for the Duchenne muscular dystrophy gene product was found by selection of conserved sequences cloned from genomic walks at both loci, each revealing the same huge messenger RNA (14 kb) in fetal skeletal muscle (Monaco *et al.*, 1986; Burghes *et al.*, 1987). The total cDNA, cloned and first

Bakker et al.

described by Koenig and colleagues (1987) was shown to involve over 60 exons (Hoffman *et al.*, 1987a; Koenig *et al.*, 1987, 1988; Monaco *et al.*, 1988), and extends over more than 2.0 million base pairs of genomic DNA (Van Ommen *et al.*, 1987; Burmeister *et al.*, 1988; see Figure 1D).

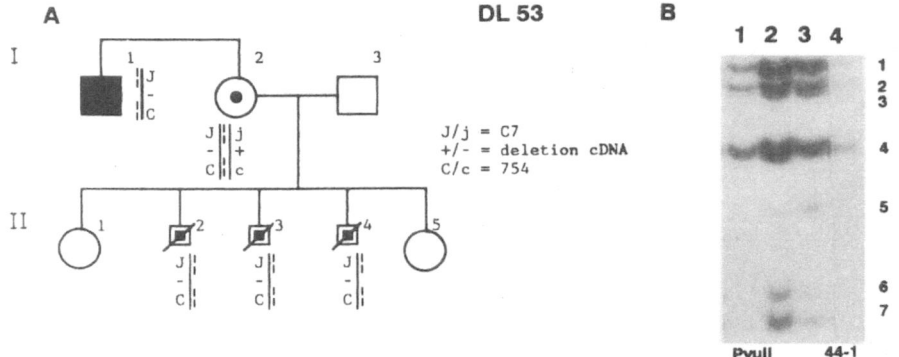

Figure 2 (A) Partial pedigree of DL 53, three male fetuses were diagnosed to be affected by the use of flanking markers. (B) Southern blot result of family DL 53, showing a cDNA deletion on a *Pvu*II digest for cDNA probe 44-1 (cDNA 8). Bands 3, 5, 6 and 7 are missing in the patient's DNA (lane 1), the same deletion is present in the DNA of the abortion material of the fetuses (lane 4 DNA from II,2)

Using Southern blots of genomic digests of DNA from Duchenne muscular dystrophy patients several laboratories found deletions for part of the coding sequences (in about 60% of the cases). Similar data, plus about 10% duplications, are observed using Field Inversion Gel Electrophoresis (FIGE) (den Dunnen *et al.*, 1987; and our own unpublished observations). Using the method of cell-mediated chromosome transfer, Wapenaar and coworkers (1988) succeeded in producing a set of chinese hamster cell-lines containing parts of the short arm of the human X-chromosome. From one of these cell-lines a probe, P20, was isolated which detects 36% of the deletions in Duchenne muscular dystrophy patients. The location of the P20 'deletion hotspot' is in a large intron in the distal half of the Duchenne muscular dystrophy gene and overlaps with the deletion hotspot described by Koenig and colleagues (1987) using cDNA probes. In Figure 1E, the distribution of the deletions and duplications within the Duchenne muscular dystrophy gene of 92 patients (79 Duchenne and 13 Becker muscular dystrophy) studied in Leiden is depicted clearly showing the non-random distribution of deletions.

A muscle-specific membrane-associated protein of 400 kDa was detected by Hofman and coworkers (1987b) using antibodies, raised against the fusion protein products of parts of the cDNA which proved to be absent in muscle biopsies of Duchenne muscular dystrophy patients. The product of the Duchenne muscular dystrophy gene, now called 'dystrophin', opens the way to expression studies, which may lead to a better understanding of the phenotypic differences between Becker and Duchenne muscular dystrophies as suggested by Monaco and coworkers (1988) and defining the function of this protein.

DIAGNOSTIC PROCEDURE

The standard procedure for carrier detection and prenatal diagnosis, which we described in 1986 has been applied on most of our 200 Duchenne and Becker muscular dystrophy families. Since August 1987 the procedure has been extended by using the Duchenne muscular dystrophy cDNA probes (kindly provided by Drs Kunkel and Worton). Table 1 shows the extended procedure currently applied. Stage 1 consists of digestion with seven restriction enzymes and hybridization with eight RFLP detecting probes (together giving a 50% chance of informative markers on both sides of the gene) and two cDNA probes, XJ10 and 44.1 (available from the American Type Culture Collection as cDNA 8), (together giving a 40% chance of detecting a structural rearrangement). Depending on the results of stage I, additional steps from stage II and III are selected until the mutation (deletion or duplication) is detected, or informative flanking markers allow a reliable diagnosis for possible carriers and fetuses at risk. After testing all the cDNA probes for deletions (on at least two different digests, to rule out possible cDNA RFLPs) and all flanking markers described to date, more than 90% of the cases have yielded conclusive results. Both Forrest and coworkers (1987) and Darras and coworkers (1988) have described the use of cDNA probes as initial step in the diagnostic service for Duchenne muscular dystrophy and they used the RFLP markers only in those cases where no mutation was found. We have distinctively chosen a combined use of cDNAs and markers on either side of this huge gene, to achieve the most effective diagnostic procedure. In doing so we have, apart from saving time, an independent check on (the haplotype of) the X-chromosome at risk while diagnosing carriers on the basis of intensity differences of one or more X-ray bands.

Most problems were encountered when no material from the index patient was available in combination with insufficient information from other family members. For deletion detection in a female carrier good quality blots are essential, because one has to compare the intensities of the bands to estimate the copy number. The difference between one or two copies is relatively easy to detect but differences between two and three copies, or sometimes three or four copies, in case of a duplication or comigrating bands can be very difficult. Therefore, in the absence of an index patient i.e. not knowing which of the over 60 exon bands needs close examination, deletions or duplications are easily missed in female carriers. If DNA of the patient is available, but the mutation not detectable, a crossover event between flanking RFLPs may occasionally hamper diagnosis. Interpreting blot results requires independent examination by at least two qualified persons before the results are sent to the genetic counsellor.

Table 1 Diagnostic (extended) procedure

| Stage | cDNA probes or RFLP markers used | | | Restriction |
	Proximal side	DMD region	Distal side	enzymes used
Stage I Initial blots		cDNA XJ10		*Eco*RI
		cDNA 44-1		*Hind*III
	OTC			*Msp*I
	<u>754</u>		<u>99.6</u>	*Pst*I
		<u>87-1–</u>	<u>C7</u>	*Eco*RV
			<u>D2</u>	*Pvu*II
		87-15/XJ1.1		*Taq*I
Stage II Re-use blots		If deletion found:		
		cDNA XJ10		*Hind*III (+other)
		cDNA 44-1		*Eco*RI (+other)
		No deletion found:		
		cDNA 47-4		*Eco*RI
		cDNA 63-1,2		*Hind*III
		P20		*Eco*RV
	<u>754-11</u>		<u>782</u>	*Eco*RI
		87-1		*Msp*I
	CX5.7			*Msp*I
		XJ2.3		*Taq*I
		87-8		*Taq*I
	<u>L1.28</u>		<u>RC8</u>	*Taq*I
			<u>B24</u>	*Msp*I
		J66-HI		*Pst*I
Stage III Re-use blots		If deletion found:		
		cDNA 47-4		*Hind*III (+other)
		cDNA 63-1,2		*Eco*RI (+other)
		No deletion found:		
		cDNA 30-2		*Eco*RI
		cDNA 30-1		*Hind*III
		cDNA 63-3,4		*Eco*RI
		cDNA 63-5		*Hind*III
Additional blots		<u>87-1/15</u>		*Xmn*I
			pXUT23	*Bgl*II
		87-8		*Bst*NI
		87-1		*Bst*XI
		Jbir		*Bam*HI

DMD = Duchenne muscular dystrophy
The probe name is underlined when it can be used in a combined hybridization (eg. 87-1 and C7)

THREE YEARS OF PRENATAL DIAGNOSES

All the Dutch requests for DNA analysis for Duchenne and Becker muscular dystrophies (carrier detection and prenatal diagnosis) come to us through any one of the seven Genetic Counselling Units in the Netherlands. The Netherlands have 14 million inhabitants and the yearly birth rate is 180 000, approximately 90 000 males. Hence about 30 Duchenne muscular dystrophy males (20 familial and 10 sporadic) are expected to be born yearly when no prenatal diagnosis is performed.

Prenatal diagnosis for Duchenne muscular dystrophy was first described in early 1985 (Bakker *et al.*, 1985). We will use some of the families first studied then to demonstrate how much the diagnostic procedures have changed over the intervening years.

Family I (DL53), presented with a situation in which the female partner was diagnosed as a carrier because of elevated creatine kinase concentrations. The presence of the Duchenne muscular dystrophy region of the chromosome at risk was inferred from the results using the closest flanking markers C7 and 754. The presence of a double crossover between the more distant flanking markers underscored the need for using the closest flanking markers which then just became available. The male fetus, diagnosed using chorionic villus sampling, carried the mutant X-chromosome. The parents decided for therapeutic termination of this pregnancy. The abortion was performed in the twelfth week of gestation. In January 1986 and in August 1986 subsequent male progressive pregnancies were terminated, because of similar high Duchenne muscular dystrophy risk. However, by the time the third 'male' pregnancy occurred another informative RFLP, pERT87, was available and this significantly reduced the chance of an undetected double recombinant from 1% with the previous markers to less then 0.25%. Finally, a pregnancy investigated in February 1987 showed a female fetus which was not further analysed and a daughter was born (see pedigree Figure 2A). Some months later a deletion was detected in the Duchenne muscular dystrophy gene of the index patient using cDNA probe 44.1 (cDNA 8). All three aborted male fetuses have since been confirmed to be affected, carrying the same deletion as the index patient (see Figure 2B, lane 1 DNA of the patient and lane 4 DNA isolated from abortion material of the first terminated pregnancy). Thus, in this family a future prenatal diagnosis has become relatively easy and without the risk of loss of information due to a recombination between flanking markers.

In another family (DL 15, Figure 3), DNA analysis was performed to determine the carrier status of four sisters at risk. Both parents, two healthy brothers and an affected nephew were available for study. Using flanking markers (pD2 and 754) and one informative pERT87 probe, two (II,2 and II,3) of the four sisters were shown to have a low (<1%) carrier risk while the others (II,7 and II,8) had a high carrier risk (<98%). Since both females were informative for the flanking probes 99-6 and 754, prenatal diagnosis was possible. In July 1986 chorionic villi of a male pregnancy of II,7 were analysed and a crossover was detected between 99-6 and 754. Thus the Duchenne muscular dystrophy risk for this male fetus was high and the parents decided to have the pregnancy terminated. One year later the same woman was again pregnant with a male fetus. This fetus was shown to have a low

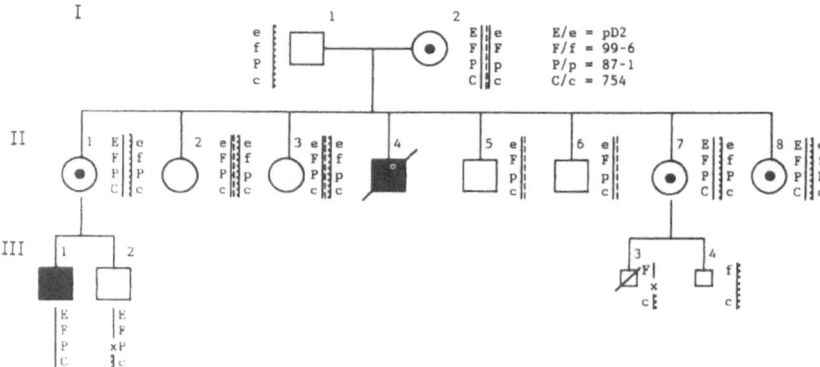

Figure 3 Pedigree of family DL 15. DNA analysis allowed carrier detection using flanking markers for four daughters at risk. II,2 and II,3 are normal, inheriting the same X-chromosome (!) as the two healthy brothers. II,7 and II,8 are carriers of the same Duchenne muscular dystrophy (DMD) X-chromosome which II,1 has transmitted to her affected son. Prenatal diagnosis on fetus III,3 revealed a crossover between 754 and 99-6, although III,2 is normal and carries a similar crossover. The risk for this fetus was estimated to be approximately 50%, if both 754 and 99-6 have a genetic distance of 10 centimorgan to an average DMD mutation. A second pregnancy, turned out to be a male fetus with a low (<1%) risk for DMD carrying the grandmaternal X-chromosome (:). A healthy boy was born

(<1.5%) risk for Duchenne muscular dystrophy, carrying the grandpaternal alleles for both 99-6 and 754 (see Figure 3). Recently a healthy boy was born from this pregnancy, based on normal creatine kinase concentrations, determined both in umbilical cord blood at delivery and in blood taken at 3 weeks of age. Now we have tested all the cDNA probes on the DNA of the index patient in this family and no deletion or duplication could be detected in the affected chromosome. Long-range electrophoretic analysis will have to be performed on large molecular weight DNA (as described by den Dunnen and coworkers (1987) to identify possible aberrant bands due to rearrangements undetected thus far. In this family we remain dependent, for the time being, on the use of flanking or intragenic RFLP markers. Thus, we are left with the chance of approximately 20% of detecting a crossover between flanking markers in a next pregnancy and with a 1.5% chance of false negative detection due to a double crossover in the remaining 80% of apparent non-recombinants. Since the chance of a single intragenic crossover event is approximately 5%, informative intragenic markers (of genomic or cDNA origin) will further reduce the chance on false negatives. Finally, any observed crossover in one of the family members may narrow down the possible mutation site and will from then on become a marker flanking the mutation in subsequent diagnoses.

In family BL16, a large four-generation family with Becker muscular dystrophy, carrier detection for three sisters at risk was performed. In Figure 4A part of the pedigree is shown. The mother, an obligate carrier, is informative for the flanking markers C7 and 754 and for pERT87-1 and XJ1.1. One daughter (II,1) has inherited the Becker muscular dystrophy X-chromosome while the other two have the normal X-chromosome. The carrier daughter in turn is informative for the flanking markers pD2 and OTC and for the markers pERT87 and XJ1.1, allowing reliable prenatal diagnosis in 75% of pregnancies (25% chance of a crossover between pD2 and OTC). Although the intragenic markers pERT87 and XJ1.1 are informative and thus useful in confirming non-recombinants, their use would have been futile in case of a crossover, since the position of this specific mutation relative to XJ1.1 and pERT87 was until recently unknown. Darras and coworkers (1987) have described a case of prenatal diagnosis in which a false negative pregnancy resulted in an affected male. This was directly attributable to uncertainty about the relative position of the observed crossover event, relative to the Duchenne muscular dystrophy mutation. Fortunately, the new probe P20 (Wapenaar *et al.*, 1988) detected a deletion within the Becker muscular dystrophy gene of the patient, see

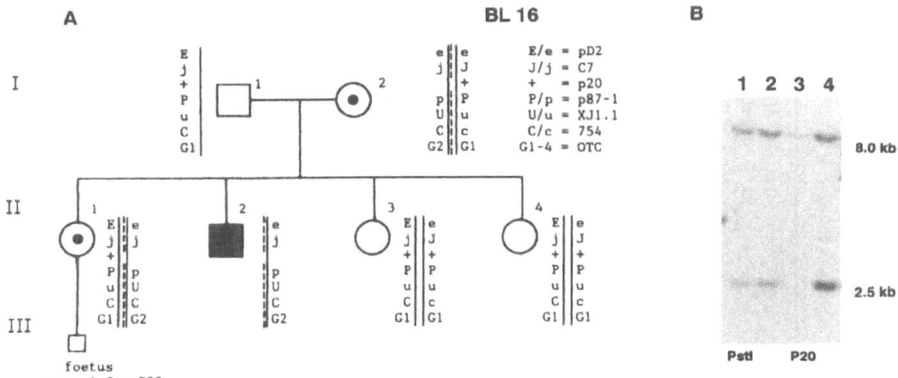

Figure 4 (A) A partial pedigree of a Becker muscular dystrophy family BL16. Initially flanking markers were used for carrier detection of the three daughters at risk. II,1 was shown to be a carrier, she inherited the same maternal X-chromosome as patient II,2. The two other daughters are normal having the other maternal X. Later a deletion for probe P20 was found in the patient's DNA. Both mother and the carrier sister were shown to carry the deletion. A male fetus was diagnosed to be normal carrying the non-deleted X-chromosome. (B) Southern blot result of prenatal diagnosis in family BL16, showing on *Pst*I digested DNA of the patient II,2 a deletion for 2.5 kb band of P20. Both the mother I,1 and sister II,1, respectively lanes 1 and 2, show a reduced hybridization signal for the 2.5 kb band. The male fetus (lane 4) was not deleted for this P20 band, and was therefore not at risk. A healthy boy was born

Figure 4B, and the carrier status of the mother (lane 1) and the daughter (lane 2) could be directly confirmed by the virtue of their heterozygosity for the P20-deletion (compare the intensities of the upper band, which is not deleted, to the lower band). In June 1987 the carrier daughter was pregnant with a male fetus and chorionic villi were analysed using P20. No deletion was found (see lane 4) and the male fetus was diagnosed to be normal. The pregnancy was continued and a healthy boy was born.

Table 2 Accuracy of Duchenne muscular dystrophy (DMD) diagnosis by means of DNA analysis

No.	Duchenne/ Becker family	DMD status mother (carrier risk) Before	After analysis	Diagnosis of fetus (DMD risk)		Analytical accuracy	Closest used informative flanking markers and intragenic probes	Pregnancy terminated or continued outcome (diagnosis confirmed)
1	DL 53	(>50%, CK)	carrier	DMD	(>99%)	>99%	754 and C7	terminated (confirmed)
2	DL 57	(33%)	normal[a]	NA	(<1%)	>99%	754 and C7	born, CK levels normal
3	DL 56	(>50%, CK)	carrier	NA	(<1%)	>99%	754 and pD2	born, CK levels normal
4	DL 61	(33–66%)	(33–66%)	NA	(<1%)	>99%	754 and C7	born, CK levels normal
5	DL 62	(33%)	(>33%)	AR	(+5%)	—	crossover L1.28 and C7	terminated (normal)[b]
6	DL 72	(50%)	(50%)	NA	(>1%)	>99%	754 and 99.6	born, CK levels normal
7	DL 75	(50%)	normal[a]	NA	(<1%)	>98%	L1.28 and C7	born, CK normal
8	DL 77	(8%)	(8%)[a]	AR	(+8%)	—	pXUT23, no other markers	terminated
9	DL 79	(50%)	(50%)[a]	AR	(25%)	—	754, 99-6 (phase DMD-X?)	terminated (normal)
10	DL 84	(13%)	normal[a]	NA	(<1%)	>99%	754 and pD2	born, CK levels normal
11	DL 89	(>50%,CK)	carrier	AR	(90%)	90%	754 (phase distal ?)	terminated (confirmed)
12	DL 92	(66%)	(66%)	AR	(60%)	—	cross over pERT87 and pD2	terminated
13	DL 93	(33%)	normal[a]	NA	(<1%)	>99%	754, pERT87 and 99-6	born, CK levels normal
14	DL 94	(20%)	normal[a]	NA	(<1%)	>99%	754 and 99-6	born, CK levels normal
15	BL 5	(25%)	(25%)	AR	(>25%)	>99%	754 and 99-6	terminated
16	DL 98	(33%)	(66%)	AR	(+60%)	—	crossover pERT87 and pD2	terminated
17	DL 99	(33%)	normal[a]	NA	(<1%)	>99%	754, pERT87, C7	born, CK normal
18	DL 102	(33%)	normal[a]	NA	(<1%)	>99%	754, pERT87, 99.6	born, CK normal
19	DL 106	(50%)	normal[a]	NA	(<1%)	>99%	754, pERT87, C7	born, CK normal
20	DL 113	(66%)	(66%)	AR	(+50%)	—	crossover 87 and C7	terminated
21	DL 80	(33%)	(33%)	NA	(<1%)	>99%	754, pERT87, pD2	born, CK normal
22	DL 73	(33%)	(33%)	AR	(30%)	>99%	OTC, pERT87, 99-6	terminated (confirmed)
23	DL 53	carrier (DNA)	carrier	DMD	(>99%)	>99%	754, pERT87, C7	terminated (confirmed)
24	DL 13	(50%)	(50%)	NA	(<1%)	>99%	754, pERT87, pD2	born, CK normal (SIDS)[c]
25	DL 43	carrier	carrier	NA	(>3%)	>97%	pERT87, C7	born, CK normal
26	DL 15	(>50%, CK)	carrier	AR	(25%)	—	crossover 754 and 99.6	terminated

Table 2 (continued) Accuracy of Duchenne muscular dystrophy (DMD) diagnosis by means of DNA analysis

No.	Duchenne/ Becker family	DMD status mother (carrier risk) Before	DMD status mother After analysis	Diagnosis of fetus (DMD risk)	Analytical accuracy	Closest used informative flanking markers and intragenic probes	Pregnancy terminated or continued outcome (diagnosis confirmed)
27	DL 120	(50%)	(25%)	AR (16%)	—	crossover 754 and pXUT23	terminated
28	DL 108	(33%)	(33%)	AR (33%)	>99%	754, pERT87, C7	terminated
29	DL 134	(50%)	(50%)	NA (<1%)	>99%	754, pERT87, pD2	born, CK normal
30	DL 142	(50%)	(50%)	AR (>10%)	—	no inf. distal marker	terminated
31	DL 144	(50%)	normal[a]	NA (<1%)	>99%	OTC, pERT87, C7	born, CK normal
32	DL 53	carrier	carrier	DMD (>99%)	>99%	754, pERT87, C7	terminated
33	DL 108	(33%)	(33%)	NA (<1%)	>99%	754, pERT87, C7	born, CK normal
34	DL 147	carrier (CK)	carrier (CK)	NA (<1%)	>99%	754, XJ1.1, pD2	born, CK normal
35	DL 73	(33%)	(33%)	AR (33%)	>99%	OTC, pERT87, 99-6	terminated
36	DL 157	(25%)	(50%)	AR (50%)	>99%	754, pERT87, C7	born, CK normal
37	DL 55	(50%)	normal[a]	NA (<1%)	>99%	(deletion) pERT87	terminated
38	DL 107	(33%)	carrier	AR (90%)	90%	754	terminated
39	BL 5	(25%)	(25%)	AR (12.5%)	—	crossover 754 and 99-6	born, CK normal
40	DL 15	carrier (CK)	carrier	NA (<1%)	>99%	754, 99-6	terminated
41	DL 8	carrier	carrier	DMD (>99%)	>99%	754, pERT87, 99-6	born, CK normal
42	BL 16	(50%)	carrier	NA (<1%)	>99%	(deletion) p20	terminated
43	DL 135	(33%)	(33%)	AR (33%)	>99%	OTC, pERT87, 99-6	terminated
44	DL 208	carrier	carrier	DMD (>99%)	>99%	deletion cDNA 63-2	terminated
45	DL 193	(50%)	(50%)	NA (<1%)	>99%	754 and 99-6	born
46	DL 73	(50%)	(50%)	AR (50%)	>99%	OTC, pERT87, 99-6	terminated
47	DL 181	(33%)	(33%)	AR (33%)	95%	only pERT87 informative	terminated, (MCA)[e]
48	DL 182	(33%)	(33%)	AR (33%)	>99%	—[d]	terminated, normal
49	DL 129	(66%)	(5%, GM)	AR (5%)	—	754, 99-6	terminated
50	DL 114	(33%)	carrier	DMD (>99%)	>99%	deletion 30-2	pregnancy continued
51	DL 159	(50%)	carrier	NA (<2%)	>98%	OTC, 99-6	pregnancy continued
52	DL 160	(50%)	normal[a]	NA (<1%)	>99%	deletion cDNA	terminated
53	DL 220	(50%)	(30%)	AR (30%)	>99%	C7, 99-6	terminated

NA = not affected; AR = at risk of DMD; DMD = affected.
[a]In these cases prenatal diagnosis had not been necessary or possible if the family material had been sent before the start of the pregnancy.
[b]A deletion for pERT 87-42 was later found in the index patient and not in the abortion material.
[c]The child died at seven days, sudden infant death syndrome (SIDS).
[d]Due to too little villus material and technical failure of the diagnosis, no conclusion was possible about the absence or presence of the deletion.
The parents decided not to have a second test on amniotic fluid and opted for abortion.
[e]The aborted fetus showed multiple congenital abnormalities.

Over the last 3 years, 110 pregnancies at risk for Duchenne muscular dystrophy have been referred to us for prenatal diagnosis. Direct chromosome analysis on chorionic villi, performed in one of the four prenatal cytogenetic laboratories in the Netherlands, showed 55 female and 53 male fetuses, while two pregnancies ended in a spontaneous abortion before sampling of the villi.

Although we always receive a villus sample for DNA preparation, the analysis is continued only in the case of a male embryo. DNA of the female fetuses is stored because we do not analyse female fetal material for Duchenne muscular dystrophy carrier risk unless specifically requested. The outcome of the 53 prenatal diagnoses performed is shown in Table 2 and summarized in Table 3.

Table 3   Duchenne muscular dystrophy: Diagnosis Summary

Prenatal diagnosis	108
Male fetuses:	53 (in 47 families; three Becker)
Affected (>99%)	6
High risk (<98%)	23
Terminated	29 (affected+high risk)
Continued:	24
born	22
affected	0

In the 47 families 53 prenatal diagnoses were performed using: flanking markers in 42 cases ($7\times$loss of information due to recombinant) often combined with internal marker; no informative flanking markers were present in six cases; there was deletion detection in six cases, five during the last year.

At this moment: in 16 out of the 47 prenatal diagnosis families a deletion or duplication has been found, allowing highly reliable diagnosis.

In 92 families a mutation has been detected (11 duplications): see Figure 1E and F.

PITFALLS

Not only should one always be aware of the risk of mixing up samples when handling so many DNA digestions but nature has also provided a number of pitfalls which should be kept in mind.

Non-paternity

The use of many X-chromosome specific RFLP probes in a large number of families, as presented here, inevitably confronts one with the detection of RFLP-alleles that do not fit in the expected Mendelian inheritance pattern: for instance, a daughter being homozygous for one or more alleles, while the supposed father has another allele. Usually we confirm this observation by testing the DNA samples with hypervariable probes (fingerprinting using the probes 33-15 or 33-6 described by Jeffreys *et al.*, 1985). Using RFLP probes we encountered non-paternity in about 5% of cases, which is a lower estimate, because we do not test paternity in all families and consequently will miss all those cases in which a son is from another father.

Karyotypic abnormalities

In Duchenne muscular dystrophy family DL159 we came across an apparently normal male, being heterozygous for a number of X-probes. After having ruled out mixing up of the samples, we hybridized a Y-chromosome specific probe. This was positive as well. Chromosome analysis subsequently confirmed that this male was indeed a Klinefelter (46XXY) carrying the Duchenne muscular dystrophy mutation and having all the characteristics of a carrier (Hennekam, personal communication).

Gonadal mosaicism

One-third of the Duchenne muscular dystrophy patients result from a 'new' mutation. Therefore a large proportion of the patients are isolated cases. Due to the non-meiotic origin of the Duchenne muscular dystrophy mutations (Bakker *et al.*, 1987; Darras and Francke, 1987; Bakker *et al.*, 1989) germline mosaicism in both male and female gametes generates a considerable recurrence risk for transmission of apparent new Duchenne muscular dystrophy mutations (which may be as high as 14% from our own data). An example of this phenomenon is shown in Figure

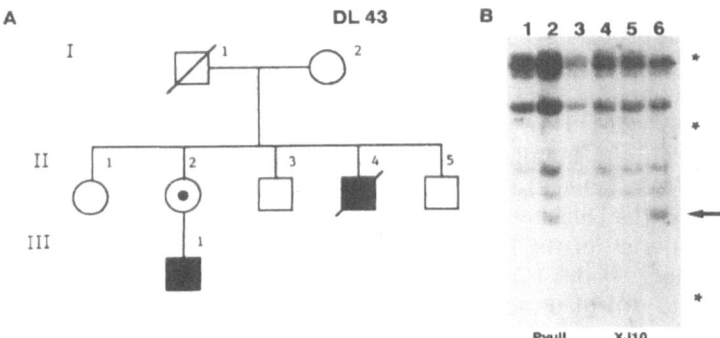

Figure 5 (A) A partial pedigree of family DL 43. Two affected children, a diseased Duchenne muscular dystrophy son and a carrier daughter, of a somatic normal mother (I,2): see (B). Using flanking markers two out of four meioses showed a recombination event (data not shown). (B) A cDNA deletion was detected in patient III,1 using cDNA probe XJ10 on several digests. The hybridization on a *Pvu*II digest reveals an altered band (junction fragment) in the DNA of the patient III,1 (lane 7) and in the DNA of his mother II,2 (lane 3) but not in the DNA of the grandmother (lane 1). It is most likely that this grandmother is carrying a gonadal mosaic for this mutation

5. A mother twice transmitted a Duchenne muscular dystrophy deletion mutation (detected using the cDNA probe XJ10), while she herself was not carrying this mutation in her somatic cells (lymphocytes). Therefore, it is imperative to test all subsequent pregnancies of mothers of isolated patients, as well as to perform a carrier detection for all sisters of the index patient and for sisters of carriers of apparent new mutations.

NEW DEVELOPMENTS

Since the detection of Duchenne muscular dystrophy mutations has become more feasible, the mutation has been found in approximately 60% of patients and neonatal screening for Duchenne muscular dystrophy has now become relevant. As reported by Greenberg and colleagues (1988) five out of 18 000 newborn males were found to be affected with either Duchenne or Becker muscular dystrophy on the basis of high creatine kinase concentration determined in dried blood samples collected on filter paper. In three cases a mutation was detected in the Duchenne muscular dystrophy gene by testing with cDNA probes and P20. Because isolated Duchenne muscular dystrophy patients are usually not diagnosed before the age of 4–5 years, currently further affected boys are often born to new-mutation carrier females. Thus, neonatal screening followed by confirmative DNA analysis in newborn males at risk presents a new development of great value, preventing the birth of more affected boys in the same sibship. In addition, in the immediate future more refined DNA analysis, combined with protein studies, should permit a much more precise prediction on the anticipated course of the disease in these cases.

Recently, exciting new possibilities for the DNA diagnosis of genetic disorders have been described. The Polymerase Chain Reaction (PCR) technique has opened an entire new era of DNA diagnosis, especially for disorders in which a limited number of mutations are present, such as the β-thallasaemias. For Duchenne muscular dystrophy, a large gene with many different mutations (each mutation is different on the molecular level), it seems at first sight impracticable to use the PCR technique for mutation detection, because one would need to test many points within this huge gene. However, Chelly and coworkers (1988) recently reported a method reducing the complexity of this problem by amplification of the mRNA. Using total RNA, isolated from muscle biopsies, cDNA was synthesized from a specific point in the Duchenne muscular dystrophy mRNA sequence and then used as starting material for the PCR reaction to detect aberrations in this part of the mRNA sequence. If this is applicable to other points in the mRNA as well, only a limited set (5–10) of these PCR reactions would permit the monitoring of the whole sequence. Combined with the finding of the same authors that the Duchenne muscular dystrophy gene is detectably transcribed, albeit in three to four orders of magnitude less efficient, in any unrelated tissue studied (white blood cells, fibro-blasts and placenta), it is not difficult to predict that the diagnostic field for Duchenne muscular dystrophy is in for a new round of technical improvements in the immediate future.

ACKNOWLEDGEMENTS

We wish to thank Drs A. J. v. Essen, B. Hamel, H. Brunner, E. Ippel, C. Schander, Ch. de Die-Smulders, F. Los, H. Oorthuis and many more Dutch clinicians for referring the Duchenne muscular dystrophy families; Drs Kunkel and Worton for supplying the cDNA probes and Dr Wapenaar for probe P20.

This work was financially supported by the Dutch Preaventie Fonds, Grant No.

28.878, and by the Muscular Dystrophy Group of Great Britain and Northern Ireland.

REFERENCES

Bakker, E., Hofker, M. H., Goor, N., Mandel, J. L., Davies, K. E., Kunkel, L. M., Willard, H. F., Fenton, W. A., Sandkuyl, L. Majoor-Krakauer, D. van Essen, A. J., Jahoda, M., Sachs, E. S., van Ommen, G. J. B. and Pearson, P. L. Prenatal diagnosis and carrier detection of Duchenne muscular dystrophy with closely linked RFLP's. *Lancet* 1 (1985) 655–658

Bakker, E., Bonten, E. J., de Lange, L. F., Veenema, H., Majoor-Krakauer, Hofker, M. H., van Ommen, G. J. B., Pearson, P. L. DNA probe analysis for carrier detection and prenatal diagnosis of Duchenne muscular dystrophy: A standard diagnostic procedure. *J. Med. Genet.* 23 (1986) 573–580

Bakker, E., Van Broeckhoven, Ch., Bonten, E. J., Van de Vooren, M. J., Veenema, H., Van Hul, W., Van Ommen, G. J. B., Vandenberghe, A. and Pearson, P. L. Germline mosaicism and Duchenne muscular dystrophy mutations. *Nature*, 328 (1987) 554–556

Bakker, C., Veenema, H., den Dunnen, J. T., Van Breechhoven, C., Grootschalten, P. M., Bouten, E. J., van Ommen, G. J. B. and Pearson, P. L. Germinal mosaicism increases the recurrence risk for "new" DMD mutations. *J. Med. Genet.* (1989) in press

Boyd, Y., Buckle, V., Holt, S., Munro, E., Hunter, D., and Graig, I. Muscular dystrophy in girls with X:autosome translocations. *J. Med. Genet.* 23 (1986) 484–490

Bullock, D. G., McSweeney, F. M., Whitehead, T. P. and Edwards, J. H. Serum creatine kinase activity and carrier status for Duchenne muscular dystrophy. *Lancet* 2 (1979) 1151

Burghes, A. H. M., Logan, C., Hu, X., Belfall, B., Worton, R. G., and Ray, P. N. A cDNA clone from the Duchenne/Becker muscular dystrophy gene. *Nature* 328 (1987) 434–437

Burmeister, M., Monaco, A. P., Gillard, E. F., van Ommen, G. J. B., Affara, N. A., Ferguson-Smith, M. A., Kunkel, L. M. and Lehrach, H. A 10-megabase physical map of human Xp21, including the Duchenne muscular dystrophy gene. *Genomics* 2 (1988) 189–202

Chelly, J., Kaplan, J. C., Maire, P., Gautron, S. and Kahn, A. Transcription of the dystrophin gene in human muscle and non-muscle tissues. *Nature* 333 (1988) 858–860

Darras, B. T., Harper, J. F., and Francke, U. Prenatal diagnosis and carriers with DNA probes in Duchenne's muscular dystrophy. *N. Engl. J. Med.* 316 (1987) 985–992

Darras, B. T. and Francke, U. A partial deletion of the muscular dystrophy gene transmitted twice by an unaffected male. *Nature* 329 (1987) 556–558

Darras, B. T., Koenig, M., Kunkel, L. M. and Francke, U. Direct method for prenatal diagnosis and carrier detection in Duchenne/Becker muscular dystrophy using the entire dystrophin cDNA. *Am. J. Med. Genet.* 29 (1988) 713–726

Davies, K. E., Pearson, P. L., Harper, P. S. *et al.* Linkage analysis of two cloned DNA sequences flanking the Duchenne muscular dystrophy locus on the short arm of the human X-chromosome. *Nucl. Acids Res.* 11 (1983) 2303–2312

Dunnen, J. T. den, Bakker, E., Klein Breteler, E. G., Pearson, P. L., and van Ommen, G. J. B. Direct detection of more than 50% of the Duchenne muscular dystrophy mutations by field inversion gels. *Nature* 329 (1987) 640–642

Emery, A. E. H. Duchenne muscular dystrophy. In: Motulski, A. G., Harper, P. S., Bobrow, M. and Scriver, C. (Eds.) *Oxford Monographs on Medical Genetics, No. 15*, Oxford University Press, Oxford, 1987

Francke, U., Ochs, H. D., de Martinville, B. *et al.* Minor Xp21 chromosome deletion in a male associated with expression of Duchenne muscular dystrophy, chronic granulomatous disease, retinitis pigmentosa and McLeod syndrome. *Am. J. Hum. Genet.* 37 (1985) 250–267

Forrest, S. M., Cross, G. S., Thomas, N. S. T., Harper, P. S., Smith, T. J., Read, A. P., Mountford, R. C., Geirsson, R. T. and Davies, K. E. Effective strategy for prenatal prediction of Duchenne and Becker muscular dystrophy. *Lancet* 1 (1987) 1294–1296

Greenberg, C. R., Rohringer, M., Jacobs, H. K., Averill, N., Nylen, E., van Ommen, G. J. B., and Wrogemann, K. Gene studies in newborn males with Duchenne muscular dystrophy detected by neonatal screening. *Lancet* 2 (1988) 425–427

Hoffman, E. P., Monaco, A. P., Feener, C. C., and Kunkel, L. M. Conservation of the Duchenne muscular dystrophy gene in mice and humans. *Science* 238 (1987a) 347–350

Hoffman, E. P., Brown, R. H., Kunkel, L. Dystrophin: The protein product of the Duchenne muscular dystrophy locus. *Cell* 51 (1987b) 919–928

Jeffreys, A. J., Wilson, V., and Thein, S. L. Individual-specific 'fingerprints' of human DNA. *Nature* 316 (1985) 76–79

Kedes, L. H. The Duchenne dystrophy gene: A great leap forward on the long march. *Trends Genet.* 1 (1985) 205–209

Kingston, H. M., Harper, P. S., Peason, P. L., Davies, K. E., Williamson, R., and Page, D. Localization of the gene for Becker muscular dystrophy. *Lancet* 2 (1983) 1200

Koenig, M., Hoffman, E. P., Bertelson, C. J., Monaco, A. P., Feener, C. and Kunkel, L. M. Complete cloning of the Duchenne muscular dystrophy (DMD) cDNA and preliminary genomic organization of the DMD gene in normal and affected individuals. *Cell* 50 (1987) 509–517

Koenig, M., Monaco, A. P., and Kunkel, L. M. The complete sequence of dystrophin predicts a rod-shaped cytoskeletal protein. *Cell* 53 (1988) 219–228

Kunkel, L. M., Monaco, A. P., Middlesworth, W. *et al.* Specific cloning of DNA fragments from the DNA from a patient with an X-chromosome deletion. *Proc. Natl. Acad. Sci. USA* 82 (1985) 82 4778–4782

Kunkel, L. M. and co-authors. Analysis of deletions in DNA from patients with Becker and Duchenne muscular dystrophy. *Nature* 322 (1986) 73–77

Monaco, A. P., Bertelson, C. J., Middlesworth, W. *et al.* Detection of deletions spanning the Duchenne muscular dystrophy locus using a tightly linked DNA segment. *Nature* 316 (1985) 845–848

Monaco, A. P., Neve, R. L., Colletti-Feener, C. A., Bertelson, C. A., Kurnit, D. M. and Kunkel, L. M. Isolation of candidate cDNAs for portions of the Duchenne muscular dystrophine gene. *Nature* 323 (1986) 646–650

Monaco, A. P., Bertelson, C. J., Liechti-Gallati, S., Moser, H. and Kunkel, L. M. An explanation for the phenotypic differences between patients bearing partial deletions of the DMD locus. *Genomics* 2 (1988) 90–95

van Ommen, G. J. B., Bertelson, C., Ginjaar, H. B., Den Dunnen, J. T., Bakker, E., Chelly, J., Matton, M., Van Essen, A. J., Bartley, J., Kunkel, L. M. and Pearson, P. L. Long-range genomic map of the Duchenne muscular dystrophy (DMD) gene: Isolation and use of J66 (DXS268), a distal intragenic marker. *Genomics* 1 (1987) 329–336

Ray, P. N., Belfall, B., Duff, C. *et al.* Cloning of the breakpoint of an X;21 translocation associated with Duchenne muscular dystrophy. *Nature* 318 (1985) 672

Verellen-Dumoulin, C. H., Freund, M., de Meyer, R. *et al.* Expression of an X-linked muscular dystrophy in a female due to translocation involving Xp21 and non-random inactivation of the normal X-chromosome. *Hum. Genet.* 67 (1984) 115–119

Wapenaar, M. C., Kievits, T., Hart, K. A., Abbs, S., Blonden, L. A. J., Den Dunnen, J. T., Grootscholten, P. M., Baaker, E., Verellen-Dumoulin, C., Bobrow, M., van Ommen, G. J. B. and Pearson, P. L. A deletion hot spot in the Duchenne muscular dystrophy gene. *Genomics* 2 (1988) 101–108

J. Inher. Metab. Dis. 12 Suppl. 1 (1989) 191–201

Prospects for Gene Therapy Now and in the Future

R. J. AKHURST

Duncan Guthrie Institute for Medical Genetics, Yorkhill Hospital, Glasgow G3 8SJ, UK

Summary: Advances in gene technology and cell biology have supplied the means to undertake human gene therapy in the near future. Techniques have been developed for the efficient introduction of gene sequences into the pluripotential stem cells of the haematopoietic system and our increased understanding of gene-regulatory mechanisms should allow therapeutic gene expression levels to be obtained.

Gene therapy should, at present, be termed gene supplementation since it will involve the addition of corrective genes to the host cell genome. It may only be used to treat recessively inherited disorders. Prospects for the future include the use of homologous recombination to correct or replace defective genes, allowing the treatment of dominantly inherited diseases.

Technological advances in molecular and cellular biology have lead to a wealth of information with respect to human genetics. Over one third of the human genome has been molecularly mapped and many DNA sequences showing restriction fragment length polymorphisms (RFLPs) are now available allowing their use for genetic linkage studies within families. We have gained an understanding of the molecular nature of a variety of single gene defects which cause disease and of the complex systems controlling the regulated expression of these genes. The stage is now set for this technology to be applied as a therapeutic tool.

Gene therapy, at present better termed gene supplementation, is the correction of genetic defects by addition of a normal gene copy into selected cells or organs of a diseased individual. Gene supplementation has already been used successfully in the correction of genetic disorders in the mouse (Readhead *et al.*, 1987). More advanced gene therapy, namely the replacement or correction of a defective gene, which could be used to treat dominantly inherited disorders such as Huntington's chorea, is still beyond our current technological capabilities.

GERM-LINE *VERSUS* SOMATIC CELL GENE THERAPY

The construction of transgenic strains of animals carrying foreign genes within the germ-line is now a successful and routine procedure in many laboratories (Hogan *et al.*, 1986). In most people's opinion, however, introduction of genes into the

Journal of Inherited Metabolic Disease. ISSN 0141–8955. Copyright © SSIEM and Kluwer Academic Publishers, PO Box 55, Lancaster, UK.

human germ-line should be forbidden since it would alter the genetic make-up of subsequent generations. Fortunately, this approach is technically not feasible since the efficiency of gene-transfer into mammalian zygotes is very low. Only 1–2% of mouse eggs microinjected with DNA will produce viable transgenic animals and there is no way of screening for such successful events at early embryonic stages.

The application of molecular techniques to genetic analysis of *in vitro* fertilized human embryos should be limited to preimplantation diagnosis. DNA from a single cell may now be amplified enzymatically in the test-tube, producing large enough quantities to enable standard molecular diagnostic techniques to be performed (Higuchi *et al.*, 1988). Theoretically this type of diagnosis could be carried out on DNA isolated from a single biopsied blastomere from a preimplantation embryo allowing the genotyping and selection of such embryos before transfer back into the mother. This is far more efficient and, though raising some ethical questions, it is certainly a more acceptable approach to 'correction' of genetic defects than germ-line gene therapy.

CANDIDATES FOR SOMATIC GENE THERAPY

Human diseases which could be candidates for gene therapy must obey certain criteria. First, they should be simple genetic disorders which represent single gene defects. They should also be recessive in nature since, at present, gene supplementation will be the chosen approach. More obviously the affected gene must have been molecularly cloned and characterized with respect to its structure and expression.

Ideally the genetic defect should affect a tissue which is easily amenable to genetic manipulation. At present, the most likely human tissues to be used in gene therapy are bone marrow or skin. These are the only cell-types which can be extracted from the body, grown and manipulated *in vitro*, and successfully retransplanted back into the patient. Correction of a genetic disease could possibly be successful using these tissues even if the defective gene product is not normally expressed here, provided that the gene product in question is a soluble extracellular factor or is freely permeable across cellular membranes. It has been suggested, for example, that haemophilia B could be remedied by transfer of the factor IX gene into the skin cells of a haemophiliac (Brownlee, 1988). The clotting factor would then enter the blood stream by diffusion. One would only need to attain levels of factor IX in the blood stream which are 10% those of normal physiological concentrations (Table 1). The advantage of using the skin as a vehicle for gene therapy is that the transplant may be easily monitored for any deleterious effects gene insertion might have on the host tissue, e.g. leading to neoplasia.

Ideally gene therapy would be attempted with genes which do not require a high degree of regulation. Adenosine deaminase, purine nucleoside phosphorylase and hypoxanthine–guanine phosphoribosyl transferase, the absence of which cause severe combined immunodeficiency, severe immunodeficiency and Lesch–Nyhan disease, respectively, would all be good candidates since they are fairly ubiquitously expressed. It would also be desirable if the gene-product were to be therapeutic at

Table 1 Candidate diseases for human gene therapy

Disease	Gene affected	Cells affected	Tissue specificity of expression	Level of expression required	Other therapies available
Immunodeficiency	Purine nucleoside phosphorylase	Lymphocytes	No	1–5% normal	Bone-marrow transplant
SCID	Adenosine deaminase	Lymphocytes	No	1–5% normal	Bone-marrow transplant
Lesch–Nyhan	Hypoxanthine–guanine phosphoribosyl transferase	Most cells esp. basal ganglia	Basal ganglia?	Normal levels?	No therapy
Thalassaemia	α- and β-globin gene loci	Red blood cells	High specificity required	Precise regulation required	Blood transfusion Bone-marrow transplant
Haemophilia A	Factor VIII	Hepatocytes	No	10% normal	Exogenous supply of missing factor
Haemophilia B	Factor IX				
Phenylketonuria	Phenylalanine hydroxylase	Hepatocytes	?	1–5% normal	Therapeutic diet during infancy

severely reduced concentrations since a major problem with gene transfer is obtaining high gene expression levels. Adenosine deaminase and purine nucleoside phosphorylase would both fit this criterion since the corresponding diseases can be corrected by enzymatic levels 20–100-fold lower than physiological enzyme concentrations (Table 1).

A large family of disorders which could be amenable to gene therapy are the thalassaemias, caused by defects in the α- and β-globin gene loci. However, these genetic diseases are far more complex to tackle than those mentioned above because of the need for highly tissue-specific gene expression and very precisely regulated levels of the appropriate gene products within the red blood cell. Nevertheless, recent advances in our understanding of globin gene expression now make this a viable prospect for the future (see below and Grosveld *et al.*, 1987; Dzierzak *et al.*, 1988).

A final consideration when selecting diseases as candidates for gene therapy is the severity of the disease and the availability of alternative conventional therapies for disease management. Phenylketonuria, caused by a deficiency of phenylalanine hydroxylase, could be a good candidate for gene therapy since the gene has been cloned and the defect is correctable by much reduced levels of the enzyme. However, the disease is clinically manageable by screening newborns for hyper-phenylalaninaemia and the use of therapeutic diets at an early age. It is debatable whether there is a need for gene therapy in this case.

There is no dispute that both severe combined immunodeficiency and purine nucleoside phosphorylase deficiency are severe clinical conditions, affected individuals rarely living beyond childhood. The only current therapy available to these individuals is bone-marrow transplantation from a suitable histocompatible donor. The advantages that gene therapy could offer over conventional bone-marrow transplant is the immediate availability of a suitable bone-marrow donor (the patient himself), the certainty that there will be no graft rejection and the absence of any possible graft-*versus*-host disease.

APPROACHES TO GENE TRANSFER

Due to the availability and easy manipulation of bone-marrow cells in culture, these are considered to be the prime targets for gene transfer and subsequent gene therapy. I will therefore focus on the attempts at introduction of genes into this cell type. The haematopoietic system consists of a heterogeneous population of cells including pluripotent stem cells, progenitor cells, and mature cells such as erythrocytes, megakaryocytes, lymphocytes, etc. To introduce genes in a stable heritable manner, and to ensure that all of the cell types are genetically modified, it will be essential to target gene transfer to the pluripotential stem cell. However, this cell type only contributes a very minor portion of the total blood cell population (0.01%) and, as yet, has not been defined in any way (Williams *et al.*, 1984). It is therefore essential to have a very efficient gene delivery system.

Various approaches to gene transfer have been taken including microinjection of DNA (Hogan *et al.*, 1986), calcium phosphate precipitation (Hogan *et al.*, 1986), electroporation (Chu *et al.*, 1987) and the use of retroviral vectors (Williams *et al.*, 1984). Of these, the only efficient and practical approach is that of retroviruses. Using this type of vector a theoretical infection efficiency of 100% can be obtained, although in practice this is nearer 10–20% for bone marrow cells (Williams *et al.*, 1984). Additionally, the retrovirus normally integrates into the host genome as a single copy of known structure and with the gene of interest intact. During physical or chemical methods of gene transfer the genes are often rearranged and integrate as multiple copies in tandem array.

The available retroviral vectors are based on naturally occurring murine retroviruses such as the Moloney murine leukaemia virus (MoMLV). The virus is composed of a single-stranded RNA genome packaged inside a glycoprotein envelope, the latter specifying host range. During the viral life cycle the genome is reverse-transcribed to produce a double-stranded DNA copy which integrates at random into the host genome. The resulting 'provirus' then expresses viral products from transcription signals which are found in the long terminal repeats at the

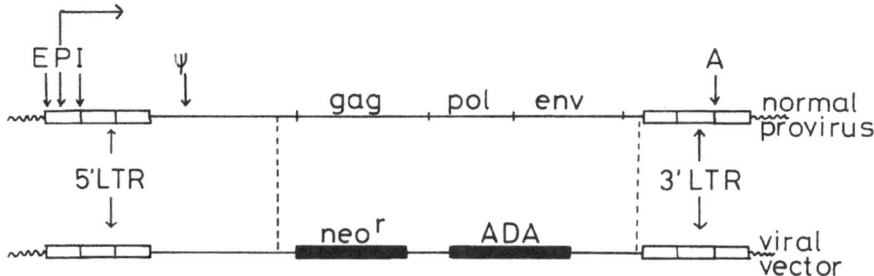

Figure 1 Structures of the Moloney murine leukaemia virus and derivative retroviral vector: LTR, long terminal repeat; E, enhancer; P, promotor: I, transcription start signal; ψ, packaging signal; A, polyadenylation site

termini of the virus (Figure 1). It can also transcribe genomic RNA which is packaged into viral particles. The viral genome normally encodes three gene products, the group specific antigen (*gag*), reverse transcriptase (*pol*) and the envelope gene (*env*), all of which are required in *trans* for viral replication and packaging of the genome into viral particles. At the 5' end of the viral genome is a DNA sequence, ψ, which is required in *cis* for packaging viral transcripts into viral particles. The long terminal repeats and ψ sequence are the only functions required to produce an integrating vector. The viral genes, *gag*, *pol* and *env* can all be deleted and replaced with exogenous DNA. This resultant defective virus is still capable of replicating and integrating into the host genome but can only produce infective viral particles with the aid of a helper virus to supply the *gag*, *pol* and *env* functions.

Various packaging cell lines have been developed by introducing a helper provirus which lacks the ψ sequence into the cellular genome. The advantage of this cell system is that infective, defective retroviral vectors can be generated at high titre without contamination with the helper virus. The ψ⁻ helper virus provides

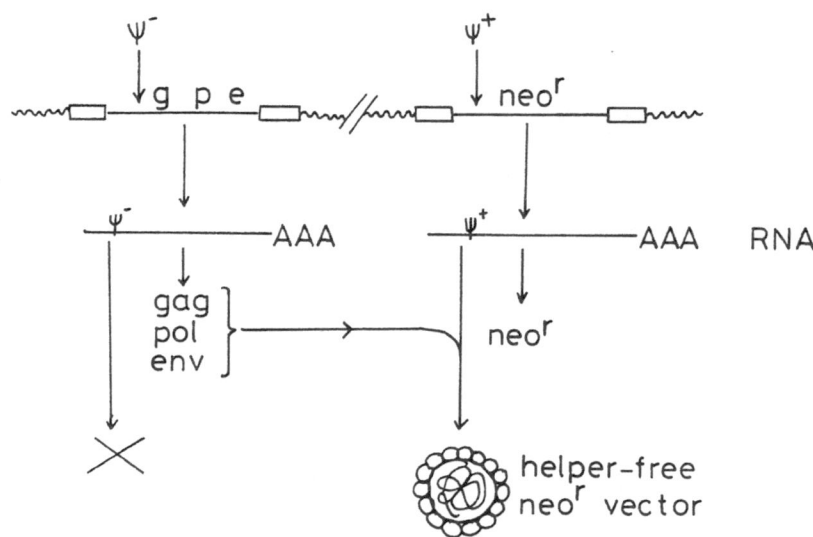

Figure 2   Packaging of a retroviral vector using a ψ⁻ packaging cell line. The cell line possesses a provirus encoding viral genes, *gag*(g), *pol*(p) and *env*(e), but no ψ packaging signal. The viral particles can thus only package transcripts in *trans* from another provirus possessing the ψ sequence

all the packaging functions for the defective recombinant retrovirus but cannot package its own viral genome due to lack of the ψ sequence (Figure 2). The host range of the resultant viral particles is determined by the *gag* gene function of the helper virus and thus by choice of packaging cell line. Such cell lines are available giving both species-specific (Mann *et al.*, 1983) and amphotrophic (broad host-range) virus particles (Hock and Miller, 1986).

The strategy for gene delivery and subsequent gene therapy of bone marrow cells involves the engineering of a recombinant virus *in vitro* to carry the gene of interest in an expressible form and a drug resistance gene, such as neomycin resistance. The naked viral DNA is then transfected into a packaging line using physical or chemical techniques and transfectants are screened for by virtue of the drug resistance marker carried within the viral genome. The packaging cell line will then produce high titres of infective viral particles containing the recombinant retroviral genome. The viral particles are used for *in vitro* infection of bone-marrow cells which have been isolated from the patient. The genetically-modified bone-marrow cells are subsequently re-injected intravenously back into the patient who may have been treated by chemotherapy or irradiation to ablate defective stem cells, allowing for the expansion of the new stem cell population. This protocol has been successfully used on mice *in vivo* for the stable introduction and expression of genes encoding neomycin resistance (Williams *et al.*, 1984), hypoxanthine–guanine phosphoribosyl transferase (Miller *et al.*, 1984) and human beta-globin (Dzierzak *et al.*, 1988) into the self-perpetuating bone-marrow population.

To achieve efficient infection the recipient cell must be in the process of dividing. Normally, at any one time, only 10% of stem cells will be mitotically active. Lemischka and colleagues (1986) pretreated mice with 5' fluorouracil prior to bone-marrow isolation to enrich for primitive stem cells and to increase the fraction of those cells which are mitotically active from 10 to 100%. Using this treatment they achieved a 50% infection efficiency. Whether the benefits of such chemotherapy for humans would outweigh the side-effects has to be considered. In fact, using genetic markers, Lemischka and colleagues (1986) found that, at any one time, only one or a few stem cells account for the majority of mature haematopoietic cells derived from the marrow. Coupled with the finding that, in some cases (such as adenosine deaminase and hypoxanthine–guanine phosphoribosyl transferase), normal stem cells could have a selective advantage over genetically defective ones (Parkman, 1986), this implies that a 10–20% stem cell infection efficiency may be sufficient for successful gene therapy. It also implies that chemotherapy or ir-radiation prior to transplantation of genetically-manipulated bone-marrow cells may not be essential in all cases.

A prospect for the future would be the development of retroviral vectors showing tissue-specificity of infection. Provided that highly efficient infection protocols were available this might allow the direct application of virus *in vivo* by intravenous injection. Not only would this bypass the need for tissue transplantation, but may allow the transfer of genes to other cell types, such as the liver or nervous tissue, opening up the possibility of treating many other diseases. At this stage, however, our state of knowledge concerning the detrimental effects of retrovirus vectors and the efficiencies with which infection can be obtained make this route inadvisable and unlikely.

THE PROBLEM OF GENE EXPRESSION

It has now been established that efficient means exist for the introduction of new genetic material into the progenitor stem cells of the bone marrow and that, for the most part, these sequences are stably maintained and propagated. However a major obstacle to gene therapy is obtaining expression levels from the exogenous gene sequence adequate for therapeutic value and, in some cases such as the thalassaemias, obtaining highly regulated gene expression in terms of tissue-speci-ficity and precise quantity.

Fortunately, as previously discussed, several genetic diseases can be corrected by supplementing enzyme levels to only a fraction of the normal physiological state (Table 1). In addition, if the gene product is freely diffusible, tissue-specificity of expression is not required. It is for this reason that most current attention in gene therapy has been focussed on severe combined immunodeficiency and Lesch–Nyhan disease (Williams *et al.*, 1986; Chang *et al.*, 1987). Recent advances in the design of retroviral expression vectors and in our understanding of eukaryotic gene regulation make the possibility of tackling more complex diseases, such as the thalassaemias, a feasible prospect. The early retroviral constructs often used constitutive promotors, such as the viral long terminal repeats or thymidine kinase promotor to drive the transcription of a full-length cDNA encoding the gene product of interest (Williams *et al.*, 1986; Chang *et al.*, 1987). These constructs were clearly not designed to obtain lineage- or stage-specific gene expression since none of the *cis*-regulatory elements required for tissue-specific expression were included. More recently, Dzierzak and colleagues (1988) introduced a human β-globin gene into mouse bone-marrow cells *in vivo*. They demonstrated that not only could they obtain a highly efficient permanent engraftment of genetically altered cells, but that appropriate lineage-specific gene expression of the new β-globin gene was achieved. This gene was only expressed at significant levels in the erythroid lineage. Their strategy was simple, namely, instead of using a cDNA sequence they utilized the complete genomic β-globin gene including both 5' and 3' flanking sequences which are known to possess tissue-specific gene enhancers. Unfortunately although lineage-specific gene expression occurred, the level of expression achieved was only 4% that of the endogenous level. The explanation for this may be supplied by the recent findings of Grosveld and colleagues (1987) who have identified two new *cis*-acting elements located 50 kb upstream and 20 kb downstream of the beta-globin gene locus and which are essential for high level expression of the genes in that locus. If these elements had been included in Dzierzak's constructs it is possible that physiological β-globin gene expression levels would have been obtained. Whether such regulatory sequences so far removed from the gene also exist at other genetic loci remains to be seen.

One approach towards optimizing the level and specificity of gene expression has been the use of self-inactivating retroviral vectors (Yu *et al.*, 1986). It was thought that the viral long terminal repeats, which possess viral enhancers and promotors, may interfere with the transcription of genes carried within the viral vector. Consequently new vectors were designed with deletions in the 3' long terminal repeat which effectively removes all of the viral transcriptional control machinery from the provirus. This strategy was utilized by Dzierzak and colleagues (1988) and did indeed appear to enhance the lineage-specificity of expression, though not the prevalence, of transcripts. In addition to the advantages for gene expression, these self-inactivating retroviral vectors give an added safety component for the use of retroviral vectors (see below).

Bearing in mind that genetic loci are extremely complex in terms of gene regulation, one would ideally seek to integrate the corrective gene into the defective gene locus itself. This might then automatically provide the appropriate distant regulatory controls for gene expression. Going one step further, it would be most useful if the defective gene could be replaced or corrected precisely. This would open up the possibility of treating dominantly inherited diseases by gene therapy. Needless to say, steps toward this end have already been taken and homologous recombination between transfected DNA and its homologous chromosomal locus has been obtained *in vitro* (Thomas *et al.*, 1986; Smithies *et al.*, 1985). The frequency of these events, however, is still far too low for the technique to be applied to gene therapy *in vivo*, only 10^{-3}–10^{-2} cells integrating exogenous DNA actually undergo a homologous recombination event. Additionally it is impossible to predict whether homologous recombination will result in single or double reciprocal recombination or in gene conversion, nor whether it will result in correction of the chromosomal gene or the incoming DNA (Thomas *et al.*, 1986; Smithies *et al.*, 1985). Furthermore, during the process of homologous recombination there are frequent events leading to the introduction of novel mutations within the chromosomal gene (Thomas and Cappechi, 1986), certainly an undesirable event for gene therapy. Of course, these are early days, advances in gene technology can be very rapid and these problems may soon be overcome.

To correct a genetic defect by homologous recombination it will be essential to know the precise molecular nature of the defect so that the appropriate gene construct may be designed. This might limit its applicability to diseases which are genetically homogenous in the population, such as sickle-cell anaemia or cystic fibrosis. Diseases such as Duchenne muscular dystrophy, which has a very large gene locus and is very heterogenous in nature, will probably not be amenable to such approaches.

RISK ASSESSMENT

With the introduction of any new clinical technique it is imperative to evaluate the safety and effectiveness of the new therapy using animal models before utilizing the technique in humans. Though detailed studies can be carried out on the safety of retroviruses both *in vitro* and with animal models, there are no known non-human models available for the diseases under question with which to assess effectiveness. Since the diseases under consideration, such as severe combined immuno deficiency and Lesch–Nyhan, are quite severe and there are few alternative therapies one may consider that clinical trials would be justifiable (Robertson, 1986).

There are two major safety considerations when using retroviral vectors. First, recombination events could occur within the cell to produce a new infective, possibly harmful, virus from a defective retroviral vector. This could be brought about by recombination with the helper provirus in the packaging cell line or, more seriously, recombination with an endogenous defective provirus within the recipient's genome. The former event is much more likely and should be tackled by strict quality control on the producer cell-line at regular intervals to check that only defective viral particles are generated. The second type of event is highly unlikely since all retroviral vectors in use at present are based on murine viruses which show no homology to human retroviruses.

A second possibility is that the site of retroviral integration could be deleterious to the recipient genome. Again this is unlikely; activation of oncogenes by insertion of the viral long terminal repeat within such a gene locus can be avoided by the use of the self-inactivating retroviral vectors (Yu *et al.*, 1986). The risk of losing an essential genetic function by viral integration is low since the locus of integration would normally be heterozygous when undertaking somatic cell gene therapy.

For certain diseases it will be essential to regulate gene expression very precisely (Table 1). Incorrect expression levels could be just as deleterious to the patient as the disease for which therapy is being sought. It is thus a major advantage of the current approaches to gene therapy that the patients cells are initially treated outside the body and can be fully assessed before re-inoculation.

In conclusion, it appears that we should be optimistic about the prospects for using human gene therapy to cure recessive genetic disorders in the near future. The possibility that dominantly inherited disorders will be treated by gene therapy should not be ruled out at this stage as advances are made in our understanding of homologous recombination. There are still, however, several ethical issues to be considered before the gene therapy approach should be implemented (Walters, 1986) and the guidelines set out by various regulatory bodies should be firmly adhered to at all times.

REFERENCES

Brownlee, G. G. Towards gene therapy for haemophilia B. *MRC News* 39 (1988) 14–15

Chang, S. M. W., Wager-Smith, K., Tsao, T. Y., Henkel-Tigges, J., Vaishnav, S. and Caskey, C. T. Construction of a defective retrovirus containing the human hypoxanthine phosphoribosyltransferase cDNA and its expression in cultured cells and mouse bone marrow. *Mol. Cell. Biol.* 7 (1987) 854–865

Chu, G., Hayakawa, H. and Berg, F. Electroporation for the efficient transfection of mammalian cells with DNA. *Nucl. Acids Res.* 15 (1987) 1311–1326

Dzierzak, E. A., Papayannopoulou, T. and Mulligan, R. C. Lineage-specific expression of a human β-globin gene in murine bone marrow transplant recipients reconstituted with retrovirus-transduced stem cells. *Nature* 331 (1988) 35–41

Grosveld, F., van Assendelft, G. B., Greaves, D. R. and Kollias, G. Position-independent, high-level expression of the human β-globin gene in transgenic mice. *Cell* 51 (1987) 975–985

Higuchi, R., von Beroldingen, C. H., Sensabaugh, G. F. and Erlich, H. A. DNA typing from single hairs. *Nature* 332 (1988) 543–546

Hock, R. A. and Miller, A. D. Retrovirus-mediated transfer and expression of drug resistance genes in human haematopoietic progenitor cells. *Nature* 320 (1986) 275–277

Hogan, B., Costantini, F. and Lacy, E. *Manipulating the Mouse Embryo: A laboratory manual*, Cold Spring Harbor Laboratory, 1986

Lemischka, I. R., Raulet, D. H. and Mulligan, R. C. Developmental potential and dynamic behaviour of haematopoietic stem cells. *Cell* 45 (1986) 917–927

Mann, R., Mulligan, R. C. and Baltimore, D. Construction of a retrovirus packaging mutant and its use to produce helper-free defective retrovirus. *Cell* 33 (1983) 153–159

Miller, A. D., Echner, R. J., Jolly, D. J., Friedmann, T. and Verma, I. M. Expression of a retrovirus encoding human HPRT in mice. *Science* 225 (1984) 630–632

Parkman, R. The application of bone-marrow transplantation to the treatment of genetic diseases. *Science* 232 (1986) 1373–1378

Readhead, C., Popko, B., Takahashi, N., Shine, H. D., Saavedra, R. A., Sidman, R. L. and Hood, L. Expression of a myelin basic protein gene in transgenic shiverer mice: Correction of the dysmyelinating phenotype. *Cell* 48 (1987) 703–712

Robertson, M. Desperate appliances. *Nature* 320 (1986) 213–214

Smithies, O., Gregg, R. G., Boggs, S. S., Koralewski, M. A. and Kucherlapati, R. S. Insertion of DNA sequences into the human chromosomal β-globin locus by homologous recombination. *Nature* 317 (1985) 230–234

Thomas, K. R. and Cappechi, M. R. Introduction of homologous DNA sequences into mammalian cells induces mutations in the cognate gene. *Nature* 324 (1986) 34–38

Thomas, K. R., Folger, K. R. and Capecci, M. R. High frequency targeting of genes to specific sites in the mammalian genome. *Cell* 44 (1986) 419–428

Walters, L. The ethics of human gene therapy. *Nature* 320 (1986) 225–227

Williams, D. A., Lemischka, I. R., Nathan, D. G. and Mulligan, R. C. Introduction of new genetic material into pluripotent haematopoietic stem cells of the mouse. *Nature* 310 (1984) 476–480

Williams, D. A., Orkin, S. H. and Mulligan, R. C. Retrovirus-mediated transfer of human adenosine deaminase gene sequences into cells in culture and into murine hematopoietic cells *in vivo*. *Proc. Natl. Acad. Sci USA* 83 (1986) 2566–2570

Yu, S-F., von Ruden, T., Kantoff, P. W., Garber, C., Seiberg, M., Ruther, U., Anderson, W. F., Wagner, E. F. and Gilboa, E. Self-inactivating retroviral vectors designed for transfer of whole genes into mammalian cells. *Proc. Natl. Acad. Sci. USA* 83 (1986) 3194–3198

J. Inher. Metab. Dis. 12 Suppl. 1 (1989) 202–206

Prenatal Diagnosis of Disorders of Galactose Metabolism

J. B. HOLTON, J. T. ALLEN and M. G. GILLETT
Department of Clinical Chemistry, Southmead Hospital, Bristol BS10 5NB, UK

Summary: Of three clinically significant galactose disorders, there is only a real need and experience of prenatal diagnosis in classical galactosaemia. Prenatal diagnosis for this disorder may be carried out by galactose-1-phosphate uridyl transferase assay in cultured amniotic fluid cells or in chorionic villus biopsies and by galactitol estimation in amniotic fluid supernatant. Although the long-term outcome of patients treated on a galactose-restricted diet is recognized to be unsatisfactory, prenatal diagnosis is only rarely performed with a view to terminating the affected pregnancy.

There are three clinically significant disorders of galactose metabolism (Dunger and Holton, 1987); these are, galactokinase deficiency (EC 2.7.1.6, McKusick 23020), classical galactosaemia or galactose-1-phosphate uridyl transferase (transferase) deficiency (EC 2.7.7.10, McKusick 23040) and uridine diphosphate galactose-4-epimerase (epimerase) deficiency (EC 5.1.3.2, McKusick 23035). Although all the disorders are amenable to prenatal diagnosis, there is very little experience except for transferase deficiency.

GALACTOKINASE DEFICIENCY

Prenatal diagnosis of galactokinase deficiency is possible by enzyme assay in cultured amniotic fluid cells. Table 1 summarizes the experience in our laboratory measuring galactokinase in cultured amniotic fluid cells and skin fibroblasts employing a method which is a modification (A. Fensom, personal communication) of a red cell enzyme assay (Beutler and Matsumoto, 1973). Although a positive case

Table 1 Galactokinase activity in cultured amniotic fluid cells and skin fibroblasts

Cell type	Origin of cells	Galactokinase activity	
Amniotic fluid	Controls ($n = 6$)	39.3–55.5	(full range)
	Prenatal diagnosis	44.6	(N/N)
Skin fibroblasts	Unaffected sibling	30.2	(N/GK)

Enzyme activity is expressed in $\mu mol\,(mg\;protein)^{-1}h^{-1}$.
N/N = normal homozygote levels on postnatal red cells; N/GK = normal/galactokinase deficient heterozygote on red cells.

Journal of Inherited Metabolic Disease. ISSN 0141–8955. Copyright © SSIEM and Kluwer Academic Publishers, PO Box 55, Lancaster, UK.

was not examined, it seems reasonably established that a successful diagnosis could be made by this means. It is likely that prenatal diagnosis could be achieved by measuring galactitol in amniotic fluid supernatant, as in transferase deficiency (see later). However, it would be essential to confirm the feasibility of this method by investigating a positive pregnancy.

TRANSFERASE DEFICIENCY

Most prenatal diagnoses for classical galactosaemia have been performed using the assay of transferase in cultured amniotic fluid cells by a number of similar techniques (Monk and Holton, 1976). This assay is extremely robust and can distinguish clearly not only an abnormal and unaffected pregnancy but also a galactosaemic heterozygote and a galactosaemic/Duarte mixed heterozygote fetus, the last of these having about 10–15% of mean normal enzyme activity. This degree of discrimination is important, since families in whom one parent is a galactosaemic/ Duarte heterozygote and the other is a normal galactosaemic heterozygote are not uncommon. The offspring in such families could be true cases of classical galactosaemia or galactosaemic/Duarte mixed heterozygotes, and the significance with respect to terminating a pregnancy would be different in these two cases.

Allen and colleagues (1980) reported that galactitol, a reduction product of galactose, accumulated in the liver of a galactosaemic fetus, along with galactose and galactose-1-phosphate, and raised levels were detected in amniotic fluid. The observation led to a method of prenatal diagnosis for transferase deficiency, measuring galactitol in amniotic fluid supernatant using a gas chromatograph with a flame ionisation detector (Allen *et al.*, 1981). Subsequently the method has been made more accurate and precise by the use of gas chromatography with mass spectrometric detection (unpublished observation). The galactitol method has been used in our laboratory in 24 pregnancies at risk for classical galactosaemia (Table 2). It differentiated affected and unaffected pregnancies quite clearly and has the

Table 2 Prenatal diagnosis of transferase deficiency by galactitol estimation in amniotic fluid supernatant

Method	Cases	Number	Galactitol (range)
Gas chromatography/flame ionisation	Controls	20	0.6–2.2
	N/N	9	0.5–1.8
	N/G	2	0.8–1.0
	G/G	4	14.0–18.7
Gas chromatography/mass spectrophotometry	Controls	6	<1.0
	N/N	1	<1.0
	N/G	4	1.4–1.6
	G/G	4	6.7–10.6

Galactitol values are in $\mu mol\, L^{-1}$.
N/N = normal fetus confirmed; N/G = normal/galactosaemic heterozygote fetus confirmed; G/G = galactosaemic fetus confirmed.

Table 3   First-trimester diagnoses for transferase deficiency in European laboratories[a]

Total number of diagnoses by chorionic villus biopsy			10
Negative results	7	Positive results	3
Results confirmed	6	Results confirmed	2
Pregnancies terminated	1 (trisomy)	Pregnancies terminated	3

[a]Bristol, Brussels, Copenhagen, London, Lyon, Munich and Rotterdam

advantage of a result being obtainable within a hour or two after the amniocentesis compared with a time of around 2 weeks by the method using cultured cells. There is a suggestion that heterozygotes might be distinguished from normal by the more refined method, but more cases would be needed to establish this.

More recently, the transferase method was adapted to assay the enzyme directly on chorionic villus biopsies, and the first successful diagnoses by this means were reported by Kleijer and colleagues (1986). A questionnaire sent out to seven European laboratories known to be involved in prenatal diagnosis of galactosaemia, in order to assess the present level of experience using chorionic villus for this purpose, revealed that only 10 diagnostic tests had been performed up to the beginning of June this year (Table 3). Of these, eight results had been verified by some other means, two out of the three positive results being in this category.

EPIMERASE DEFICIENCY

A method for prenatal diagnosis of epimerase deficiency has been reported (Gillett *et al.*, 1983) using enzyme assay on cultured amniotic fluid cells. Since the disorder appears to be extremely rare there has been no incentive to develop a method on chorionic villus biopsies.

THE NEED FOR PRENATAL DIAGNOSIS OF GALACTOSE DISORDERS

The only consistent clinical abnormality associated with *galactokinase deficiency* is cataract. This problem resolves rapidly with the early introduction of a galactose-restricted diet and, therefore, there seems no real need for a prenatal diagnosis in the majority of cases. It may be justified, and has been used, however, when the social circumstances of the family indicate that a low galactose diet would not be maintained in the child.

The obvious reason for performing prenatal diagnosis for *transferase deficiency*, as with other disorders, is with the object of terminating affected pregnancies. There are, however, other possible reasons which will be discussed later. The justification for aborting a galactosaemic fetus is questioned by many because it is seen as a treatable condition, although it has been known for a number of years that the intellectual outcome is poor even with early and carefully controlled dietary treatment (Donnell *et al.*, 1980; Sardharwalla, 1980). At least one authority in this disease has stated that prenatal diagnosis is justifiable (Komrower, 1982). A recent large-scale study (Buist *et al.*, 1988) has revealed that the numbers of patients with developmental delay and the degree to which they are affected is far greater than earlier imagined; specific speech abnormality and ovarian dysfunction are now recognized as major problems. Growth retardation and neurological abnormalities occur, but less frequently.

There is no comprehensive data on the numbers of and reasons for carrying out prenatal diagnosis for galactosaemia but it seems probable that only a small proportion of them are undertaken with a view to terminating affected pregnancies. This is consistent with the finding (Table 3) that so few diagnoses are done by chorionic villus biopsy because, although the technique has many advantages, the increased risk of obtaining the specimen could only be justified if termination is being considered. Amongst the reasons why so few diagnoses are done with possible abortion in mind, a lack of understanding or of acceptance of the real facts about the long-term outcome in galactosaemia on the part of the counsellor must be important; but it is also obvious that counselling the parents is particularly difficult when the index child in the family is alive and being enthusiastically treated. In this connection it is noteworthy that series of prenatal diagnoses for galactosaemia contain a preponderance of families in which the index child succumbed in the neonatal period (Holton and Raymont, 1980), although there is no inherent reason why prenatal diagnosis is more necessary in this group.

Other reasons which are encountered for wanting to do a prenatal diagnosis for galactosaemia include: (1) the wish of parents to have foreknowledge of another affected child; (2) the relative ease with which a prenatal diagnosis can be made in comparison to a definitive postnatal diagnosis, with a view to very early treatment in positive cases; (3) to determine whether maternal galactose restriction is required during pregnancy. The first two of these reasons do not justify obtaining a specimen for prenatal diagnosis but if amniotic fluid is available for some other purpose it would be perfectly reasonable to perform a galactitol estimation since this is an extremely simple, reliable and cheap method of diagnosis. With regard to maternal galactose restriction, available biochemical evidence suggests that this will not confer any advantage on the fetus (Irons *et al.*, 1985). In addition, preliminary analysis of data from the previously mentioned galactosaemia survey indicates that there may be little or no benefit to the long-term progress of the baby (N. Buist, personal communication). Therefore, this does not seem a good reason for prenatal diagnosis.

Only two cases of clinically affected *epimerase deficiency* have been reported (Holton *et al.*, 1981; Sardharwalla *et al.*, 1987) and both were maintained on what were considered to be appropriate galactose-restricted diets for the condition. At the age of 7 years, the former patient had an IQ of 85 and severe sensorineural deafness (R. McFaul, personal communication). The latter child was assessed to have serious developmental delay and bilateral sensorineural deafness at the age of 2 years 9 months. The similarity of the clinical picture and its nature tempts one to suggest that prenatal diagnosis might be considered in this condition but more cases are needed to confirm the prognosis in this disease. As recorded earlier, a prenatal diagnosis was made in the mother of the first child; but the reasons for this were not entirely related to the expected outcome of a case of the disorder.

ACKNOWLEDGEMENTS

We acknowledge the contributions of Y. Shin, F. Van Hoof, N. J. Brandt, A. Fensom, W. J. Kleijer and M. O. Rolland, who provided data on chorionic villus assays.

REFERENCES

Allen, J. T., Gillett, M. G., Holton, J. B., King, G. S. and Pettit, B. R. Evidence of galactosaemia *in utero*. *Lancet* 1 (1980) 603

Allen, J. T., Holton, J. B. and Gillet, M. Gas liquid chromatographic determination of galactitol in amniotic fluid for possible use in prenatal diagnosis of galactosaemia. *Clin. Chim. Acta* 110 (1981) 59–63

Beutler, E. and Matsumoto, F. A rapid simplified assay for galactokinase activity in whole blood. *J. Lab. Clin. Med.* 82 (1973) 818–821

Buist, N., Waggoner, D., Donnell, G. and Levy, H. The effect of newborn screening in galactosaemia: results of the international survey. *Abstracts of the 26th Annual Symposium of the Society for the Study of Inborn Errors of Metabolism*, 1988

Donnell, G. N., Koch, R., Fishler, K. and Ng, W. G. Clinical aspects of galactosaemia. In Burman, D., Holton, J. B. and Pennock, C. A. (Eds.) *Inherited Disorders of Carbohydrate Metabolism*, MTP Press, Lancaster, 1980, pp. 103–115

Dunger, D. B. and Holton, J. B. Disorders of carbohydrate metabolism. In Holton, J. B. (Ed.) *The Inherited Metabolic Diseases*, Churchill Livingstone, Edinburgh, 1987, pp. 18–58

Gillett, M. G., Holton, J. B. and MacFaul, R. Prenatal determination of uridine diphosphate galactose-4-epimerase activity. *Prenat. Diagn.* 3 (1983) 57–59

Holton, J. B. and Raymont, C. M. Prenatal screening for galactosaemia. In Burman, D., Holton, J. B. and Pennock, C. A. (Eds.), *Inherited Disorders of Carbohydrate Metabolism*, MTP Press, Lancaster, 1980, pp. 141–147

Holton, J. B., Gillett, M. G., MacFaul, R. and Young, R. Galactosaemia: a new severe variant due to uridine diphosphate galactose-4-epimerase deficiency. *Arch. Dis. Child.* 56 (1981) 885–887

Irons, M., Levy, H. L., Pueschel, S. and Castree, K. Accumulation of galactose-1-phosphate in the galactosaemic fetus despite maternal milk avoidance. *J. Pediatr.* 107 (1985) 261–263

Komrower, G. M. Galactosaemia – thirty years on. The experience of a generation. *J. Inher. Metab. Dis.* 5 Suppl. 2 (1982) 96–104

Kleijer, W. J., Janse, H. C., van Diggelen, O. P., Macek, M., Hajek, Z., Gillett, M. and Holton, J. B. First-trimester diagnosis of galactosaemia. *Lancet* 1 (1986) 748

Monk, A. M. and Holton, J. B. Galactose-1-phosphate uridyl transferase in cultured cells. *Clin. Chim. Acta* 73 (1976) 537–546

Sardharwalla, I. B. In Burman, D., Holton, J. B. and Pennock, C. A. (Eds.) *Inherited Disorders of Carbohydrate Metabolism*, MTP Press, Lancaster, 1980, p. 151

Sardharwalla, I. B., Wraith, J. E., Bridge, C., Fowler, B. and Roberts, S. A. A patient with severe type of epimerase deficiency galactosaemia. *Abstracts of the 25th Annual Symposium of the Society for the Study of Inborn Errors of Metabolism*, 1987, p. 91

J. Inher. Metab. Dis. 12 Suppl. 1 (1989) 207–214

Prenatal and Postnatal Diagnosis of Menkes Disease, an Inherited Disorder of Copper Metabolism

T. Tønnesen and N. Horn

The John F. Kennedy Institute, Gl. Landevej 7, DK-2600 Glostrup, Denmark

Summary: 105 patients with Menkes disease have been diagnosed from ^{64}Cu-uptake studies in fibroblasts. These results are presented together with chase results following removal of ^{64}Cu from the medium for 16 Menkes patients. Second-trimester prenatal diagnosis has been performed in 80 pregnancies with male karyotype. These ^{64}Cu-uptake results show some overlap between the upper end of the normal range and the lower end of the Menkes range. Results are presented to show that a combination of ^{64}Cu-uptake and chase results offers a better diagnostic potential than ^{64}Cu-uptake *per se*. Chorionic villus copper values from 53 first-trimester prenatal diagnoses are presented. Maternal deciduum from some of these pregnancies contain similar high amounts of copper as found in the chorionic villus samples from affected fetuses. ^{64}Cu-uptake in cultured chorionic villi from affected fetuses and unaffected fetuses is not discriminatory. Chase results seem however to offer a better diagnostic potential.

Menkes disease (McKusick 30940) is an inherited syndrome of copper metabolism transmitted as an X-linked recessive trait. Patients show specific copper deficiency symptoms, such as lack of keratinization and pigmentation of hair, degenerative changes of the elastic tissue in the aorta and blood vessels, and scorbutic changes (Danks *et al.*, 1972). In addition, progressive psychomotor retardation with seizures and temperature instability are seen and the affected males rarely survive for more than 3 years.

The disturbance of copper metabolism is characterized by increased copper accumulation in multiple cell types in the body and in culture (Horn, 1976; Goka *et al.*, 1976; Beratis *et al.*, 1978; Camakaris *et al.*, 1980), and this provides a useful diagnostic marker. Incorporation of labelled copper into cultured amniotic fluid cells is routinely used for second-trimester prenatal diagnosis (Horn, 1981). Determination of the amount of copper in chorionic villi has now been used in more than 50 first-trimester prenatal diagnoses (Horn *et al.*, 1985; Tønnesen *et al.*, 1985, 1987a, 1989).

207

Journal of Inherited Metabolic Disease. ISSN 0141–8955. Copyright © SSIEM and Kluwer Academic Publishers, PO Box 55, Lancaster, UK.

MATERIALS AND METHODS

^{64}Cu-*uptake studies:* ^{64}Cu-uptake in amniocytes, fibroblast cultures and cultured chorionic villi was measured as described by Horn (1981). A 24-h chase was performed by removal of the ^{64}Cu-containing medium and determination of the ^{64}Cu remaining after 24 h subsequent growth in unlabelled medium.

Cultivation of chorionic villi: Cultures were established from the chorionic villus samples as described by Søndergaard and colleagues (1985) or by other standard methods.

Copper measurement: Copper was determined by neutron activation analysis as previously described (Tønnesen, *et al.*, 1987a).

RESULTS

Postnatal diagnosis

Our first contact with a family affected by Menkes disease is very often a request for a biochemical verification of a clinical suspicion of Menkes disease. An example of a typical positive diagnosis is shown in Table 1. The ^{64}Cu-uptake in the tested patient is significantly higher than that of the controls. Using this method we have diagnosed more than 105 patients with Menkes disease from many different countries. The ^{64}Cu-uptake results obtained so far are shown in Table 2.

Table 1 A positive diagnosis of Menkes disease by measuring ^{64}Cu-uptake in fibroblast cultures

	$^{64}Cu^a$
D.L. Exp. I	93.2
Exp. II	88.2
Control $(n = 1)$	17.4
Menkes $(n = 1)$	92.7
Reference values:	
Controls XX $(n = 20)$	18.9 (11.5 – 26.7)
Controls XY $(n = 21)$	21.1 (9.0 – 33.3)
Menkes $(n = 105)$	72.1 (34.3 – 135.1)

[a] ^{64}Cu values are expressed in ng (mg protein)$^{-1}$ (20 h)$^{-1}$; reference values are means with 95% limits in parentheses

In most cases of Menkes disease the ^{64}Cu-uptake is significantly higher than that of the controls but occasionally we obtain values inside the normal range, when several experiments are performed on the same patient. An additional diagnostic parameter is determination of the ^{64}Cu-retention after 24 h in unlabelled medium (Table 2). The fibroblasts from patients with Menkes disease retain significantly more ^{64}Cu than the controls.

Table 2 An additional diagnostic parameter for Menkes disease: 'chase' results

	^{64}Cu retained after 24 h in unlabelled medium (%)
Menkes patients	
(34, 16)[a]	53.0 – 84.2
Median	65.3
(2.5; 97.5) percentiles[b]	52.5 – 79.8
Normal males	
(17, 6)[a]	13.4 – 23.1
Median	15.9
(2.5; 97.5) percentiles[b]	13.1 – 21.3

[a] The first number in the parentheses is the total number of experiments; the second is the number of individuals tested.
[b] The percentiles have been determined by interpolation from the cumulative curves

Second-trimester prenatal diagnosis

After having established a diagnosis of Menkes disease in the index-patient, the family in question can be offered a prenatal diagnosis in subsequent pregnancies. So far we have performed 80 second-trimester prenatal diagnoses on fetuses of male karyotype (Table 3).

20 affected males have been diagnosed and in 18 of these cases the diagnosis was confirmed from placental copper measurements or ^{64}Cu-uptake in fetal fibroblasts. In the last two cases no material was available for these confirmatory analyses. As seen from Table 3 the lower end of the range from affected fetuses and the upper end of the control range overlap. This will make ^{64}Cu-uptake values in diagnostic samples in this region difficult to interpret.

As seen from Table 4, amniotic fluid cells from affected fetuses retain much more ^{64}Cu after a 24 h chase than both unaffected males and control males. A

Table 3 ^{64}Cu-uptake into amniotic fluid cells: male fetuses

	$^{64}Cu^a$		
	Range	(2.5; 95.7) percentiles	Median
Affected males (72; 20)[b]	26.2–95.0	28.2–76.5	45.5
Unaffected males (147; 60)	5.8–36.1	7.4–25.0	14.7
Control males (138; 99)	5.8–30.2	7.4–26.9	15.3

[a] ^{64}Cu values are expressed in ng (mg protein)$^{-1}$(20 h)$^{-1}$; percentiles are as shown in footnote to Table 2.
[b] Numbers in parentheses are as defined for Table 2

Table 4   'Chase' results for amniotic fluid cells: male fetuses

| | ^{64}Cu retained after 24h in unlabelled medium (%) | |
	Range	Median
Affected males (19, 6)[a]	43.6–88.0	60.9
Unaffected males (18, 10)	11.8–32.8	21.0
Control males (13, 11)	11.4–27.8	20.9

[a] Numbers in parentheses are as defined in Table 2

combination of ^{64}Cu-uptake and chase is thus a very good combination, when second-trimester diagnoses are performed.

First-trimester prenatal diagnosis

Since the initial discovery that trophoblast tissues could accumulate high amounts of copper we have performed more than 53 first-trimester prenatal diagnoses and diagnosed five affected fetuses. The results of these copper analyses are shown in Figure 1. There is a clear discrimination between the copper results obtained from affected males and unaffected males. No overlap has been observed between control results and those of affected male fetuses. In three cases of female karyotype copper results above the control range were observed. We take this as an indication of carrier status in these fetuses. In two of these cases supplementary analyses (^{64}Cu-uptake in fibroblasts, copper determination in placenta) showed these females to be carriers. In the third case lack of material has made a confirmation impossible.

In eleven at-risk pregnancies, where chorionic villus material was obtained, the copper content in maternal deciduum was determined as well (Figure 2). In five pregnancies, in obligate carriers, low copper values in maternal deciduum was seen. In three pregnancies, in obligate carriers, significantly increased quantities of copper were found. These values are in the same range as chorionic villus copper content from fetuses affected with Menkes disease (Figure 1). In one pregnancy in an obligate carrier both one normal value and two significantly increased values were observed. In two additional pregnancies in high-risk women, one maternal deciduum had significantly increased copper content and the other was normal. The copper contents in the chorionic villus samples diagnosed the three male fetuses in pregnancy 3, 4 and 5 to be affected. In the other eight pregnancies the prenatal diagnosis gave a normal result.

We have also measured ^{64}Cu-uptake in cultured chorionic villi in a search for a possible supplement to the direct copper determination in chorionic villus samples. This was meant to help avoid false-positive results due to exogenous copper contamination. As can be seen from the results presented in Table 5, interpretation of ^{64}Cu-uptake results in a diagnostic case is impossible. The range of affected males, unaffected males and controls overlap extensively. By performing 24-h chase experiments, the individual culture serves as its own control. The retention values for the affected males are outside the range for the unaffected males and the controls.

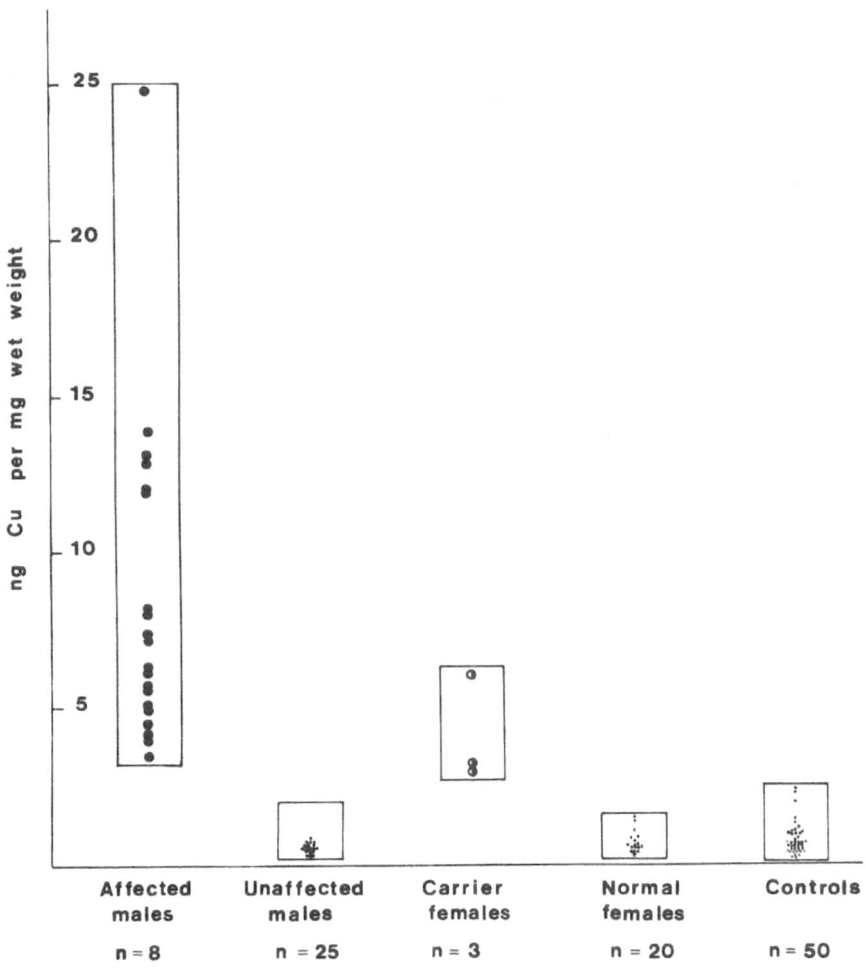

Figure 1 Copper values obtained from chorionic villus samples: these were taken with either Portex catheters or Dyonics biopsy forceps. For case 8 (Tønnesen *et al.*, 1987a) only the value obtained after abortion is shown. Two chorionic villus samples taken transabdominally have been included, since the corresponding controls were inside the control range. Two chorionic samples from female fetuses which were taken with silver and aluminium cannulae, respectively (Tønnesen *et al.*, 1987a) have not been included. For three of the affected fetuses chorionic samples were prepared at abortion after a second-trimester prenatal diagnosis

DISCUSSION

Postnatal diagnosis

Until now we have diagnosed 105 patients with Menkes disease from ^{64}Cu-uptake in fibroblast cultures. In none of these cases have chase results been necessary to

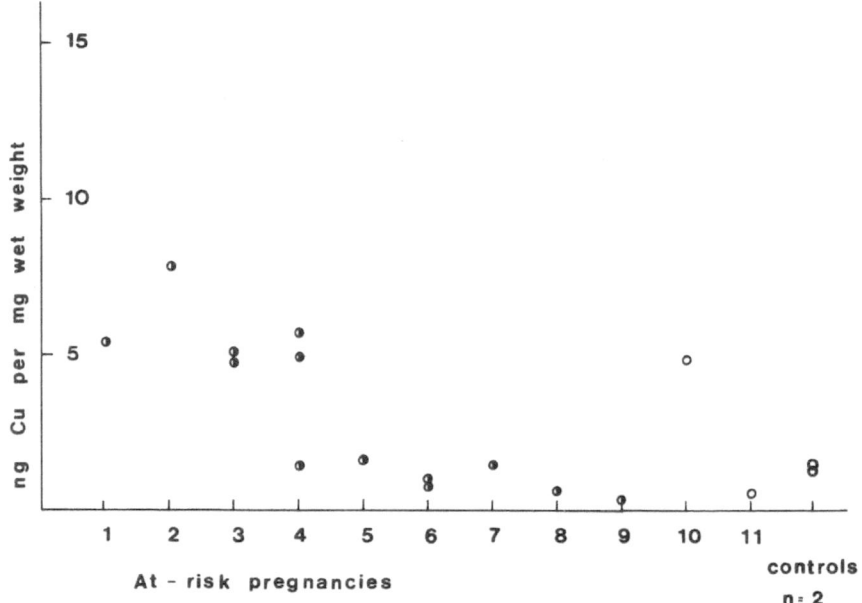

Figure 2 Copper in maternal deciduum: the deciduum was prepared simultaneously with the chorionic villus samples in all but pregnancies 3, 4, 5 and 6. In pregnancies 3 and 5 maternal deciduum was prepared at abortion after a second-trimester prenatal diagnosis; in pregnancies 4 and 6 maternal deciduum was prepared after normal birth. (◑) obligate carrier; (○) high risk carrier

Table 5 ^{64}Cu uptake and 'chase' results for cultured chorionic villi

	^{64}Cu uptake[a]	^{64}Cu retained after 24 h in unlabelled medium (%)
Affected males (4, 2)		
Range	40.5–106.5	48.4–72.5
Median	78.2	61.7
Unaffected males (8, 4)		
Range	21.7–156.8	13.4–48.3
Median	45.5	23.0
Controls (10, 6)		
Range	9.4–108.9	12.0–47.7
Median	30.1	22.3

[a] ^{64}Cu values are expressed in $ng\,(mg\ protein)^{-1}(20\,h)^{-1}$
[b] Numbers in parentheses are as defined in Table 2

evaluate the ^{64}Cu-uptake results. At present we are diagnosing 10–14 new patients each year. In only five cases received over the years have we been unable to verify the clinical suspicion due to a normal ^{64}Cu-uptake. The genetic centres sending us the cases are thus very good at selection of their material. In two cases post-mortem diagnosis was performed by direct copper measurement on other tissues, as no fibroblasts were available (Tønnesen *et al.*, 1986, 1987b). Unfortunately, not all possible cases of Menkes disease are diagnosed, as we sometimes receive requests for prenatal diagnoses in possible Menkes families with a deceased index patient. In such cases with very incomplete clinical information, no fibroblasts available from the index patient and no family history indicating X-linked inheritance, a normal result of a prenatal investigation in a male fetus is not enough to eliminate the suspicion of a disease similar to that of the index patient.

Second-trimester prenatal diagnosis

It is quite obvious that a combination of ^{64}Cu-uptake results and chase results offers a much better diagnostic potential than the ^{64}Cu results *per se*. However, prenatal diagnosis should not be performed later than the 17th week of gestation, as ^{64}Cu-uptake in amniocytes tends to normalize from the 18th week (Horn, 1983). Before the introduction of the chase both one false-negative and one false-positive diagnosis occurred (Horn, 1985). In one case intrauterine death occurred at the 21st week of gestation, while the prenatal diagnosis was still in progress. The ^{64}Cu-uptake was within normal limits but the amniocytes showed extremely poor growth, and the amniocentesis was performed at the 18th week of gestation. A high copper content of a placental sample showed the fetus to be affected (Horn, 1985). In one case a borderline ^{64}Cu-uptake was seen in a poorly growing culture. The amniotic fluid copper was found to be above the 95% probability limit for the control group. A therapeutic abortion was performed in this dubious case but the placental copper content was found to be low and proved the fetus to be unaffected (Horn, 1985). Since the introduction of the chase, it should be possible to avoid false-negative and false-positive diagnoses. A ^{64}Cu value of 31.2 ng (mg protein)$^{-1}$ (20 h)$^{-1}$ in an affected fetus gave a retention value of 65.7%, which is in the range of patients with Menkes disease. A male control gave a value of 36.3 ng (mg protein)$^{-1}$ (20 h)$^{-1}$, the retention value was 23.3%, which is in the normal range.

First-trimester prenatal diagnosis

The direct copper determination on chorionic villus samples in first-trimester offers a good alternative to second-trimester prenatal diagnoses. However two warnings have to be given: (a) an identically prepared control is necessary to reduce the impact of exogenous copper contamination from the sampling equipment (Tønnesen *et al.*, 1987a); (b) a careful removal of maternal decidnum from the chorionic villus sample is mandatory, as copper contents as high as in chorionic villus samples from affected fetuses have been observed (Figure 2).

^{64}Cu-uptake in cultured chorionic villi by itself is not a good diagnostic marker. Different amounts of metallothionein induced by the hormones in the specific growth media for cultured chorionic villi is the possible cause of this variation. Chase experiments on cultured chorionic villi might be a usable diagnostic marker but further experiments are needed to verify this point.

ACKNOWLEDGEMENTS

We wish to thank numerous colleagues for their help in referring Menkes patients and 1st and 2nd trimester prenatal diagnoses to our institute.

This work was supported by the Danish Medical Research Council (grant 12-4670; 12-4672; 12-5573, and 12-6546), the Foundation of 1870, the Sick-benefit Association's Health Foundation (H/36-86) and the Research Foundation of the Queen Louise Children's Hospital.

REFERENCES

Beratis, N. G., Price, P., La Badie, G. and Hirschhorn, K. ^{64}Cu metabolism in Menkes and normal cultured skin fibroblasts. *Pediatr. Res.* 12 (1978) 699–702

Camakaris, J., Danks, D. M., Ackland, L., Cartwright, E., Borger, P. and Cotton, R. G. H. Altered copper metabolism in cultured cells from human Menkes' syndrome and mottled mouse mutants. *Biochem. Genet.* 18 (1980) 117–131

Danks, D. M., Campbell, P. E., Stevens, B. J., Mayne, V. and Cartwright, E. Menkes kinky hair syndrome. An inherited defect in copper absorption with widespread effects. *Pediatrics* 50 (1972) 188–201

Goka, T. J., Stevenson, R. E., Hefferan, P. M. and Howell, R. R. Menkes disease: A biochemical abnormality in cultured human fibroblasts. *Proc. Natl. Acad. Sci. USA* 73 (1976) 604–606

Horn, N. Copper incorporation studies on cultured cells for prenatal diagnosis of Menkes' disease. *Lancet* 1 (1976) 1156–1158

Horn, N. Menkes X-linked disease: Prenatal diagnosis of hemizygous males and heterozygote females. *Prenat. Diagn.* 1 (1981) 107–120

Horn, N. Menkes' X-linked disease: Prenatal diagnosis and carrier detection. *J. Inher. Metab. Dis.* 6 suppl. 1 (1983) 59–62

Horn, N. Prenatal Diagnosis of Menkes Disease. In Gladtke, E., Heimann, G., Lombeck, I. and Eckert, I. (Eds.) *Spurenelemente. Stoffwechsel, Ernährung, Imbalancen, Ultra-Trace-Elemente*, Georg Thieme Verlag, Stuttgart, 1985, pp. 67–72

Horn, N., Søndergaard, F., Damsgaard, E. and Heydorn, K. Prenatal diagnosis of Menkes disease by direct copper analysis of trophoblast tissue. In Fraccaro, M., Simoni, G. and Brambati, B. (Eds.) *First Trimester Fetal Diagnosis*, Springer-Verlag, Heidelberg, 1985, pp. 251–255

Søndergaard, F., Kristensen, M. and Tommerup, N. High resolution chromosomes from first trimester trophoblast cultures. *Prenat. Diagn.* 5 (1985) 291–294

Tønnesen, T., Horn, N., Søndergaard, F., Mikkelsen, M., Boué, J., Damsgaard, E. and Heydorn, K. Measurement of copper in chorionic villi for first-trimester diagnosis of Menkes' disease. *Lancet* 1 (1985) 1038–1039

Tønnesen, T., Müller-Schauenburg, G., Damsgaard, E. and Horn, N. Copper measurement in a muscle biopsy. A possible method for postmortem diagnosis of Menkes disease. *Clin. Genet.* 29 (1986) 258–261

Tønnesen, T., Horn, N., Søndergaard, F., Jensen, O. A., Gerdes, A-M., Girard, S. and Damsgaard, E. Experience with first trimester prenatal diagnosis of Menkes disease. *Prenat. Diagn.* 7 (1987a) 497–509

Tønnesen, T., Silengo, M., Gerdes, A-M., Hansen, J. C., Reske-Nielsen, E., Franceschini, F. and Horn, N. Postmortem Menkes diagnosis from carrier testing of female relatives. *Clin. Genet.* 32 (1987b) 393–397

Tønnesen, T., Gerdes, A-M., Damsgaard, E., Miny, P., Holzgreve, W., Søndergaard, F. and Horn, N. First trimester diagnosis of Menkes disease: intermediate copper values in chorionic villi from three affected male fetuses. *Prenat. Diagn.* 9 (1989) 159–165

J. Inher. Metab. Dis. 12 Suppl. 1 (1989) 215–230

Disorders of Mitochondrial β-Oxidation: Prenatal and Early Postnatal Diagnosis and their Relevance to Reye's Syndrome and Sudden Infant Death

R. J. POLLITT
University Department of Paediatrics, The Children's Hospital, Sheffield S10 2TH, UK

Summary: There are still many problems with the diagnosis and classification of inherited disorders of mitochondrial β-oxidation. At present only the acyl-CoA dehydrogenase step of the β-oxidation spiral has been explored in any detail and a large number of patients have disorders that cannot be properly characterized. β-Oxidation defects may present in a wide variety of ways, the most dramatic being acute encephalopathy with hepatic involvement (atypical Reye's syndrome) or 'sudden' death. Investigations may include urinary and plasma organic acids, metabolic stress tests and assays of overall metabolic pathways or of specific enzymes in cultured fibroblasts, lymphocytes, or other material. Early postnatal diagnosis presents particular difficulties but in medium-chain acyl-CoA dehydrogenase deficiency the diagnosis may be apparent from careful examination of urine. There is as yet little general experience in prenatal diagnosis of this group of disorders except for glutaric aciduria type II. Single prenatal diagnoses of medium-chain acyl-CoA dehydrogenase deficiency and of an incompletely characterized defect of medium-chain fatty acid oxidation have been performed.

Most of the early-discovered organic acidurias were due to defects in the catabolism of the carbon skeletons of various amino acids. Patients with such disorders usually show consistent and grossly abnormal urinary organic acid patterns though, as was later recognized, a minority exhibit clearcut abnormalities only intermittently, usually during some crisis brought about by infection or other metabolic stress. In the late 1970s, a number of patients with intermittent dicarboxylic aciduria were described where again the abnormality was only apparent at times of metabolic stress. Once attention was focussed on the need to collect urine specimens for metabolic investigations at an appropriate time in relation to the illness being investigated, it became evident that disorders of the mitochondrial pathway for the β-oxidation of fatty acids, most of which produce only intermittent organic acidurias, are relatively common. They can present with a wide spectrum of symptoms, ranging from hypotonia, failure to thrive, and episodic hypoglycaemia, through to

Journal of Inherited Metabolic Disease. ISSN 0141–8955. Copyright © SSIEM and Kluwer Academic Publishers, PO Box 55, Lancaster, UK.

atypical Reye's syndrome and sudden infant death. The tendency of subjects with β-oxidation defects to suffer sudden catastrophic attacks makes prompt recognition of such individuals particularly important. However, the diagnosis of such disorders can present difficulties and it is important that these are appreciated before the more specific problems of prenatal or early postnatal diagnosis are considered. The inborn errors of mitochondrial fatty acid oxidation have recently been reviewed comprehensively by Vianey-Liaud and colleagues (1987) and also by Turnbull and colleagues (1988). The present review recapitulates this material only to the extent that it is relevant to the specific problems under consideration.

BASIC BIOCHEMISTRY

The oxidation of long-chain fatty acids is an important energy-producing pathway in many tissues, particularly muscle and, during starvation, liver. Fatty acids are oxidized as their coenzyme-A (CoA) esters, the process involving a sequence of reactions (Sherratt, 1988) which result in the production of acetyl-CoA and the CoA ester of the chain-shortened fatty acid (Figure 1). The sequence is then repeated until the fatty acid is converted entirely to acetyl-CoA. During starvation the acetyl-CoA produced by this process in the liver is used in the production of free acetoacetic and 3-hydroxybutyric acids (ketone bodies) which serve as a fuel in peripheral tissues, including brain. The inability to produce ketone bodies in response to starvation is one of the hallmarks of the fatty acid oxidation defects and is the basis of the diagnostic fasting test (see below).

The only disorders of mitochondral β-oxidation that are presently well character-ized (Table 1) affect the acyl-CoA dehydrogenase step of the spiral. Specific defects of short-chain (Amendt *et al.*, 1987; Coates *et al.*, 1988), medium-chain (Coates *et al.*, 1985; Treem *et al.*, 1986) and long-chain acyl-CoA dehydrogenases (Hale *et al.*, 1985; Treem *et al.*, 1986) have been described. A common electron-transfer chain is used by these three dehydrogenases and also by the branched-chain acyl-CoA dehydrogenases and by glutaryl-CoA dehydrogenase. Defects in this chain result in loss of functional activity of all these enzymes simultaneously even though the enzymes proteins themselves are present in normal amounts and show normal activity *in vitro* if an appropriate electron-acceptor is supplied. Glutaric aciduria type II is an example of this type of disorder and may be due to deficiency of either electron-transfer flavoprotein or of electron-transfer flavoprotein dehydrogenase (Frerman and Goodman, 1985a; Ikeda *et al.*, 1986). The basic defect in a further type of multiple dehydrogenation disorder, ethylmalonic-adipic aciduria (Mantagos *et al.*, 1979), is not fully characterized.

In all the disorders of β-oxidation the CoA esters of monocarboxylic fatty acids accumulate within the mitochondria. These esters and the corresponding free acids undergo a wide variety of secondary reactions, particularly conjugations and $(\omega-1)$- and ω-oxidations. ω-Oxidation results eventually in the production of even-chain dicarboxylic acids which may, in turn, be converted to mono-CoA esters and then chain-shortened by β-oxidation. The importance of peroxisomes in chain-shortening of dicarboxylic acids has been recognized for some years. The role of mitochondria

Table 1 **Provisional classification of disorders of mitochondrial β-oxidation**

Type	Site of defect	Major urinary metabolites[a]
Acyl-CoA dehydrogenase deficiencies		
	Long-chain acyl-CoA dehydrogenase	C_{6-12} dicarboxylic acids
	Medium-chain acyl-CoA dehydrogenase	C_{6-10} dicarboxylic acids Hexanoylglycine Suberylglycine Octanoylcarnitine 5-Hydroxyhexanoic acid
	Short-chain acyl-CoA dehydrogenase	?Ethylmalonic acid
Multiple acyl-CoA dehydrogenation deficiencies		
Glutaric aciduria type II	Electron transfer flavoprotein / Electron transfer flavoprotein dehydrogenase	Glutaric acid 2-Hydroxylglutaric acid Branched-chain acylglycines Adipic and other dicarboxylic acids
Ethylmalonic-adipic aciduria	Unknown	Ethylmalonic acid C_{6-10} dicarboxylic acids Glutaric acid Branched-chain acylglycines
Pseudo-(acyl-CoA dehydrogenase deficiencies)		
Long- and medium-chain	Unknown	Adipic and other dicarboxylic acids
Short-chain	Unknown	Ethylmalonic acid
Hydroxydicarboxylic acidurias		
Reye type Cirrhotic type	Possibly 3-hydroxyacyl-CoA dehydrogenases or medium/ long-chain thiolase	C_{6-10} dicarboxylic acids C_{6-12} 3-hydroxydicarboxylic acids
Others		
	Systemic carnitine palmitoyl transferase deficiency	None reported
	Carnitine transport defect	None reported

[a]Usually excreted intermittently except in ethylmalonic-adipic aciduria (very variable) and glutaric aciduria type II

is more difficult to assess but recent experiments on riboflavin-deficient rats suggest that mitochondrial β-oxidation of dicarboxylic acids may be quite active under certain physiological conditions (van Hoof *et al.*, 1988). This pathway results in the production of succinyl-CoA and thus would contribute to anaplerosis of the tricarboxylic acid cycle and provide a route for the conversion of fat to glucose. Blockage of this route in multiple dehydrogenation deficiency and probably also in medium-chain acyl-CoA dehydrogenase deficiency could well contribute to the tendency to fasting hypoglycaemia seen in these disorders.

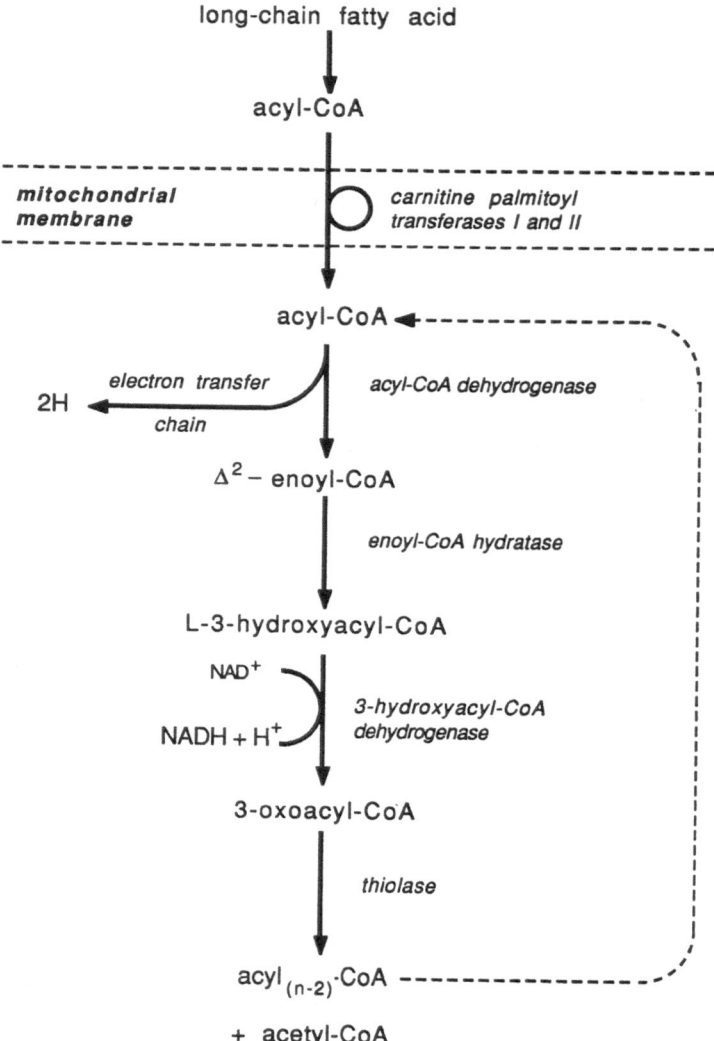

Figure 1 Outline of the mitochondrial β-oxidation pathway

CLINICAL PRESENTATION

Most patients with glutaric aciduria type II (deficiency of electron-transfer flavo-protein or its dehydrogenase) present with severe illness soon after birth, and indeed such babies may show various congenital abnormalities. Ethylmalonic-adipic aciduria and the long, medium or short-chain acyl-CoA dehydrogenase deficiencies share a spectrum of clinical presentation, though with different emphases in the different conditions. The most common, medium-chain acyl-CoA de-hydrogenase deficiency, can produce chronic problems with failure to thrive and hypotonia, often associated with secondary carnitine deficiency. More often, though, patients with this deficiency remain well except for acute episodes of metabolic decompensation with hypoglycaemia as a prominent feature. Such episodes may be recurrent but are often isolated and usually triggered by infection. A mild attack may be passed off as a febrile convulsion. More severe episodes may develop into a condition similar to Reye's syndrome, with marked hepatic involvement. Such severe attacks are sometimes so rapid in their evolution that the resultant fatality is classified as a sudden infant death. At the other end of this spectrum, many subjects with medium-chain acyl-CoA dehydrogenase deficiency remain completely asymptomatic. Long-chain acyl-CoA dehydrogenase deficiency seems in general to be more severe than medium-chain acyl-CoA dehydrogenase deficiency and more likely to lead to death in early infancy. Cardiomegaly and a tendency to cardiac arrest have been noted. In the few cases of ethylmalonic-adipic aciduria reported in detail there has been a tendency to failure to thrive, with acute Reye-like episodes superimposed.

DIAGNOSIS

Urinary metabolites

The first indication of the presence of a β-oxidation defect often comes in the course of routine investigation of urinary organic acids. Though the pattern of metabolites excreted in any given disorder may be very variable, and the patterns in different disorders show many similarities, it is still possible to obtain considerable diagnostic information by careful examination using gas chromatography–mass spectrometry. The urinary metabolites arising in specific defects are surveyed in some detail by Vianey-Liaud and colleagues (1988) and are summarized in Table 1.

The diagnosis of glutaric aciduria type II does not normally present any difficulty as the urine contains very large quantities of glutaric acid and usually other characteristic metabolites including the glycine conjugates of branched-chain fatty acids. The organic acid profile in ethylmalonic-adipic aciduria is extremely variable, sometimes strongly resembling that seen in medium-chain acyl-CoA dehydrogenase deficiency, while on other occasions tending to a picture like glutaric aciduria type II with moderate excretion of isovalerylglycine. In remission, patients with ethylmalonic-adipic aciduria show a slight to moderate ethylmalonic aciduria as the only abnormality (Dusheiko *et al.*, 1979; Green *et al.*, 1985; Gregersen *et al.*, 1986) and the diagnosis may easily be missed.

Medium and long-chain acyl-CoA dehydrogenase deficiencies produce intermittent organic acidurias with prominent abnormalities only when the patient is under some form of metabolic stress. There is a striking even-chain dicarboxylic aciduria during metabolic crisis but it is usually not possible to distinguish between the two disorders on the basis of the dicarboxylic acid pattern. The long-chain dicarboxylic acids (formed from the longer-chain fatty acids in long-chain acyl-CoA dehydrogenase deficiency, are poorly excreted in the urine and there is extensive secondary chain-shortening of the dicarboxylic acids resulting in a tendency for adipic acid to be the predominant species in both conditions. The presence of other metabolites such as hexanoylglycine, suberylglycine or phenylpropionylglycine in medium-chain acyl-CoA dehydrogenase deficiency may serve to make a preliminary distinction. Reports on the organic aciduria in short-chain acyl-CoA dehydrogenase deficiency (Amendt *et al.*, 1987; Coates *et al.*, 1988) are conflicting but ethylmalonic acid would be expected as the characteristic metabolite.

Metabolites in blood and other fluids

There has been rather little interest in the examination of organic acids in blood in this group of disorders as the dicarboxylic acids are present in relatively small amounts compared to the monocarboxylic acids and this creates analytical problems. Free octanoic, decanoic and *cis*-4-decenoic acids are present in unusually high concentrations in plasma in medium-chain acyl-CoA dehydrogenase deficiency during crisis (see Table 3 in Vianey-Liaud *et al.*, 1988). This may be a particularly useful investigation where urine is not available, for example in cases of sudden death. Eye-fluid, which is often collected routinely during paediatric *post-mortem* examination, has been used to diagnose glutaric aciduria type II (Bennett *et al.*, 1987a) but there is no information at present whether it would reflect the more rapidly-evolving abnormalities of medium or long-chain acyl-CoA dehydrogenase deficiency, for example.

Stress and loading tests

Patients with defective oxidation of fatty acids show a reduced tolerance to fasting, developing a hypoketotic hypoglycaemia leading eventually, if the fast is prolonged, to a general collapse of mitochondrial functions. Controlled fasting, under close medical supervision, may be used as a diagnostic investigation. As the fast progresses, glycogen stores become depleted, blood glucose concentration falls and there is a mobilization of free fatty acids. An inadequate ketogenic response, with abnormally high free fatty acid to 3-hydroxybutyric acid ratio in plasma, will be seen in patients with systemic carnitine palmitoyl-transferase deficiency, most β-oxidation defects or 3-hydroxy-3-methylglutaryl-CoA lyase deficiency (which has a quite distinctive organic aciduria and will not be confused with these other disorders). It seems unlikely that patients with short-chain acyl-CoA dehydrogenase deficiency or other defects in the oxidation of short-chain fatty acids will show this response but there is no practical experience of this at present. There is an understandable reluctance on the part of clinicians to undertake such tests. They are not without danger to the patient and must be carefully supervised, with intravenous glucose ready in case of sudden collapse. Fasting may also need to be prolonged to produce an unequivocal result (either a marked ketosis or incipient hypoglycaemia), particularly in older patients. Nevertheless this is the only test that can detect these disorders as a group and will give positive results in patients with as yet unclassified conditions of the type discussed below.

Urine collected towards the end of a prolonged fast may show dicarboxylic aciduria and the other characteristic features discussed above and this may be important in refining the diagnosis. Fat loading tests using triglycerides rich in unsaturated long-chain fatty acids are being developed to try to produce such organic acid abnormalities without recourse to fasting. Medium-chain triglycerides should not be given as the results are difficult to interpret and the test is intrinsically dangerous for medium-chain acyl-CoA dehydrogenase deficiency patients. The phenylpropionic acid load test (Rumsby *et al.*, 1986; Seakins and Rumsby, 1988) is claimed to be specific for medium-chain acyl-CoA dehydrogenase deficiency and appears to be well tolerated. It has been successfully used in a baby of 10 weeks of age. Carnitine loading may also be used to reveal this deficiency (Roe *et al.*, 1986) and other disorders during the asymptomatic period but analysis of acyl-carnitines requires special chromatographic techniques or fast atom bombardment mass spectrometry.

In vitro **tests**

The ability of intact cultured fibroblasts to metabolize individual fatty acids can readily be assessed using appropriate radio-labelled substrates. The simplest assays determine the release of $^{14}CO_2$ from $[1-^{14}C]$-fatty acids, palmitate or oleate, octanoate and butyrate being used to assess long-, medium- and short-chain fatty acid metabolism, respectively, while $[U-^{14}C]$palmitate or, better, $[16-^{14}C]$palmitate can give an estimate of the overall activity of the β-oxidation spiral. These assays have been criticized on the grounds that much of the $[^{14}C]$acetyl-CoA generated is incorporated into other metabolites and only a fraction of the label is released as $^{14}CO_2$. With long-chain substrates it is possible to measure perchloric-acid-soluble products as an alternative but both tests lead to essentially similar conclusions and for diagnostic purposes there seems little to choose between them. The production of ^3H_2O from $[9,10(n)-^3H]$palmitate (Moon and Rhead, 1987) or from $[9,10(n)-^3H]$myristate (Manning, Olpin, Pollitt and Webley, unpublished) provide the basis for simple and sensitive assays for determining the overall activity of the upper portion of the β-oxidation spiral and will detect long-chain acyl-CoA dehydrogenase deficiency or both this and medium-chain acyl-CoA dehydrogenase deficiency, respectively, as well as multiple dehydrogenation defects.

Specific assays for the individual acyl-CoA dehydrogenases are available. For small amounts of material, such as cultured fibroblasts, the only practicable approach is to use the native fluorescence of electron-transfer flavoprotein (Frerman and Goodman, 1985b; Coates *et al.*, 1985; Hale *et al.*, 1985). For larger amounts of tissue, such as those acquired at post-mortem examination, the electron-transfer flavoprotein may be linked to another acceptor such as dichlorophenolindophenol to give a more convenient assay. Electron-transfer flavoprotein and electron-transfer flavoprotein dehydrogenase may also be assayed in cultured fibroblasts (Frerman and Goodman, 1985a). Unfortunately none of these assays is at present suitable for the routine clinical chemistry laboratory as they all require components such as purified electron-transfer flavoprotein or purified medium-chain acyl-CoA dehydrogenase which are difficult and time-consuming to prepare. It is possible to determine other enzymes of the β-oxidation pathway in cultured fibroblasts and it will not be long before further specific defects are characterized (see below).

Unclassified disorders

A substantial proportion of the patients who are suspected of having some disorder of fatty acid oxidation on the basis of urinary organic acid findings and/or the occurrence of episodes of hypoketotic hypoglycaemia do not have any of the known disorders. Some of these patients have organic acid profiles resembling those of specific acyl-CoA dehydrogenase deficiencies. Their cultured fibroblasts may show a chain-length specific deficit in the production of $^{14}CO_2$ from labelled fatty acids but normal acyl-CoA dehydrogenase activities are found using specific electron-transfer flavoprotein-linked assays. Such disorders may, for the sake of convenience, be described as pseudo-(acyl-CoA dehydrogenase deficiencies). A case of pseudo-(short-chain acyl-CoA dehydrogenase deficiency) has been well documented (Bennett *et al.*, 1985; Coates *et al.*, 1988) and pseudo-(long-chain acyl-CoA dehydrogenase deficiency) appears to be quite common. In practice, many patients with non-specific intermittent dicarboxylic acidurias are not investigated at the enzyme level.

A more distinctive type of intermittent dicarboxylic aciduria, in which the unsubstituted and mono-unsaturated dicarboxylic acids are accompanied by comparable amounts of 3-hydroxydicarboxylic acids, is seen fairly regularly and has accounted for nearly a quarter of the total dicarboxylic acidurias encountered by the Sheffield gas chromatography–mass spectrometry reference service over the past 5 years. The majority of such 'hydroxydicarboxylic aciduria' patients have presented with hypoglycaemia or Reye-like episodes (Riudor *et al.*, 1986) which were sometimes fatal. In some cases where cultured fibroblasts have been examined with appropriate techniques (e.g. using [9,10-^{3}H]palmitate or myristate) they show diminished activity of the β-oxidation pathway (unpublished). Such patients may be deficient in some chain-length specific 3-hydroxyacyl-CoA dehydrogenase or possibly thiolase (Pollitt *et al.*, 1987). A few patients showed progressive cirrhosis of the liver and died within the first year of life (Pollitt *et al.*, 1987; Kelley and Morton, 1988). The diagnostic specificity of hydroxydicarboxylic aciduria is still to be determined. There appears to be both clinical and biochemical heterogeneity within the group and it is possible that in some instances hydroxydicarboxylic aciduria is secondary to some primary defect unconnected with fatty acid metabolism.

REYE'S SYNDROME

A number of inherited metabolic diseases produce, in some patients at least, episodes that satisfy the criteria originally used to define Reye's syndrome. β-Oxidation defects are particularly prominent in this group, though the crises in medium-chain and long-chain acyl-CoA dehydrogenase deficiencies differ from those of 'true' Reye's syndrome in clinical details and in the histochemical and ultrastructural changes in hepatic mitochondria (Treem *et al.*, 1986). Nevertheless, the realization that patients who have had a Reye's syndrome-like episode may be suffering from some permanent underlying disorder and have a high risk of further life-threatening episodes has led to the retrospective re-examination of such patients

J. Inher. Metab. Dis. 12 Suppl. 1 (1989)

or, where the attack has been fatal, their surviving sibs. A number of cases of medium-chain acyl-CoA dehydrogenase deficiency have been uncovered in this way. However, where specific methods such as the phenylpropionic acid loading test are used in such investigations the incidence of inherited metabolic disorder will be underestimated since conditions such as the hydroxydicarboxylic acidurias will, presumably, not be detected.

There have been contradictory reports of urinary organic acid abnormalities in Reye's syndrome. It seems quite plausible that the generalized loss of mitochondrial function and the high levels of circulating free fatty acids found in Reye's syndrome would lead to dicarboxylic aciduria similar to that seen in long-chain acyl-CoA dehydrogenase deficiency. Such dicarboxylic acidurias and the simultaneous accumulation in plasma of various long-chain dicarboxylic acids have been reported in a large series with Reye's syndrome by Tonsgard (1985, 1986) though the possibility of underlying inherited metabolic disease was not explicitly excluded in these patients. A marked hydroxydicarboxylic aciduria and other unusual findings in a case of Reye's syndrome have been interpreted in terms of loss of activity of multiple mitochondrial enzymes by Tracey *et al.* (1987). If such marked dicarboxylic acidurias can indeed arise in acquired mitochondrionopathies then the recognition of those patients with inherited β-oxidation defects is even more difficult than we have so far realized.

SUDDEN INFANT DEATH

Inherited disorders of fatty acid oxidation have also been much discussed in relation to sudden infant death (Anonymous, 1986). Sudden infant death, with an incidence of approximately 1 in 500 live births, is much more common than Reye's syndrome and is a complex and multifactorial problem. The situation is confused by an unfortunate terminology arising from the concept that there is a clinical syndrome, the Sudden Infant Death Syndrome, of babies dying from natural causes in the post-neonatal period and where no cause of death can be found at necropsy. This concept was developed in the USA in the early 1960s as a means of reducing distress in parents whose children have been found dead unexpectedly. Such a diagnosis has seductive simplicity and its availability must tend to discourage thorough necropsy examination which, in any case, may well be performed by a general pathologist with no special training in paediatric pathology. Under these circumstances sudden infant death syndrome will encompass deaths caused by disorders of fatty acid oxidation but as part of a large and heterogeneous group in which the incidence of inherited metabolic disease is probably too low to justify detailed biochemical investigation.

A converse situation may arise where a specialized paediatric autopsy service is available. Some paediatric pathologists accept that, in the absence of an obvious terminal disease, an explanation for sudden infant death should be sought in terms of multiple aetiologies, whereby factors which, though often rather subtle and insufficient in themselves to cause death, can do so in combination. Thus the paediatric pathologist when conducting a post-mortem examination may try to assess the amount of metabolic disturbance present at death, the developmental state of various organs and whether there is any congenital anatomical deformity, and whether there is any evidence of atopy. The incidence of 'true' sudden infant death syndrome decreases dramatically with this approach and babies dying as a result of inherited metabolic disease are likely to be eliminated from this category. Thus, in selecting cases for biochemical investigation it is better to avoid using terms such as sudden infant death, sudden infant death syndrome, or cot death and to concentrate on clinical and pathological criteria which might point more directly to a metabolic causation of death. In the case of fatty acid oxidation defects, fatty infiltration of the muscles or the liver are important signs; particularly microvesicular panlobular fatty infiltration of the liver for acute crises in medium-chain and long-chain acyl-CoA dehydrogenase deficiencies and related disorders, more massive fatty infiltration, often including the heart, in more chronic disorders such as glutaric aciduria type II.

There is some controversy as to the proportion of life-threatening episodes and sudden infant deaths attributable to fatty acid oxidation defects (Harpey *et al.*, 1986, 1987; Bennett *et al.*, 1986). Differing methods of patient selection and the use of non-specific diagnostic criteria may give rise to widely differing estimates of frequency. A systematic approach to this problem has been attempted by the Sheffield group. A retrospective study of material collected at autopsy from 200 consecutive sudden infant deaths identified 14 with severe diffuse microvesicular panlobular fatty infiltration of the liver. In nine cases sufficient stored material (liver or heart muscle) was available for specific enzyme assays, leading to the diagnosis of three cases of medium-chain and one of long-chain acyl-CoA dehydrogenase deficiency (Howat *et al.*, 1985; Allison *et al.*, 1988a). In two of the cases of medium-chain acyl-CoA dehydrogenase deficiency the diagnosis was confirmed by the subsequent birth of affected siblings while in the third case a small amount of urine, collected post-mortem, contained high concentrations of dicarboxylic acids as expected. It is worth noting that in all four of these cases there had been a prodromal illness with diarrhoea and vomiting and it was only the rapid evolution of illness, leading to death, that had been 'sudden'. There is clearly a continuum between the Reye's type of presentation and sudden infant death.

Though the small numbers in this study leave a high degree of statistical uncertainty as to the true contribution of β-oxidation defects to unexpected death in infancy, the results suggest that detailed enzymological investigation of the relatively few cases with severe diffuse panlobular microvesicular fatty infiltration of the liver should be instituted as a routine. Some caveats are necessary, however. Reliance on highly specific assays for the currently well-characterized conditions will lead to an underestimate of the overall frequency of fatty acid oxidation defects and there is a danger that in specific cases unjustified reassurances may be given, when in fact other siblings are at risk with hydroxydicarboxylic aciduria or some other as yet uncharacterized type of β-oxidation defect. Another problem is that panlobular microvesicular fatty infiltration of the liver is part of the picture of Reye's syndrome and can also occur as a non-specific result of prolonged terminal illness. As noted above, a generalized loss of mitochondrial enzymes occurs in liver during Reye's syndrome and this may well extend to the acyl-CoA dehydrogenases. This phenomenon should be easily detectable provided that more than one enzyme is being assayed. Potentially more serious is the selective loss of long-chain acyl-CoA dehydrogenase found in the liver of a child who had experienced a severe and prolonged terminal illness. This liver showed fatty infiltration as might be expected but urine collected post-morten did not show significant dicarboxylic aciduria. Long-chain acyl-CoA dehydrogenase activity in heart muscle from this child was within the normal range (Bennett *et al.*, 1989). This example shows the importance of thorough and systematic autopsy procedures with collection and preservation of material (including cryopreservation of skin samples for subsequent culture of fibroblasts) for biochemical investigation should this be indicated by the histopathological findings (Emery *et al.*, 1988).

PRENATAL DIAGNOSIS

Glutaric aciduria type II has been the subject of a number of successful prenatal diagnoses. With cultured amniotic fluid cells CO_2 release assays are used to give an overall measure of oxidation of labelled fatty acid substrates (Mitchell *et al.*, 1983; Niederwieser *et al.*, 1984; Bennett *et al.*, 1984) rather than the more difficult specific measurements of electron-transfer flavoprotein or its dehydrogenase. Glutaric acid is present in amniotic fluid at approximately ten times normal concentrations and may readily be measured by gas chromatography–mass spectrometry (Jakobs *et al.*, 1984).

There is rather little in the way of practical experience in prenatal diagnosis of other disorders of mitochondrial β-oxidation. One may predict that the conditions that have been clearly characterized at enzyme level will all be detectable by direct enzyme assay in cultured amniotic fluid cells or chorionic villus biopsy whereas analysis of metabolites in amniotic fluid will provide useful information only in disorders where there is an abnormal organic aciduria in the unstressed state (Table 2).

Table 2 Possible approaches to prenatal diagnosis

	Amniotic fluid metabolites	*Overall assay*[a]	*Specific assay*[b]
Acyl-CoA dehydrogenase deficiencies	−	+	+ +
Glutaric aciduria type II	+ +	+ +	(+ +)
Ethylmalonic-adipic aciduria	(? +)	(? +)	x
Pseudo-(acyl-CoA dehydrogenase deficiencies)	−	+	x
Hydroxydicarboxylic acidurias	(−)	(+)	x

[a]For example $^{14}CO_2$ release or ^3H_2O formation from appropriately labelled substrates.
[b]Specific assay of the defective enzyme or protein concerned: x indicates that the basic defect(s) in these groupings have not been identified.
− indicates that a method is not applicable; + and + + indicate that a method is usable with a lesser or greater degree of reliability, respectively; ratings in parentheses are speculative

Using the specific electron-transfer flavoprotein-linked assay it is possible to measure the specific long, medium, and short-chain acyl-CoA dehydrogenases in cultured amniotic fluid cells. Medium-chain acyl-CoA dehydrogenase deficiency has been diagnosed following amniocentesis at 14–15 weeks of pregnancy using this assay (Bennett *et al.*, 1987b). Amniotic fluid dicarboxylic acid concentrations were within the normal range. $^{14}CO_2$-release assays or similar non-specific methods may also be used but these often show high residual activity in medium-chain acyl-CoA dehydrogenase deficiency and there is a degree of overlap between the normal and affected ranges. The activities shown in the CO_2-release assay using [1-^{14}C]octanoate are similar in the epithelial and fibroblastoid types of cultured amniotic fluid cells (Allison *et al.*, 1988b).

The non-specific nature of the $^{14}CO_2$ release assays can be turned to advantage to perform prenatal diagnosis even when the exact nature of the disorder being sought is in doubt. Thus, in the family described by Bennett *et al.* (1984), the diagnosis of a fatty acid oxidation disorder was made on the basis of a much reduced production of $^{14}CO_2$ from [1-^{14}C]palmitate by cultured fibroblasts of the index case, who died at 32 h of age. The same disorder was diagnosed prenatally in the mother's next pregnancy, using the same assay on cultured amniotic fluid cells. The pregnancy was allowed to proceed and it was only subsequent investigation of the resulting baby that enabled the disease in question to be diagnosed as glutaric aciduria type II.

A similar non-specific assay, the release of $^{14}CO_2$ from [1-^{14}C]octanoate was used for prenatal diagnosis of a disorder of medium-chain fatty acid oxidation by Bennett *et al.* (1987c). This disorder was believed at the time to be medium-chain acyl-CoA dehydrogenase deficiency as in fibroblasts the defect in CO_2 release was confined to the oxidation of fatty acids of medium chain-length. However, the urine of the index case during crisis did not contain detectable excess of hexanoylglycine or suberylglycine. Despite the well-recognized variability of the urinary organic acid patterns in these disorders this raises the question as to whether this patient in fact had some other, as yet uncharacterized, defect of medium-chain fatty acid oxidation, a pseudo-(medium-chain acyl-CoA dehydrogenase deficiency).

The unpredictable clinical course of some of the β-oxidation defects causes problems when counselling parents over the risks to future affected offspring and considering with them the option of prenatal diagnosis with termination of an affected pregnancy. In a family that has already experienced a case of neonatal glutaric aciduria type II the case for prenatal diagnosis may seem clear. Intermediate degrees of morbidity are seen in diagnosed cases of long-chain acyl-CoA dehydrogenase deficiency, ethylmalonic-adipic aciduria and in some families with medium-chain acyl-CoA dehydrogenase deficiency. At the other extreme, seen in medium-chain acyl-CoA dehydrogenase deficiency in particular, many completely asymptomatic cases are known, even in families where a child has died of the disease. One might expect that in such families one could easily forestall the development of acute attacks in other affected children by simple prophylactic measures and give a firm guarantee against serious misadventure. Unfortunately this does not seem to be entirely the case and there remains a fairly high risk of fatality even in diagnosed cases of medium-chain acyl-CoA dehydrogenase deficiency. Given these circumstances some parents will wish to opt for prenatal diagnosis and termination of affected pregnancies, even for medium-chain acyl-CoA dehydrogenase deficiency, as they may feel unable to cope with the anxiety of bringing up a child at risk in this way, particularly if a previous affected child died suddenly without warning.

EARLY POSTNATAL DIAGNOSIS

Enzymatic methods of diagnosis can be applied to samples taken soon after birth in exactly the same way as to samples taken later in life. As fibroblasts, the mainstay of such investigations, take some while to grow this introduces considerable delay. Leukocytes or lymphocytes can be used for some specific assays to overcome this delay (e.g. Coates *et al.*, 1985) as well as with the less reliable CO_2 release assays. Placenta might be a useful tissue for enzme assay but this has not been systematically explored.

Urinary organic acids provide the other obvious means of rapid early diagnosis. Glutaric aciduria type II may normally be detected by analysis of urinary organic acids soon after birth, though in exceptional cases the abnormal metabolite excretion may take some while to develop. The diagnosis might also be missed under abnormal feeding regimes with low protein and fat content (Bennett *et al.*, 1984). This disease often presents with severe symptoms in the first weeks of life and even the routine monitoring of acid–base status while the results of more definitive investigations are awaited may be sufficient to suggest the diagnosis in a baby at risk.

Disorders characterized by intermittent organic acidurias (i.e. the majority of the β-oxidation defects) may be more difficult to detect. The metabolic stress of the perinatal period, with its switch from carbohydrate-based to fat-based energy production, causes some actual and pseudo-(long-chain acyl-CoA dehydrogenase deficiency) patients to show severe symptoms but, rather surprisingly, it is rare for medium-chain acyl-CoA dehydrogenase deficiency patients to do so at this age. Formal fasting tests would be difficult to administer in the neonatal period and might in any case be expected to be particularly hazardous. However, the sudden switch to fat utilization may result in informative urinary organic acid patterns without fasting. Patients with medium-chain acyl-CoA dehydrogenase deficiency have shown characteristic profiles during the first days of life, with suberic acid exceeding adipic acid and the presence of hexanoylglycine, suberylglycine or both in the urine. Such abnormalities may be seen in random non-fasting urine samples for several months (Bennett *et al.*, 1987b; Downing *et al.*, 1989). Transient abnormalities may also be seen in other disorders of β-oxidation during the first week of life but interpretation is complicated by the fact that a (benign) generalized dicarboxylic aciduria is seen fairly frequently in the newborn period (Downing *et al.*, 1989). Thus, in attempting to pick out newborn babies with specific fatty acid oxidation defects it is essential to consider the pattern of the organic aciduria rather than the concentrations of specific components. Benign neonatal generalized dicarboxylic acidurias can be quite striking and, in a minority of babies, persist for several weeks. In one such patient, who was beng followed up because of a serious congenital heart defect, the dicarboxylic aciduria, which had been slowly decreasing over several weeks became very prominent again when she experienced a period of semi-fasting during the course of a gastrointestinal infection. This phenomenon makes it very difficult to assess the significance of mild to moderate dicarboxylic acidurias in the early months of life.

PROSPECT

Increased clinical awareness of disorders of mitochondrial fatty acid oxidation in both their chronic and acute presentations will lead to increasing demands for diagnostic services. The development of clinically applicable assays for the remaining steps of the β-oxidation pathway should resolve much of the present uncertainty surrounding this group of disorders and provide means of prenatal diagnosis and early postnatal recognition of new cases in families known to be at risk. However, there will continue to be major problems in the recognition of affected individuals in the community at large, not least because of the transient nature of the more readily detectable metabolic disturbances. Routine diagnosis will continue to rely heavily upon careful interpretation of urinary organic acid profiles as a preliminary to selecting the most appropriate specific investigations.

ACKNOWLEDGEMENTS

I should like to thank the numerous colleagues in Sheffield and elsewhere whose work has contributed to my appreciation of the subjects under review and who have generously shared information and materials with me over the years. I am a member of the external scientific staff of the Medical Research Council.

REFERENCES

Allison, F., Bennett, M. J., Variend, S. and Engel, P. C. Acyl-coenzyme A dehydrogenase deficiency in heart tissue from infants who died unexpectedly with fatty change in the liver. *Br. Med. J.* 296 (1988a) 11–12

Allison, F., Barnes, I. C. S. and Bennett, M. J. The oxidation of octanoic acid by amniotic fluid cells; The effect of cell type and passage number. *Prenat. Diagn.* 8 (1988b) 397–398

Amendt, B. A., Greene, C., Sweetman, L., Cloherty, J., Shih, V., Moon, A., Teel, L. and Rhead, W. J. Short-chain acyl-CoA dehydrogenase deficiency. Clinical and biochemical studies in two patients. *J. Clin. Invest.* 79 (1987) 1303–1309

Anonymous. Sudden infant death and inherited disorders of fat oxidation. *Lancet* 2 (1986) 1073–1075

Bennett, M. J., Curnock, D. A., Engel, P. C., Shaw, L., Gray, R. G. F., Hull, D., Patrick, A. D. and Pollitt, R. J. Glutaric aciduria type II: Biochemical investigation and treatment of a child diagnosed prenatally. *J. Inher. Metab. Dis.* 7 (1984) 57–61

Bennett, M. J., Gray, R. G. F., Isherwood, D. M., Murphy, N. and Pollitt, R. J. Diagnosis and biochemical investigation of a patient with a short-chain fatty acid oxidation defect. *J. Inher. Metab. Dis.* 8 Suppl. 2 (1985) 99–100

Bennett, M. J., Variend, S. and Pollitt, R. J. Screening siblings for inborn errors of fatty acid metabolism in families with a history of sudden infant death. *Lancet* 2 (1986) 1470

Bennett, M. J., Pollitt, R. J., Land, J. M., Turner, M. J. and Cheetham, C. H. Lethal multiple acyl-CoA dehydrogenase deficiency with dysmorphic features. *J. Inher. Metab. Dis.* 10 (1987a) 95–96

Bennett, M. J., Allison, F., Pollitt, R. J., Manning, N. J., Gray, R. G. F., Green, A., Hale, D. E. and Coates, P. M. Prenatal diagnosis of medium-chain acyl-CoA dehydrogenase deficiency in family with sudden infant death. *Lancet* 1 (1987b) 440–441

Bennett, M. J., Allison, F., Lowther, G. W., Gray, R. G. F., Johnston, D. I., Fitzsimmons, J. S., Manning, N. J. and Pollitt, R. J. Prenatal diagnosis of medium-chain acyl-coenzyme A dehydrogenase deficiency. *Prenat. Diagn.* 7 (1987c) 135–141

Bennett, M. J., Allison, F., Pollitt, R. J. and Variend, S. Fatty acid oxidation defects as causes of unexpected death in infancy. In Coates, P. M. (Ed.) *Enzymes of Fatty Acid Oxidation and Their Genetic Defects.* Alan R. Liss, New York, 1989

Coates, P. M., Hale, D. E., Stanley, C. A., Corkey, B. E. and Cortner, J. A. Genetic deficiency of medium-chain acyl coenzyme A dehydrogenase: Studies in cultured skin fibroblasts and peripheral mononuclear leukocytes. *Pediatr. Res.* 19 (1985) 671–676

Coates, P. M., Hale, D. E., Finocchiaro, G., Tanaka, K. and Winter, S. C. Genetic deficiency of short-chain acyl-coenzyme A dehydrogenase in cultured fibroblasts from a patient with muscle carnitine deficiency and severe skeletal muscle weakness. *J. Clin. Invest.* 81 (1988) 171–175

Downing, M., Rose, P., Bennett, M. J., Manning, N. J. and Pollitt, R. J. Generalized dicarboxylic aciduria: A common finding in neonates. *J. Inher. Metab. Dis.* 12 Suppl. 2 (1989) 321–324

Dusheiko, G., Kew, M. C., Joffe, B. I., Lewin, J. R., Mantagos, S. and Tanaka, K. Recurrent hypoglycemia associated with glutaric aciduria type II in an adult. *N. Engl. J. Med.* 301 (1979) 1405–1409

Emery, J., Howat, A. J., Variend, S. and Vawter, G. F. Investigation of inborn errors of metabolism in unexpected infant death. *Lancet* 2 (1988) 29–31

Frerman, F. E. and Goodman, S. I. Deficiency of electron transfer flavoprotein or electron transfer flavoprotein: ubiquinone oxidoreductase in glutaric acidemia type II fibroblasts. *Proc. Natl. Acad. Sci. USA* 82 (1985a) 4517–4520

Frerman, F. E. and Goodman, S. I. Fluorimetric assay of acyl-CoA dehydrogenase in normal and mutant human fibroblasts. *Biochem. Med.* 33 (1985b) 38–44

Green, A., Marshall, T. G., Bennett, M. J., Gray, R. G. F. and Pollitt, R. J. Riboflavin responsive ethylmalonic-adipic aciduria. *J. Inher. Metab. Dis.* 8 (1985) 67–70

Gregersen, N., Christensen, M. F., Christensen, E. and Kølvraa, F. Riboflavin responsive multiple acyl-CoA dehydrogenase deficiency. Assessment of three years of riboflavin treatment. *Acta Paediatr. Scand.* 77 (1986) 676–681

Hale, D. E., Batshaw, M. L., Coates, P. M., Frerman, F. E., Goodman, S. I., Singh, I. and Stanley, C. A. Long-chain acyl coenzyme A dehydrogenase deficiency: an inherited cause of non-ketotic hypoglycemia. *Pediatr. Res.* 19 (1985) 666–671

Harpey, J.-P., Charpentier, C. and Paterneau-Jouas, M. Sudden infant death syndrome and inherited disorders of fat metabolism. *Lancet* 2 (1986) 1332

Harpey, J.-P., Charpentier, C. and Paterneau-Jouas, M. Fatty acid oxidation defects and sudden infant death. *Lancet* 1 (1987) 163

Howat, A. J., Bennett, M. J., Variend, S., Shaw, L. and Engel, P. C. Defects in the metabolism of fatty acids in the sudden infant death syndrome. *Br. Med. J.* 290 (1985) 1771–1773

Ikeda, Y., Keese, S. M. and Tanaka, K. Biosynthesis of electron-transfer flavoprotein in a cell-free system and in cultured human fibroblasts. Defect in the α-subunit synthesis is a primary lesion in glutaric aciduria type II. *J. Clin. Invest.* 78 (1986) 997–1002

Jakobs, C., Sweetman, L., Wadman, S. K., Duran, M., Saudubray, J.-M., and Nyhan, W. L. Prenatal diagnosis of glutaric aciduria type II by direct chemical analysis of dicarboxylic acids in amniotic fluid. *Eur. J. Pediatr.* 141 (1984) 153–157

Kelley, R. I. and Morton, H. 3-Hydroxyoctanoic aciduria: Identification of a new organic acid in the urine of a patient with non-ketotic hypoglycemia. *Clin. Chim. Acta* 175 (1988) 19–26

Mantagos, S., Genel, M. and Tanaka, K. Ethylmalonic-adipic aciduria. In vivo and in vitro studies indicating deficiency of activities of multiple acyl-CoA dehydrogenases. *J. Clin. Invest.* 64 (1979) 1580–1589

Mitchell, G., Saudubray, J.-M., Benoit, Y., Rocchiccioli, F., Charpentier, C., Ogier, H. and Boué, J. Antenatal diagnosis of glutaric aciduria type II. *Lancet* 1 (1983) 1099

Moon, A. and Rhead, W. J. Complementation analysis of fatty acid oxidation disorders. *J. Clin. Invest.* 79 (1987) 59–64

Niederwieser, A., Steinmann, B., Exner, U., Neuheiser, F., Redweik, U., Wang, M., Rampini, S. and Wendel, U. Multiple acyl-CoA dehydrogenase deficiency (MADD) in a boy with non-ketotic hypoglycemia, hepatomegaly, muscle hypotonia and cardiomyopathy. Detection of *N*-isovalerylglutamic acid and its monoamide. *Helvet. Paediatr. Acta* 38 (1983) 9–26

Pollitt, R. J., Losty, H. and Westwood, A. 3-Hydroxydicarboxylic aciduria; A distinctive type of intermittent dicarboxylic aciduria of possible diagnostic significance. *J. Inher. Metab. Dis.* 10 Suppl. 2 (1987) 266–269

Riudor, E., Ribes, A., Boronat, M., Sabado, C., Dominguez, C. and Ballabriga, A. A new case of C_6–C_{14} dicarboxylic aciduria with favourable evolution. *J. Inher. Metab. Dis.* 9 Suppl. 2 (1986) 297–299

Roe, C. R., Millington, D. S., Maltby, D. A. and Kinnebrew, P. Recognition of medium-chain acyl-CoA dehydrogenase deficiency in asymptomatic siblings of children dying of sudden infant death or Reye-like syndromes. *J. Pediatr.* 108 (1986) 13–18

Rumsby, G., Seakins, J. W. T. and Leonard, J. V. A simple screening test for medium-chain acyl CoA dehydrogenase deficiency. *Lancet* 2 (1986) 467

Seakins, J. W. T. and Rumsby, G. The use of phenylpropionic acid as a loading test for medium-chain acyl-CoA dehydrogenase deficiency. *J. Inher. Metab. Dis.* 11 Suppl. 2 (1988) 221–224

Sherratt, H. S. A. (ed.) The enzymology of β-oxidation. *Biochem. Soc. Trans.* 16 (1988) 409–427

Tonsgard, J. H. Urinary dicarboxylic acids in Reye's syndrome. *J. Pediatr.* 107 (1985) 79–84

Tonsgard, J. H. Plasma dicarboxylic acids in Reye's syndrome. *J. Pediatr.* 109 (1986) 440–445

Tracey, B. M., Chalmers, R. A., Mehta, A., English, N., Purkiss, P., Valman, H. B. and Stacey, T. E. Studies on abnormal metabolic function in Reye's syndrome. *J. Inher. Metab. Dis.* 10 Suppl. 2 (1987) 263–265

Treem, W. L., Witzleben, C. A., Piccoli, D. A., Stanley, C. A., Hale, D. E., Coates, P. M. and Watkins, J. B. Medium-chain and long-chain acyl CoA dehydrogenase deficiency: Clinical, pathologic and ultrastructural differentiation from Reye's syndrome. *Hepatology* 6 (1986) 1270–1278

Turnbull, D. M., Shepherd, I. M. and Aynsley-Green, A. Inherited defects of mitochondrial fatty acid oxidation. *Biochem. Soc. Trans.* 16 (1988) 424–427

van Hoof, F., Vamecq, J., Draye, J.-P. and Veitch, K. The catabolism of medium- and long-chain dicarboxylic acids. *Biochem. Soc. Trans.* 16 (1988) 423–424

Vianey-Liaud, C., Divry, P., Gregersen, N. and Mathieu, M. The inborn errors of mitochondrial fatty acid oxidation. *J. Inher. Metab. Dis.* 10 Suppl. 1 (1987) 159–198

J. Inher. Metab. Dis. 12 Suppl. 1 (1989) 231–246

Gene Mapping of Mineral Metabolic Disorders

R. V. THAKKER[1], K. E. DAVIES[2] and J. L. H. O'RIORDAN[3]
[1]Division of Molecular Medicine, Clinical Research Centre, Watford Road, Harrow, Middlesex HA1 3UJ; [2]Nuffield Department of Clinical Medicine, John Radcliffe Hospital, Oxford; [3]The Middlesex Hospital, London W1, UK

Summary: Recent advances in the techniques of molecular biology and cytogenetics have enabled the localization of several mutant genes which result in disorders of phosphate, calcium, magnesium and water homeostasis. Thus, the genes causing X-linked hypophosphataemic rickets, Lowe's syndrome, Di George syndrome, X-linked recessive hypoparathyroidism, multiple endocrine neoplasia Type I, primary hypomagnesaemia and X-linked nephrogenic diabetes insipidus have been mapped. The molecular and genetic studies which localized these disease genes are described and the implications of this gene mapping in genetic counselling and in further elucidation of the mineral metabolic defects are discussed.

In recent years, there have been important advances in the techniques of molecular biology and human genetics which have facilitated the chromosomal localization of genes. This chromosomal localization of genes, which is also referred to as 'gene mapping' has two major applications. Firstly, the mapping of a disease gene locus with genetic markers permits genetic counselling, where appropriate, of affected families (Pembrey, 1986). In addition, this localization of a disease gene locus represents the first step towards defining the genetic abnormality and subsequently characterizing the gene product, i.e. the protein (Ruddle, 1984). This approach called 'reverse genetics' is of particular importance in the investigation of inherited disorders whose primary biochemical defect is unknown. A recent example of the success of this type of approach is the localization and subsequent identification of the genetic and protein abnormalities which lead to Duchenne muscular dystrophy (Davies *et al.*, 1983; Koenig *et al.*, 1987; Hoffman *et al.*, 1987). These methods have also been used to investigate the molecular basis of inherited mineral metabolic disorders, and several mutant genes have recently been localized (Table 1).

In this review the mapping of the genetic abnormalities which cause inherited disorders of phosphate, calcium, magnesium and water homeostasis will be described. The clinical disorders which will be discussed are: X-linked hypophosphataemic rickets and Lowe's syndrome in which there is a defect in the renal tubular transport of phosphate; hypoparathyroidism and Di George syndrome in which hypocalcaemia is a feature and multiple endocrine neoplasia type I in which

231

Table 1 Inheritance and chromosomal localization of some mineral metabolic disorders

Mineral homeostasis	Disease	Inheritance	Chromosomal localization
Phosphate	Hypophosphataemic rickets	X-linked dominant	Xp22.31–p21.3
	Lowe's syndrome	X-linked recessive	Xq24–q26
Calcium	Hypoparathyroidism	Autosomal dominant	?
		Autosomal recessive	?
		and X-linked recessive	Xq26–q27
	Di George syndrome	Autosomal dominant	22q11
	Multiple endocrine neoplasia Type I	Autosomal dominant	11q
Magnesium	Primary hypomagnesaemia	X-linked recessive	Xp22
Water	Nephrogenic diabetes insipidus	X-linked recessive	Xq28

hypercalcaemia occurs; primary hypomagnesaemia in which there is a failure of intestinal absorption of magnesium; and nephrogenic diabetes insipidus in which there is an abnormality in water conservation.

DISORDERS OF PHOSPHATE HOMEOSTASIS

The mutant genes for two inherited disorders of phosphate homeostasis, X-linked hypophosphataemic (vitamin D resistant) rickets and Lowe's syndrome, have been mapped by genetic linkage studies of affected families. X-linked hypophosphataemic rickets is dominantly inherited and is due to a single renal proximal tubular transport defect for phosphate, whereas Lowe's syndrome is inherited as an X-linked recessive disorder and is due to multiple renal proximal tubular transport defects for bicarbonate, phosphate and amino acids. The X-linked hypophosphataemic rickets gene has been localized on the short arm of the X-chromosome whereas the Lowe's syndrome gene has been localized on the long arm of the X-chromosome (for reviews, see Davies *et al.*, 1987; Thakker and O'Riordan, 1988).

X-linked hypophosphataemic rickets

Clinical and biochemical features: Albright and colleagues (1937) recognized that some patients with rickets did not respond to therapy with normal doses of vitamin D but did respond to large doses of vitamin D and called this condition vitamin D-resistant rickets. The most common form of vitamin D-resistant rickets occurred in early life and was associated with a low serum phosphate, and was therefore called hypophosphataemic (vitamin D-resistant) rickets (Winters *et al.*, 1958). The incidence of hypophosphataemic (vitamin D) resistant rickets, which is the commonest inherited form of metabolic rickets, has been estimated as 1 in 20 000 live births (Burnett *et al.*, 1964). The disorder is clinically characterized by growth retardation and childhood rickets which is unresponsive to physiological doses of vitamin D. Untreated this results in dwarfism, osteomalacia and bone deformities in the adult. In addition, extraskeletal ossification, limitation of joint mobility, deafness and occasionally spinal cord compression may develop. Affected individuals have hypophosphataemia due to renal tubular defect. Treatment consists of large doses of vitamin D or its active metabolite calcitriol and oral phosphate supplements.

The first familial occurrence of vitamin D-resistant rickets was described in a mother, her son and her daughter (Christensen, 1941). Skeletal deformities were used to ascertain the affected phenotype and an autosomal dominant mode of inheritance was proposed. However, it was observed that the severity of skeletal deformities varied and that some females had no evidence of rickets but were hypophosphataemic. When hypophosphataemia was used as the discriminant, an X-linked dominant mode of inheritance was established (Winters *et al.*, 1958; Graham *et al.*, 1959; Burnett *et al.*, 1964). The variability in female patients, which is expected in an X-linked disease could be explained by the Lyon hypothesis, which states that one of the X-chromosomes in a pair is randomly inactivated in each cell of the early female embryo (Lyon, 1974). Thus a female hypophosphataemic patient is a mixture of cells some of which have an active normal X-chromosome and some of which have an active 'hypophosphataemic' X-chromosome. The relative proportions of each cell type vary from female to female and this would determine the variable expression of the X-linked hypophosphataemic rickets gene in females. Support for this came from phosphate infusion studies in hypophosphataemic patients and normals. These demonstrated that hypophosphataemic males (hemizygotes) had decreased maximum tubular capacity for reabsorbing phosphate ($TmPO_4$), while hypophosphataemic females (heterozygotes) had a $TmPO_4$ which was intermediate between that of normals and hypophosphataemic males (Glorieux *et al.*, 1972). The site of this renal phosphate transport defect has been localized to the brush border membrane of the proximal convoluted tubule (Tenenhouse *et al.*, 1978) though the nature of the phosphate transport defect and possible transport proteins involved still need to be defined. These studies of renal phosphate transport mechanisms have been facilitated by investigating hypophosphataemic mouse models (for review see Thakker and O'Riordan, 1988).

Hypophosphataemic mouse models: Hyp and Gyro: Two hypophosphataemic mouse models have been described and are called *Hyp* and *Gyro*. The *Hyp* mouse was described first when mutant male mice were observed to have shortened trunk and limbs in association with hypophosphataemia (Eicher *et al.*, 1976). The mutant was called *hypophosphataemia* and allocated the gene symbol *Hyp*. The second model to be described was called *Gyro* as the mutant mice exhibited circling behaviour in addition to the hypophosphataemia (Lyon *et al.*, 1986). In the *Gyro* mice both hearing and the vestibular apparatus are defective. Genetic studies of the *Hyp* and *Gyro* mice revealed that both mutations were dominant and X-linked. In addition, classical linkage studies localized the *Hyp* and *Gyro* loci to the distal part of the mouse X-chromosome. Close similarities of features were observed between the human disorder X-linked hypophosphataemic rickets and the *Hyp* mice, but no human equivalent of the *Gyro* mutation has been established (for review, see Thakker and O'Riordan, 1988).

The homology between the mouse model *Hyp* and human X-linked hypophosphataemic rickets gives some clue to the location of the hypophosphataemic rickets gene in man. This is possible because genes that are X-linked in any one mammalian species are X-linked in all other mammals (Ohno, 1967). Analogies between the mouse and human X-chromosomes require careful interpretation as the mouse X-chromosome is not subdivided into a short and long arm like its human counterpart. However the mouse and human X-chromosomes are related by multiple rearrangements of blocks of homologous genes (Buckle *et al.*, 1984, 1985). In the mouse, the hypophosphataemic rickets gene locus has been mapped to the distal end of the X-chromosome and is located proximal to the steroid sulphatase gene locus but distal to the α-galactosidase locus. If the hypophosphataemic rickets gene was located on the same homologous segment as the steriod sulphatase gene locus, then its position would be on the short arm in man (situation 1, Figure 1). If however, the hypophosphataemic rickets gene was located on the same homologous segment as the α-galactosidase gene, then its position would be on the long arm in man (situation 2, Figure 1). In order to study these comparative maps and to localize the human hypophosphataemic rickets gene, genetic markers spanning the short and long arms of the human X-chromosome are required. Such genetic markers are available (Figure 2) through the advances in recombinant DNA technology (Botstein *et al.*, 1980; White *et al.*, 1985; Davies, 1985), and were used to map the human hypophosphataemic rickets gene (Mächler *et al.*, 1986; Read *et al.*, 1986; Thakker *et al.*, 1986).

Mapping of the human X-linked hypophosphataemic rickets gene: Cloned human X-chromosome sequences, which reveal restriction fragment length polymorphism (RFLPs) were used in linkage studies of affected families to map the hypophosphataemic rickets gene. These RFLPs are the result of variations in the DNA sequence in individuals and may lead to the presence or absence of a cleavage site for a restriction endonuclease. RFLPs are useful genetic markers for linkage studies as they are inherited in a Mendelian manner and their inheritance can be followed together with a disease in an affected family. The inheritance of hypophosphataemic rickets and the RFLPs obtained with probe 99.6 are shown in a study of family B/85 (Figure 3). Analysis of this pedigree reveals that the inheritance of the disease is associated with inheritance of the 25 kb allele in all the children with one exception (*). This one exception is the heterozygous daughter II.5 who has inherited a recombinant gamete, in which the disease locus is no longer linked to the 25 kb allele (A) but has become linked to the 11 kb allele (a). Such recombination would occur during maternal meiosis, when the two X-chromosomes become closely apposed and crossing over of genes may result. The frequency of recombination between two genes is related to the distance between those two genes. Genes that are further apart will recombine more frequently than genes that are close together on the same chromosome, i.e. linked genes. Thus, by studying such recombination events in family studies, the distance between two genes and the probability that they are linked can be ascertained (Morton, 1955; Ott, 1974).

J. Inher. Metab. Dis. 12 Suppl. 1 (1989)

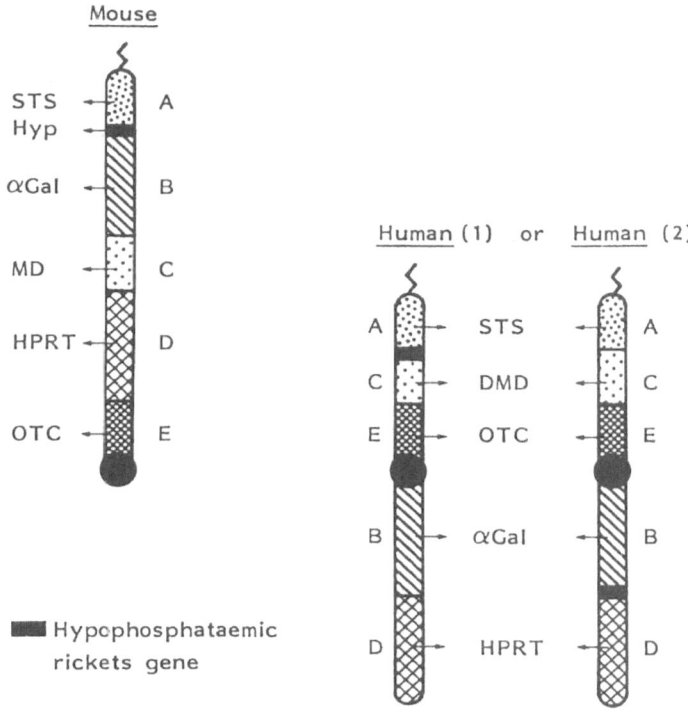

Figure 1 Schematic relationship between mouse and human X-chromosome maps used as a model to predict the sites of the hypophosphataemic rickets gene in man. The human X-chromosome is divided into a short and a long arm whereas the mouse X-chromosome is not. The locations of the steroid sulphatase gene (STS), α-galactosidase gene (αGal) muscular dystrophy gene (MD/DMD), hypoxanthine–guanine phosphoribosyltransferase gene (HPRT), ornithine transcarbamylase gene (OTC), pairing segment (⌇) and centromere (●) are shown for both species. The murine hypophosphataemic rickets gene (*Hyp*) has been localized to the distal end of the mouse X-chromosome. On the basis of homologies between mouse and human X-chromosomes, two possible locations (1) and (2) for the hypophosphataemic rickets gene (▬) in man can be postulated. Genetic linkage studies subsequently indicated that situation (1) is correct. (Reproduced from Thakker and O'Riordan, 1988)

The distance between two genes is expressed as a recombination fraction (θ), which is equal to the number of recombinants divided by the total number of offspring resulting from double heterozygotes within a family. The value of the recombination fraction ranges from 0 to 0.5; a value of zero indicates that the genes are very closely linked while a value of 0.5 indicates that the genes are far apart. A recombination fraction of 0.1 (10%) relates to a genetic map distance of 10 centiMorgans (cM) and is on average equivalent to 10 million base pairs. The probability that the two loci are linked is expressed as a 'LOD score' which is $\log_{10}$ of the odds ratio favouring linkage. A LOD score of +3, which indicates a probability in favour of linkage of 1000 to 1, establishes linkage between two loci

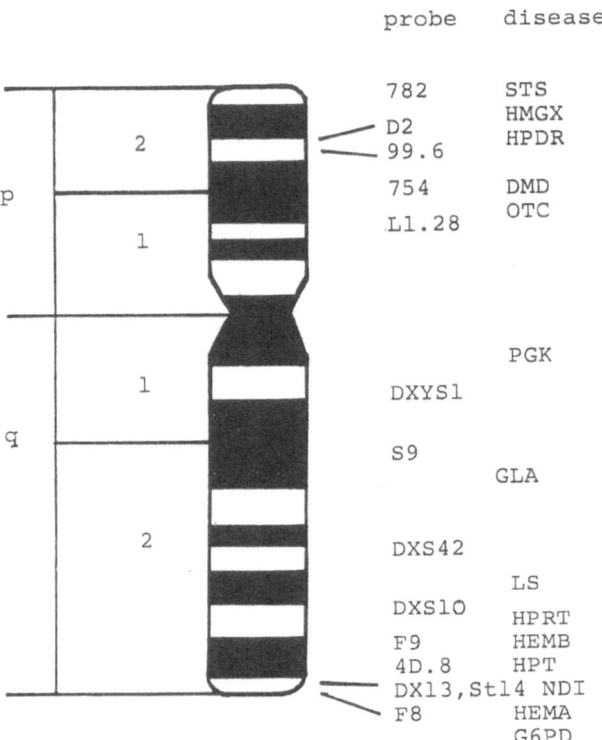

probe   disease

782   STS
         HMGX
D2   HPDR
99.6
754   DMD
L1.28   OTC

         PGK
DXYS1
S9
         GLA
DXS42
         LS
DXS10
         HPRT
F9   HEMB
4D.8   HPT
DX13,St14 NDI
F8   HEMA
         G6PD

Figure 2 Map of some clinically useful DNA probes on the human X-chromosome and their relations to the loci of some X-linked diseases. The X-chromosome with Giemsa bands is schematically represented and the DNA probe is shown juxtaposed to its region of origin. These DNA probes are cloned human X-chromosome sequences. The regions from which each DNA probe is derived is ascertained by hybridization *in situ*, or by somatic cell hybrids. The human X-chromosome is divided into a short arm (p) and a long arm (q). The X-linked disease loci shown are: steroid sulphatase (STS), hypomagnesaemia (HMGX), hypophosphataemic rickets (HPDR), Duchenne muscular dystrophy (DMD), ornithine transcarbamylase (OTC), phosphoglycerate kinase (PGK), α-galactosidase (GLA), Lowe's syndrome (LS), hypoxanthine–guanine phosphoribosyl transferase deficiency (HPRT), haemophilia B (HEMB), hypoparathyroidism (HPT), nephrogenic diabetes insipidus (NDI), classical haemophilia–factor VIII deficiency (HEMA) and glucose-6-phosphate dehydrogenase deficiency (G6PD)

and a LOD score of −2, indicating a probability against linkage of 100 to 1, is taken to exclude linkage between two loci.

The results of linkage analysis from 16 families, in whom hypophosphataemic rickets had been inherited in an X-linked dominant manner in three or more generations, are shown in Figure 4. A total of 189 family members, 95 of whom were affected (61 females, 34 males) and 94 of whom were unaffected (34 females, 60 males) were studied with X-linked genetic markers (Thakker *et al.*, 1987).

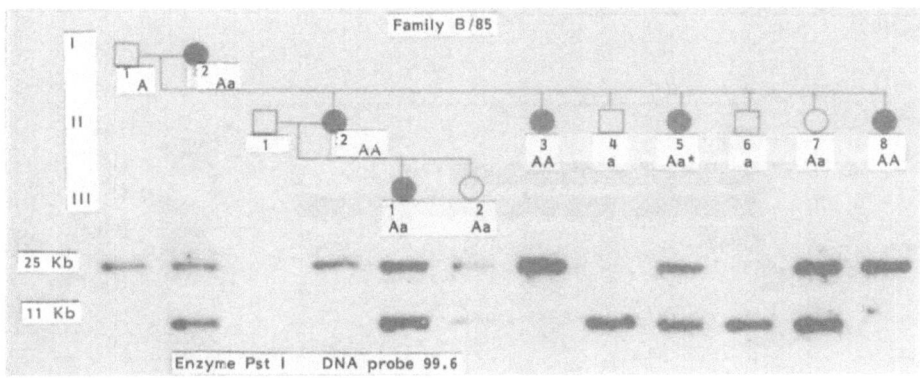

Figure 3 Pedigree of family segregating for X-linked hypophosphataemic rickets and short-arm RFLP locus 99.6. Autoradiograph obtained with probe 99.6 hybridized to 5 μg genomic DNA digested with enzyme *Pst*I. The family is drawn so that each member appears above his or her RFLP pattern. The affected grandmother (I.2) is heterozygous (Aa) in having one 25 kb allele (designated 'A') and one 11 kb allele (designated 'a'). Two unaffected sons (II.4 and II.6) are homozygous for the 11 kb allele and three affected daughters (II.2, II.3 and II.8) are homozygous for the 25 kb allele. This suggests that the disease is segregating with the 25 kb allele 'A' and not with the 11 kb allele 'a'. Of the two heterozygous daughters one is unaffected (II.7) and the other (II.5*) is affected. Both these sisters have inherited the 25 kb allele from the father (I.1) and the 11 kb allele from the mother (I.2), and both sisters have the same genotype but different phenotypes. This difference has arisen because the affected daughter (II.5) has inherited a recombinant gamete. □ normal male, ○ normal female, ■ affected male, ● affected female, * recombinant (Reproduced from Thakker, 1988)

Linkage between hypophosphataemic rickets and the 99.6 loci was established with a peak LOD score = 7.35, θ = 0.09, indicating a probability in favour of linkage in excess of 10 million to 1. Linkage was also established between the hypophosphataemic rickets gene locus and the D2 locus, peak LOD score = 4.77, θ = 0.16, indicating a probability in favour of linkage in excess of 10,000 to 1. All other X-linked RFLP loci gave negative or low LOD scores although many of these are also on the short arm of the chromosome. Furthermore, an analysis of multi-point crossovers established that the hypophosphataemic rickets gene locus was situated distal to the 99.6 locus but proximal to the D2 locus. The distance between the hypophosphataemic rickets gene and the nearest genetic marker locus 99.6 is 9 centiMorgans. This corresponds to approximately 9 million base pairs between the two loci and further studies are in progress to characterize the gene abnormality more fully. The two genetic markers 99.6 and D2 have been previously localized by hybridization *in situ* to the short arm of the X-chromosome in the region Xp22.31–p21.3, and the results demonstrating the linkage between the disease gene and these genetic markers mapped the hypophosphataemic rickets gene locus on the short arm of the X-chromosome distal to the Duchenne muscular dystrophy locus but proximal to the steroid sulphatase gene locus (Figure 2). This location

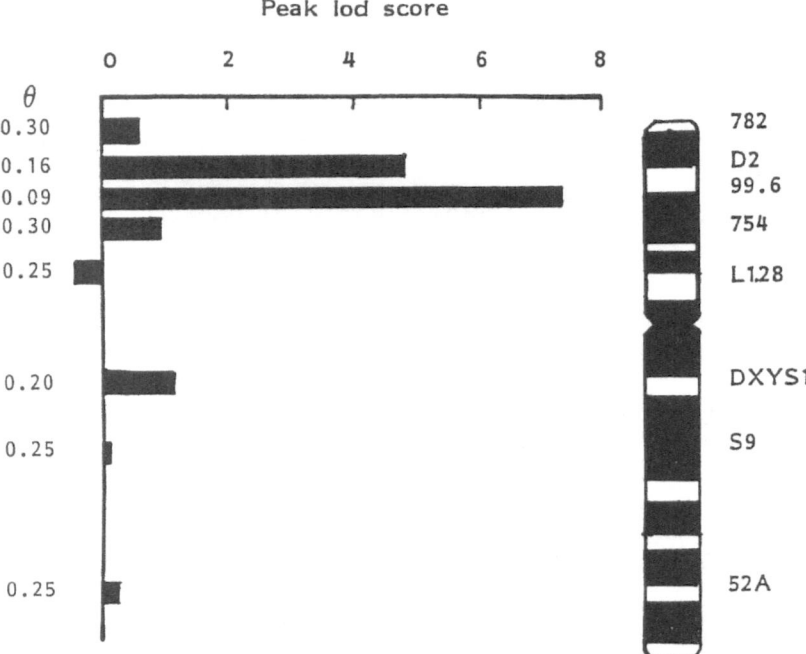

Figure 4 Linkage studies in X-linked hypophosphataemic rickets. Results of linkage analysis of 16 families with eight X-linked genetic markers. The bar represents the peak LOD score (LOD score = $\log_{10}$ odds favouring linkage/odds favouring non-linkage) between hypophosphataemic rickets and the genetic marker, whose position is shown on the X-chromosome, while θ is the recombination fraction at which the peak LOD score was obtained. A LOD score of +3 establishes linkage. The peak LOD score between hypophosphataemic rickets and the short-arm X-linked marker 99.6 is 7.35, indicating a probability in excess of 10 million to 1 in favour of linkage. The distance between the hypophosphataemic rickets locus and 99.6 locus is θ = 0.09, indicating a distance of 9 centiMorgans which is equivalent to 9 million base pairs. (Reproduced from Thakker and O'Riordan, 1988)

of the hypophosphataemic rickets gene in man is consistent with the first of the two locations predicted from a consideration of homologies between human and mouse X-chromosomes (Figure 1).

The human hypophosphataemic gene has been localized on the short arm of the X-chromosome (Xp22.31–p21.3), by using the techniques of molecular genetics. This mapping of the gene regulating phosphate excretion will help to further elucidate the genetic abnormality and biochemical defects causing this disorder of phosphate homeostasis.

Lowe's syndrome

Lowe's syndrome is a rare disorder which is characterized by congenital cataracts, mental retardation, muscular hypotonia, rickets, and defective proximal tubular reabsorption of bicarbonate, phosphate and aminoacids (Lowe *et al.*, 1952). It is also referred to as the oculo-cerebro-renal syndrome. The disease is nearly always confined to males, who may die in childhood, and family studies have confirmed the X-linked recessive inheritance (Abbassi *et al.*, 1968; Pallisgaard *et al.*, 1971). It has been reported that female carriers who have normal neurological and renal function can be identified in 80% of cases by micropunctate cortical lens opacities (Gardner *et al.*, 1976; Johnston *et al.*, 1976). The basic biochemical defect remains unknown and genetic counselling has been limited. The Lowe's syndrome gene has now been mapped to the distal part of the long arm of the X-chromosome at Xq24–q26, by using RFLPs in linkage studies (Silver *et al.*, 1987). The probability in favour of linkage between Lowe's syndrome and the long-arm genetic markers DXS10 and DXS42 exceeded one million to 1 and 100000 to 1, respectively. The Lowe's syndrome gene locus is proximal to the hypoxanthine–guanine phosphoribosyl transferase gene locus (Figure 2). This location of the Lowe's syndrome gene locus to Xq24–Xq26 by linkage studies is consistent with the observation of a female in whom the disease arose *de novo* due to a balanced X/3 translocation involving a break point at Xq25 (Hodgson *et al.*, 1986). The mapping of the Lowe's syndrome gene will not only help in genetic counselling, but defining the gene abnormality will help in the characterization of the defect in renal phosphate transport.

DISORDERS OF CALCIUM HOMEOSTASIS

The mutant genes for three inherited disorders of calcium homeostasis, which are X-linked hypoparathyroidism, Di George syndrome and multiple endocrine neoplasia type I have been mapped. Linkage studies were used to localize the X-linked hypoparathyroid gene to Xq26–q27 and the multiple endocrine neoplasia type I gene to 11q, and a combination of cytogenetic, *in situ* hybridization and deletion mapping studies were used to localize the gene causing Di George syndrome to 22q11.

Hypoparathyroid disorders

Hypoparathyroidism, which is characterized by a low serum calcium concentration due to parathyroid hormone deficiency, may occur as part of a complex autoimmune disorder, or as an isolated endocrinopathy, or in association with developmental abnormalities, e.g. Di George syndrome. Most cases are sporadic but familial occurrences of these disorders have also been reported and studies have been undertaken to define the genetic abnormalities in this heterogenous group of metabolic disorders. Autosomal dominant, autosomal recessive, and X-linked recessive forms of hypoparathyroidism have been reported (McKusick, 1988).

Autosomal forms: Hypoparathyroidism can occur in association with autoimmune disorders of the thyroid and adrenal glands and pernicious anaemia, which may be associated with HLA B8. However, no linkage or association between this type of hypoparathyroidism and the HLA loci which are located on the short arm of chromosome 6 has been established (Proto *et al.*, 1985). In some patients hypoparathyroidism occurs in the absence of autoimmune or development disorders and the possibility that mutations in or near the parathyroid hormone gene may cause this *isolated* form of hypoparathyroidism has been explored. Human parathyroid hormone is encoded by a single gene located on the short arm of chromosome 11 (Naylor *et al.*, 1983) and two high frequency RFLPs have been reported (Schmidtke *et al.*, 1984). These RFLPs were used in linkage studies of affected families with *isolated* hypoparathyroidism, and the results did not demonstrate linkage between the parathyroid hormone gene locus and the disease (Ahn *et al.*, 1986; Schmidtke *et al.*, 1986). Furthermore, it was observed that there was no absence of the parathyroid hormone gene or abnormal restrictions patterns to suggest recognizable deletions, insertions or rearrangements in the DNA of affected individuals. This data suggests that the primary molecular defect leading to this form of familial *isolated* hypoparathyroidism is not located in the PTH gene itself.

Hypoparathyroidism can occur in association with congenital abnormalities, for example in Di George syndrome. In this disorder there is a failure of development of the derivatives of the third and fourth pharyngeal pouches with resulting absence or hypoplasia of the parathyroid glands and thymus. Affected individuals suffer from hypocalcaemia and from severe infections resulting from immunodeficiency which is due to thymic aplasia. An autosomal dominant inheritance of Di George syndrome has been observed (Rohn *et al.*, 1984) and an association between the syndrome and deletion of the proximal part of the long arm of chromosome 22 has also been reported (de la Chapelle *et al.*, 1981; Kelley *et al.*, 1982). Molecular mapping studies using *in situ* hybridization have been undertaken to further define this deletion (Cannizaro and Emmanuel, 1985). The Di George syndrome deletion breakpoint was found to be proximal to the locus for the immunoglobulin lambda polypeptide constant region but distal to the locus for the DNA probe D22S9. Furthermore, Southern blot and densitometric analysis has revealed that D22S9 is deleted in cell lines from patients with Di George syndrome. These closely mapping markers will help in characterizing the Di George syndrome gene, which is of importance in the development of the parathyroid glands.

X-linked recessive forms: X-linked recessive hypoparathyroidism has been reported in two multigeneration families (Peden, 1960; Whyte and Weldon, 1981). Only males were affected and suffered from infantile onset of epilepsy and hypocalcaemia, which appears to be due to parathyroid hypoplasia (Whyte *et al.*, 1986). Linkage studies in these families have localized the X-linked hypoparathyroid gene to Xq26–Xq27 (Thakker *et al.*, 1988) Figure 2. Defining this gene locus will open the way for elucidating the factors controlling the development and activity of the parathyroid gland.

Multiple endocrine neoplasia type I

Multiple endocrine neoplasia type I is characterized by the occurrence of hormone-secreting tumours of the parathyroid glands, the pancreatic islet cells and the pituitary gland. Hypercalcaemia due to parathyroid gland overactivity occurs in 95% of all multiple endocrine neoplasia type I patients (for review see Marx *et al.*,

1982). The disease may arise sporadically in patients or be inherited as an autosomal dominant condition. Tumour development may be caused by a plasma growth factor which appears to be a protein with a molecular weight of 50 000 daltons (Brandi *et al.*, 1986). Studies have been undertaken to identify the genetic abnormalities causing multiple endocrine neoplasia type I and the production of this growth factor.

A two-stage genetic mutational model has been proposed for the development of tumours in multiple endocrine neoplasia type I (Knudson *et al.*, 1973). The model is analogous to those reported for Wilms' tumour (Koufos *et al.*, 1984), retinoblastoma (Cavenee *et al.*, 1986) and multiple endocrine neoplasia type II (Mathew *et al.*, 1987) in which two recessive mutations are associated with tumorogenesis. The first mutation, which is recessive to the normal allele does not result in tumour formation but predisposes the cell to tumorogenesis. The growth of a tumour ensues only after the occurrence of the second mutation which eliminates the normal allele and thereby unmasks the altered allele of the first mutation. The genetic abnormalities causing the inherited and sporadic forms are the same but the cell types in which they occur are different. In the sporadic form both mutations occur in the somatic cells, whereas in the inherited form only the second mutation occurs in the somatic cells the first mutation having been inherited via the germinal cells.

The genetic mutations causing one type of multiple endocrine neoplasia type I tumour (insulinomas) have been identified by molecular studies in which RFLPs obtained from the patient's tumour DNA were compared to the RFLPs obtained from the same patient's leukocyte DNA (Larsson *et al.*, 1988). A loss of RFLPs (i.e. alleles) obtained with DNA probes from the short and long arms of chromosome 11 were found to occur in two insulinomas from multiple endocrine neoplasia type I patients. In addition, linkage studies of three affected families revealed linkage between the multiple endocrine neoplasia type I and human muscle phosphorylase (*PYGM*) genetic loci. The muscle phosphorylase gene had previously been localized to the long arm of chromosome 11 and this result mapped the multiple endocrine neoplasia type I gene to 11q. Further studies are required to define this disease locus and to clarify the mutational events in other multiple endocrine neoplasia type I tumours.

DISORDERS OF MAGNESIUM HOMEOSTASIS

Autosomal recessive and X-linked recessive inherited forms of hypomagnesaemia have been described. In the autosomal forms, hypomagnesaemia is probably the result of a renal tubular defect (Gitelman *et al.*, 1966; Manz *et al.*, 1978), whereas in the X-linked recessive form hypomagnesaemia seems to be due to an intestinal defect in magnesium absorption (Stromme *et al.*, 1969). Affected neonates with these disorders suffer from convulsions, tetany, a failure to thrive and non-specific dermatitis. The X-linked gene mutant in this disease may be situated on the short arm of the X-chromosome. Meyer *et al.* (1978) observed, in a girl, primary hypomagnesaemia in association with a 9/X unbalanced translocation involving the

Xp22 region. The genetic abnormalities causing this intestinal defect in magnesium absorption need to be defined further.

DISORDERS OF WATER HOMEOSTASIS

In diabetes insipidus there is an inability to concentrate urine and this results in polyuria and an excessive loss of water. Diabetes insipidus may be either due to a lack of production of arginine vasopressin, also referred to as anti-diuretic hormone, as occurs in neurohypophyseal (neurogenic) diabetes insipidus, or to insensitivity of the renal tubules to both endogenous and exogenous arginine vasopressin as occurs in nephrogenic diabetes insipidus. Autosomal dominant and X-linked recessive forms of nephrogenic diabetes insipidus have been reported. The gene causing X-linked nephrogenic diabetes insipidus has been localized and this will be discussed.

X-linked nephrogenic diabetes insipidus

McIlraith first observed in 1892 that nephrogenic diabetes insipidus may be inherited as an X-linked recessive disease. He noted that affected males presented with 'extreme thirst' and that some females were 'slightly affected'. However, male offspring of 'slightly affected' females suffered from 'extreme thirst' and that there was 'a heredity [of the disease] occurring chiefly in males on the female side of the house'. The disorder is rare and affected males present soon after birth with polyuria, fever, vomiting, dehydration, constipation and failure to thrive. Without treatment some patients die and those surviving are mentally retarded. The primary biochemical defect is unknown, although there is evidence of a defect in the arginine vasopressin receptor (Kobrinsky et al., 1985). Family linkage studies have localised the gene causing nephrogenic diabetes insipidus to Xq28 (Figure 2), by establishing linkage with the long arm markers DXS52 (Knoers et al., 1987) and F8A and DXS15 (Kambouris et al., 1988). This mapping of the disease gene will help in genetic counselling and in characterizing the defect in the arginine vasopressin receptor.

CONCLUDING REMARKS

The recent advances in molecular biology and cytogenetics have made it possible to map human disease genes. These methods have been used to localize the mutant genes causing several inborn errors of mineral metabolism. Thus the genetic abnormalities have been mapped which result in defects of: renal tubular handling of phosphate, as occurs in X-linked hypophosphataemic rickets and Lowe's syndrome; parathyroid gland development, as occurs in Di George syndrome and X-linked hypoparathyroidism; formation of endocrine tumours, as occurs in multiple endocrine neoplasia type I; absorption of magnesium, as occurs in X-linked hypomagnesaemia; and the arginine vasopressin receptor, as occurs in nephrogenic diabetes insipidus. The localization of these disease genes not only permits genetic counselling, but also opens the way to defining these genetic abnormalities and in characterizing their products of expression. This reverse genetics approach provides a unique opportunity to further elucidate the pathogenesis of these inherited mineral metabolic disorders.

REFERENCES

Abbassi, V., Lowe, C. U. and Calcagno, P. L. Oculo-cerebro-renal syndrome. *Am. J. Dis. Child.* 115 (1968) 145–168

Ahn, T. G., Antonarakis, S. E., Kronenberg, H. M., Igarashi, T. and Levine, M. A. Familial isolated hypoparathyroidism: a molecular genetic analysis of 8 families with 23 affected persons. *Medicine* 65 (1986) 73–81

Albright, F., Butler, A. M. and Bloomberg, E. Rickets resistant to vitamin D therapy. *Am. J. Dis. Child.* 54 (1937) 529–547

Botstein, D., White, R. L., Skolnick, M. and Davis, R. W. Construction of a genetic linkage map in man using restriction fragment length polymorphisms. *Am. J. Hum. Genet.* 32 (1980) 314–331

Brandi, M. L., Aurbach, G. D., Fitzpatrick, L. A., Quarto, R., Spiegel, A. M., Bliziotes, M. M., Norten, J. A., Doppman, J. L. and Marx, S. J. Parathyroid mitogenic activity in plasma from patients with familial multiple endocrine neoplasia type I. *N. Engl. J. Med.* 314 (1986) 1287–1293

Buckle, V. J., Edwards, J. H., Evans, E. P., Jonasson, J. A., Lyon, M. F., Peters, J., Searle, A. G. and Wedd, N. S. Chromosome maps of man and mouse II. *Clin. Genet.* 26 (1984) 1–11

Buckle, V. J., Edwards, J. H., Evans, E. P., Jonasson, J. A., Lyon, M. F., Peters, J. and Searle, A. G. Comparative maps of human and mouse X-chromosomes. *Cytogenet. Cell Genet.* 40 (1985) 594–595

Burnett, C. H., Dent, C. E., Harper, C. and Warland, B. J. Vitamin D resistant rickets. Analysis of 24 pedigrees with hereditary and sporadic cases. *Am. J. Med.* 36 (1964) 222–232

Cannizzaro, L. A. and Emanuel, B. S. *In situ* hybridization and translocation breakpoint mapping: II Di George syndrome with partial monosomy of chromosome 22. *Cytogenet. Cell Genet.* 39 (1985) 179–183

Cavenee, W. K., Murphree, A. L., Shull, M. M., Benedict, W. F., Sparkes, R. S., Kock, E. and Nordenskjold, M. Prediction of familial predisposition to retinoblastoma. *N. Engl. J. Med.* 314 (1988) 1201–1207

Christensen, J. F. Three familial cases of atypical late rickets. *Acta Paediatr. Scand.* 28 (1941) 247–270

Davies, K. E., Pearson, P. L., Harper, P. S., Murray, J. M., O'Brien, T., Sarfarazi, M. and Williamson, R. Linkage analysis of two cloned DNA sequences flanking the Duchenne muscular dystrophy locus on the short arm of the human X-chromosome. *Nucl. Acids Res.* 11 (1983) 2303–2312

Davies, K. E. Molecular genetics of the human X chromosome. *J. Med. Genet.* 22 (1985) 243–249

Davies, K. E., Mandel, J. L., Weissenbach, J. and Fellous, M. Report of the committee on the genetic constitution of the X and Y chromosomes, Ninth International Workshop on Human Gene Mapping, *Cytogenet. Cell Genet.* 46 (1987) 277–315

de la Chappelle, A., Herva, R., Koivisto, M. and Aula, P. A deletion in chromosome 22 can cause Di George syndrome. *Hum. Genet.* 57 (1981) 253–256

Eicher, E. M., Southard, J. L., Scriver, C. R. and Glorieux, F. H. Hypophosphataemia: Mouse model for human familial hypophosphataemic (vitamin D-resistant) rickets. *Proc. Natl. Acad. Sci. USA* 73 (1976) 4667–4671

Fibison, W. J. and Emanuel, B. S. Molecular mapping in Di George syndrome. *Am. J. Hum. Genet.* 41 (1987) A119

Gardner, R. J. M. and Brown, N. Lowe's syndrome: Identification of carrier by lens examination. *J. Med. Genet.* 13 (1976) 449–454

Gitelman, H. J., Graham, J. B. and Welt, L. G. A new familial disorder characterised by hypokalaemia and hypomagnesemia. *Trans. Assoc. Am. Physicians* 79 (1966) 221–235

Glorieux, F. H. and Scriver, C. R. Loss of a parathyroid hormone-sensitive component of phosphate transport in X-linked hypophosphataemia. *Science*, 175 (1972) 997–1000

Graham, J. B., McFalls, V. W. and Winters, R. W. Familial hypophosphataemia with vitamin D resistant rickets. II. Three additional kindreds of the sex-linked dominant type with a genetic analysis for four such families. *Am. J. Hum. Genet*, 11 (1959) 311–332

Hodgson, S. V., Heckmatt, J. Z., Hughes, E., Crolla, J. A., Dubowitz, V. and Bobrow, M. A balanced *de novo* X/autosome translocation in a girl with manifestations of Lowe syndrome. *Am. J. Med. Genet.* 23 (1986) 837–847

Hoffman, E. P., Knudson, C. M., Campbell, K. P. and Kunkel, L. M. Subcellular fractionation of dystrophin to the triads of skeletal muscle. *Nature* 330 (1987) 754–758

Johnston, S. S. and Nevin, N. C. Ocular manifestations in patients and female relatives of families with the oculocerebrorenal syndrome of Lowe. *Birth Defects: Orig. Art. Ser.* X11(3) (1976) 569–577

Kambouris, M., Dlouhy, S. R., Trofatter, J. A., Conneally, P. M. and Hodes, M. E. Localisation of the gene for X-linked nephrogenic diabetes insipidus to Xq28. *Am. J. Med. Genet.* 29 (1988) 239–246

Kelley, R. I., Zackai, E. H., Emmanuel, B. S., Kistenmacher, M., Greenberg, F. and Punnett, H. H. The association of the Di George anomalad with partial monosomy of chromosome 22. *J. Pediatr.* 101 (1982) 197–200

Knoers, N., van den Heyden, H., van Oost, B., Monnens, L., Willems, J. and Ropers, H. Tight linkage between nephrogenic diabetes insipidus and DXS52. *Cytogenet. Cell Genet.* 46 (1987) 640

Knudson, A. G., Strong, L. C. and Anderson, D. E. Heredity and cancer in man. *Progr. Med. Genet.* 9 (1973) 113–158

Kobrinsky, N. L., Doyle, J. J., Israels, E. D., Winter, J. S. D., Cheang, M. S., Walker, R. D. and Bishop, A. J. Absent factor VIII response to synthetic vasopressin analogue (DDAVP) in nephrogenic diabetes insipidus. *Lancet* 1 (1985) 1293–1294

Koenig, M., Hoffman, E. P., Bertelson, C. J., Monaco, A. P., Feener, C. and Kunkel, L. M. Complete cloning of the Duchenne muscular dystrophy (DMD) cDNA and preliminary genomic organisation of the DMD gene in normal and affected individual. *Cell* 50 (1987) 509–517

Koufos, A., Hansen, M. F., Lampkin, B. C., Workman, M. L., Copeland, N. G., Jenkins, N. A. and Cavenee, W. K. Loss of alleles at loci on human chromosome 11 during genesis of Wilms' tumour. *Nature* 309 (1984) 170–172

Larsson, C., Skogseld, B., Oberg, K., Nakamura, Y. and Nordenskjold, M. Multiple endocrine neoplasia Type 1 gene maps to chromosome 11 and is lost in insulinoma. *Nature* 332 (1988) 85–87

Lowe, C. U., Terrey, M. and MacLachlan, E. A. Organic-aciduria, decreased renal ammonia production, hydrophthalmos and mental retardation. *Am. J. Dis. Child.* 83 (1952) 164–168

Lyon, M. F. Mechanisms and evolutionary origins of variable X chromosome activity in mammals. *Proc. R. Soc. Lond.* B 1987 (1974) 243–268

Lyon, M. F., Scriver, C. R., Baker, L. R. I., Tenenhouse, H. S., Kronick, J. and Mandla, S. The *Gy* mutation: another cause of X-linked hypophosphataemia in mouse. *Proc. Natl. Acad. Sci. USA* 83 (1986) 4899–4903

Mächler, M., Fre, D., Gal, A., Orth, U., Wienker, T. F., Fanconi, A. and Schmid, W. X-linked dominant hypophosphataemia is closely linked to DNA markers DXS41 and DXS43 at Xp22. *Hum. Genet.* 73 (1986) 271–275

Manz, F., Scharer, K., Janka, P. and Lombeck, J. Renal magnesium wasting, incomplete tubular acidosis, hypercalciuria and nephocalcinosis in siblings. *Eur. J. Pediatr.* 128 (1978) 67–79

Marx, S. J., Spiegel, A. M., Levine, M. A., Rizzoli, R. E., Lasker, R. D., Santora, A. C., Downs, R. V. Jr. and Aurbach, G. D. Familial hypocalciuric hypercalcaemia: the relation to primary parathyroid hyperplasia. *N. Engl. J. Med.* 307 (1982) 416–426

Mathew, C. G. P., Smith, B. A., Thorpe, K., Wong, Z., Royle, N. J., Jeffreys, A. J. and Ponder, B. A. J. Deletion of genes on chromosome 1 in endocrine neoplasia. *Nature* 328 (1987) 524–526

McIlraith, C. H. Notes on some cases of diabetes insipidus with marked familial and hereditary tendencies. *Lancet* 2 (1892) 767–768

McKusick, V. A. *Mendelian Inheritance in Man.* 8th edition, Baltimore, John Hopkins University Press, 1988

Meyer, M., Mattei, J. F., Viallard, J. L., Goumy, P., Dastugue, B. and Malpuech, G. Hypocalcemie magnesodependante par trouble specifique de l'absorption du magnesium, associee a une anomalie chromosomique. *Rev. Fr. Endocr. Clin.* 19 (1978) 101–108

Morton, N. E. Sequential tests for the detection of linkage. *Am. J. Hum. Genet.* 7 (1955) 277–318

Naylor, S. L., Sakuguchi, A. Y., Szoka, P., Hendy, G. N., Kronenberg, H. M., Rich, A. and Shows, T. B. Human parathyroid hormone gene (PTH) is on the short arm of the chromosome 11. *Somat. Cell Genet.* 9 (1983) 609–616

Ohno, S. *Sex Chromosomes and Sex-linked Genes*, Springer, Berlin, Heidelberg, New York, 1967

Ott, J. Estimation of the recombination fraction in human pedigrees: efficient computation of the likelihood for human linkage studies. *Am. J. Hum. Genet.* 26 (1974) 588–597

Pallisgaard, G. and Goldschmidt, T. The oculo-cerebro-renal syndrome of Lowe in four generations of one family. *Acta Paediatr. Scand.* 60 (1971) 146–148

Peden, V. H. True idiopathic hypoparathryoidism as a sex-linked recessive trait. *Am. J. Hum. Genet.* 12 (1960) 323–337

Pembrey, M. E. Applications and limitations of direct DNA analysis in genetic prediction. *J. Inher. Metab. Dis.* 9 Suppl. 1 (1986) 38–48

Proto, G., Barberi, M., Cattalini, M. and Bertolissi, F. Transmissione autosomica dominante dell'ipoparatiroidismo idiopatico familiare. *Estrat. Minerva Endocriniol.* 10 (1985) 217–222

Read, A. P., Thakker, R. V., Davies, K. E., Mountford, R. G., Brenton, D. P., Davies, M., Glorieux, F., Harris, R., Hendy, G. N., King, A., McGlade, S., Peacock, J., Smith, R. and O'Riordan, J. L. H. Mapping of human X-linked hypophosphataemic rickets by multilocus linkage analysis. *Hum. Genet.* 73 (1986) 267–270

Rohn, R. D., Leffell, M. S., Leadem, P., Johnson, D., Rubiot, T. and Emanuel, B. S. Familial third–fourth pharyngeal pouch syndrome with apparent autosomal dominant transmission. *J. Pediatr.* 105 (1984) 47–51

Ruddle, F. H. The William Allan Memorial Award Address: Reverse genetics and beyond. *Am. J. Hum. Genet.* 36 (1984) 944–953

Schmidtke, J., Pape, B., Krenegel, U., Langenbeck, U., Cooper, D., Breyel, E. and Mayer, H. Restriction fragment length polymorphisms at the human parathyroid hormone gene locus. *Hum. Genet.* 67 (1984) 428–431

Schmidtke, J., Kruse, K., Pape, B. and Sippell, G. Exclusion of close linkage between parathyroid hormone gene and a mutant gene locus causing idiopathic hypoparathyroidism. *J. Med. Genet.* 23 (1986) 217–219

Silver, D. N., Lewis, R. A. and Nussbaum, R. L. Mapping the Lowe oculocerebrorenal syndrome to Xq24–q26 by use of restriction fragment length polymorphisms. *J. Clin. Invest.* 79 (1987) 282–285

Stromme, J. H., Nesbakken, R., Normann, T., Skjorten, F., Skyberg, D. and Johannessen, B. Familial hypomagnesemia. *Acta Paediatr. Scand.* 58 (1969) 433–444

Tenenhouse, H. S., Scriver, C. R., McInnes, R. R. and Glorieux, F. H. Renal handling of phosphate *in vivo* and *in vitro* by the X-linked hypophosphataemic male mouse; Evidence for a defect in the brush border membrane. *Kidney Int.* 14 (1978) 236–244

Thakker, R. V. Localisation of the hypophosphataemic rickets gene. *Bone* 5 (1988) 27–30

Thakker, R. V. and O'Riordan, J. L. H. Inherited forms of rickets and osteomalacia. In Martin, T. J. (Ed.) *Clinical Endocrinology and Metabolism*, Vol. 2 No. 1, *Metabolic Bone Disease*. Balliere Tindall, London (1988) pp. 157–191

Thakker, R. V., Davies, M., Davies, K. E., Hendy, G. N., McGlade, S., King, A., Read, A. P., Mountford, R. G., Kilgore, C. J., Glorieux, F., Brenton, D. P., Smith, R., Harris, R. and O'Riordan, J. L. H. Localisation of the gene causing X-linked hypophosphataemic rickets. *Q. J. Med.* 61 (1986) 1071–1072

Thakker, R. V., Read, A. P., Davies, K. E., Whyte, M. P., Weksberg, R., Glorieux, F., Davies, M., Mountford, R. G., Harris, R., King, A., Kim, G. S., Fraser, D., Kooh, S. W. and O'Riordan, J. L. H. Bridging markers defining the map positon of X-linked hypophosphataemic rickets. *J. Med. Genet.* 24 (1987) 756–760

Thakker, R. V., Davies, K. E., Whyte, M. P., Wooding, C. and O'Riordan, J. L. H. Localisation of the gene causing X-linked hypoparathyroidism to the long arm of the X-chromosome (Xq26–Xq27). *J. Bone Min. Res.* 3 (1988) S–210

White, R., Leppert, M., Bishop, D. T., Barker, D., Berkowitz, J., Brown, C., Calahan, P., Holm, T. and Jerominski, L. Construction of linkage maps with DNA markers for human chromosomes. *Nature* 313 (1985) 101–105

Whyte, M. P. and Weldon, V. V. Idiopathic hypoparathyroidism presenting with seizures during infancy: X-linked recessive inheritance in a large Missouri kindred. *J. Pediatr.* 99 (1981) 608–611

Whyte, M. P., Kim, G. S. and Kosanovich, M. Absence of parathyroid tissue in sex-linked recessive hypoparathyroidism. *J. Pediatr.* 109 (1986) 915

Winters, R. W., Graham, J. B., Williams, T. F., McFalls, V. W. and Burnett, C. H. A genetic study of familial hyophosphataemia and vitamin D resistant rickets with a review of the literature. *Medicine* 37 (1958) 97–142

J. Inher. Metab. Dis. 12 Suppl. 2 (1989) 247–256

Preface to Short Communications

This issue is devoted to selected short communications based on oral and poster presentations at the free sessions of the Annual Meeting of the Society for the Study of Inborn Errors of Metabolism held in Glasgow, 6–9th September 1988. The main topic of the symposium was pre- and perinatal diagnosis. The contributions of the invited speakers were complemented by many of the oral and poster free communications which dealt with pre- or perinatal diagnosis of specific diseases or summarized regional, national, or international experiences in offering services for a wider range of conditions. The free communications covered in addition a variety of other aspects of the study of inherited metabolic disease. Those not reported elsewhere in this issue are listed below. The book of abstracts of all free communications may be purchased from the Society for the Study of Inborn Errors of Metabolism at 15 Saint Thomas' Drive, Hatch End, Pinner, Middlesex HA5 4SX, UK, price £10, including postage.

Many of the short communications were submitted for the SSIEM Award, which is judged on the basis of the manuscript prepared for the *Journal*. This year the prize was awarded to R. Matalon, R. Kaul, J. Casanova, K. Michals, A. Johnson, I. Rapin, P. Gashkoff and M. Deanching for their paper "Aspartoacylase deficiency: the enzyme defect in Canavan disease".

With pressure on space in all scientific journals we hope that contributors and users will accept our suggestion that these papers be generated and used as short communications rather than as preliminary abstracts, at least in part. This year we have been able to accommodate less than half of those offered for publication and thus an element of appraisal is inherent in their selection. It is clear to the editors that some are preliminary communications which allow priority to be established. However, others are worthwhile additional records which are adequate in themselves as contributions to our accumulated experience and do not require additional recording.

G. M. Addison
R. A. Harkness
R. J. Pollitt

Free Communications

Experience of prenatal diagnosis by analysis of chorionic villi in approximately 100 pregnancies at risk for an inherited metabolic disorder. *E. P. Young, A. E. Whitfield and A. D. Patrick*

Journal of Inherited Metabolic Disease. ISSN 0141–8955. Copyright © SSIEM and Kluwer Academic Publishers, PO Box 55, Lancaster, UK.

Complementation analysis in peroxisomal disorders: evidence for genetic hetero-geneity within Zellweger syndrome and indications for 'peroxisomal ghosts'. *S. Brul, E. A. C. Strijland, R. J. A. Wanders, H. S. A. Heymans and R. B. H. Schutgens*

Dietary restriction of maternal lactose intake does not prevent accumulation galactitol in amniotic fluid of fetuses affected with galactosaemia. *C. Jakobs, W. J. Kleijer, H. D. Bakker, A. H. van Gennip, H. Przyrembel and M. F. Niermeijer*

X-linked recessive lipid myopathy responsive to elimination of dietary long chain fatty acids. *M. A. Nigro, J. Saad, C. H. Chang, S. Di Mauro and Z. Farooki*

The mechanism by which dietary protein restriction benefits children with inborn errors of amino acid metabolism. *G. N. Thompson, J. H. Walter, D. Halliday and J. V. Leonard*

In vivo enzyme activity in children with inborn metabolic errors. *G. N. Thompson, J. H. Walter, J. V. Leonard and D. Halliday*

International recipe book for PKU patients. *P. Portnoi and R. Stocking*

Plasma lipid levels in treated and untreated phenylketonuria patients: preliminary data. *R. Cerone, M. C. Schiaffino, G. Zignego, L. Maritano, F. Parisi, A. Cohen and C. Romano*

Investigation of the haplotype pattern of the mutant PKU allele in the Welsh gypsy population using the cDNA probe. *L. A. Tyfield, L. M. Meredith, M. J. Osborn and P. S. Harper*

Different haplotype combinations of mutant alleles at the phenylalanine hydroxy-lase locus in several affected members of one family. *L. A. Tyfield, A. L. Meredith, M. J. Osborn and P. S. Harper*

Relation between genotype and phenotype in Swedish phenylketonuria and hyper-phenylalaninaemia patients. *E. Svensson, L. Hagenfeldt and U. von Dobeln*

Congenital malformations in offspring of PKU mother: a preliminary study. *C. Romano, R. Cerone, M. T. Gandolfo, M. C. Schiaffino, G. Zignego and Caruso, U.*

Amino acid and haplotype analysis for the detection of phenylketonuria. *L. J. Mienie, J. H. Ueckermann, I. Mohr, C. H. Marais, J. Op't Hof and W. J. de Wet*

Restriction fragment length polymorphism in the phenylalanine hydroxylase locus in the Belgian population. *P. Verelst, C. Denis, M. Rossius, D. Allaer, B. Francois, J. Martial and H. Dahl*

Selenium intakes by PKU children under phenylalanine restricted diet. Correlation with selenium levels. *F. Eysckens, R. Bahadori, M. Diels, M. Callie-Bertrand, H. Deelstra and B. Francois*

Evaluation of the phenylketonuria cases seen in Istanbul Faculty of Medicine. *G. Kurdoglu, M. Demirkol, H. Songur and S. Yalvac*

Prenatal diagnosis in 6-pyruvoyltetrahydropterin synthase deficiency. *S. Biasetto, A. Ponzone, S. Ferraris, D. Delmastro and A. Niederwieser*

Progressive systemic scleroderma in an infant with atypical phenylketonuria. *M. Haktan, A. Aydin, H. Bahat, B. Tuysuz, H. H. Yazici and M. D. S. Altay*

Pattern electroretinogram, flash and pattern reversal visual evoked potentials in phenylketonuria. *E. Riva, M. Giovannini, N. Canal, G. Comi, V. Martinelli, R. Valsasina, G. Biasucci and R. Longhi*

A case of pyruvoltetrahydropterin-synthetase deficiency: response to oral BH_4 therapy. *R. Longhi, M. Giovannini, G. Biasucci, R. Valsasina, H. Ch. Curtis, N. Blau and E. Riva*

Basal ganglion calcification in hyperphenylalaninaemia due to deficiency of dihydropteridine reductase. *H. Schmidt, K. Ullrich, R. Korinthenberg, P. E. Peters and E. Harms*

RFLPs of the phenylalanine hydroxylase gene in the Italian population. *I. Diazani, L. Farinasso, P. Fortina, C. Camaschella, R. Ponzone, H. H.-M. Dahl, R. G. H. Cotton and A. Ponzone*

Incidence of PKU and other HPA in a sample of Turkish newborn population. *I. Ozalp, T. Coskun, S. Tokol, F. Guneral and G. Demircin*

Prenatal diagnosis of hereditary tyrosinaemia type I. *E. A. Kvittingen and E. K. Brodtkorb*

Expression of the gene encoding fumarylacetoacetase in acute and chronic forms of hereditary tyrosinaemia type I. *R. Beger, H. van Faassen, I. van den Berg, E. Agsteribbe, P. van der Veer, M. Hartog and E. Wiemer*

Urinary succinylacetone and the dietary treatment of tyrosinaemia, type I. *P. Purkiss, M. D. Bain, M. Jones, T. E. Stacey and R. A. Chalmers*

Methylenetetrahydrofolate reductase deficiency: *in vivo* and *in vitro* response to folate cofactors in a juvenile. *E. M. Layward, J. R. Moore and B. Fowler*

Maple syrup urine disease: a case report. *C. S. Pang and Y. T. Mak*

DNA analysis for ornithine transcarbamylase deficiency. *I. Okabe, H. Kodama, M. Yanagisawa and T. Awata*

Hyperammonaemia associated with orotic aciduria and cryptogenic cirrhosis. Primary or secondary ornithine carbamyl transferase 'deficiency?' *I. Cree, L. M. Nelson, J. A. Young, D. B. Walsh, B. Lake, J. V. Leonard and A. Westwood*

Orthotopic liver transplantation in a girl with partial ornithine carbamyl transferase deficiency. *C. Largilliere, D. Houssin, F. Gottrand, O. Bernard, C. Mathey, A. Checoury, A. Alagille and J. P. Farriaux*

Acute encephalopathic episodes in an adult patient with a mild variant form of ornithine transcarbamylase deficiency. *M. E. Haseler, D. A. Fraser, S. Krywawych and D. P. Brenton*

Argininosuccinic aciduria revealed by valproate intolerance. *C. Boujet, A. Joannard, N. Jourdil and I. Wroblewski*

Exclusion of argininosuccinic aciduria by direct analysis in chorionic villi. *A. B. Burlina, W. J. Kleijer and D. Gaburro*

Pregnancies in patients with lysinuric protein intolerance. *O. Simell, K. Parto, K. Nanto-Salonen and I. Sipila*

Neonatal treatment of urea cycle disorders and MSUD. *R. Cerone, U. Caruso, M. C. Schiaffino, S. Lupino and C. Romano*

The production of the mesaconate, an inhibitor of fumarase, from methylsuccinate contaminated in clinically used sodium benzoate. *E. Maeda, M. Matsuo, K. Saiki, H. Nakamura and T. Matsuo*

Gyrate atrophy of the choroid and retina with hyperornithinaemia: effect of dietary treatment. *W. Endres, Y. S. Shin, W. Roschinger, B. Lorenz and E. Zrenner*

The effect of newborn screening on prognosis in galactosaemia: results of the international survey. *N. Buist, D. Waggoner, G. Donnell and H. Levy*

Assay of enzymes in galactose and sorbitol metabolism in human and cow lens. *Y. S. Shin, V. Vetter, K. Schmidt, B. Lorenz and W. Endres*

Deleterious effects of lactation in a galactosaemic mother. *M. Brivet, J. P. Raymond, P. Konopka and A. Lemonnier*

Cytosolic thymidine kinase activity in galactokinase deficient fibroblasts. *J. Baptista, M. Brivet, N. Kadhom, M. Gautier and A. Lemonnier*

Atypical galactosaemia with normal enzyme activities. *G. Bracco, S. Pagliardini, A. Iavarone, G. Dotti, O. Guardamagna, I. Dianzani, S. Biasetti and A. Ponzone*

Characterisation of human liver and muscle phosphorylase b kinase. *I. van Den Berg, H. van Faassen, L. Quarles van Ufford, C. Oldenhof, J. Fernandes and R. Berger*

Mini polyacrylamide gel isoelectrofocusing of phosphorylases, phosphorylase-B-kinase and phosphoglucomutase in human tissues by Phastsystem. *Y. S. Shin, T. Miller and W. Endres*

Enzymological classification of patients with methylmalonic aciduria: basis for a clinical trial of deoxyadenosylcobalamin in a hydroxocobalamin-responsive patient. *R. A. Chalmers, M. Bain, J. Mistry, M. A. Jones, B. M. Tracey, J. C. Linnell, J. Faludy and C. Weaver*

Metronidazole reduces *in vivo* propionate production and methylmalonate excretion in methylmalonic acidaemia. *J. H. Walter, G. N. Thompson, M. Jones, D. Halliday, J. V. Leonard and R. A. Chalmers*

The disposal of substrate in methylmalonic acidaemia. *J. H. Walter, G. N. Thompson, J. V. Leonard, K. Bartlett and D. Halliday*

Identification of 3-ethyl-3-hydroxy-δ-valerolactone in urine in propionic acidaemia. *I. Fleming, S. K. Armstrong and R. J. Pollitt*

The management and long term outcome of propionic acidaemia and methylmalonic acidaemia. *T. Ohura, M. Kikuchi, J. Aikawa, S. Ishizawa, K. Hayasaka, Y. Igarashi, K. Narisawa and K. Tada*

Evidence of primary CNS 'organic acidurias'. *C. R. Roe, D. S. Gale and D. S. Millington*

Pyruvate carboxylase deficiency associated with organic aciduria. *V. Barash, O. Elpeleg, Y. Shapira, S. Yosha, B. Glick and A. Gutman*

The use of amniotic fluid in the prenatal diagnosis of pyroglutamic aciduria. *E. Erasmus, L. J. Mienie and C. J. Reinecke*

Inherited metabolic diseases amongst mentally retarded and paediatric patients. *C. J. Reinecke and J. Op't Hof*

First trimester prenatal diagnosis of propionyl-CoA carboxylase deficiency by chorionic villi biopsy. *N. Venizelos, L. Hagenfeldt, U. von Dobeln and T.-H. Bui*

Treatment of 4-hydroxybutyric acidaemia by inhibition of GABA-transaminase. *J. Jaeken, B. Francois, L. Leyssens, P. Pitance, H. Hainaut and K. Gibson*

A further case of 3-hydroxy-3-methylglutaryl-CoA lyase deficiency. Familial studies and one-year follow-up. *M. A. Vilaseca, A. Ribes, P. Briones, A. Maya, R. Baraiber and J. M. Gairi*

Cytochrome *c* oxidase activity in chorionic villi. *L. de Meirleir, W. Lissens, G. DeDobbeleer, L. Decatte, W. Foulonm and I. Liebaers*

Cytochrome *c* oxidase deficiency: diagnosed in chorionic villi. *W. Ruitenbeek, R. Sengers, M. Albani, F. Trijbels, A. Janssen, O. van Diggelen and J. Bakkeren*

The subunit pattern of defective cytochrome *c* oxidase in muscle biopts of patients wth mitochondrial myopathies. *K. M. C. Sinjorgo, J. A. Berden, P. Bolhuis, E. M. Brouwer-Kelder, A. O. Muijsers, H. R. Scholte and J. M. Tager*

^{1}H-NMR analysis of human cerebrospinal fluid in a case with MERF (myoclonus epilepsy with ragged red fibres) syndrome. *A. Federico, M. T. Dotti, G. Fabrizi, L. Manneschi, E. Gaggelli, M. P. Picchi and G. Valensin*

3-Methylglutaconic and 3-methylglutaric aciduria: estimation of 3-methyl-glutaconyl-CoA hydratase in different tissues. *H. Ibel, W. Endres, H.-B. Hadorn, K. M. Gibson and M. Duran*

3-Methylglutaconic aciduria: neonatal onset with lactic acidosis. *C. Largilliere, L. Vallee, B. Cartigny, J. P. Dubos, K. M. Gibson, J. P. Nuyts and J. P. Farriaux*

An atypical case of 3-methylglutaconic aciduria. *C. J. Reinecke, L. J. Mienie and E. Erasmus*

Isolated biotin resistant 3-methylcrotonyl CoA carboxylase deficiency presenting as a Reye's syndrome-like illness. *B. M. Layward, M. S. Tanner, R. J. Pollitt and K. Bartlett*

The contribution of protein catabolism decompensation in 3-hydroxy-3-methylglutaric aciduria. *G. N. Thompson, D. Halliday, M. Jones, J. H. Walter, R. A. Chalmers and J. V. Leonard*

Fumarase deficiency: neonatal presentation with cerebral malformation and liver disease. *V. Walker, G. A. Mills, M. A. Hall, G. H. Millward-Sadler, N. R. English and R. A. Chalmers*

Biotinidase deficiency: clinical, biochemical and therapeutical aspects. *E. Ruidor, A. Vilaseca, P. Briones, A. Ribes, J. Sune, R. Martorell, A. Macaya, M. Roig and A. Ballabriga*

Biotinidase deficiency with residual biotinidase activity. *T. S. Suormala, E. R. Baumgartner, H. Wick, S. Scheibenreiter, P. C. Clemens, S. Schweitzer, E. Harms and C. Bachmann*

A new case of holocarboxylase synthetase. *P. Briones, A. Ribes, M. A. Vilaseca, G. Rodriquez-Valcarcel, L. P. Thuy and L. Sweetman*

Prenatal diagnosis of glutaric aciduria type I using GC–MS of amniotic fluid and enzymology with oxidation of [6-^{14}C] lysine. *R. A. Chalmers, K. N. Cheng, N. R. English, M. A. Jones and W. Savage*

Neural dysfunction during hypoglycaemia corrected by restoration of normoglycaemia. *T. H. H. G. Koh, A. Aynsley-Green, M. Tarbit and J. A. Eyre*

Hepatic phosphoenol pyruvate carboxykinase deficiency in a neonate with hypoglycaemia, metabolic acidosis, hyperammonaemia and thrombocytopenia. *M. Matsuo, E. Maeda, K. Saiki, H. Nakamura, T. Matsuo, K. Koike and M. Koike*

A possible unrecognised defect in gluconeogenesis in a child with lactic aciduria. *M. Wajner, C. M. D. Wannmacher, J. C. Dutra, R. Giugliani and R. A. Chalmers*

A new multisystem syndrome of mitochondrial cytopathy, progressive cerebral calcification and recurring stroke. *M. A. Nigro, M. E. Martens and C. P. Lee*

Dicarboxylic acids in medium chain acyl-CoA dehydrogenase deficiency and sudden infant death syndrome. *L. Hagenfeldt, U. von Dobeln, N. Venizelos and J. Rajs*

Oxidation of [^{13}C]palmitate and [^{13}C]octanoate *in vivo* in children with defects in fatty acid oxidation. *G. N. Thompson, J. V. Leonard, J. H. Walter, E. E. Mathews and D. Halliday*

Are N-acyl-glycine metabolites in urine pathogenomic for medium-chain acyl-CoA deficiency? *D. J. Reijngoud, K. Niezen-Koning, T. E. Chapman, G. P. A. Smit and R. Berger*

Comments on the [9,10-^{3}H]palmitate assay for medium chain acyl-CoA dehydrogenase deficiency. *N. J. Manning, S. Olpin, R. J. Pollitt and J. Webley*

Diagnosis of medium chain acyl-CoA dehydrogenase deficiency by stable isotope dilution analysis of urinary acylglycines. *P. Rinaldo, J. J. O'Shea and K. Tanaka*

A genetic defect in carnitine transport causing primary carnitine deficiency. *C. A. Stanley, W. R. Treem, D. E. Hale and P. M. Coates*

Transport of carnitine into cells in hereditary carnitine deficiency. *B. O. Eriksson, B. Gustafson, S. Lindstedt and I. Nordin*

Excretion of 3-oxo-Δ^4-bile acids – inborn error or consequence of hepatocellular damage? *P. T. Clayton, E. Patel, R. A. Carruthers and A. M. Lawson*

Lack of 3-β-hydroxy-Δ^5-steroid dehydrogenase/isomerase in fibroblasts from a child with giant cell hepatitis and urinary excretion of 3-β-hydroxy-Δ^5-bile acids. *M. Buchmann, E. A. Kvittingen, H. Nazer, P. T. Clayton, J. Sjovall and I. Bjorkhem*

Osteoporosis and cerebrotendinous xanthomathosis: a pathological study. *R. Nuti, G. Martini, R. Righi, F. Lore, M. T. Dotti and A. Federico*

Juvenile Gaucher disease: brain lipid composition in a Spanish case without β-glucocerebrosidase deficiency and massive intraneuronal lipid storage. *T. Pampols, M. Giros, A. Chabas, M. Pineda, I. Ferrer and T. Vanier*

Normal liver rhodanese activity in two patients with Leber's hereditary optic atrophy. *R. Pallini, P. Di Natale, C. Alessandrini, M. T. Dotti, P. Vivrea, G. C. Guazzi and A. Federico*

Tay–Sachs carrier detection in Manchester by automated ion-exchange chromatography of white cell extracts. *A. Cooper, C. E. Hatton, I. B. Sardharwalla, M. Super and S. Simon*

Prenatal diagnosis of sialic acid storage disease. *B. D. Lake, E. P. Young and K. Nicolaides*

A case of nephrosialidosis on CAPD therapy for four years. *J. Nishimoto, K. Inui, H. Tsukamoto, M. Taniike, M. Midorokawa, S. Okada and H. Yabuuchi*

Oligosaccharide metabolism in cultured skin fibroblasts from a patient with beta-mannosidosis. *C. Hatton, A. Cooper and I. B. Sardharwalla*

Application of a flow-chart for the investigation of lysosomal storage diseases in 105 high-risk patients. *R. Giuglianoi, M. L. Barth, S. L. Goldenfum, R. Munarski, A. Folberg, M. Jackson, C. M. Vimal and A. H. Fensome*

Lysosomal storage diseases in Greece. Laboratory experience. *H. Michelakakis, S. Tsagarakis, E. Dimitriou, C. Soulpis and S. Giouroukos*

Biochemical differences in two families with juvenile Sandhoff's disease. *A. Cooper, C. E. Hatton and I. B. Sardharwalla*

Prenatal diagnosis of type II mucopolysaccharidosis 'Hunter' disease. *R. Dumoulin, G. Mandon, I. Maire and P. Guibaud*

Enhanced β-adrenergic transmission in fibroblasts of patients with Zellweger Syndrome. *H. Toplak, U. Honegger, A. Hermetter, F. Paltauf and U. N. Wiesmann*

Peroxisomal disorders caused by an impairment in peroxisomal β-oxidation. Clinical characteristics, biochemical detection and prenatal diagnosis. *R. J. A. Wanders, C. W. T. van Roermund, M. J. A. van Wijland, R. B. H. Schutgens, P. G. Barth, H. van den Bosch, J. M. Tager and A. W. Schram*

Prenatal dagnosis of Zellweger syndrome by determination of trihydroxy-copro-stanic acid in amniotic fluid. *F. Stellaard, C. Jakobs, S. A. Langelaar, R. M. Kok, W. J. Kleijer and R. B. H. Schutgens*

Two new cases of Pseudozellweger's (Zellweger-like) syndrome. Differential diagnosis from Zellweger's syndrome. *R. G. F. Gray, M. M. Honeyman, R. B. H. Schutgens, R. J. A. Wanders and A. Green*

L-Pipecolic acid oxidase in human liver: identification of an enzyme not previously demonstrated in mammals and its deficiency in the Zellweger syndrome. *R. J. A. Wanders, G. J. Romeyn, R. B. H. Schutgens, H. van den Bosch and J. M. Tager*

Complementation analysis in classical Refsum's disease. *O. H. Skjeldal, B. T. Poll-Thé, O. Stokke and J. M. Saudubray*

Unequivocal carrier detection and prenatal diagnosis of inherited diseases. An example demonstrated with α_1-antitrypsin deficiency. *C. Newton, N. Kalsheker, A. Graham, J. Riley, S. Powell, A. Gammack and A. Markham*

Dot-blot analysis of α-1-antitrypsin variants by biotinylated allele specific oligo-nucleotides after sequence specific amplification. *N. Gregersen, K. B. Petersen, J. Koch, S. Kolvraa, G. B. Petersen and L. Bolund*

Investigation of the enzyme activity associated with the microvillar membrane fraction of amniotic fluid from pregnancies with cystic fibrosis. *E. Gracey, D. A. Aitken, J. A. M. Maatouk, G. W. Graham and J. M. Connor*

Steroid sulphatase expressions in hair roots. *D. A. Aitken, J. R. W. Yates and M. A. Ferguson-Smith*

Scottish experience in carrier detection and early prenatal diagnosis of X-linked muscular dystrophies. *W. G. Lanyon, E. O'Hare, S. Loughlin, A. McWhinnie, J. Lambert, A. Findlay, A. Cooke, D. A. Aitkin and J. M. Connor*

A case of adenosine deaminase deficiency and severe combined immunodeficency disease diagnosed prenatally using chorionic villi and fetal blood. *D. A. Aitken, D. M. Gilmore, P. J. Batstone, J. McIver, C. Swindlehurst and M. J. Whittle*

α-1-Fetoprotein in neonates. *H. M. May, J. D. Stevenson, D. Farquharson and A. McWhinnie*

Chorionic villus sampling at Birmingham Maternity Hospital and Birmingham Children's Hospital: biochemical disorders. *J. McCormack, R. G. F. Gray, A. Green, W. McKenzie and J. Newton*

Cytochrome *c* oxidase in muscle of two patients with Menke's disease. *D. C. Davidson, D. Isherwood, M. J. Jackson and R. D. Griffiths*

Menke's disease. Acute oral loading tolerance tests with copper and ionphores. *D. C. Davidson, D. M. Isherwood, R. Griffiths and M. Jackson*

Thyroid metabolism in the newborn: low Apgar score and euthyroxinaemic hyper-thyrotropinaemia. *P. C. Clemens, S. Neumann and C. Plettner*

Plasma and CSF amino acid levels in neonates with perinatal anoxia. *J. Lambarda-ridis, Ch. Kostalos, S. Sevastiadou, A. Thalassinos and H. Michelakakis*

Diagnosis of the causes of developmental delay and cerebral palsy. *R. A. Harkness, I. Laing and J. K. Brown*

Detection of β-thalassaemia using a neonatal screening programme for sickle cell disease. *P. D. Griffiths, A. Green and P. J. Darbyshire*

Myoglobinuria with transient acute renal failure in patients with fatty acid oxidation defects in muscle. *S. Krywawych, R. Stephenson, C. Kingswood, J. Round and D. P. Brenton*

Adenine phosphoribosyl transferase deficiency in a Pakistani boy. *G. M. Addison, H. A. Simmonds and I. D. Ward*

Evaluation of an *in situ* technique for sexing interphase nuclei from chorion villus samples using X and Y centromeric probes. *L. Murer, M. Murer-Orlando and J. Crolla*

Maternal PKU: foetal blood and tissue amino acid concentrations in mid-trimester. *B. Fowler, J. Horner, J. E. Wraith and I. B. Sardharwalla*

In vivo and *in vitro* B_{12} responsiveness in methymalonic acidaemia. *B. Merinero, C. Perez-Cerda, M. J. Garcia, A. Jimenez, P. Sanz, C. Hernandez and M. Ugarte*

Biotin metabolism in nervous cells culture. *P. Rodriguez-Pombo, J. Belloque and M. Ugarte*

Adrenoleukodystrophy: two cases with different phenotypic expression? *S. Stockler, F. Ebner and B. Molzer*

Decreased endocytosis of labelled LDL in cultured fibroblasts with impaired peroxisomal plasmalogen biosynthesis: a consequence of decreased membrane fluidity? *W. Erwa, B. Pertl, E. Paschke, G. M. Klostner, A. Hermetter and F. Paltauf*

Measurement of cystine in leukocyte suspensions in cystinosis patients using deuterium labelled cystine and isotope dilution GC/MS. *T. E. Chapman, S. Kuipers, I. E. Mulder, D.-J. Reijngoud, R. Berger and W. van Luyk*

Molecular analysis of steroid sulphatase deficiency. *A. Ballabio, R. Carrozzo, G. Parenti, A. Gil, M. Zollo, M. G. Persico, N. Affara, M. A. Ferguson-Smith and G. Andria*

α-N-Acetylgalactosaminidase deficiency, a new lysosomal storage disease. *O. P. van Diggelen, D. Schindler, R. Willemsen and W. J. Kleijer*

A new method for the determination of urinary orotate excretion. *A. Cracco, V. Ferrari, G. Giordano, N. Dussini, L. Chiandetti and F. Zacchello*

A baby with cardiomyopathy cured by thiamine. *H. D. Bakker, A. H. van Gennip, H. R. Scholte and I. E. M. Luyt-Houwen*

The inheritance of the galactosaemia allele in three families. *H. D. Bakker, A. H. van Gennip, N. G. G. M. Abeling, J. R. Rajnherc and C. van der Heiden*

Sarcosinaemia in a patient with Usher's syndrome. *E. Christensen, N. Jacob Brandt and T. Rosenberg*

O-Phosphohydroxylysinuria. A possible newborn error of metabolism. *L. Dorland, M. Duran, P. K. de Bree, G. R. Smith, A. Horvath, A. S. Tibosch and S. K. Wadman*

Pitfall in the diagnosis of mild multiple acyl-CoA dehydrogenase deficiency. *B. T. Poll Thé, A. Lombes, A. Pellet, C. Charpentier, M. Paturneau Jouas, C. Jakobs and J. M. Saudubray*

Complementation analysis of peroxisomal disorders and classical Refsum disease. *B. T. Poll Thé, O. H. Skjeldall, O. Stokke, F. Damaugre and J. M. Saudubray*

Genetic hypomagnesaemia. *D. P. Brenton, T. B. Weir, R. Street and J. C. Kingswood*

Potential use of RFLP technique in genetic counselling in familial hypophosphataemic rickets. *E. Pronicka, E. Popowska and M. Krajewska-Walasek*

Mitochondrial myopathies. Isolation of cDNA clones coding for nuclear encoded subunits of human cytochrome *c* oxidase. *J. W. Taanman, J. A. Schrage-Tabak, H. de Vries, R. Berger and E. Agsteribbe*

First trimester diagnosis of Wolman's disease. *W. J. Kleijer, O. P. van Diggelen, H. von Koskull and P. Ammala*

Juvenile Sandhoff disease. *C. Rittey, J. Stephenson, G. Besley, A. Weir, R. Logan and J. Tolmie*

Inborn errors of fatty acid metabolism in Reye's syndrome. *C. Rittey, J. Stephenson, R. J. Pollitt, C. Roe and R. Logan*

An improved method for the measurement of plasma carnitine and its derivatives and its application to the investigation of inherited metabolic disorders. *A. K. M. J. Bhuiyan, A. Aynsley-Green, J. V. Leonard and K. Bartlett*

Quantitative analysis of urinary acyl-carnitines by high performance liquid chromatography. *A. K. M. J. Bhuiyan, A. Aynsley-Green, J. V. Leonard and K. Bartlett*

J. Inher. Metab. Dis. 12 Suppl. 2 (1989) 257–259

Short Communication

15 Years of Prenatal Diagnosis of Inherited Metabolic Diseases: the Lyon Experience

G. Mandon and M. Mathieu

Laboratoire de Biochimie, Centre d'Etude des Maladies Métaboliques, Hôpital Debrousse, 69322 Lyon Cédex 05, France

Our centre, located in the Children's Hospital of Lyon, has been devoted to the study of inherited metabolic diseases for 30 years (Divry *et al.*, 1988). The field of our study concerns mainly carbohydrate inborn errors (glycogenoses, fructose and galactose metabolism), lysosomal storage diseases, amino acidopathies, organic acidurias, disorders of nucleotide and nucleic acid metabolism and, more recently, peroxisomal diseases and mitochondrial cytopathies.

Beside postnatal diagnosis and neonatal screening of curable diseases we have been involved in prenatal diagnosis of non-curable inborn errors since 1973 (Mathieu *et al.*, 1978).

MATERIALS AND METHODS

From 1973 until 1985, we used only amniotic fluid from around the 17th week of amenorrhea (Divry *et al.*, 1988). Since 1985 we have been working more and more with chorionic villi obtained between the 9–11th week (Guibaud *et al.*, 1986).

Amniotic fluid: Amniotic fluid cells are separated by gentle centrifugation. Some biochemical analyses are performed directly on the supernatant. Cells are cultivated in Ham F 10 medium supplemented with fetal calf serum 10% and Ultroser G (IBF) 1%, with antibiotics. Usually, the cells are grown for two or three weeks before analysis. They are harvested by trypsinization, then placed in the appropriate medium (saline, buffer, etc.) depending on the analysis performed.

Chorionic villi: Fetal tissue is separated from maternal decidua (when necessary) under a microscope, then, in most cases, directly analysed. At the same time, some villi are planted in the culture medium with the help of chicken plasma as adhesion factor. They are grown for two or three weeks before being harvested for confirmative biochemical analysis.

Whichever cells are used (amniotic or chorionic cells), they are always compared for the analysis with cells of familial index cases (usually skin fibroblasts) kept frozen in our cell strains bank (Zabot *et al.*, 1978; Mathieu *et al.*, 1986). After analysis, they are frozen in the same way as a further control after birth or abortion depending on the issue.

Journal of Inherited Metabolic Disease. ISSN 0141–8955. Copyright © SSIEM and Kluwer Academic Publishers, PO Box 55, Lancaster, UK.

Mandon and Mathieu

Table 1 Prenatal diagnoses achieved to June 1988

Diseases	Amniotic fluid		Chorionic villi		Total Affected	
	Total	Affected	Total	Affected	Total	Affected
Neurolipidoses						
GM I Gangliosidosis (Landing)	8	1	—	—	8	1
GM II Gangliosidosis Tay Sachs	3	0	1	0	4	0
Sandhoff	10	0	3	1	13	1
Gaucher	4	0	2	1	6	1
Metachromatic leucodystrophy	23	7	2	1	25	8
Fabry	—	—	1	0	1	0
Oligosaccharidoses						
α-Mannosidosis	2	1	—	—	2	1
Mucolipidosis II and III	2	1	—	—	2	1
Mucopolysaccharidoses						
MPS I (Hurler)	18	6	7	1	25	7
MPS II (Hunter)	16	0	6	1	22	1
MPS III A (San Filippo)	2	0	1	0	3	0
MPS III B (San Filippo)	2	0	—	—	2	0
MPS IV A (Morquio)	2	1	—	—	2	1
MPS IV B (Morquio)	1	0	—	—	1	0
MPS VII (β-glucuronidase)	1	0	—	—	1	0
Aminoacidopathies and organic aciduria						
MSUD	5	0	1	0	6	0
Methylmalonic aciduria	3	0	—	—	3	0
Propionic aciduria	7	1	—	—	7	1
Glutaric aciduria I	1	0	—	—	1	0
Tyrosinaemia I	6	1	—	—	6	1
Homocystinuria	5	1	—	—	5	1
Cystinosis	4	2	2	1	6	3
Citrullinaemia	1	0	—	—	1	0
Combined SO-XO deficiency	1	1	6	1	7	2
Glycogenoses and carbohydrates						
GSD type II Pompe	9	3	4	1	13	4
GSD type III	6	0	1	1	7	1
Phosphorylase activator	1	0	—	—	1	0
Galactosaemia	5	3	2	1	7	4
Purine metabolism						
Lesch Nyhan	5	1	1	0	6	1
Disorder of immune defense systems						
Adenosine deaminase deficiency	3	0	—	—	3	0
Peroxysomal diseases						
Zellweger	—	—	4	0	4	0
Refsum	—	—	1	0	1	0
Others						
Wolman's disease	—	—	1	0	1	0
Xeroderma pigmentosum	3	1	2	1	5	2
Hypophosphatasia	7	3	—	—	7	3
Cystic fibrosis	112	23	5	1	117	24
Total	278	67	53	12	331	69

RESULTS

Three hundred and thirty-one diagnoses have been made, corresponding to 36 different diseases: 278 used amniotic fluid (either supernatant or cultivated cells) and 53 used chorionic villi (either direct analysis (45) or cultivated (8)).

Sixty-nine fetuses have been found to be affected. At the present time, no false diagnosis has been observed. The results are summarized in Table 1.

Most of the index cases and fetal cells (cultivated skin fibroblasts, amniotic fluid cells and trophoblasts) are kept frozen in our cell strains bank.

Cystic fibrosis diagnosis is made either by intestinal enzyme activities in amniotic fluid or by DNA analysis of chorionic villi.

CONCLUSIONS

From our experience, for most diseases, chorionic villi are to be preferred to amniotic fluid cells since the diagnosis is made at an earlier stage of pregnancy and direct analysis eliminates problems due to culture conditions (for example Pompe's disease). However some direct analyses have to be confirmed with cultivated trophoblasts (mucopolysaccharidosis type I). Some diseases (for example, mucolipidoses I, II, III and xeroderma pigmentosum) need obligatory cultivated trophoblasts. The only restriction is the necessary verification of absence of maternal contamination.

REFERENCES

Divry, P., Maire, I. and Mathieu, M. Diagnostic biologique des maladies héréditaires du métabolisme du dépistage orienté à la banque de cellules mutantes. *Ann. Biol. Clin.* 46 (1988) 381–386

Guibaud, P., Mathieu, M., Mandon, G., Divry, P., Dorche, C., Dumoulin, R., Rolland, M. O. and Domenichini, Y. Etudes des villosités choriales dans le diagnostic prénatal des maladies métaboliques. *Rev. Int. Pediatr.* 163 (1986) 24

Mathieu, M., Zabot, M. T., Maire, I. and Mandon, G. Enzyme studies in cultivated amniotic cells in the field of prenatal diagnosis in metabolic diseases. In Golberg, G. M. and Wilkinson, J. H. (Eds.). *Enzymes in health and diseases*, Karger, Basel, 1978, pp. 232–237

Mathieu, M., Zabot, M. T., Mandon, G., Boyer, S., Servetti, A., Biron, A. and Messy, P. *The Human Genetic Cell Repository*, 4th Edn., H. C. Lyon, 1986

Zabot, M. T., Boyer, S., Genoud, J., Guibaud, P., Mathieu, M. and Cotte, J. Organisation et gestion informatique d'une banque cellulaire. *Ann. Biol. Clin.* 36 (1978) 230–232

J. Inher. Metab. Dis. 12 Suppl. 2 (1989) 260–262

Short Communication

A Survey on Prenatal Diagnosis of Inherited Metabolic Diseases in Japan

K. Tada[1], J. Aikawa[1], Y. Igarashi, K. Hayasaka[2], K. Narisawa[2], M. Owada[3] and T. Kitagawa[3]

Department of [1]Pediatrics and [2]Biochemical Genetics, Tohoku University School of Medicine, Sendai and [3]Department of Pediatrics, Nihon University Medical School, Tokyo, Japan

A survey for prenatal diagnosis of inherited metabolic diseases was made in 15 principal clinics for this particular field in Japan. The results were summarized in Table 1. In total, 263 cases of pregnant women at risk for 37 disorders were

Table 1 Prenatal diagnosis of inherited metabolic diseases

Disorders†	Diagnosis			
	Cases	Normal	Affected	Impossible
Tay–Sachs	50	40 (1*)	10	
Gaucher	36	27	9	
Hunter	24	18 (1*)	6	
GM$_1$ gangliosidosis	22	14	8	
Krabbe	19	15	3	1
I-cell	16	12	4	
Pompe	10	7	3	
MMA	10	7	3	
Hurler	7	5 (1*)	2	
Menkes	7	4	1	2
Nieman–Pick A	5	3	2	
MLD	5	3	2	
Lesch–Nyhan	5	3	1	1
Sandhoff	4	3	1	
PPA	4	3	1	
MSUD	4	3	1	
Sialidosis	4	3	1	
Maroteax–Lamy	3	3	0	
21-Hydroxylase	3	3	0	
Miscellaneous	25	19	6	
Total	263	195 (3*)	64	4
%	100	74.1	24.3	1.5

*erroneous diagnosis
† abbreviations: MMA, methylmalonic acidaemia; MLD, metachromatic leucodystrophy; PPA, propionic acidaemia; MSUD, maple syrup urine disease

Journal of Inherited Metabolic Disease. ISSN 0141-8955. Copyright © SSIEM and Kluwer Academic Publishers, PO Box 55, Lancaster, UK.

monitored, of which 195 cases (74.1%) were diagnosed as normal and 64 (24.3%) were diagnosed as 'affected'. Pregnancies were interrupted at the parents' wishes in all cases diagnosed as 'affected'. Except in a few cases, the aborted fetuses were examined and proved to be homozygotes of the respective disorders. In 4 cases, the diagnosis was not possible and there were three cases of erroneous diagnosis among those diagnosed as normal. These cases occurred before 1980 and were due to insufficient cell culture. The 133 prenatal diagnoses performed after 1980 were all correct. The disorders most frequently monitored were Tay–Sachs disease (50 cases), and then Gaucher disease (36), Hunter syndrome (24), GM_1 gangliosidosis (22), Krabbe disease (19), I-cell disease (16), Pompe disease (10), methylmalonic acidaemia (10), Hurler syndrome (7) and Menkes syndrome (7). 'Miscellaneous' includes argininosuccinic aciduria, galactosialidosis, citrullinaemia, adenosine deaminase deficiency, Sanfillippo B syndrome, Morquio syndrome, β-glucuronidase deficiency, pyruvate carboxylase deficiency, pyruvate decarboxylase deficiency, ornithine transcarbamylase deficiency, Zellweger syndrome, xerodermia pigmentosum, isovaleric acidaemia, methylentetrahydrofolate reductase deficiency, Wolman disease, Cockayne syndrome, dihydrobiopterin synthetase deficiency and non-ketotic hyperglycinaemia. Diagnosis was made by amniocentesis in most cases but the use of chorionic villi has gradually been increasing since 1985. Diagnosis was by determination of enzyme activity in the cultured amniotic fluid cells in most cases. DNA diagnosis was made in cases of 21-hydroxylase deficiency (congenital adrenal hyperplasia), Lesch–Nyhan syndrome and ornithine transcarbamylase deficiency. Out of 263 cases monitored, 211 (80%) were for lysosomal diseases. Tay–Sachs disease, Gaucher disease, Hunter syndrome and GM_1 gangliosiodosis showed a relatively high prevalence, accounting for approximately 24%, 17%, 11% and 10% of the total lysosomal diseases, respectively. These results are essentially similar to those of the survey of patients with lysosomal diseases in Japan (Kitagawa *et al.*, 1981) and may reflect the incidence of each disease. According to the results of a survey on the prenatal diagnosis of lysosomal diseases in West-European countries (Galjaard, 1976), Tay–Sachs disease is the most common disorder there, as well as in Japan. Gaucher disease and I-cell disease seemed to be relatively more common in Japan. In contrast, Pompe disease and cystinosis were less frequent in Japan. Hunter syndrome was found to be more frequent than Hurler syndrome in Japan whereas the reverse was true in caucasian countries.

PRENATAL DIAGNOSIS OF NON-KETOTIC HYPERGLYCINAEMIA

There has been a special need for prenatal diagnosis of non-ketotic hyperglycinaemia (NKH) which is an incurable and severe disease. The fundamental defect in NKH is known to be in the glycine cleavage system (Tada and Hayasaka, 1987). However, prenatal diagnosis using cultured amniotic fluid cells is impossible because the glycine cleavage enzyme is not manifest in cultured skin fibroblasts. In 1987, we had an opportunity to investigate retrospectively the feasibility of prenatal diagnosis of NKH by analysing the glycine cleavage system in the placenta (Hayasaka *et al.*, 1987). The fourth pregnancy of a woman was monitored. The family had one healthy child (14 years of age) and an 11-year-old severely retarded daughter with NKH. Their first-born child died of NKH at the age of 3 weeks in 1970, after a typical clinical course. An abortion was performed in 12th week of gestation, according to the parents' wish. The overall activity of the glycine cleavage system in the liver and brain of the fetus at risk for NKH was extremely low compared with that of control fetuses, and the placenta also had markedly low activity. There was no detectable activity of T protein but other components of the glycine cleavage system were not decreased. From these findings, it was confirmed that the aborted fetus was a homozygote for NKH, with a defect in T protein. These results showed the existence of the glycine cleavage system in the placenta and proves the feasibility of prenatal diagnosis of NKH by chorionic villi biopsy. Prenatal diagnosis was then performed for a pregnant woman whose previous child was affected by NKH. At the 12th week of gestation, about 20 mg chorionic villi was biopsied and was assayed for the glycine cleavage system, according to the method described previously (Hayasaka *et al.*, 1987). There was no significant difference in the activity between the fetus at risk ($4.4 \, \mu\text{mol} \, (\text{g protein})^{-1} \text{h}^{-1}$) and control fetuses ($2.5-6.0 \, \mu\text{mol} \, (\text{g protein})^{-1} \text{h}^{-1}$). Subsequently, a healthy girl was born after a full-term pregnancy. Her glycine level in plasma was found to be within normal range.

ACKNOWLEDGEMENTS

We are indebted to Drs S. Arashima, K. Oyanagi, T. Eto, M. Arima, Y. Suzuki, Y. Wada, K. Suzumori, T. Orii, M. Sudo, S. Okada, G. Isshiki, T. Sugawa, K. Takeshita, F. Yamashita and I. Matsuda for their co-operation in performing this survey. This work was supported by Grants from the Ministry of Health and Welfare and from the Ministry of Education, Science and Culture, Japan.

REFERENCES

Galjaard, H. European experience with prenatal diagnosis of congenital disease: A survey of 6121 cases. *Cytogenet. Cell Genet.* 16 (1976) 453–467

Hayasaka, K., Tada, K., Fueki, N., Takahashi, I., Takebayashi, T. and Baumgartner, R. Feasibility of prenatal diagnosis of nonketotic hyperglycinemia: Existence of the glycine cleavage system in placenta. *J. Pediatr.* 110 (1987) 124–126

Kitagawa, T., Arima, M., Eto, Y., Tarui, S., Yabuuchi, H., Tada, K., Kusumoki, T., Suzuki, Y. and Orii, T. The survey of lysosomal storage disease in Japan. *Annual Report of the Study on Chronic Diseases in Children.* The Ministry of Public Health and Welfare, Japan, 1981, pp. 11–24

Tada, K. and Hayasaka, K. Nonketotic hyperglycinemia: Clinical and biochemical aspects. *Eur. J. Pediatr.* 146 (1987) 221–227

J. Inher. Metab. Dis. 12 Suppl. 2 (1989) 263–266

Short Communication

Prenatal Diagnosis of Inherited Metabolic Disease by Chorionic Villus Analysis: The Edinburgh Experience

G. T. N. BESLEY and D. M. BROADHEAD
Department of Paediatric Biochemistry, Royal Hospital for Sick Children, Edinburgh EH9 1LF, UK

Prenatal diagnosis of inherited metabolic disease is possible when suitable samples of fetal material are available and when these samples express a clear biochemical abnormality that is specific to that disorder. In the past, tests have been carried out by enzyme assay on cultured amniotic fluid cells and/or analysis of amniotic fluid for metabolites. These tests, carried out late into pregnancy (16 weeks plus), cause much anxiety and added risks to mothers. With the advent of first trimester chorionic villus sampling, tests may now be carried out directly on chorionic villus samples (CVS) with results available in a matter of days (Poenaru, 1987; Sachs *et al.*, 1988). The advantages to those at risk are obvious but like many new techniques specific problems may arise.

MATERIALS AND METHODS

During the last 3 years, we have carried out 36 prenatal diagnoses on CVS. Samples were collected into sterile tissue culture fluid containing approximately 10 units heparin mL^{-1}, cleaned and sent in tissue culture medium, usually overnight, to the laboratory. On receipt, clean and viable samples were selected under a dissecting microscope, washed in isotonic saline and either assayed immediately or frozen at $-70°C$. Other pieces were set up for culture (Besley *et al*, 1988) and direct chromosome analysis.

All diagnoses were carried out by enzyme assay of whole tissue homogenates with or without sonication. Standard methods of enzyme assay were used and reference activities were always measured in parallel.

RESULTS AND DISCUSSION

Chorionic villus samples were analysed from 36 pregnancies at risk for 14 different inherited metabolic disorders. A total of nine affected fetuses were identified (Figure 1), although in one case, (Niemann–Pick type C) confirmation was established by Dr Marie Vanier (Lyon), from cholesterol esterification studies (Vanier *et al.*, 1988).

Of the 36 diagnoses undertaken, 29 were carried out by direct enzyme analysis

Journal of Inherited Metabolic Disease. ISSN 0141–8955. Copyright © SSIEM and Kluwer Academic Publishers, PO Box 55, Lancaster, UK.

of fresh CVS. In four samples there was insufficient material for direct analysis and diagnosis was therefore made on cultured CVS cells. In three of these chromosome analysis revealed a 46,XY karyotype, indicating that they were fetal in origin. The fourth was 46,XX and because maternal cell contamination could not be excluded, the diagnosis was confirmed by amniocentesis.

Diagnosis or confirmation was carried out on cultured villus cells in 31/36 cases. Two samples from abroad arrived frozen and were therefore not cultured, and in three samples culture was either not attempted or not successful. During the last 2 years all CVS have been successfully cultured. Confirmation on cultured amniotic fluid cells was carried out on seven samples only and all were biochemically unaffected.

In our experience, CVS had residual activities of less than 10% of controls from fetuses affected with the following conditions: GM1-gangliosidosis, GM2-gangliosidosis variant (Besley *et al.*, 1987), Krabbe, Gaucher (Besley *et al.*, 1988), Niemann–Pick, Hurler–Scheie and Zellweger syndrome. In the Hunter fetus, iduronate sulphatase activity was 11% in CVS but only 2% in fetal skin fibroblasts. A similar observation was made by Kleijer *et al.* (1984) who suggested this might arise from a maternal source or from other sulphatases. In any event, interpretation will be aided by chromosome analysis in this X-linked disorder.

In the fetus with Niemann–Pick type C, normal activities of sphingomyelinase and β-glucosidase were found in fresh CVS but partial deficiencies in cultured CVS, similar to the enzyme pattern common in affected fibroblasts. Confirmation of this diagnosis required specific studies elsewhere (Vanier *et al.*, 1988). The one case of propionic acidaemia shown (Figure 1) was, in fact, strictly a placental biopsy taken at 19 weeks gestation following diagnostic amniocentesis. It is included for information, and emphasises the use of propionyl-CoA carboxylase assay over the less reliable incorporation studies (Chadefaux *et al.*, 1988). Only one case of Zellweger syndrome was diagnosed in our series where dihydroxyacetone phosphate acyl transferase activity was measured. Although this enzyme is not partially deficient in carriers, care should be taken to avoid low protein levels in the assay leading to non-linearity.

In 3/31 cultured villus samples there was clear evidence of maternal cell contamination. This high level is clearly worrying but similar to the 13% reported by Williams *et al.* (1987). One case was a Gaucher fetus with trisomy 21 (Besley *et al.*, 1988), and in another approx. 50% 46,XX cells grew from a 46,XY direct preparation. These two CVS were of excellent quality and no contamination was expected. In the third, the quality of the original CVS was poor and the result was confirmed by amniocentesis. The importance of back-up cytogenetic studies was also emphasized by the 45,X/46,Xi(Xq) mosaic found in an amniotic cell culture used to exclude Hunter disease following a diagnosis on CVS culture which was reported as 46,XX. This sample may also have suffered maternal contamination.

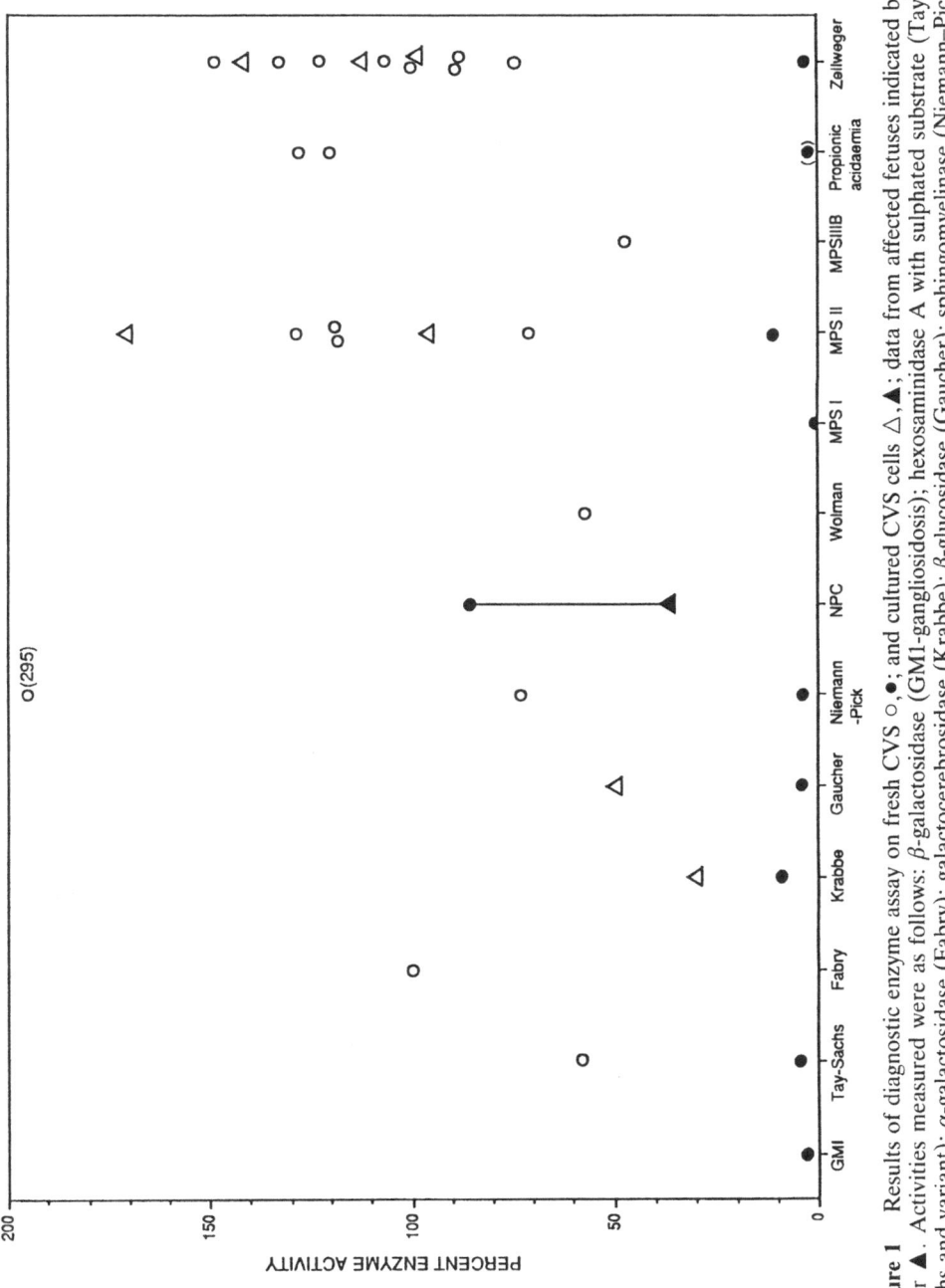

Figure 1 Results of diagnostic enzyme assay on fresh CVS ○, ●; and cultured CVS cells △, ▲; data from affected fetuses indicated by ● or ▲. Activities measured were as follows: β-galactosidase (GM1-gangliosidosis); hexosaminidase A with sulphated substrate (Tay–Sachs and variant); α-galactosidase (Fabry); galactocerebrosidase (Krabbe); β-glucosidase (Gaucher); sphingomyelinase (Niemann–Pick and type C variant); acid esterase (Wolman); α-iduronidase (MPS I); iduronate sulphatase (MPS II); α-N-acetyl glucosaminidase (MPS IIIB), propionyl-CoA carboxylase (propionic acidaemia); dihydroxyacetone phosphate acyl transferase (Zellweger)

ACKNOWLEDGEMENTS

We thank many colleagues who referred samples to us, in particular Dr W. A. Liston who also provided many controls. We are also most grateful to Mrs Eleanor Cochrane for cell culture and Dr Lynn Hendry for cytogenetic studies.

REFERENCES

Besley, G. T. N., Broadhead, D. M. and Young, J. A. GM2-gangliosidosis variant with altered substrate specificity: evidence for α-locus genetic compound. *J. Inher. Metab. Dis.*, 10 (1987) 403–404

Besley, G. T. N., Ferguson-Smith, M. E., Frew, C., Morris, A. and Gilmore, D. H. First trimester diagnosis of Gaucher disease in a fetus with trisomy 21. *Prenat. Diagn.* 8 (1988) 471-474

Chadefaux, B., Augereau, C., Rabier, D., Rocchicciolo, F., Boue, J., Oury, J. F. and Kamoun, P. Prenatal diagnosis of propionic acidemia in chorionic villi by direct assay of propionyl-CoA carboxylase. *Prenat. Diagn.* 8 (1988) 161-164

Kleijer, W. J., van Diggelen, O. P., Janse, H. C., Galjaard, H., Dumez, Y. and Boue, J. First trimester diagnosis of Hunter syndrome on chorionic villi. *Lancet* 2 (1984) 472

Poenaru, L. First trimester prenatal diagnosis of metabolic diseases. A survey in countries in the European Community *Prenat. Diagn.* 7 (1987) 333-341

Sachs, E. S., Jahoda, M. G. J., Kleijer, W. J., Pijpers, L. and Galjaard, H. Impact of first trimester chromosome, DNA, and metabolic studies on pregnancies at high genetic risk: experience with 1000 cases. *Am. J. Med. Genet.* 29 (1988) 293-303

Vanier, M. T., Wenger, D. A., Comly, M. E., Rousson, R., Brady, R. O. and Pentchev, P. G. Niemann–Pick disease group C: clinical variability and diagnosis based on defective cholesterol esterification. A collaborative study on 70 patients. *Clin. Genet.* 33 (1988) 331-348

Williams, J., Medearis, A. L., Chu, W. H., Kovacs, G. D. and Kaback, M. M. Maternal cell contamination in cultured chorionic villi: comparison of chromosome Q-polymorphisms derived from villi, fetal skin, and maternal lymphocytes. *Prenat. Diagn.* 7 (1987) 315-322

J. Inher. Metab. Dis. 12 Suppl. 2 (1989) 267–270

Short Communication

Prenatal Diagnosis of Inherited Metabolic Disorders by Stable Isotope Dilution GC-MS Analysis of Metabolites in Amniotic Fluid: Review of Four Years Experience

C. Jakobs

Department of Pediatrics, Free University Hospital Amsterdam, De Boelelaan 1117, 1007 MB Amsterdam, The Netherlands

The direct chemical analysis of metabolites excreted by the fetus using cell-free amniotic fluid obtained at 12–18 weeks of pregnancy offers the advantage of rapid and reliable prenatal diagnosis. This method can only be used when unambiguous discrimination is achieved between normal levels of a metabolite and the elevated levels observed in affected cases. This technique is particularly well suited for prenatal diagnosis of organic acidurias in which high concentrations of specific metabolites accumulate in urine. Similarly, abnormal metabolites produced by the fetus can accumulate in amniotic fluid since this is partially derived from fetal urine (Sweetman, 1984).

Currently, the method of choice for measurement of metabolites in amniotic fluid is stable isotope dilution gas chromatography–mass spectrometry with selected ion monitoring (GC–MS–SIM). In this procedure, an analogue of the compound to be detected, labelled with stable isotopes, is included as a carrier as well as an internal standard, preventing inaccuracy due to loss by adsorption of the compound being analysed. This method provides high sensitivity and specificity, excellent precision and reproducibility with very low concentrations of metabolites. This cannot be achieved by GC or GC–MS alone. Sensitivity is increased further by using the GC–MS in the chemical ionization (CI) or electron capture negative ion (ECNI) mode. In addition, this method is rapid, providing the final result within 1–2 days.

This communication reports 4 years of experience of prenatal monitoring of 76 pregnancies 'at risk' for the following 6 disorders: methylmalonic acidaemia, propionic acidaemia, glutaric aciduria type II, tyrosinaemia type I, isovaleric acidaemia and galactosaemia. For all characteristic metabolites, normal values have been determined and the ranges in the samples from affected fetuses are presented.

Journal of Inherited Metabolic Disease. ISSN 0141–8955. Copyright © SSIEM and Kluwer Academic Publishers, PO Box 55, Lancaster, UK.

MATERIALS AND METHODS

Cell-free amniotic fluid samples from pregnancies 'at risk' were received lyophilized or frozen in dry ice and were stored at −20°C prior to analysis. The 'at risk' samples ($n = 76$) were referred from the following countries: France ($n = 23$), The Netherlands ($n = 17$), USA ($n = 8$), Italy ($n = 6$), German F. R. ($n = 5$), United Kingdom ($n = 4$), Czechoslovakia ($n = 4$), Belgium ($n = 3$), Finland ($n = 2$), and Austria, Spain, Poland and South Africa ($n = 1$).

To confirm the validity of the prenatal diagnosis of a disorder by metabolite measurement, enzymatic analysis of cultured amniocytes was performed whenever possible.

The procedures used for the quantitation of the different metabolites in amniotic fluid have been described before in detail. Methylmalonic acid and methylcitric acid were measured as described by Sweetman *et al.* (1982) and glutaric acid by the method of Jakobs *et al.* (1984a) with the introduction of [^{2}H$_4$]glutaric acid as internal standard. Succinylacetone and galactitol were determined as described by Jakobs *et al.* (1988a and 1984b, respectively) and the procedure used for isovalerylglycine was according to Hine *et al.* (1986).

RESULTS AND DISCUSSION

The results of prenatal monitoring of 76 pregnancies 'at risk' for the 6 conditions listed above are summarized in Table 1 which also includes normal values of the characteristic metabolites. For the conditions where the number of affected fetuses is greater than 3, the mean and range of affected values are given; otherwise only

Table 1 Stable isotope dilution analysis of metabolites (μmol/L) in amniotic fluid

Disease (metabolite)	Controls mean±SD (n) (range)	At risk	
		Affected mean (n) (range)	Unaffected mean (n) (range)
Propionic acidaemia (methylcitrate)	0.30±0.10 (20) (0.15–0.50)	6.04 (4) (5.30–6.62)	0.39 (10) (0.19–0.63)
Methylmalonic acidaemia (methylmalonic acid)	0.30±0.13 (20) (0.08–0.46)	41.2 (5) (10.1–71.6)	0.40 (14) (0.12–0.80)
Glutaric aciduria type II (glutaric acid)	0.90±0.18 (20) (0.69–1.17)	12.3; 14.5 (2)	1.05 (6) (0.50–1.28)
Isovaleric acidaemia (isovalerylglycine)	0.020±0.012 (10) (0.002–0.038)	—	0.010; 0.036; 0.050
Tyrosinaemia type I (succinylacetone)	0.016±0.008 (20) (0.001–0.030)	0.085; 0.70; 1.50 (3)	0.010 (15) (0.001–0.030)
Galactosaemia (galactitol)	0.80±0.15 (20) (0.44–1.20)	7.61 (4) (6.35–9.21)	0.72 (10) (0.50–1.21)

the individual concentrations are shown. In all 76 cases, the correct diagnosis has been obtained, based on either confirmation by enzyme assay or studies in the child at birth. For all the diseases combined, 23.7% were affected which is close to the 25% expected for autosomal recessive inheritance. The mean values for unaffected 'at risk' pregnancies and controls were similar, implying that heterozygous fetuses are not distinguished from normal.

The concentrations of methylcitrate in amniotic fluid of fetuses with propionic acidaemia were about 15 times higher than the mean of unaffected fetuses and the concentration of methylmalonic acid in pregnancies with methylmalonic acidaemia ranged from 25–180 times the unaffected mean. For both disorders, control, unaffected mean and affected mean values are in good accordance with those reported by Sweetman (1984).

Glutaric acid concentrations in pregnancies affected by glutaric aciduria type II were about 12 times higher than the unaffected mean value. It is noteworthy that this method can also be applied to glutaric aciduria type I for which the prenatal diagnosis has been previously described (Goodman *et al.*, 1980).

Our experience with isovaleric acidaemia is limited to 3 pregnancies with no affected fetus. The normal values for isovalerylglycine are very low and the use of the stable isotope labelled internal standard as a carrier to prevent adsorption losses is essential. In affected cases, Hine *et al.* (1986) report values 30–60 times greater than the levels found in their unaffected cases.

For determination of normal amounts of succinylacetone, this compound requires specific derivatization with pentafluorobenzylesters, followed by electron capture negative ionization mass fragmentography detection (Jakobs *et al.*, 1988a). For reliable prenatal diagnosis of tyrosinaemia type I, accurate determination of the control range is extremely important since the range of values in affected pregnancies varies considerably from 5–95 times higher than the mean of the unaffected cases. Distinguishing the lowest affected value might be difficult with conventional GC–MS assays.

In pregnancies affected with galactosaemia, the concentrations of the characteristic metabolite, galactitol, ranged from 9–13 times higher than the mean of the unaffected values. It should be noted that galactitol accumulation in amniotic fluid is independent of the lactose content of the diet of the mother (Jakobs *et al.*, 1988b).

In 6 cases, amniocentesis was preceded by chorionic villus biopsy. In all 3 (1 affected, 2 unaffected) cases of tyrosinaemia type I, the result of the fumarylacetoacetase (FAH) assay in chorionic villus material agreed with the result of the metabolite assay (Kvittingen *et al.*, 1986). In 2 out of 3 cases of methylmalonic acidaemia, the [14C]propionic acid incorporation assay gave false negative results in affected pregnancies which were indicated by clearly elevated methylmalonic acid accumulation in the amniotic fluid. This finding supports the study by Fowler *et al.* (1988) which showed that the [14C]propionate incorporation test is not reliable for use in intact villi.

In conclusion, prenatal diagnosis by quantitation of metabolites in amniotic fluid using stable isotope dilution GC–MS is reliable for the above mentioned disorders.

Its validity and potential is also established for many other organic acidurias (Sweetman, 1984). These are, however, specialized tests and, considering the rarity of the disorders and the ease of shipment of frozen or lyophilized amniotic fluid, it would be preferable for a few major centres to provide this prenatal diagnostic service.

ACKNOWLEDGEMENTS

I would like to express my appreciation to the many colleagues who provided the amniotic fluids, especially to Dr W. J. Kleijer, Rotterdam and to Dr K. Tanaka for providing [^{2}H$_3$]isovalerylglycine. Dr A. de Jong, Dr F. Stellaard, Mr R. Kok and Mr S. Langelaar are gratefully acknowledged for the GC–MS analysis.

REFERENCES

Fowler, B., Giles, L., Sardharwalla, I. B., Donnai, P. and Clayton, J. K. First trimester diagnosis of methylmalonic aciduria. *Prenatal Diagnosis* 8 (1988) 207–213

Goodman, S. I., Gallegos, D. A., Pullin, C. J., Halpern, B., Truscott, R. J. W., Wise, G., Wilcken, B., Ryan, E. D. and Whelan, D. T. Antenatal diagnosis of glutaric aciduria. *Am. J. Hum. Genet.* 32 (1980) 695–699

Hine, D. G., Hach, A. M., Goodman, S. I. and Tanaka, K. Stable isotope dilution analysis of isovalerylglycine in amniotic fluid and urine and its application for the prenatal diagnosis of isovaleric acidemia. *Pediatr. Res.* 20 (1986) 222–226

Jakobs, C., Sweetman, L., Wadman, S. K., Duran, M., Saudubray, J. M. and Nyhan, W. L. Prenatal diagnosis of glutaric aciduria type II by direct chemical analysis of dicarboxylic acids in amniotic fluid. *Eur. J. Pediatr.* 141 (1984a) 153–157

Jakobs, C., Warner, T. G., Sweetman, L. and Nyhan, W. L. Stable isotope dilution analysis of galactitol in amniotic fluid: An accurate approach to the prenatal diagnosis of galactosemia. *Pediatr. Res.* 18 (1984b) 714–718

Jakobs, C., Dorland, L., Wikkerink, B., Kok, R. M., de Jong, A. P. J. M. and Wadman, S. K. Stable isotope dilution analysis of succinylacetone using electron capture negative ion mass fragmentography: an accurate approach to the pre- and postnatal diagnosis of hereditary tyrosinemia type I. *Clin. Chim. Acta* 223 (1988a) 223–232

Jakobs, C., Bakker, H. D., van Gennip, A. H., Przyrembel, H., Kleijer, W. J. and Niermeijer, M. F. Dietary restriction of maternal lactose intake does not prevent accumulation of galactitol in amniotic fluid of fetuses affected with galactosemia. *Prenatal Diagnosis* 8 (1988b) 641–645

Kvittingen, E. A., Guibaud, Pr. P., Divry, P., Mandon, G., Rolland, M. O., Domenichini, Y., Jakobs, C. and Christensen, E. Prenatal diagnosis of hereditary tyrosinemia type I by determination of fumarylacetoacetase in chorionic villus material. *Eur. J. Pediatr.* 144 (1986) 597–598

Sweetman, L. Prenatal diagnosis of the organic acidurias. *J. Inher. Metab. Dis.* 7 Suppl. 1 (1984) 18–22

Sweetman, L., Naylor, G., Ladner, T., Holm, J., Nyhan, W. L., Hornbeck, C., Griffiths, J., Morch, L., Brandange, S., Gruenke, L. and Craig, J. C. Prenatal diagnosis of propionic and methylmalonic acidemia by stable isotope dilution analysis of methylcitric and methylmalonic acids in amniotic fluid. In Schmidt, H. L., Forstel, H. and Heinziger, K. (eds.) *Stable Isotopes*, Elsevier Sci. Publ. Co., Amsterdam, 1982, pp. 287–293

J. Inher. Metab. Dis. 12 Suppl. 2 (1989) 271–273

Short Communication

Prenatal Diagnosis of Propionic and Methylmalonic Acidaemia by Stable Isotope Dilution Analysis of Amniotic Fluid

J. HOLM, L. PONDERS and L. SWEETMAN*

Department of Pediatrics, University of California San Diego, La Jolla, CA 92093, USA

Stable isotope dilution gas chromatography–mass spectrometry (GC/MS) analysis of methylcitric acid in amniotic fluid for the rapid and accurate prenatal diagnosis of propionic acidaemia (McKusick 23200) and methylmalonic acidaemia (McKusick 25100) was first described in 1980 (Naylor *et al.*, 1980). This was soon followed by similar methods for the determination of methylmalonic acid in amniotic fluid for prenatal diagnosis of methylmalonic acidaemia (Trefz *et al.*, 1981; Zinn *et al.*, 1982; Sweetman *et al.*, 1982). We describe here our results for the prenatal diagnosis of 102 pregnancies at risk for either propionic acidaemia or methylmalonic acidaemia.

METHODS

Amniotic fluids from around the world were obtained at between 12 and 20 weeks of pregnancy by amniocentesis, centrifuged to remove cells for establishing cell cultures for karyotypes or back-up assay of enzymes, and the supernatant frozen and shipped frozen. Two aliquots, 1 mL and 4 mL, were analysed as has been described (Naylor *et al.*, 1980; Sweetman *et al.*, 1982). For the later analyses, 50 nmol rather than 100 nmol of each trideuterated internal standard was added and the GC/MS analysis of the methyl esters was done with wide-bore fused silica capillary columns of bonded DB-Wax, 0.53 mm (ID)×15 m or 30 m in place of packed columns.

RESULTS

The concentrations of methylmalonic acid and methylcitric acid in amniotic fluids are shown in Table 1. The mean concentration of methylcitric acid in the 47 amniotic fluids from pregnancies at risk for but not affected with propionic acidaemia, and the 32 amniotic fluids from pregnancies at risk for but not affected with methylmalonic acidaemia was the same as the normal mean. The mean concentration of

---

*Correspondence

271

Journal of Inherited Metabolic Disease. ISSN 0141–8955. Copyright © SSIEM and Kluwer Academic Publishers, PO Box 55, Lancaster, UK.

Table 1 Concentrations of methylcitric acid and methymalonic acid (μmol L^{-1}) in amniotic fluid

Subjects	Methylmalonic acid	Methylcitric acid
Normal: mean±SD (n)	0.29±0.08(9)	0.38±0.10(8)
range	0.17–0.44	0.24–0.58
At risk for propionic acidaemia:		
not affected: mean±SD (n)	—	0.38±0.18 (47)
range	—	0.11–1.10
affected: mean±SD (n)	—	7.00±1.80 (17)
range	—	4.07–10.16
At risk for methylmalonic acidaemia:		
not affected: mean±SD (n)	0.41±0.17 (29)	0.35±0.16 (32)
range	0.14–0.78	0.08–0.89
affected: mean±SD (n)	29.0±26.2 (5)	2.51±0.34 (6)
range	6.8–74.0	2.03–2.78

methylmalonic acid in the 29 amniotic fluids at risk for but not affected with methylmalonic acidaemia was only slightly higher than the normal mean. Two-thirds of the fetuses from at risk but not affected pregnancies would be expected to be heterozygotes for one of the two organic acidaemias. Therefore the normal levels of the metabolites in the amniotic fluids of these pregnancies indicate that heterozygotes are not distinguishable from normals.

Of the 64 pregnancies at risk for propionic acidaemia, 26% were found to be affected by elevation of methylcitric acid in amniotic fluid. This is close to the 25% expected for an autosomal recessive disorder. The mean concentration of methylcitric acid in these amniotic fluids was 18 times normal with a fairly small relative standard deviation of 26%. There were no differences in the levels of methylcitric acid for the different genetic complementation groups of propionic acidaemia.

Of the 38 pregnancies at risk for methylmalonic acidaemia, 16% were found to be affected by elevation of methylcitric acid and/or methylmalonic acid in amniotic fluid. This is not significantly different from the 25% expected for an autosomal recessive disorder. The mean concentration of methylcitric acid in the amniotic fluids of fetuses with methylmalonic acidaemia was somewhat less than in those with propionic acidaemia, being about seven times normal, with a small relative standard deviation of 14%. In contrast, the concentration of methylmalonic acid was much higher and had a wide range from 23 to 255 times normal. The highest concentration was found with an affected fetus at risk for a vitamin B12 unresponsive mutase defect while the lowest concentration was found with an affected fetus at risk for the *cbl*-C genetic complementation group.

DISCUSSION

Our results for 102 prenatal diagnoses of pregnancies at risk for propionic acidaemia or methylmalonic acidaemia show that stable isotope dilution GC/MS analysis of amniotic fluid is a reliable technique. Confirmation of the diagnoses by assay of enzymes in cultured amniocytes is not necessary. Although earlier prenatal diagnosis may be possible by assay of enzymes or incorporation of propionate into macromolecules in chorionic villous samples (Kleijer *et al.*, 1984), the diagnostic accuracy of this method has not been firmly established. With new techniques being developed for obtaining small amounts of amniotic fluid earlier than 12 weeks of pregnancy, the assay of metabolites may provide prenatal diagnoses almost as early as chorionic villous samples.

REFERENCES

Kleijer, W. J., Thoomes, R., Galjaard, H., Wendel, U. and Fowler, B. First-trimester (chorion biopsy) diagnosis of citrullinaemia and methylmalonic aciduria. *Lancet* 2 (1984) 1340

Naylor, G., Sweetman, L., Nyhan, W. L., Hornbeck, C., Griffiths, J., Mörch, L. and Brandänge, S. Isotope dilution analysis of methylcitric acid in amniotic fluid for the prenatal diagnosis of propionic and methylmalonic acidaemia. *Clin. Chim. Acta* 107 (1980) 175–183

Sweetman, L., Naylor, G., Ladner, T., Holm, J., Nyhan, W. L., Hornbeck, C., Griffiths, J., Mörch, L., Brandänge, S., Gruenke, L. and Craig, J. C. Prenatal diagnosis of propionic and methylmalonic acidaemia by stable isotope dilution analysis of methylcitric and methylmalonic acids in amniotic fluid. In Schmidt, H-L., Förstel, H. and Heinzinger, K. (eds.) *Stable Isotopes*, Elsevier Sci. Publ. Co., Amsterdam, 1982, pp. 287–293

Trefz, F. K., Schmidt, H., Tauscher, B., Depène, E., Baumgartner, R., Hammersen, G. and Kochen, W. Improved prenatal diagnosis of methylmalonic acidaemia: Mass fragmentography of methylmalonic acid in amniotic fluid and maternal urine. *Eur. J. Pediatr.* 137 (1981) 261–266

Zinn, A. B., Hine, D. G., Mahoney, M. J. and Tanaka, K. The stable istope dilution method for measurement of methylmalonic acid: A highly accurate approach to the prenatal diagnosis of methylmalonic acidaemia. *Pediatr. Res.* 16 (1982) 740–745

J. Inher. Metab. Dis. 12 Suppl. 2 (1989) 274–276

Short Communication

Successful First Trimester Diagnosis in a Pregnancy at Risk for Propionic Acidaemia

C. Pérez-Cerdá[1], B. Merinero[1], P. Sanz[1], A. Jiménez[1], M. J. García[1], A. Urbón[2], J. Díaz Recasens[3], C. Ramos[3], C. Ayuso[3] and M. Ugarte[1]

[1]Centro de Diagnóstico de Enfermedades Moleculares, Universidad Autónoma, Madrid 28049; [2]Servicio de Pediatria, Hospital General, Segovia; [3]Unidad de Diagnóstico Prenatal. Fundación Jiménez Diaz, Madrid 28041, Spain

Propionic acidaemia is an inborn error of amino acid metabolism caused by a deficiency of propionyl-CoA carboxylase (PCC) (EC 6.4.1.3). PCC activity has been demonstrated in several tissues including fibroblasts, amniotic fluid cells and chorionic villi (Sweetman et al., 1986). Prenatal diagnosis of propionic acidaemia can be performed by the determination of the methylcitrate level in amniotic fluid (Naylor et al., 1980), by studies of incorporation of [1-^{14}C]propionate into protein of amniocytes (Willard et al., 1976) and by direct assay of PCC activity in cultured amniotic fluid cells (Gompertz et al., 1975) or in intact chorionic villi (Chadefaux et al., 1988). We report a successful first trimester diagnosis by direct PCC assay in uncultured chorionic villi in a pregnancy at risk for propionic acidaemia.

CASE HISTORY

The first child of healthy and consanguineous parents was born at 40 weeks of gestation. Apgar score was 5 at 1 min and 2 at 5 min. He presented apnoea and bradycardia. During the first day of life, he developed metabolic acidosis and hyperammonaemia (2200 µg dL^{-1}). Exchange transfusion and peritoneal dialysis could remove the ammonia (200 µg dL^{-1}), but there was no clinical improvement. Hypotonia, seizures and a progressive neurological deterioration led to death on day 13 of life. Postmortem biochemical studies revealed hyperglycinaemia (0.62 mmol L^{-1}), elevated plasma propionic acid (12.7 mmol L^{-1}) and a high excretion of propionic acid, methyl citrate, 3-hydroxypropionic acid and propionyl glycine of 1615, 968.3, 2612 and 65 mg (g creatinine)$^{-1}$, respectively. The diagnosis of propionic acidaemia was confirmed by the reduced PCC activity in liver necropsy: 0.58±0.13 nmol CO_2 fixed (mg protein)$^{-1}$h^{-1} compared to 47.2±8.5 for the matched control. β-Methylcrotonyl-CoA carboxylase activity was within the normal range.

At the next pregnancy, the parents asked for prenatal diagnosis. It was carried out by direct enzymatic analysis in chorionic villi material at week 11 of gestation. The results showed a normal fetus. A healthy boy (V.S.C.) was born at term, and confirmatory studies demonstrated that the newborn did not suffer the disease.

274

Journal of Inherited Metabolic Disease. ISSN 0141–8955. Copyright © SSIEM and Kluwer Academic Publishers, PO Box 55, Lancaster, UK.

METHODS

Plasma and urine organic acids were analysed by gas-chromatography, and amino acids were quantified by conventional automated ion-exchange chromatography.

Lymphocytes were isolated from whole blood after 1:2 dilution with phoshate-buffered saline by centrifugation, using commercially available lymphocyte separation medium (Hystopaque, Sigma). Chorionic villus sampling was performed under real-time ultrasound by rigid cannula. Maternal decidua tissue was meticulously separated under the microscope. Then the villi were kept in culture medium with 10% fetal calf serum (FCS) at room temperature until examination. For the $[1-^{14}C]$propionate incorporation (Willard *et al.*, 1976), the tissue was incubated for 8 h in Puck solution containing 15% FCS, $1 \mu Ci \mu L^{-1}$ $[1-^{14}C]$propionate and $0.8 \mu Ci \mu L^{-1}$ $[4,5-^3H]$leu. For carboxylase assay (Weyler *et al.*, 1977), the tissue was resuspended in $0.02 \text{ mol } L^{-1}$ Tris-HCl, $0.025 \text{ mmol } L^{-1}$ EDTA, $0.83 \text{ mmol } L^{-1}$ reduced glutathione, pH 7.8, and disrupted by sonication three times for 5 s and then assayed immediately.

RESULTS AND DISCUSSION

Prenatal diagnosis by direct analysis of chorionic villus tissue was performed in 48 h. The incorporation of $[1-^{14}C]$propionate into protein in three chorionic tissue fragments was normal (Table 1). The incorporation of $[4,5-^3H]$leucine into villous

Table 1 Enzymatic studies: pre- and postnatal diagnosis

A. Incorporation of ^{14}C from $[1-^{14}C]$propionate and ^3H from $[4,5-^3H]$leucine into cell protein: measured as nano-atoms $(\text{mg protein})^{-1}(10 h)^{-1}$

Chorionic villi	^{14}C	^3H	*Ratio* $^{14}C/^3H$ $(\times 10^3)$
Propositus (V.S.C.)	2.6	10.4	250
Control			
range $(n=4)$	1.0–3.2	8.8–17.4	113–250

B. Propionyl-CoA carboxylase (PCC), β-methylcrotonyl-CoA carboxylase (β-MCCC) and pyruvate carboxylase (PC) activities: measured as pmol Co_2 fixed $(\text{mg protein})^{-1} \text{min}^{-1}$

	PCC	*β-MCCC*	*PC*
Chorionic villi:			
propositus (V.S.C.)	3307	667	1237
matched control	2200	521	1045
Lymphocytes:			
neonate (V.S.C.)	1200	409	47
control			
range $(n=3)$	503–1116	369–479	25–62

For controls in both (A) and (B) n = number of specimens assayed. Each value is the mean of at least duplicate determinations

protein was simultaneously measured as a control of general metabolic activity, and was found to be normal. These results were confirmed by direct PCC assay in other villus fragments, which also showed normal activity (Table 1). Amniotic fluid was not available. A healthy boy was born at term and the prediction of an unaffected fetus was confirmed by the normal level of propionic acid and its metabolites in plasma and urine and by a normal PCC activity in isolated lymphocytes from peripheral blood (Table 1).

Recently, prenatal diagnosis of propionic acidaemia has been performed by direct PCC assay in chorionic villi (Chadefaux *et al.*, 1988). These authors reported discrepancies between [1-^{14}C]propionate incorporation into protein and PCC activity in affected fetuses. In our studies, we have found similar results by both methods in intact chorionic villi, excluding propionic acidaemia in a fetus at risk for this disease. We suggest that a direct assay of PCC activity on uncultured chorionic tissue is a reliable method for prenatal diagnosis of propionic acidaemia due to a high PCC activity and to the short time required for obtaining the results.

REFERENCES

Chadefaux, B., Augereau, C., Rabier, D., Rochiccioli, F., Boue, J., Oury, J. F. and Kamoun, P. Prenatal diagnosis of propionic acidemia in chorionic villi by direct assay of propionyl-CoA carboxylase. *Prenat. Diagn.* 8 (1988) 161–164

Gompertz, D., Goodey, P. A., Thom, H., Russell, G., Johnston, A. W., Mellor, D. H., Maclean, M. W., Ferguson-Smith, M. E. and Ferguson-Smith, M. A. Prenatal diagnosis and family studies in a case of propionic acidemia. *Clin. Genet.* 8 (1975) 244–255

Naylor, G., Sweetman, L., Nyhan, W. L., Hornbeck, C., Griffiths, J., Morch, L. and Brandage, S. Isotope dilution analysis of methylcitric acid in amniotic fluid for the prenatal diagnosis of propionic and methylmalonic acidemia. *Clin. Chim. Acta* 107 (1980) 175–183

Sweetman, F. R., Gibson, K. M., Sweetman, L., Nyhan, W. L., Chin, H., Swartz, W. and Jones, O. W. Activity of biotin-dependent and GABA metabolizing enzymes in chorionic villus samples: Potential for 1st trimester prenatal diagnosis. *Prenat. Diagn.* 6 (1986) 187–193

Weyler, W., Sweetman, L., Maggio, D. C. and Nyhan, W. L. Deficiency of propionyl-CoA carboxylase in a patient with methylcrotonylglycinuria. *Clin. Chim. Acta* 76 (1977) 321–323

Willard, H. F., Ambani, L. M., Hart, A. C. Mahoney, M. J. and Rosenberg, L. E. Rapid prenatal and postnatal detection of inborn errors of propionate, methylmalonate and cobalamin metabolism. *Hum. Genet.* 34 (1976) 277–283

J. Inher. Metab. Dis. 12 *Suppl.* 2 (1989) 277–279

Short Communication

First Trimester Prenatal Exclusion of Glutaryl-CoA Dehydrogenase Deficiency (Glutaric Aciduria Type 1)

E. CHRISTENSEN

Section of Clinical Genetics, University Department of Paediatrics, Rigshospitalet 4062, Blegdamsvej 9, 2100 Copenhagen, Denmark

Glutaryl-CoA dehydrogenase (GDH: EC 1.3.99.7) deficiency, glutaric aciduria type 1 (GA1; McKusick 23167) is an autosomal recessively inherited inborn error of lysine and tryptophan catabolism. The first case was described in the USA by Goodman *et al.* in 1975. Up to now about 16 patients have been described in the literature (Amir *et al.*, 1987) but the author is aware of 30 other cases from a region including only Europe and Israel.

Most patients with GA1 develop within the first years of life a severe debilitating dystonia and choreoathetosis. Although the clinical symptoms in this disease can vary from the very severe form, leading to inability to speak and walk, to a form without clinical symptoms even within the same sibship (Amir *et al.*, 1987), prenatal diagnosis is requested by the parents in subsequent pregnancies in most families with a child with GA1.

Prenatal diagnosis of GA1 has been performed previously on cultured amniotic fluid cells (AFC) and by measuring glutaric acid concentration in amniotic fluid (Goodman *et al.*, 1980, and Christensen, unpublished results).

We have investigated four pregnancies at risk for GA1 by measuring GDH activity directly on chorionic villi biopsied at 9–10 weeks of gestation. In two cases GDH activity was determined on cultured chorionic cells as well.

METHODS

Control chorionic villus samples (CVS) were obtained from normal pregnancies terminated by legal first trimester abortion. Chorionic villus sampling in the pregnancies at risk for GA1 was performed under ultrasound guidance by transcervical aspiration, in cases 1, 2 and 4, and by the transabdominal route in case 3. The chorionic villi were dissected immediately from the obtained samples under stereo microscope and washed twice in HBSS.

The villi were used directly for GDH determination by the previously published method (Christensen, 1983). In cases 1 and 4, parts of the villi were cultured and GDH activity was determined on the cultured cells as well. Cells were released from the villi by mincing the tissue carefully with scissors and treating with a solution of 0.05% trypsin and 0.02% EDTA. Cells were cultured in a medium

277

Journal of Inherited Metabolic Disease. ISSN 0141–8955. Copyright © SSIEM and Kluwer Academic Publishers. PO Box 55, Lancaster, UK.

containing 2% Ultroser G serum substitute, 5% fetal calf serum, $2 \, \mathrm{mmol \, L}^{-1}$ glutamine in a basal medium of Ham's F12 and RPMI-1640 in a ratio of one to one. For prevention of microbial growth, penicillin and streptomycin were added to a final concentration of 100 IU per mL and $0.1 \, \mathrm{mg \, mL}^{-1}$, respectively.

RESULTS

Normal GDH activities were found in uncultured CVS from four pregnancies at risk for GA1. In the two at-risk pregnancies also studied by enzyme assay using

Table 1   Glutaryl-CoA dehydrogenase activity

Tissue	Uncultured sample	Cultured cells
Fibroblast controls	—	5.0 ± 1.6 ($n = 51$)
CVS controls	3.5 ± 1.6 ($n = 8$)	9.1 ± 1.8 ($n = 10$)
CVS from fetus at risk for GA1:		
case 1	5.0	3.0
case 2	3.5	—
case 3	3.0	—
case 4	1.3	7.5

Values for controls are means±SD; enzyme activity is expressed in μmol (g protein)$^{-1}$h^{-1}

cultured chorionic cells, normal GDH activities were found as well (see Table 1). These results indicated that all four cases were either normal homozygotes or heterozygotes for GA1 deficiency, i.e. the fetuses were not affected by GA1.

In accordance with the enzymatic results, the pregnancies in cases 2, 3 and 4 resulted in healthy infants. The pregnancy in case 1 resulted in a spontaneous abortion after 25 weeks gestation. GDH activities in liver tissue and cultured skin fibroblasts from the aborted fetus were 32 and 4.0 μmol (g protein)$^{-1}$h^{-1}, respectively. These normal GDH activities confirmed the results obtained on chorionic tissue that the fetus in case 1 was unaffected.

DISCUSSION

GA1 can be diagnosed prenatally after amniocentesis, as described by Goodman *et al.* (1980), using gas chromatography–mass spectrometry in the selected ions mode or by measuring GDH activity in cultured AFC. Glutaric acid concentration in amniotic fluid can be measured shortly after the amniocentesis has been performed. The result of the prenatal diagnosis can then be available after about 14 weeks gestation. This is far better than the determination of GDH activity in cultured AFC, where you have to include about 3 weeks of culture time before the enzyme assay can be performed; 17–18 weeks of gestation have elapsed before the result of the prenatal diagnosis in this case. However, determination of GDH activity directly on a CVS gives you the result of prenatal diagnosis as early as

9–10 weeks gestation, 4 weeks before the results of amniotic fluid glutaric acid determination and 8 weeks before determination of GDH in AFC are possible.

Although we have not yet identified an affected fetus it seems possible to use the assay for GDH activity directly on CVS for first trimester prenatal diagnosis of GA1.

REFERENCES

Amir, N., Elpeleg, O., Shalev, R. S. and Christensen, E. Glutaric aciduria type I: Clinical heterogeneity and neuroradiologic features. *Neurology* 37 (1987) 1654–1657

Christensen, E. Improved assay of glutaryl-CoA dehydrogenase in cultured cells and liver: application to glutaric aciduria type I. *Clin. Chim. Acta* 129 (1983) 91–97

Goodman, S. I., Markey, S. P., Moe, P. G., Miles, B. S. and Teng, C. C. Glutaric aciduria; a 'new' disorder of amino acid metabolism. *Biochem. Med.* 12 (1975) 12–21

Goodman, S. I., Gallegos, D. A., Pullin, C. J., Halpern, B., Truscott, R. J. W., Wise, G., Wilcken, B., Ryan, E. D. and Whelen, D. T. Antenatal diagnosis of glutaric acidemia. *Am. J. Hum. Genet.* 32 (1980) 695–699

J. Inher. Metab. Dis. 12 Suppl. 2 (1989) 280–282

Short Communication

Early Prenatal Diagnosis in Two Pregnancies at Risk for Glutaryl-CoA Dehydrogenase Deficiency

E. HOLME[1], M. KYLLERMAN[2] and S. LINDSTEDT[1]

[1]*Department of Clinical Chemistry, Gothenburg University, Sahlgren's Hospital, S-413 45 Gothenburg;* [2]*Department of Pediatrics II, Gothenburg University, East Hospital, S-416 85 Gothenburg, Sweden*

Glutaryl-CoA dehydrogenase (EC 1.3.99.7) participates in the degradative pathways of lysine and tryptophan. Deficiency of this enzyme is the primary defect of glutaric aciduria I (McKusick 23167) (Goodman *et al.*, 1975). Most children with this disorder develop a severe dyskinetic–dystonic syndrome with a sudden onset often precipitated by an infection (Brandt *et al.*, 1978).

Glutaryl-CoA dehydrogenase deficiency is expressed in several tissues, e.g. leukocytes, fibroblasts and amniotic fluid cells (Christensen and Brandt, 1978), which have been used for successful prenatal diagnosis (Goodman *et al.*, 1980).

This prompted a trial of early prenatal diagnosis by chorionic villus biopsies in two pregnancies at risk for glutaryl-CoA dehydrogenase deficiency.

CASE HISTORIES

Family 1: A girl (T.E. born 18.3.77) was born to healthy non-consanguineous parents. A severe dyskinetic–dystonic syndrome developed at 10 months of age. A diagnosis of glutaric aciduria was suspected clinically, although the excretion of glutaric acid in urine was only occasionally above the reference limit. The diagnosis was confirmed by determination of glutaryl-CoA dehydrogenase activity in fibroblasts and leukocytes. At the second pregnancy a chorionic villus biopsy was performed in the 9th gestational week.

Family 2: The index case, a girl (J. E. born 19.1.75) has been described (Kyllerman and Steen, 1977). She is the first child of healthy non-consanguineous parents. At 12 months of age a respiratory tract infection precipitated a severe dyskinetic–dystonic syndrome. Glutaric aciduria and deficient fibroblast glutaryl-CoA dehydrogenase were found. At the second pregnancy a chorionic villus biopsy was performed in the 11th gestational week.

METHODS

Chorionic villus samples were collected by the vaginal route. Control samples were taken after informed consent from patients subjected to legal abortion.

Journal of Inherited Metabolic Disease. ISSN 0141-8955. Copyright © SSIEM and Kluwer Academic Publishers, PO Box 55, Lancaster, UK.

Glutaryl-CoA dehydrogenase activity was estimated from the production of $^{14}CO_2$ from [$1,5^{14}C$]glutaryl-CoA essentially as described by Christensen and Brandt (1978). Homogenates of chorionic-villus samples or trypsinized cultured cells were incubated for 30 min at 37°C. The concentration of glutaryl-CoA was $0.075 \, \text{mmol} \, L^{-1}$ and of FAD $0.1 \, \text{mmol} \, L^{-1}$.

RESULTS

Residual enzyme activity in fibroblasts of 9% of the control mean was found in the index case of the first family. No residual enzyme activity was found in fibroblasts in the index case of the second family (Table 1).

Table 1 Glutaryl-CoA dehydrogenase activity in two pregnancies at risk for deficiency, in family index cases and in controls

	Chorionic villus biopsy	Cultured chorionic villus cells	Amniotic fluid cells	Fibroblasts from the children
Index case 1 (T.E.)	—	—	—	8.6
Index case 2 (J.E.)	—	—	—	<1
Pregnancy 1	56	84	—	85
Pregnancy 2	77	—	98	110
Controls				
mean	112 ($n = 12$)	114 ($n = 4$)		95 ($n = 22$)
range	70–160	99–132		61–152

Values are glutaryl-CoA dehydrogenase activity in $\text{pmol (mg protein)}^{-1} \text{min}^{-1}$.

The normal range of glutaryl-CoA dehydrogenase activity in chorionic villus samples was of the same magnitude as in fibroblasts. Glutaryl-CoA dehydrogenase was not deficient in any of the pregnancies although the activity was slightly below the normal range in pregnancy 1. The activity in cultured cells from that biopsy was normal. In the second pregnancy amniotic fluid cells were also analyzed and found to be normal. Fibroblast analysis from the two babies was in accordance with the prenatal measurements (Table 1). The pregnancies in both families resulted in healthy children, who developed normally during a 2-year follow-up period.

CONCLUSION

Glutaryl-CoA dehydrogenase deficiency is expressed in fibroblasts and amniotic fluid cells (Christensen and Brandt, 1978; Goodman *et al.*, 1980). The concordance in enzyme activities between the chorionic villus material and fibroblasts strongly suggests that chorionic villus samples can be used for prenatal diagnosis of glutaryl-CoA dehydrogenase deficiency. However, final evaluation of chorionic villus sampling in prenatal diagnosis of glutaryl-CoA dehydrogenase deficiency must await experience from pregnancies with affected fetuses.

ACKNOWLEDGEMENT

This work was supported by a grant from the Swedish Medical Research Council (03X-585).

REFERENCES

Brandt, N. J., Brandt, S., Christensen, E., Gregersen, N. and Rasmussen, K. Glutaric aciduria in progressive choreo-athetosis. *Clin. Genet.* 13 (1978) 77–80

Christensen, E. and Brandt, N. J. Studies on glutaryl-CoA dehydrogenase in leukocytes, fibroblasts and amniotic fluid cells. The normal enzyme and the mutant form in patients with glutaric aciduria. *Clin. Chim. Acta* 88 (1978) 267–276

Goodman, S. I., Markey, S. P., Moc, P. G., Miles, B. S. and Teng, C. C. Glutaric aciduria: a 'new' inborn error of amino acid metabolism. *Biochem. Med.* 12 (1975) 12–21

Goodman, S. I., Gallegos, D. A., Pullin, C. J., Halpern, B., Truscott, R. J. W., Wise, G., Wilcken, B., Ryan, E. D. and Whelan, D. T. Antenatal diagnosis of glutaric acidemia. *Am. J. Hum. Genet.* 32 (1980) 695–699

Kyllerman, M. and Steen, G. Intermittently progressive dyskinetic syndrome in glutaric aciduria. *Neuropädiatrie* 8 (1977) 397–404

J. Inher. Metab. Dis. 12 Suppl. 2 (1989) 283–285

Short Communication

First Trimester Prenatal Diagnosis of 3-Hydroxy-3-Methylglutaric Aciduria

R. A. Chalmers, J. Mistry, R. Penketh and I. R. McFadyen

Perinatal and Child Health, MRC Clinical Research Centre, Harrow, UK

3-Hydroxy-3-methylglutaric aciduria (McKusick 24645) is a disorder of L-leucine metabolism and of ketone body biosynthesis caused by deficient activity of 3-hydroxy-3-methylglutaryl (HMG) CoA lyase. The disorder is characterized bio-chemically by increased tissue and urinary concentrations of several organic acids and clinically by recurrent severe and potentially lethal episodes that resemble Reye's syndrome, with non-ketotic hypoglycaemia, metabolic acidosis and encepha-lopathy.

We have previously briefly reported (Chalmers *et al.*, 1985) the early prenatal diagnosis of this condition at 16 weeks gestation using gas-chromatography–mass spectometry (GC/MS) of amniotic fluid supernatant, with confirmatory enzymology on cultured amniocytes. Termination of an affected fetus at that time allowed study of chorionic villus tissue at 17–18 weeks gestation. Chorionic villus HMG-CoA lyase activity in tissue from the terminated pregnancy was 0.87 nmol HMG-CoA removed (mg protein)$^{-1}$ min^{-1} compared to control values of 7.47–8.63, these results indicating the potential suitability of chorionic villus biopsy for prenatal diagnosis at 9–10 weeks gestation.

We now report here the first trimester prenatal diagnosis of HMG-CoA lyase deficiency in two unrelated families at risk for this condition.

PATIENTS AND METHODS

Patients: The first family studied (Q) had one previous affected female child (Greene *et al.*, 1984) with one normal older sibling. Prenatal diagnosis in a subsequent pregnancy using GC/MS and enzymology had shown an affected fetus and the pregnancy was terminated (see above; Chalmers *et al.*, 1985).

The second family studied (S) had presented with dizygotic twin siblings with HMG-CoA lyase deficiency (Stacey *et al.*, 1985). Subsequent to this the mother had one spontaneous abortion and one unaffected female baby. In the latter pregnancy, analysis of placental tissue showed HMG-CoA lyase activities of 3.39 ± 0.69 ($n = 8$) compared to controls of 8.04 ± 0.49 ($n = 6$), consistent with an heterozygous baby.

In both the present studies, chorionic villus biopsy was carried out at 9–10 weeks gestation and the villi assayed directly for HMG-CoA lyase activity.

Journal of Inherited Metabolic Disease. ISSN 0141–8955. Copyright © SSIEM and Kluwer Academic Publishers, PO Box 55, Lancaster, UK.

Methods: Chorionic villi were separated out from the biopsy tissue under a microscope and were placed in Eagle's minimum essential medium containing penicillin and streptomycin and 200 units of heparin.

Samples of the chorionic villi (approx. 15 mg) were taken and homogenized by hand in a glass homogenizer in 250 μL of a 'lysis' buffer (10 mmol L^{-1} Tris-HCl, pH 7.4) and the homogenate sonicated for 10 s. 10 μL of the sonicate was diluted tenfold and used for protein determination by a standard method. 50 μL aliquots of the sonicate (containing approximately 200 μg protein) were used for the HMG-CoA lyase assay. Similar procedures were used for assays on cultured skin fibroblasts using the cell pellet from a 75 cm^2 Falcon flask.

HMG-CoA lyase was measured by mixing 50 μL sonicate with 100 μL 'assay buffer' (containing 20 μmol Tris, pH 8.2, 1 μmol dithiothreitol, 0.4 mg Triton X-100, 2 μmol MgCl$_2$), preincubated at 30°C for 10 min and the reaction started by addition of 50 μL *RS*[3–^{14}C glutaryl]HMG-CoA solution (40 nmol per 36 nCi). The assay mixture was incubated for 10 min at 30°C, 40 μL aliquots removed into scintillation vials containing 100 μL 6 mol L^{-1} HCl, the aliquots dried at 95°C for 30 min, the residues dissolved in 250 μL water, 10 mL ethanol/toluene/PPO/POPOP scintillator added and the radioactivity determined in a β-counter. Results were expressed as nmol HMG-CoA removed (mg protein)$^{-1}$ min^{-1}.

RESULTS

Results of direct assays for HMG-CoA lyase activity in the chorionic villi are shown in Table 1.

The results in Mrs Q were consistent with a heterozygous fetus and the pregnancy

Table 1 HMG-CoA lyase activity in chorionic villus tissue in pregnancies at risk for 3-hydroxy-3-methylglutaric aciduria, in chorionic villi and other fetal tissue obtained at termination and in cultured fetal fibroblasts and controls

A. First trimester prenatal diagnoses		
Mrs Q	2.48±0.92	($n = 5$)
Control values	7.02±1.55	($n = 10$)
Mrs S	0.24; 0.21	($n = 2$)
Control values	7.51±1.37	($n = 17$)
Fibroblasts 'S' index case	0.43±0.16	($n = 4$)
Control fibroblasts	4.01±0.93	($n = 9$)
B. Fetal tissue from termination of 'S' pregnancy		
Mrs S chorionic villi	0	(triplicate assays)
Mrs S fetal tissue	0.24±0.42	(range 0–0.73)
Control termination chorionic villi	5.31±1.42	($n = 7$)
Cultured fetal fibroblasts from 'S' pregnancy	0.11±0.16	(range 0–0.48)
		($n = 9$)
Control fetal fibroblasts	1.78±0.43	($n = 5$)
Control fibroblasts	2.92±0.34	($n = 9$)

3-Hydroxy-3-methylglutaryl-CoA lyase activity expressed in nmol HMG-CoA removed (mg protein)$^{-1}$ min^{-1}; values are means±SD; n = number of assays, each in triplicate

was allowed to continue. Unfortunately the mother spontaneously aborted 1 week later and the diagnosis was unconfirmed.

The results in Mrs S were consistent with a homozygous fetus (affected) and the pregnancy was terminated at 11 weeks gestation. The diagnosis was confirmed immediately in chorionic villus tissue and other fetal tissue obtained at termination (Table 1). Fetal fibroblasts were cultured from the terminated fetus and assay of HMG-CoA lyase activity confirmed the diagnosis made.

DISCUSSION

These results show that reliable first trimester prenatal diagnosis of 3-hydroxy-3-methylglutaric aciduria may be made by direct enzyme assay on chorionic villi obtained at 9–10 weeks gestation. The results were obtained on the day of biopsy or within a maximum of 2 days from biopsy. This allows a repeat biopsy to be made if essential and permits early termination of an affected pregnancy and early reassurance of the parents where the fetus is unaffected. The results in the Q family (and in the S family at term) indicate that heterozygous fetuses may also be distinguished by this assay in chorionic tissue.

REFERENCES

Chalmers, R. A., Tracey, B. M., Mistry, J., Stacey, T. E., McFadyen, I. R. and Madigan, M. J. The prenatal diagnosis of 3-hydroxy-3-methylglutaric aciduria by GC-MS and enzymology on cultured amniocytes and on chorionic villi. *Pediatr. Res.* 19 (1985) 1075

Greene, C. L., Cann, H. M., Robinson, B. M., Gibson, K. M., Sweetman, L., Holm, J. and Nyhan, W. L. 3-Hydroxy-3-methylglutaric aciduria. *J. Neurogenet.* 1 (1984) 165–173

Stacey, T. E., de Sousa, C., Tracey, B. M., Whitelaw, A., Mistry, J., Timbrell, P. and Chalmers, R. A. Dizygotic twins with 3-hydroxy-3-methylglutaric aciduria; unusual presentation, family studies and dietary management. *Eur. J. Pediatr.* 144 (1985) 177–181

J. Inher. Metab. Dis. 12 Suppl. 2 (1989) 286–288

Short Communication

Enzymatic Prenatal Diagnosis of Primary Hyperoxaluria Type 1: Potential and Limitations

C. J. Danpure[1], P. J. Cooper[2], P. R. Jennings[1], P. J. Wise[1], R. J. Penketh[3] and C. H. Rodeck[3]

Divisions of [1]Inherited Metabolic Diseases, and [2]Clinical Cell Biology, Clinical Research Centre, Harrow, Middlesex HA1 3UJ, UK; [3]Institute of Obstetrics & Gynaecology, Queen Charlotte's Maternity Hospital, London W6 0XG, UK

Primary hyperoxaluria type 1 (PH1; McKusick 25990) is an autosomal recessive inborn error of glyoxylate metabolism which leads to excessive synthesis of oxalate and glycolate. The low solubility of calcium oxalate causes all the pathological manifestations of the disease, namely urolithiasis, nephrocalcinosis and systemic oxalosis. Attempts to diagnose PH1 prenatally, by measuring oxalate and glycolate in amniotic fluid, have not been successful, presumably because the placental clearance of these metabolites from the fetal circulation is much greater than the renal clearance. Alternatively, it is possible that PH1 is not expressed metabolically in the fetus.

However, the discovery that PH1 is caused by a deficiency of the hepatic peroxisomal enzyme alanine:glyoxylate aminotransferase (AGT) (Danpure and Jennings, 1986), has enabled us to diagnose prenatally two fetuses, each at a 25% risk of being affected with PH1, by measuring AGT activity in fetal liver biopsies obtained in the second trimester (Danpure *et al.*, 1988, 1989a). The liver of one fetus had a marked deficiency of AGT enzyme activity and AGT immunoreactive protein (affected), while the other had normal amounts of AGT enzyme activity and immunoreactive protein (unaffected) (Table 1). These prenatal diagnoses were confirmed, in the first case, by re-assay of the liver recovered from the abortus, and, in the second case, by the birth of a healthy baby with normal plasma and urinary oxalate levels.

Although the results of these two particular prenatal diagnoses were unambiguous, the potential for confusion exists because of the enzymic heterogeneity found in PH1. For example, although most PH1 patients have no AGT enzyme activity or immunoreactive protein, some have partial deficiencies of both activity and protein, while others have normal levels of AGT protein but are completely deficient in enzyme activity (Danpure and Jennings, 1988; Wise *et al.*, 1987). Although most (24/27) of these patients could be diagnosed unequivocally by measuring AGT enzyme activity alone, a small minority could easily be confused with asymptomatic heterozygotes, because they have similar levels of enzyme activity (30–50% of the normal level). In at least one of these patients, as well as

286

Journal of Inherited Metabolic Disease. ISSN 0141–8955. Copyright © SSIEM and Kluwer Academic Publishers, PO Box 55, Lancaster, UK.

Table 1   **Heterogeneity in AGT enzyme activity, immunoreactive protein and subcellular distribution in fetal and non-fetal livers**

	AGT enzyme activity[a]	*AGT immuno-reactive protein*[b]	*AGT subcellular distribution*[c]
Fetal livers			
Fetuses at risk:			
unaffected (21 weeks)	1.15	++	P
affected (24 weeks)	0.16	−	−
Controls (17–21 weeks, $n = 9$)	1.14–1.61	++	P(3)
Non-fetal livers			
PH1 patients ($n = 27$)	0.27–2.78	−,+,++,+++	−(13),P(1),M(3)
PH1 heterozygote	2.00	++	P
Controls ($n = 16$)	3.25–8.99	++,+++	P(4)
Experimental limitations			
Amount of tissue required	5 mg (radiochemical microassay)	1–5 mg	<1 mg (EM immunocytochemistry)
	20 mg (spectrophotometric assay)		100 mg (density gradient centrifugation)
Time taken	1 day	2 days	4 days

PH1 refers to hyperoxaluric patients with total or partial AGT deficiency. The more mildly-affected patients may not have significant hyperglycolic aciduria. PH1 heterozygotes are asymptomatic.

[a]*AGT enzyme activity* is expressed as $\mu mol\,(mg\ protein)^{-1}h^{-1}$ and is not corrected for crossover from glutamate:glyoxylate aminotransferase (GGT) as there is not enough material from fetal liver biopsy to perform the assay. GGT accounts for about 0.1–0.3 units of AGT activity in fetal livers and about 0.3–0.7 units in non-fetal livers. Fetal (17–21 weeks) liver AGT activity is only about one third of the activity in post-natal (≥ 2 days) liver. The fetal livers were assayed by a radioactive micromethod (Allsop *et al.*, 1987). The non-fetal livers were assayed by a spectrophotometric method (Danpure and Jennings, 1988).

[b]*AGT immunoreactive protein* was measured by SDS-PAGE and immunoblotting (Wise *et al.*, 1987). The values represent the amount of immunoreactive material with a molecular weight of 40 kDa (− = none, +++ = most).

[c]*Subcellular distribution* was determined by sucrose gradient centrifugation together with enzyme assay (Danpure and Jennings, 1988) and immunoblotting, or by protein A-gold immunocytochemistry (Cooper *et al.*, 1988). P = peroxisomal, M = mitochondrial, − = absent. Numbers in parentheses are number of livers in which the subcellular distribution was studied.

in two others with much lower enzyme activities, the PH1 appears to be caused, at least in part, by a mislocalization of AGT into the mitochondria rather than the peroxisomes (Table 1) (Danpure *et al.*, 1989b).

    Fetuses with this latter variant of PH1 could be misdiagnosed unless the intra-cellular location of AGT is identified. Unfortunately, the amount of material provided by fetal liver biopsy (5–20 mg) is not enough to carry out conventional subcellular fractionation (e.g. sucrose gradient centrifugation). However, the intra-cellular distribution of immunoreactive AGT protein, but not enzyme activity, can be determined at the electron-microscopic level on less than 1 mg of tissue by protein A-gold post-embedding immunocytochemistry (Cooper *et al.*, 1988). Such a procedure was able to distinguish clearly between an asymptomatic PH1 hetero-zygote, possessing peroxisomal AGT, and a PH1 patient, possessing mitochondrial AGT, even though both had about 30% of normal AGT activity (Danpure *et al.*, 1989b).

Despite the wide range of phenotypic expression of PH1, in molecular as well as clinical terms, the risk of erroneous prenatal diagnosis is likely to be small if a combination of enzyme assay, immunoblotting and immunocytochemistry is used.

REFERENCES

Allsop, J., Jennings, P. R. and Danpure, C. J. A new micro-assay for human liver alanine: glyoxylate aminotransferase. *Clin. Chim. Acta* 170 (1987) 187–194

Cooper, P. J., Danpure, C. J., Wise, P. J. and Guttridge, K. M. Immunocytochemical localization of human hepatic alanine: glyoxylate aminotransferase in control subjects and patients with primary hyperoxaluria type 1. *J. Histochem. Cytochem.* 36 (1988) 1285–1294

Danpure, C. J. and Jennings, P. R. Peroxisomal alanine: glyoxylate aminotransferase deficiency in primary hyperoxaluria type 1. *FEBS Lett.* 201 (1986) 20–24

Danpure, C. J. and Jennings, P. R. Further studies on the activity and subcellular distribution of alanine:glyoxylate aminotransferase in the livers of patients with primary hyperoxaluria type 1. *Clin. Sci.* 75 (1988) 315–322

Danpure, C. J., Jennings, P. R., Penketh, R. J., Wise, P. J. and Rodeck, C. H. Prenatal exclusion of primary hyperoxaluria type 1. *Lancet.* 1 (1988) 367

Danpure, C. J., Jennings, P. R., Penketh, R. J., Wise, P. J., Cooper, P. J. and Rodeck, C. H. Fetal liver alanine:glyoxylate aminotransferase and the prenatal diagnosis of primary hyperoxaluria type 1. *Prenat. Diag.* 9 (1989a) in press

Danpure, C. J., Cooper, P. J., Wise, P. J. and Jennings, P. R. An enzyme trafficing defect in two patients with primary hyperoxaluria type 1: peroxisomal alanine:glyoxylate aminotransferase rerouted to mitochondria. *J. Cell Biol.* (1989b) in press

Wise, P. J., Danpure, C. J. and Jennings, P. R. Immunological heterogeneity of hepatic alanine:glyoxylate aminotransferase in primary hyperoxaluria type 1. *FEBS Lett.* 222 (1987) 17–20

J. Inher. Metab. Dis. 12 Suppl. 2 (1989) 289–291

Short Communication

First Trimester Diagnosis of Glycogen Storage Disease Type II and Type III

Y. S. Shin, M. Rieth, J. Tausenfreund and W. Endres

Universitäts Kinderklinik, Lindwurmstrasse 4, D8 München 2, FRG

Prenatal diagnosis of glycogen storage disease (GSD) type II and type III (McKusick 23230 and 23240) has been performed by enzyme assay in cultivated amniotic fluid cells. We have also performed prenatal diagnosis by amniocentesis in about 30 at risk pregnancies for glycogen storage diseases. Recently, we have reported a case of first-trimester diagnosis of GSD type II using uncultured chorionic villous sampling (Grubisic *et al.*, 1986). In this report, we describe further cases of first-trimester diagnosis of GSD type II in 8 pregnancies using chorionic villi, as well as one case of GSD type III.

Sampling of chorionic villi and assay of acid α-glucosidase in villi and in leukocytes using specific antibodies were performed by the procedures described previously (Shin *et al.*, 1985). The assay of amyloglucosidase in villi was done as in erythrocytes with a Sephadex G-50 column for the separation of glycogen from glucose (Shin *et al.*, 1984).

Table 1 First trimester diagnosis of glycogen storage disease type II

Sample no.	Week of gestation	Enzyme activity (nmol min^{-1} (mg protein)$^{-1}$)	Diagnosis	Outcome
1	9	2.22	N or HE	HE*
2	11	5.90	N or HE	N*
3	10	0	HO	HO
4	10	7.37	N or HE	N*
5	11	0	HO	HO
6	11	2.65	N or HE	HE*
7	9	3.04	N or HE	HE*
8	9	1.65	N or HE	—
Normal range ($n = 21$)		3.0–12.0		

* acid glucosidase activity in leukocytes in the normal range or the heterozygous range
N, normal; HE, heterozygote; HO, homozygote
Homozygote states were diagnosed by the assay of aborted fetal samples (case 3) or of autopsy samples (case 5)

Table 1 shows results of first-trimester diagnosis of GSD type II. For 2 cases where no acid α-glucosidase activity was found in chorionic villi, the enzyme deficiency was found in fetal tissues (case 3) and in postmortem samples (case 5). It is also interesting to note that all cases where the activity in villi lay below the

Journal of Inherited Metabolic Disease. ISSN 0141-8955. Copyright © SSIEM and Kluwer Academic Publishers, PO Box 55, Lancaster, UK.

normal range were found to have the heterozygous value in leukocytes after birth (cases 1, 6 and 7). The pregnancy for case 8 is now in progress.

These results indicate that the method of first-trimester diagnosis by chorionic villous sampling is not only easier and prompt, but also accurate and appropriate for heterozygote detection in comparison with that by amniocentesis.

A further advantage for this technique is a larger quantity of the applicable materials without the necessity of culturing which may cause contamination by other cells.

Table 2 Prenatal diagnosis of glycogen storage disease type III

Sample	Gestational age (weeks)	Amyloglucosidase activity (nmol min^{-1}(mg protein)$^{-1}$)
Chorionic villi		
Patient	11	0
Controls ($n = 22$)	8–12	0.15–0.74
Placental biopsy		
Patient	18	0–0.01
Controls ($n = 3$)	20–23	0.30–1.07
Fetal liver		
Patient	23	0.01 (1.0)*
Controls ($n = 3$)	18–22	0.30–1.00 (0.3–0.6)*

* glycogen content in liver (g per 100 g wet tissues). The glycogen content in cardiac muscle of the patient was 2.8, that in kidney 0.23, in spleen 0.28 and in skeletal muscle 0.69

In Table 2, the prenatal diagnosis of a case of GSD type III is summarized. The first child of consanguineous Turkish parents was diagnosed as suffering from GSD type IIIa at the age of 1 month. He showed an enlarged heart, hypoglycaemic tendency and hepatosplenomegaly since birth. According to the parents' wish, prenatal diagnosis was performed first by chorionic villous sampling which showed a pathological result. Since this was our first case of first-trimester diagnosis for this disease, amniocentesis and placental biopsy were performed as well at the 18th week of gestation. The pregnancy was terminated and the diagnosis was confirmed by analysing fetal tissues. What was especially significant, in view of the clinical manifestation, was that there was, already at the 23rd week of gestation distinctly increased glycogen content in cardiac muscles, contrary to that in other tissues.

In conclusion, first-trimester diagnosis is possible for various glycogen storage diseases, such as type II and III. The only enzyme system for which the activity is not measurable in chorionic villi is glucose-6-phosphatase. Branching enzyme, glycogen synthetase, phosphorylases, phosphorylase b-kinase and UDP-glucose pyrophosphorylase are expressed in chorionic villi and the activities are readily determined. However, further studies concerning tissue-specific isozymes are necessary in order to apply chorionic villous sampling safely to diagnosis of the respective enzyme deficiencies.

ACKNOWLEDGEMENTS

This work is supported in part by the Deutsche Forschungs gemeinschaft Grant, Sh 17/1-1.

REFERENCES

Grubisic, A., Shin, Y. S., Meyer, W., Endres, W., Becker, U. and Wischerath, H. First trimester diagnosis of Pompe's disease (glycogenosis type II) with normal outcome: Assay of acid α-glucosidase in chorionic villous biopsy using antibodies. *Clin. Genet.* 30 (1986) 298–302

Shin, Y. S., Ungar, R., Rieth, M. and Endres, W. A simple assay for amylo-1, 6-glucosidase to detect heterozygotes for glycogenosis type III in erythrocytes. *Clin. Chem.* 30 (1984) 1717–1718

Shin, Y. S., Endres, W., Unterreithmeier, J., Rieth, M. and Schaub, J. Diagnosis of Pompe's disease using leukocytes preparations. Kinetic and immunological studies of 1,4-α-glucosidase in human fetal and adult tissues and cultured cells. *Clin. Chim. Acta* 148 (1985) 9–21

J. Inher. Metab. Dis. 12 Suppl. 2 (1989) 292–294

Short Communication

First Trimester Prenatal Diagnosis of Glycogen Storage Disease Type III

I. Maire, G. Mandon and M. Mathieu
Laboratoire de Biochimie, Hôpital Debrousse, 69322 Lyon Cédex 05, France

Glycogen storage disease (GSD) type III (McKusick 23240) is an autosomal recessive disorder due to a deficiency of glycogen debranching enzyme (Illingworth *et al.*, 1956). This enzyme presents a transferase activity: oligo α-1,4-glucan-α-1,4 glucan-4-glycosyltransferase (EC 2.4.1.25) and a hydrolytic activity: amylo-1,6-glucosidase (EC 3.2.1.33); both activities have been located on the same macromolecule. Debranching enzyme deficiencies have been reported in muscle, liver, leukocytes, erythrocytes and fibroblasts. Generally, the course of the disease seems rather mild, in spite of some difficulties in long-term outcome (De Parscau *et al.*, 1988); but, in some cases, an unusually severe course in a previous child leads the parents to request a prenatal diagnosis for a further pregnancy. We have previously reported the possibility of prenatal diagnosis of GSD type III using cultured amniotic fluid (AF) cells (Maire and Mathieu, 1986) and the feasibility of the diagnosis using chorionic villi (CV) has been suggested by Van Diggelen *et al.* (1985). We report here the first trimester prenatal diagnosis of an affected case.

MATERIALS AND METHODS

Biological material: Leukocytes from controls and the patient Diane GU (referred by Pr. Odièvre, Paris) were isolated from 10 ml heparinized blood. Contaminating red blood cells were destroyed by hypotonic shock at $+4°C$. Cells were used immediately or stored overnight at $+4°C$ suspended in NaCl, 0·9%.

CV biopsy was performed between 10 and 11 weeks of amenorrhoea by transcervical biopsy under ultrasound guidance (Pr. Thoulon, Hotel Dieu, Lyon). Maternal decidua were separated from villi under the microscope. CV were seeded after dissection in chicken plasma on plastic flasks containing Ham F10, supplemented with fetal calf serum, Ultroser G (IBF–France) 1% and antibiotics. Fetal skin fibroblasts were grown similarly and normal CV were obtained from elective abortion at 9–10 weeks of amenorrhoea.

Enzyme activity measurement: Debranching enzyme activity was measured by a method derived from Brown *et al.* (1978) comparing hydrolytic activities at pH 6·4 on phosphorylase limit dextrin of glycogen and glycogen as substrates. The sensitivity of the assay was increased by fluorescent measurement of NADPH formed from released glucose through hexokinase and glucose-6-phosphate dehydrogenase reactions.

Journal of Inherited Metabolic Disease. ISSN 0141–8955. Copyright © SSIEM and Kluwer Academic Publishers, PO Box 55, Lancaster, UK.

RESULTS

Results are summarized in Table 1. Deficiency of debranching enzyme was confirmed in the index case's leukocytes. Uncultured CV revealed an affected fetus; the results were confirmed on cultured CV and fetal skin fibroblasts taken after therapeutic abortion.

Table 1 Type III Glycogenosis prenatal diagnosis combined assay using limit dextrin (LD) and glycogen (G) hydrolysis

	Debranching enzyme activity (nmol glucose min^{-1}(mg protein)$^{-1}$)		
	LD	*G*	*LD–G*
Leukocytes			
Controls range (*n*=20)	0.39–1.06	0.08–0.35	+0.30–0.80
mean value	0.70	0.16	+0.55
Diane GU	**0.02**	0·36	**−0.34**
Uncultured chorionic villi			
Controls range (*n*=8)	1.55–3.79	0.95–3.05	+0.20–1.30
mean value	2.37	1.76	+0.61
Control	1.42	0.75	+0.67
'At risk' cells	**1.33**	1.57	**−0.24**
Cultured chorionic villi			
Control	0.84	0.55	+0.29
'At risk' cells	**0.22**	0.30	**−0.08**
Fetal fibroblasts			
Control	0.59	0.40	+0.19
Fetus GU	**0.28**	0.35	**−0.07**

DISCUSSION AND CONCLUSION

The diagnosis was first assessed by a different method using erythrocytes (C. Baussan and Pr. Lemonnier, Paris); for this reason, we wished to verify the accuracy of the method used for prenatal diagnosis on patient's leukocytes.

This method depends on the fact that glycogen debranching enzyme is the only glucosidase which acts more rapidly in reaction conditions on phosphorylase limit dextrin of glycogen than on glycogen itself, and using the difference between activities on the two substrates avoids the interference of α-glucosidase as demonstrated by Van Diggelen *et al.* (1985). It is noticeable (Table 1) that this acid maltase activity is particularly high in uncultured CV.

This case demonstrates the reliability of chorionic villi as a convenient fetal biological material for the prenatal diagnosis of GSD type III.

REFERENCES

Brown, D., Waindle, L. and Illingworth Brown, B. The apparent activity in vivo of the lysosomal pathway of glycogen catabolism in cultured human skin fibroblasts from patients with type III glycogen storage disease. *J. Biol. Chem.* 253 (1978) 5001–5011

De Parscau, L., Guibaud, P. and Odièvre, M. Evolution à long terme des glycogénoses hépatiques: étude rétrospective de 76 observations. *Arch. Franç. Pediatr.* 45 (1988) 641–645

Illingworth, B., Cori, G. and Cori, C. Amylo-1,6-glucosidase in muscle tissue in generalized storage disease. *J. Biol. Chem.* 218 (1956) 123–129

Maire, I. and Mathieu, M. Possible prenatal diagnosis of type III glycogenosis. *J. Inher. Metab. Dis.* 9 (1986) 89–91

Van Diggelen, O., Janse, H. and Smit, G. Debranching enzyme in fibroblasts, amniotic fluid cells and chorionic villi: pre- and postnatal diagnosis of glycogenosis type III. *Clin. Chim. Acta* 149 (1985) 129–134

J. Inher. Metab. Dis. 12 Suppl. 2 (1989) 295–298

Short Communication

Prenatal Diagnosis of Atypical Phenylketonuria

N. Blau[1]*, A. Niederwieser[1]†, H. Ch. Curtius[1], L. Kierat[1],
W. Leimbacher[1], A. Matasovic[1], F. Binkert[2], H. Lehmann[3],
D. Leupold[3], O. Guardamagna[4], A. Ponzone[4], H. Schmidt[5],
T. Coskun[6], I. Özalp[6], R. Giugliani[7], G. Biasucci[8] and
M. Giovannini[8]

[1]*Division of Clinical Chemistry, Department of Pediatrics, [2]Institute of Genetics,
University of Zurich, Zurich, Switzerland; [3]Department of Pediatrics, University
of Ulm, FRG; [4]Department of Pediatrics, University of Torino, Italy;
[5]Department of Pediatrics, University of Heidelberg, FRG; [6]Institute of Child
Health, Department of Pediatrics, Nutrition and Metabolism, Hacettepe
University, Ankara, Turkey; [7]Department of Medical Genetics, Hospital of Porto
Alegre, Brazil; [8]Department of Pediatrics, University of Milano, Italy*

Atypical phenylketonuria (PKU) is a group of very rare and severe diseases caused by tetrahydrobiopterin (BH_4) deficiency (Niederwieser and Curtius, 1987). So far three inborn errors of metabolism are known to cause BH_4 deficiency, defects in: GTP cyclohydrolase I (GTPCH); 6-pyruvoyl tetrahydropterin synthase (PPH_4S); and dihydropteridine reductase (DHPR) (Blau, 1988). Recently a new form of atypical PKU with unusual 7-iso-biopterin excretion in the urine of patients was described (Curtius *et al.*, 1988). Prenatal diagnosis of BH_4 deficiency can be achieved mainly by measurement of pterin metabolites in amniotic fluid and of enzyme activities in cultured fluid cells and fetal blood (Blau *et al.*, 1987).

We performed the prenatal diagnosis of DHPR deficiency in two cases (one diagnosed as homozygote and one as heterozygote), and of PPH_4S deficiency in four cases (one diagnosed as homozygote, one as heterozygote, and two as normal). Our results suggest that measurement of neopterin and biopterin by HPLC in amniotic fluid is adequate. But it is recommended that diagnosis should be confirmed by enzyme measurements.

MATERIALS AND METHODS

Pterins in amniotic fluid collected by amniocentesis at 16–18 weeks of gestation were measured after oxidation with manganese dioxide and subsequent deproteinization with trichloracetic acid, by HPLC (Niederwieser *et al.*, 1986). 5-Hydroxyindole-acetic acid and homovanillic acid in amniotic fluid were measured by HPLC with

*Correspondence: Dr Nenad Blau, Med. Chem. Abteilung, Universitäts-Kinderklinik, Steinwiesstr. 75, 8032 Zürich, Switzerland
†Deceased

Journal of Inherited Metabolic Disease. ISSN 0141–8955. Copyright © SSIEM and Kluwer Academic Publishers, PO Box 55, Lancaster, UK.

an ESA Coulochem 5100A electrochemical detector. The separation was achieved on a Hypersil 3MOS (150×4.6 mm) column (HPLC Technology, UK) using a 20 mmol L^{-1} potassium phosphate buffer, pH 3.0, containing 0.5 mmol L^{-1} heptan-sulphonic acid, 0.12 mmol L^{-1} EDTA, 0.28% (v/v) perchloric acid, and 15% (v/v) methanol as the mobile phase. The flow rate was 0.7 mL min^{-1} and the analytical cell (Model 5011) was adjusted to 0.45 V(+) with a response time of 2 s. Amino acids were measured using a Biotronic ion-exchange amino acid analyser. DHPR activity was measured in amniocyte extracts obtained after 21 days of culturing. Lysed cells were passed through a small Sephadex-G25 column and assayed as described previously (Arai *et al.*, 1982). DHPR activity in fetal erythrocytes and liver was measured by the same method. PPH$_4$S activity was measured in fetal erythrocytes obtained from an umbilical vessel under ultrasonographic monitoring. The HPLC method is based on the measurement of BH$_4$ derived from dihydroneop-terin triphosphate (substrate) in the presence of NADPH, magnesium, and sepiap-terin reductase (Niederwieser *et al.*, 1986).

RESULTS AND DISCUSSION

Prenatal diagnosis of all three variants of atypical PKU is possible by measurement of neopterin and biopterin in amniotic fluid. In PPH$_4$S deficiency high neopterin and low biopterin were measured and the percentage of biopterin was very low (case 3). The percentage of biopterin = $100 \times$ biopterin/(neopterin + biopterin). In DHPR deficiency high biopterin and normal neopterin were measured and the percentage of biopterin was increased (case 1). In GTPCH deficiency low neopterin and low biopterin would be expected, and the percentage of biopterin will be normal. However, so far no case of prenatal diagnosis of GTPCH has been described. Measurement of the neurotransmitter metabolites 5-hydroxyindoleacetic acid and homovanillic acid in amniotic fluid was less informative. In almost all cases normal values were found. The same is true for phenylalanine and tyrosine in amniotic fluid. Both amino acids were found in normal concentrations in all cases investigated. Measurement of enzyme activities is important for confirmation of pathological pterin patterns in amniotic fluid. DHPR activity can be measured in fetal erythrocytes and cultured amniocytes, as well as in liver biopsy material. Measurement of PPH$_4$S activity can be routinely performed only in fetal erythro-cytes because the enzyme is not expressed in amniotic fluid cells. In both cases it should be proved that the blood is really fetal by the Kleihauer test. Measurement of GTPCH activity is not possible in erythrocytes and amniocytes because this enzyme is not expressed in these cells. However, measurement of activity can be performed in stimulated mononuclear white blood cells and in liver biopsy (Blau *et al.*, 1987).

In Table 1 we summarize the findings of the patients investigated.

Case 1: Prenatal diagnosis was performed in a mother whose first DHPR deficient child died at the age of 3 years. A high percentage of biopterin was found in amniotic fluid when compared with controls. In cultured amniotic fluid cells as well as in fetal erythrocytes no activity was detectable. In fetal serum a very high percentage of biopterin (74%) was found. All these results indicated that the fetus

Table 1 Pterins, neurotransmitter metabolites and amino acids in amniotic fluid, and DHPR and PPH_4S activity in amniocytes and erythrocytes

Fetus at risk	Weeks of gestation	Amniotic fluid							DHPR activity in amniocytes (% of controls)	PPH_4S activity in erythrocytes (% of controls)	Diagnosis
		N (nmol L^{-1})	B (nmol L^{-1})	%B	5HIAA (nmol L^{-1})	HVA (nmol L^{-1})	Phe (µmol L^{-1})	Tyr (µmol L^{-1})			
DHPR deficiency											
Case 1 (Milano)	17	36	56	61	67	185	61	75	<1		Homozygote
Case 2 (Ankara)	21	70	16	19	nd	nd	54	39	48		Heterozygote
PPH_4S deficiency											
Case 3 (Brazil)	19	136	2	1.3	nd	nd	51	34		<1	Homozygote
Case 4 (Torino)	16	51	9	11	69	92	55	45		nd	Heterozygote
Case 5 (Torino)	17	33	15	31	124	117	70	58		247	Normal
Case 6 (Ulm)	20	38	11	22	100	109	45	56		194	Normal
Normal values	16–21	16–40	6–21	17–54	32–135	50–144	<120	<109	100	100	

B = biopterin; N = neopterin; 5HIAA = 5-hydroxyindoleacetic acid; HVA = homovanillic acid; %B = B100/(N+B); nd = not determined

was DHPR deficient. After abortion and autopsy no DHPR activity was detected in the liver.

Case 2: In a family with a DHPR deficient child, a heterozygote fetus with DHPR deficiency was diagnosed (Blau *et al.*, 1987). Measurement of pterins in amniotic fluid showed quite normal neopterin and biopterin content. In the cultured amniocytes about 50% activity was found. After the birth, diagnosis was confirmed by the assay of DHPR activity in erythrocytes.

Case 3: In a first case of prenatal diagnosis of PPH_4S deficiency (Niederwieser *et al.*, 1986) amniocentesis was performed at 19 weeks of gestation. We investigated amniotic fluid and fetal blood. In the amniotic fluid high neopterin and low biopterin concentrations were found when compared with normal controls. The percentage of biopterin was very low. PPH_4S activity was extremely low in fetal erythrocytes, although fetal controls showed two to three fold higher PPH_4S activities than adult controls. Diagnosis of PPH_4S deficiency was confirmed by measurement of enzyme activity in fetal liver after abortion.

Case 4: In a family with a PPH_4S deficient child the father was found to be a heterozygote for PPH_4S deficiency, whereas the mother proved to be normal. Differentiation between homozygotes and heterozygotes of PPH_4S deficiency is possible by measurement of enzyme activity in erythrocytes and pterins in urine of the parents. In amniotic fluid obtained at 16 weeks of gestation normal neopterin and biopterin concentrations were found. The percentage of biopterin was slightly decreased indicating that the fetus might be a heterozygote of PPH_4S deficiency or even normal.

Cases 5 and 6: In both families at risk for PPH_4S deficiency normal pterin patterns were found in amniotic fluid. Diagnosis was confirmed by measurement of PPH_4S activity in fetal blood.

ACKNOWLEDGEMENTS

We are grateful to W. Staudenmann and Dr G. Schoedon for technical assistance. This work was supported by the Swiss National Science Foundation, project No. 3.395-0.86.

REFERENCES

Arai, N., Narisawa, K., Hayakawa, H. and Tada, K. Hyperphenylalaninemia due to dihydropteridine reductase deficiency: Diagnosis by enzyme assays on dried blood spots. *Pediatrics* 70 (1982) 426–430

Blau, N., Niederwieser, A., Curtius, H. Ch., Leimbacher, W., Kierat, L., Matasovic, A., Staudenmann, W. and Özalp, I., Prenatal diagnosis of tetrahydrobiopterin deficiency. In Curtius, H. Ch., Blau, N. and Levine, R. (eds.) *Unconjugated Pterins and Related Biogenic Amines*, Walter de Gruyter, Berlin, 1987, pp. 237–246

Blau, N. Inborn errors of pterin metabolism. *Annu. Rev. Nutr.* 8 (1988) 185–209

Curtius, H. Ch., Kuster, Th., Matasovic, A., Blau, N. and Dhondt, J. L. Primapterin, anapterin, and 6-oxo-primapterin, three new 7-substituted pterins in a patient with hyperphenylalaninemia. *Biochem. Biophys. Res. Commun.* 153 (1988) 715–721

Niederwieser, A., Shintaku, H., Hasler, Th., Curtius, H. Ch., Lehmann, H., Guardamagna, O. and Schmidt, H. Prenatal diagnosis of 'dihyrobiopterin synthetase' deficiency, a variant form of phenylketonuria. *Eur. J. Pediatr.* 145 (1986) 176–178

Niederwieser, A. and Curtius, H. Ch. Tetrahydrobiopterin biosynthetic pathway and deficiency. *Enzyme* 38 (1987) 302–311

J. Inher. Metab. Dis. 12 Suppl. 2 (1989) 299–300

Short Communication

First Trimester Prenatal Diagnosis of Wolman Disease

A. Iavarone[1], G. Dolfin[2], G. Bracco[1], M. Zaffaroni[3], M. R. Gallina[3] and G. Bona[3]
[1]*Ospedale Infantile Regina Margherita, Piazza Polonia 94, 10126 Torino;*
[2]*Ospedale Ostetrico-Ginecologico S. Anna, Torino;* [3] *Istituto di Puericultura –*
Clinica Pediatrica II, Università di Torino, Italy

Wolman disease (WD; McKusick 27800) is a rare metabolic disorder with autosomal recessive inheritance. Pathologically, it is characterized by intracellular triglyceride and cholesteryl ester storage caused by absence of lysosomal acid lipase activity. This deficiency has been demonstrated in a variety of tissues from patients affected by WD, including liver, spleen, cultured skin fibroblasts and amniotic fluid cells (Patrick and Lake, 1973; Cortner *et al.*, 1976; Kryiakides *et al.*, 1972), but only recently, in a few cases, in chorionic villi (Gatti *et al.*, 1988).

We report here our experience with first trimester prenatal diagnosis (propositus) during an at-risk pregnancy, and some comments on the relative efficacy of the tests.

CASE REPORT

D. L. D. (index case) was the first child of unrelated parents, both coming from the same Sicilian town of 10 000 inhabitants. She was affected by WD: diagnosis was clinically and roentgenologically suspected (liver and spleen enlargement, failure to thrive, bilateral calcification of the adrenals), and biochemically confirmed (see Results for enzyme measurements). The baby died at age 6 months because of liver failure.

A second pregnancy was monitored: chorionic villi (at 10 weeks gestation) and amniotic fluid (at 16 weeks) were sampled. Cytogenetical analysis was performed. Acid lipase activity was measured on chorionic villi and on cultured amniotic cells, using both artificial and ^{14}C-labelled natural substrates (Coates *et al.*, 1979; Burton *et al.*, 1980).

RESULTS AND DISCUSSION

Acid lipase activity in chorionic villi and in cultured amniotic cells was in accordance with a non-affected (possibly heterozygous) fetus. The pregnancy was continued and the correctness of prenatal diagnosis was confirmed on cord-blood lymphocytes. Results of enzyme measurements are shown in Table 1.

Journal of Inherited Metabolic Disease. ISSN 0141–8955. Copyright © SSIEM and Kluwer Academic Publishers, PO Box 55, Lancaster, UK.

Table 1   Acid lipase activity $(nmol\,(mg\;protein)^{-1}\,h^{-1})$ with different substrates

	Fibroblasts	Chorionic villi	Amniotic cells	Lymphocytes
Index case	0.1 (1.4%)[a]	—	—	—
	113 (11%)[c]	—	—	209 (15%)[c]
Propositus	*	0.89 (49%)[a]	4.5 (63%)[b]	14.8 (60%)[b]
	*	361 (83%)[c]	377 (40%)[c]	803 (57%)[c]
Controls: mean	6.9[a]	1.82[a]	7.1[b]	24.6[b]
range	5.8–8.2	1.52–2.33	5.7–11.3	20.6–31.0
mean	1244[c]	432[c]	949[c]	1400[c]
range	600–1709	390–476	667–1512	848–1779

* Not yet available.
Substrates: [a] [^{14}C]cholesteryl oleate; [b] [^{14}C]triolein; [c] 4-methylumbelliferyl oleate.

In order to obtain reliable results, acid lipase activity was measured both on chorionic villi and on cultured amniotic fluid cells. For this same reason, all measurements were made both with artificial and ^{14}C-labelled natural substrates.

Our data indicate that direct enzyme analysis of chorionic villi is as satisfactory as analysis of cultured amniotic cells. Moreover, assay methods used for cultured amniotic cells have adequate sensitivity when applied to chorionic villi. First trimester prenatal diagnosis of WD thus seems possible.

Although the fluorometric assay of acid lipase is simpler and less time-consuming than the assay employing radiolabelled substrates, our data show that enzyme activity measured with 4-methylumbelliferyl-oleate (4-MUO) does not always accurately reflect activity measured with either [^{14}C]cholesteryl oleate or [^{14}C]tri-olein (Table 1). This discrepancy suggests the need for extreme caution in interpreting results of assays performed using 4-MUO, or even the need to always confirm these results with more sensitive radiometric assays.

REFERENCES

Burton, B. K., Emery, D. and Mueller, H. W. Lysosomal acid lipase in cultivated fibroblasts: characterization of enzyme activity in normal and enzymatically deficient cell lines. *Clin. Chim. Acta* 101 (1980) 25–32

Coates, P. M., Cortner, J. A., Hoffman, M. and Brown, S. A. Acid lipase activity of human lymphocytes. *Biochem. Biophys. Acta* 572 (1979)225-234

Cortner, J. A., Coates, P. M., Swoboda, E. and Schnatz, J. D. Genetic variation of lysosomal acid lipase *Pediatr. Res.* 10 (1976) 927-932

Gatti, R., Borrone, C., Filocamo. M., Stroppiano, N., Lituania, M., Cordone, M. and Durand, P. Diagnosi prenatale delle malattie metaboliche – Esperienza relativa a 220 casi. *Riv. Ital. Pediatr.* 14 (1988) 196-202

Kryiakides, E. C., Paul, B., and Balint, J. A. Lipid accumulations and acid lipase deficiency in fibroblasts from a family with Wolman's disease, and their apparent correction *in vitro*. *J. Lab. Clin. Med.* 80 (1972) 810-816

Patrick, A. D. and Lake, B. D. Wolman disease, In Hers G. and Van Hoof (eds.) *Lysosomes and Storage Diseases*. Academic Press, New York, 1973, pp. 453-473

J. Inher. Metab. Dis. 12 Suppl. 2 (1989) 301–304

Short Communication

Prenatal Diagnosis of Zellweger Syndrome by Direct Visualization of Peroxisomes in Chorionic Villus Fibroblasts by Immunofluorescence Microscopy

R. J. A. Wanders[1], E. A. C. Wiemer[2], S. Brul[2], R. B. H. Schutgens[1], H. van den Bosch[3] and J. M. Tager[2]
[1]*Department of Pediatrics, University Hospital Amsterdam, AMC, Meibergdreef 9, 1105 AZ Amsterdam;* [2]*Laboratory of Biochemistry, University of Amsterdam, P.O. Box 20151, 1000 HA Amsterdam;* [3]*Laboratory of Biochemistry, University of Utrecht, Padualaan 8, 3584 CH Utrecht, The Netherlands*

Goldfischer and coworkers (1973) were the first to describe the absence of morphologically distinguishable peroxisomes in liver and kidney tubule cells of patients with the cerebro-hepato-renal (Zellweger) syndrome (McKusick 21410). In recent years it has become clear that peroxisomes are also (virtually) absent in patients with neonatal adrenoleukodystrophy (McKusick 20237), infantile Refsum disease and hyperpipecolic acidaemia (McKusick 23940), at least in the four patients described in the literature (see Wanders *et al.*, 1988, for discussion). The (virtual) absence of peroxisomes in these patients is associated with a generalized loss of peroxisomal functions as reflected in the accumulation of very long-chain fatty acids, bile acid intermediates, pipecolic acid and phytanic acid in plasma from the patients.

Using a technique which makes use of digitonin to selectively permeabilize the cell, we established earlier that in chorionic villus fibroblasts catalase is contained in subcellular particles (peroxisomes) as in skin fibroblasts (Wanders *et al.*, 1986). Based upon this finding we have now developed a sensitive method which allows direct visualization of peroxisomes in cultured chorionic villus fibroblasts by immunofluorescence microscopy using an anti-(catalase) antiserum, thus providing a simple method for prenatal diagnosis of Zellweger syndrome or any of the other peroxisome deficiency disorders.

MATERIALS AND METHODS

The procedure for staining cultured chorionic villus fibroblasts with the anti-(catalase) antiserum was as follows: cells grown on coverslips were washed three times with phosphate-buffered saline (PBS) and incubated for 20 min with 2% (w/v) paraformaldehyde in PBS containing 0.2% (v/v) Triton X-100 (PBS/Triton).

Journal of Inherited Metabolic Disease. ISSN 0141-8955. Copyright © SSIEM and Kluwer Academic Publishers, PO Box 55, Lancaster, UK.

Subsequently, the coverslips were washed three times with PBS/Triton, and incubated for 10 min in PBS containing 0.2% (v/v) Triton X-100 and 0.1 mol L $^{-1}$ NH$_4$Cl in order to block free aldehyde groups. After this the coverslips were extensively washed with PBS and either stored in PBS plus sodium azide and protease inhibitors or stained immediately with the anti-(catalase) antiserum according to the following protocol. Fixed cells on coverslips were incubated for 30 min in a 30 μL drop of PBS containing 10 mg mL^{-1} bovine serum albumin (BSA) and a 1:250 dilution of the primary anti-(catalase) antiserum. Next, the coverslip was washed three times with PBS and incubated for 30 min in PBS-bovine serum albumin containing a 1:100 dilution of biotinylated donkey anti-(rabbit) IgG. After washing the coverslip three times with PBS, it was finally incubated for 30 min in a 1:100 dilution of streptavidin-fluorescein isothiocyanate in PBS–bovine serum albumin. The coverslip was washed extensively with PBS and mounted on a microscope slide in a mounting medium consisting of nine volumes of glycerol, one volume of PBS containing 1 mg mL^{-1} *p*-phenylenediamine. The coverslip was sealed with nail varnish and examined in a Leitz fluorescence microscope with a No. 4 blue filter (excitation maximum: 466 nm, emission maximum 530 nm).

Biotinylated donkey anti-(rabbit) IgG (biotin-DAR) and streptavidin-fluorescein isothiocyanate (streptavidin-FITC) were from Amersham (UK). Anti-(bovine liver catalase) antiserum was prepared as described before (Tager *et al.*, 1985).

RESULTS

We recently developed an indirect immunofluorescence labelling technique to visualize microperoxisomes in cultured human skin fibroblasts using an anti-(catalase) antiserum and a biotin–streptavidin signal enhancement step (Wiemer *et al.*, 1988). In control cells a punctate fluorescence pattern was observed. In Zellweger fibroblasts, however, in which catalase is normally active but localized in the cytosolic compartment rather than in peroxisomes as is the case in control fibroblasts (Wanders *et al.*, 1984), no punctate fluorescence was observed.

Figures 1A and 1B show a similar picture in cultured chorionic villus fibroblasts from a control and Zellweger patient, respectively. Indeed, when control chorionic villus fibroblasts were immunolabelled with anti-(catalase), a punctate pattern of fluorescence was observed (Figure 1A), whereas in chorionic villus fibroblasts from a Zellweger patient, fluorescence was diffuse (Figure 1B). Accordingly, there was a deficient dihydroxyacetone phosphate acyltransferase activity, a deficient *de novo* plasmalogen biosynthesis, a deficiency of particle-bound catalase, a deficient C26:0 β-oxidation activity as well as an elevated C26:C22 ratio in these fibroblasts (see Wanders *et al.*, 1987).

In summary, the results described in this paper indicate that prenatal diagnosis of the Zellweger syndrome, or any of the other peroxisome deficiency disorders, can be done by direct visualization of peroxisomes in chorionic villus fibroblasts by the immunofluorescence technique described here. Alternatively, visualization of peroxisomes can occur by means of the diaminobenzidine staining procedure (Roels

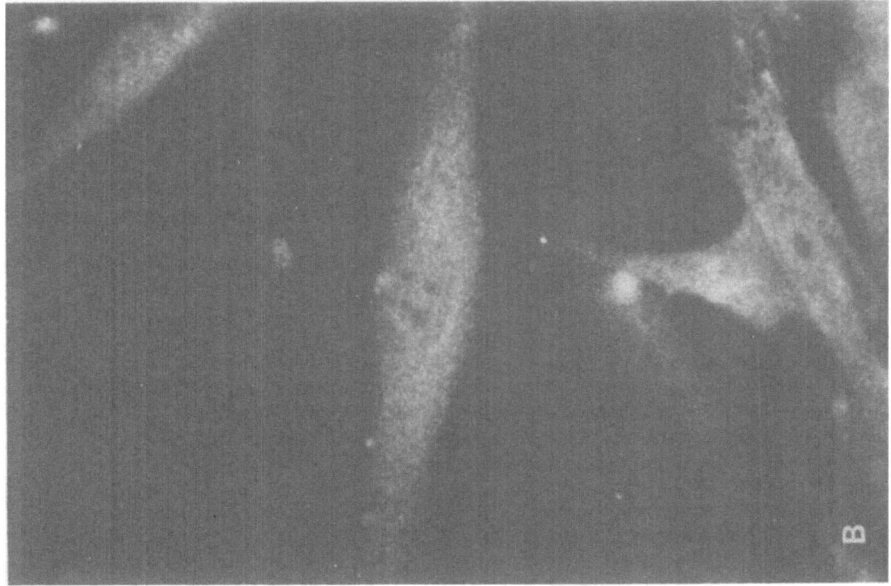

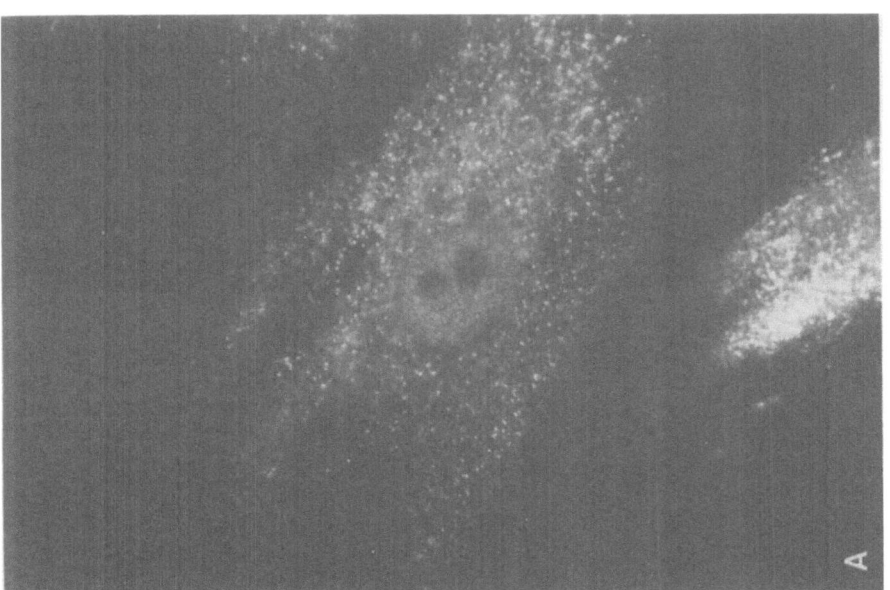

Figure 1 Visualization of peroxisomes using indirect immunofluorescence. Chorionic villus fibroblasts from a control (A) and a Zellweger fetus (B) were processed for immunofluorescence microscopy using an anti-(catalase) antiserum as described in Methods

et al., 1987). Experiments are underway to establish whether the procedure can also be applied directly to chorionic biopsy material.

ACKNOWLEDGEMENTS

The research reported in this paper was supported by a grant from the Netherlands Foundation for Medical Health Research (MEDIGON) and the Princess Beatrix Fund (The Hague, The Netherlands). The authors are grateful to Paula Zwaal for preparation of the manuscript.

REFERENCES

Goldfischer, S., Moore, C. L., Johnson, A. B., Spiro, A. J., Valsamis, M. P., Wisniewski, H. K., Ritch, R. H. Norton, W. T., Rapin, I. and Gartner, L. M. Peroxisomal and mitochondrial defects in the cerebro-hepato-renal syndrome. *Science* 182 (1973) 62–64

Roels, T., Verdonck, V., Pauwels, M., Lissens, W. and Liebaerts, I. Visualisation of peroxisomes and plasmalogens in first trimester chorionic villus. *J. Inher. Metab. Dis.* 10 Suppl. 2 (1987) 349-354

Tager, J. M., ten Harmsen van de Beek, W. A. H., Wanders, R. J. A., Hashimoto, T., Heymans, H. S. A., van den Bosch, H., Schutgens, R. B. H. and Schram, A. W. Peroxisomal β-oxidation enzyme proteins in the Zellweger syndrome. *Biochem. Biophys. Res. Commun.* 126 (1985) 1269–1275

Wanders, R. J. A., Kos, M., Roest, B., Meijer, A. J., Schrakamp, G., Heymans, H. S. A., Tegelaers, W. H. H., van den Bosch, H., Schutgens, R. B. H. and Tager, J. M. Activity of peroxisomal enzymes and intracellular distribution of catalase in Zellweger syndrome. *Biochem. Biophys. Res. Commun.* 123 (1984) 1054–1061

Wanders, R. J. A., Schrakamp, G., van den Bosch, H., Tager, J. M., Moser, H. W., Moser, A. E., Aubourgh, P., Kleyer, W. J. and Schutgens, R. B. H. Pre- and postnatal diagnosis of the cerebro-hepato-renal (Zellweger) syndrome via a simple method directly demonstrating the presence or absence of peroxisomes in cultured skin fibroblasts, amniocytes or chorionic villous fibroblasts. *J. Inher. Metab. Dis.* 9 Suppl. 2 (1986) 317–320

Wanders, R. J. A., van Wijland, M. J. A., van Roermund, C. W. T., Schutgens, R. B. H., van den Bosch, H., Tager, J. M., Nijenhuis, A. and Tromp, A. Prenatal diagnosis of Zellweger syndrome by measurement of very long-chain fatty acid (C26:0) β-oxidation in cultured chorionic villous fibroblasts: implications for early diagnosis of other peroxisomal disorders. *Clin. Chim. Acta* 165 (1987) 303–310

Wanders, R. J. A., Heymans, H. S. A., Schutgens, R. B. H., Barth, P. G., van den Bosch, H. and Tager, J. M. Peroxisomal disorders in neurology (Review). *J. Neurol. Sci.* 88 (1988) 1–39

Wiemer, E. A. C., Brul, S., Just, W. W., van Driel, R., Brouwer-Kelder, E. M., Van den Berg, M., Schutgens, R. B. H., van den Bosch, H., Schram, A. W., Wanders, R. J. A. and Tager, J. M. Presence of peroxisomal membrane proteins in liver and fibroblasts from patients with the Zellweger syndrome and related disorders: evidence for the existence of peroxisomal ghosts. *Eur. J. Cell. Biol.* submitted for publication

J. Inher. Metab. Dis. 12 Suppl. 2 (1989) 305–307

Short Communication

Prenatal Diagnosis of Cystic Fibrosis: Experience of Two Complementary Methods

D. Bozon, I. Maire, A. Vialle, G. Mandon, P. Guibaud and R. Gilly

Centre d'Etudes des Maladies Métaboliques, Hôpital Debrousse, 69322 Lyon Cédex 05, France

Cystic fibrosis (CF; McKusick 21970) is a common and severe autosomal recessive single gene disorder affecting one in 2000–2500 Caucasians. A prenatal test for one in four at-risk pregnancies is based on reduced levels of microvillar intestinal enzymes (MVE) in amniotic fluid (AF) due to intestinal obstruction in affected fetuses (Brock, 1983).

In 1985, the discovery of a linkage with DNA markers mapped on chromosome 7 established the locus on chromosome 7. The availability of close DNA probes (MetD, MetH, KM19, XV2C, J3.11) (White *et al.*, 1985; Wainwright *et al.*, 1985; Estivill *et al.*, 1987) tightly linked to the CF gene allows the use of restriction fragment length polymorphism (RFLP) analysis for prenatal diagnosis and heterozygote detection in one in four at-risk families with an alive affected child.

MATERIALS AND ASSAYS

Microvillar enzyme assays: The amniotic fluids were sampled between 17 and 18.5 weeks of amenorrhoea. γ-Glutamyl transpeptidase (GGT) and leucine aminopeptidase (LAP) were measured following classical spectrophotometric kinetic methods. Alkaline phosphatase and its isoenzymes were determined using 4-methylumbelliferyl phosphate in the absence or presence of specific inhibitors (L-phenylalanine (Phe), L-homoarginine (Homo) and bromotetramisole (BTM)).

DNA analysis: For DNA analysis, the affected individuals, parents and all available siblings were sampled. DNA was extracted from blood, cultured amniotic cells or chorionic villi using standard protocols. After extraction, 8 µg of DNA were digested by restriction enzymes and analysed by Southern blotting using Zetaprobe membranes (Biorad). All samples were analysed for five RFLP: MetD: *Taq*I; MetH: *Taq*I; KM19: *Pst*I; XV2C: *Taq*I; J3.11:*Msp*I.

RESULTS

Analysis of microvillar enzymes in amniotic fluids: GGT, LAP and ALP isoenzymes were measured in 70 at-risk amniotic fluids. An abnormal low content of microvillar enzymes and intestinal ALP isoenzyme is indicative of a CF fetus. We elected to consider values (for GGT, LAP, ALP, Phe inhibition) below the first

Journal of Inherited Metabolic Disease. ISSN 0141–8955. Copyright © SSIEM and Kluwer Academic Publishers, PO Box 55, Lancaster, UK.

percentile as abnormal and values from the first to the 5th as inconclusive. Values above the 99th percentile for Homo and BTM inhibition are considered as abnormal and values from the 95th to the 99th are considered as inconclusive.

To date, no false negative has been found; 22 fetuses were found to be affected (i.e. 31%). In all cases, when it could be verified, a meconium ileus with a raised albumin content was found.

DNA analysis: So far, prenatal diagnosis by DNA typing on chorionic villi has been attempted in seven informative families. In two cases, the direct analysis was not possible because of sampling problems (only maternal tissue in one case and a biopsy below 3 mg in the other case). Among the five other cases, three were found homozygous normal and two heterozygous carriers (Table 1).

Table 1 Prenatal diagnosis by DNA typing

Chorionic villus biopsies		Results	MVE control
Attempted	*Successful*		
7	5	Normal homozygous 3	
		Heterozygous 2	1* (not affected)

*Control by MVE required because, in the nuclear family, only one child: the index case

Furthermore, 14 prenatal diagnoses performed by MVE analysis in AF were controlled by DNA analysis using cultured AF cells or fetal fibroblasts. Among the nine unaffected fetuses diagnosed by MVE, DNA analyses were confirmative and revealed six normal homozygous and three heterozygous carriers. Among the six affected fetuses diagnosed by MVE assay, four were completely confirmative one was inconclusive (the father presented the same chromosome haplotypes), and in one case there was a discrepancy between the two methods (affected MVE assay and heterozygous by DNA typing) (Table 2).

Table 2 MVE analysis prenatal diagnosis

MVE Analysis		Control by DNA typing in AF cells	
Pregnancies studied	*Results*	*Pregnancies controlled*	*Results*
70	22 affected	6	1 unaffected 1 partially informative 4 confirmative
	48 unaffected	9	6 normal homozygous 3 heterozygous carrier

DISCUSSION

For MVE analysis, the choice of sampling time is important as the enzyme activities are changing with the gestational age: the enzyme assay data can be within the limits of the normal range at 16 weeks and fall to the abnormal range by 17 or 18 weeks of amenorrhoea; an early inconclusive sampling must be verified by a second one later. In our experience, no false negative has been reported until now; but all samplings were made after ultrasound dating and the gestational age was expressed in terms of biparietal diameter (38–40 mm).

False positives remain the major problem: in our experience, out of about 300 normal amniotic fluids tested as controls, four were found in the abnormal range: three of them gave birth to normal children, one could not be found – so the false positive rate can be estimated at about 1.3%. Among the false positives in our at-risk families, figure chromosomal abnormalities such trisomy 21 (two cases in our series). Furthermore, we found the proportion of affected fetuses to be 31%, which is higher than the expected rate of 25%; this finding has been reported by others (Brock *et al.*, 1988). Besides the previously reported chromosomal abnormalities, 'true' false positives have been demonstrated by DNA typing in two cases: one in a one in four at-risk pregnancy and another one in a relative of an affected child (the fetus presented the same haplotypes as one of its non-affected sisters). In both cases, a meconial ileus was found at autopsy as well as increased albumin content in the meconium.

CONCLUSION

MVE analysis false positives may be related to the fact that enzymes are not excreted normally in AF in some cases of transient meconial ileus without cystic fibrosis. For this reason, MVE analysis must be restricted to one in four at-risk families. But the method remains worthwhile in those either non-informative (10% in our experience) or without any alive affected child.

REFERENCES

Brock, D. Amniotic fluid alkaline phosphatase isoenzymes in early prenatal diagnosis of cystic fibrosis. *Lancet* 2 (1983) 941–943

Brock, D., Clarke, H. and Barron, L. Prenatal diagnosis of cystic fibrosis by microvillar enzyme assay on a sequence of 258 pregnancies. *Hum. Genet.* 78 (1988) 271–275

Estivill, X., Farrall, M., Scambler, P., Bell, G., Hawley, K., Lench, N., Bates, G., Kruyer, H., Frederick, P., Stanier, P., Watson, E., Williamson, R. and Wainwright, B. A candidate for the cystic fibrosis locus isolated by selection for methylation free islands. *Nature* 326 (1987) 840–845

Wainwright, B., Scambler, P., Schmidtke, J., Watson, E., Law, H. Y., Farrall, M., Cooke, H., Eiberg, H. and Williamson, R. Localization of cystic fibrosis locus to human chromosome 7 cen-q22. *Nature* 318 (1985) 384–385

White, R., Woodward, S., Leppert, M., O'Connel, P., Hoof, M., Herbst, J., Lalouel, J. M., Dean, M. and Van de Woude, G. A closely linked genetic marker for cystic fibrosis. *Nature* 318 (1985) 382–384

J. Inher. Metab. Dis. 12 Suppl. 2 (1989) 308–310

Short Communication

Prenatal Diagnosis of Cystic Fibrosis Using Closely Linked DNA Probes

W. Lissens[1], M. Vercammen[1], W. Foulon[2], L. De Catte[2], I. Dab[3], A. Malfroot[3], M. Bonduelle[1] and I. Liebaers[1]

Departments of [1]Medical Genetics, [2]Gynecology and Obstetrics and [3]Pediatrics, University Hospital, Vrije Universiteit Brussel, Brussels, Belgium

Cystic fibrosis (CF; McKusick 21970) is a common autosomal recessive disease in the Caucasian population with an incidence of approximately 1 in 1600 live births and a carrier frequency of 1 in 20. The biochemical pathology of CF is unknown, but recent work has implicated anion transport across membranes as the physiological basis of the disease (Li *et al.*, 1988).

During the past few years, genetic linkage between the CF locus and several polymorphic DNA markers on chromosome 7q22-31 has been demonstrated (Estivill *et al.*, 1987; Tsui *et al.*, 1985; Wainwright *et al.*, 1985; White *et al.*, 1985). We have used six of these markers to study 55 Belgian families, with at least one CF child, for carrier detection and prenatal diagnosis. In this communication, we report the results of first trimester prenatal diagnosis for pregnancies in four families.

METHODS

Chorionic villus sampling was performed by aspiration with a Portex catheter, under continuous ultrasound guidance, at 9 to 11 weeks of gestation. A minimum amount of 5 mg pure villous tissue was obtained. The average yield was 4 μg of DNA per mg wet tissue.

DNA extraction from chorionic villi or whole blood and Southern blot analysis of DNA has been described (Farrall *et al.*, 1986). Results were obtained within one week after chorionic villus sampling. The probes J3.11, metH, 7C22, XV-2C and KM19 were used. J3.11 detects an *Msp*I polymorphism with alleles 4.2 kb (A1) and 1.8 kb (A2); metH, metD and XV-2C, *Taq*I polymorphisms with alleles 7.0 kb (B1) and 4.2 kb (B2), 5.0 kb (C1) and 4.0 kb (C2) and 2.1 kb (D1) and 1.4 kb (D2), respectively; 7C22 an *Eco*RI polymorphism with alleles 7.2 kb (E1) and 5.1 kb (E2); KM19 a *Pst*I polymorphism with alleles 7.6 kb (F1) and 6.8 kb (F2). The recombination fractions at maximal lod scores for linkage between CF and the probes are: J3.11 – 0.003, metH and metD – 0.004 (Beaudet *et al.*, 1986), 7C22 – 0.025 (Farrall *et al.*, 1987). The probes XV-2C and KM19 are in a region less than 50 kb away from the CF gene (Estivill *et al.*, 1987). The most likely order of probes versus CF is J3.11–CF–KM19–XV-2C–met–7C22 (Lathrop *et al.*, 1988).

Journal of Inherited Metabolic Disease. ISSN 0141-8955. Copyright © SSIEM and Kluwer Academic Publishers, PO Box 55, Lancaster, UK.

RESULTS AND DISCUSSION

The four families described in this study are from a group of 55 Belgian CF families requesting haplotype analysis with linked DNA probes for carrier detection and/or prenatal diagnosis. Using six restriction fragment length polymorphisms (RFLPs), these families were all fully informative allowing the phase of the normal and the CF alleles of both parents to be traced (unpublished data).

Table 1   First trimester prenatal diagnosis of cystic fibrosis in four families

		RFLP alleles* of:				
Family	Polymorphism	Father	Mother	CF child	Fetus at risk	Diagnosis
1	J3.11/MspI	A1A2	A1A2	A1A2	A1A2	CF
	metH/TaqI	B2B2	B2B1	B2B1	B2B1	
2	metD/TaqI	C2C1	C2C1	C2C2	C2C1	Carrier
	7C22/EcoRI	E2E1	E1E1	E2E1	E2E1	
	XV-2C/TaqI	D1D2	D1D1	D1D1	D1D1	
3	J3.11/MspI	A1A2	A1A2	A1A1	A1A2	Carrier
	metH/TaqI	B1B2	B1B1	B1B1	B1B1	
	metD/TaqI	C1C1	C2C1	C1C2	C1C1	
	7C22/EcoRI	E2E1	E1E1	E2E1	E2E1	
	KM19/PstI	F2F1	F1F1	F2F1	F2F1	
4	J3.11/MspI	A2A2	A1A2	A2A1	A2A2	Carrier
	metH/TaqI	B2B1	B1B1	B2B1	B2B1	
	metD/TaqI	C1C1	C1C2	C1C1	C1C2	
	XV-2C/TaqI	D1D2	D1D1	D1D1	D1D1	
	KM19/PstI	F2F1	F2F1	F2F2	F2F1	

*For CF carriers, the allele segregating with CF is given in the first position, except for family 1 where the J3.11/MspI CF alleles of the parents could not be determined.

The results of prenatal diagnosis in these four families are given in Table 1. Every informative RFLP was studied for each family. In family 1, DNA analysis indicated an affected fetus. At the moment of diagnosis (February 1986), only probes J3.11 and metH were available. The probability of the fetus being affected is 98·4%. Pregnancy was terminated after genetic counselling without attempting to confirm the diagnosis by microvillar enzyme testing. In the other three families, fetuses were diagnosed as carriers; in each case, the paternal CF allele was inherited. The inaccuracy of the predictions, due to possible recombination during meiosis, is less than 1%. One pregnancy (family 2) resulted in live birth at normal term and the child was found to be healthy. One pregnancy (family 3) is still in progress, while the other pregnancy (family 4) unfortunately resulted in a spontaneous abortion at 18 weeks of gestation.

As long as the basic molecular defect in CF is unknown, prenatal diagnosis through RFLP analysis will be of considerable interest for the prevention of the disease. Results are obtained before the second trimester of pregnancy and are highly reliable. The number of families that will be informative for diagnosis is high: in our laboratory all 55 families are fully informative. A major disadvantage of RFLP diagnosis is that the parents and at least one living CF child must be available for haplotyping. The isolation of the CF gene will circumvent this problem and allow screening for carriers in the population.

ACKNOWLEDGEMENTS

We would like to thank R. Williamson, P. Scambler and G. Vande Woude for providing the probes. This work was supported by a grant to W. L. from the Belgian NFWO/Cystic fibrosis foundation.

REFERENCES

Beaudet, A., Bowcock, L., Buchwald, M., Cavalli-Sforza, M., Farrall, M., King, M., Klinger, K., Lalouel, J. M., Lathrop, G., Naylor, S., Ott, J., Tsui, L., Wainwright, B., Watkins, P., White, R. and Williamson, R. Linkage of cystic fibrosis to two tightly linked DNA markers: joint report from a collaborative study. *Am. J. Hum. Genet.* 39 (1986) 681–693

Estivill, X., Farrall, M., Scambler, P., Bell, G., Hawley, K., Lench, N., Bates, G., Kruyer, H., Frederick, P., Stanier, P., Watson, E., Williamson, R. and Wainwright, B. A candidate for the cystic fibrosis locus isolated by selection for methylation-free islands. *Nature* 326 (1987) 840–845

Farrall, M., Law, H., Rodeck, C., Warren, R., Stanier, P., Super, M., Lissens, W., Scambler, P., Watson, E., Wainwright, B. and Williamson, R. First-trimester prenatal diagnosis of cystic fibrosis with linked DNA probes. *Lancet* 1 (1986) 1402–1405

Farrall, M., Lathrop, M., Spence, J., Bowcock, A., Klinger, K. and Tsui, L. Further data on linkage between cystic fibrosis and 7C22. *Am. J. Hum. Genet.* 41 (1987) 286–287

Lathrop, G., Farrall, M., O'Connell, P., Wainwright, B., Leppert, M., Nakamura, Y., Lench, N., Kruyer, H., Dean, M., Park, M., Vande Woude, G., Lalouel, J. M., Williamson, R. and White, R. Refined linkage map of chromosome 7 in the region of the cystic fibrosis gene. *Am. J. Hum. Genet.* 42 (1988) 38–44

Li, M., McCann, J., Nairn, A., Greengard, P. and Welsh, M. Cyclic AMP-dependent protein kinase opens chloride channels in normal but not cystic fibrosis airway epithelium. *Nature* 331 (1988) 358–360

Tsui, L., Buchwald, M., Barker, D., Braman, J., Knowlton, R., Schumm, J., Eiberg, H., Mohr, J., Kennedy, D., Plavsic, N., Zsiga, M., Markiewicz, D., Akotts, G., Brown, V., Helms, C., Gravius, T., Parker, C., Reddiger, K. and Keller, M. Cystic fibrosis locus defined by a genetically linked polymorphic DNA marker. *Science* 230 (1985) 1054–1057

Wainwright, B., Scambler, P., Schmidtke, J., Watson, E., Law, H. Y., Farrall, M., Cooke, H., Eiberg, H. and Williamson, R. Localisation of cystic fibrosis locus to human chromosome 7 cen-q22. *Nature* 318 (1985) 384–385

White, R., Woodward, S., Leppert, M., O'Connell, P., Hoff, M., Herbst, J., Lalouel, J., Dean, M. and Vande Woude, G. A closely linked genetic marker for cystic fibrosis. *Nature* 318 (1985) 382–384

J. Inher. Metab. Dis. 12 Suppl. 2 (1989) 311–314

Short Communication

Plasma Amino Acids During the First 24 Hours of Life: Feasibility of Early Diagnosis in the Newborn at Risk of Amino Acid Disorders

U. Caruso, R. Cerone, A. R. Fantasia, M. C. Schiaffino, G. Zignego and C. Romano
University Department of Pediatrics; G. Gaslini Institute, Via 5 maggio, 39 – 16149 Genova, Italy

Availability of early diagnosis and early treatment is fundamental to the prevention of neurological damage in patients affected by metabolic disorders with neonatal expression.

While plasma amino acid (AA) measurements accordingly provide fundamental clues to early diagnosis of inborn errors of AA metabolism, more information concerning the trends of plasma AA levels in the first 24 h of life may prove useful. Therefore 27 healthy newborns (control subjects) and five newborns at risk of amino acid disorders were studied, testing plasma AA levels in cord blood and during the first 24 h of life.

PATIENTS AND CONTROLS

Plasma AA levels were measured in cord blood and at 6, 12 and 24 h of life in all patients and in control subjects. The control specimens came from a pilot screening programme for aminoacidopathies (Caruso *et al.*, 1984; Cerone *et al.*, 1988): all normal newborns were also routinely tested day 4 (plasma AA) and day 15 (urine amino acids) of life; they did not present any clinical manifestations at 6 months of life. Of the five patients, one was at risk of urea cycle disorder (UCD); three of maple syrup urine disease (MSUD); and one of phenylketonuria (PKU).

MATERIALS AND METHODS

Cord and venous blood, collected in lithium heparinized plastic tubes and immediately centrifuged to separate plasma from red cells, was deproteinized with 2.2% sulphosalicylic acid in water (1/1, v/v). Clear supernatant was kept frozen at $-20°C$ until analysis. All analyses were performed using ion-exchange chromatography (Carlo Erba 3A29 and 3A30 equipped with 0.4×20 and 0.4×12 cm stainless steel columns. All specimens were obtained from subjects (normal and at risk) in basal and in conventional conditions of nutrition and care.

Journal of Inherited Metabolic Disease. ISSN 0141-8955. Copyright © SSIEM and Kluwer Academic Publishers, PO Box 55, Lancaster, UK.

Table 1 Plasma amino acids during the first 24h of life in five at-risk newborns and in 27 control subjects

Patient	Sex	At-risk of	Specimen taken[a]	Val	Ile	Leu	Gln	Cit	Tyr	Phe	Final diagnosis
L.M.	F	MSUD	Cord	389	133	253					MSUD
			12h	323	191	324					
			24h	176	126	259					
G.R.	F	MSUD	Cord	117	55	411[b]					Not affected
			12h	62	30	125					
			24h	47	17	111					
G.D.	M	MSUD	Cord	252	71	147	533	10	70	75	Not affected
			12h	110	35	73	725	6	60	68	
			24h	89	30	71	624	10	62	58	
C.D.	M	UCD	Cord	145	41	74	365	6	54	244[c]	CPS deficiency
			12h	129	40	69	698	Trace	102	87	
			24h	115	34	63	1653	Absent	46	54	
P.R.	F	PKU	Cord	284	62	101	566	6	43	221[c]	PKU
			12h	136	45	70		18	46	324	
			24h	90	35	47			61	402	
Controls			Cord	123–341	30–100	71–226	317–551	10–36	52–91	58–109	
			6h	90–311	70–99	74–189	439–566	8–19	57–80	53–90	
			12h	94–300	31–98	55–208	383–664	10–26	52–122	49–104	
			24h	109–348	34–63	56–163	338–802	7–24	51–120	48–100	

Values are expressed in μmol L^{-1}; concentrations not specified are not available
[a] Specimens taken were cord blood and at 6, 12 and 24h of life
[b] Not explicable
[c] Maternal hyperphenylalaninaemia

RESULTS AND DISCUSSION

In the control population a progressive reduction of total AA plasma levels was observed (average values in μmol L^{-1} were: cord, 3893; at 6 h, 3434; at 12 h, 3556; at 24 h, 3212) and a more relevant reduction of essential AA levels (reported as percentage of total AA level) especially in the last specimen (cord, 33%; 6 h, 32%; 12 h, 30%; 24 h, 24%). Similarly the branched chain AA (BCAA)/aromatic AA and Phe/Tyr ratios were clearly lower at 24 h than in cord blood or at 6 h. Cys was present only in traces in cord blood and increases slowly to an average of 6.55 μmol L^{-1} at 24 h. The results for at-risk newborns are compared with the results in controls subjects in Table 1.

Patient L.M. is the second newborn of a family group at risk of MSUD (Romano *et al.*, 1985); the firstborn is affected. The diagnosis of MSUD in L.M. was prenatal. In this patient BCAA (specially Ile and Leu) were strongly increased at 12 and 24 h, whereas BCAA plasma levels are decreasing in normal newborns. On the basis of these data it was possible to start treatment from the 6th hour of life. The diagnosis of MSUD was confirmed by enzymatic assay on cultured fibroblasts (Kleijer, Rotterdam). In contrast, in the other two patients at risk of MSUD the BCAA pattern was comparable with the pattern observed in normal newborns. MSUD was excluded, in agreement with the results of prenatal enzymatic studies.

Patient C.D. was the third born (after two neonatal deaths and two spontaneous abortions) of a hyperphenylalaninaemic mother, who received a low Phe diet at conception (Romano *et al.*, 1986). The diet and the metabolic conditions were strictly controlled (plasma Phe levels under 300 μmol L^{-1}), but the early death of the first two babies and the main clinical manifestations presented were clearly suggestive of an inborn error of metabolism in its severe neonatal form; fetal damage in maternal PKU appeared untenable. In this patient Gln markedly increased and Cit decreased until it reached zero at 24 h when hyperammonaemia and clinical manifestations were not yet present. The diagnosis of carbamyl phosphate synthetase deficiency, proposed on the basis of these results and the absence of orotic aciduria, was confirmed by enzymatic assay on liver cells (Bachmann, Berne). The Phe level in cord blood was high, according with the maternal hyperphenylalaninaemia, but decreased immediately to normal values.

The last patient, P.R., sister of a PKU firstborn, daughter of a PKU mother (in strict dietary and biochemical control from the 11th week of pregnancy) and of a PKU heterozygote father (Romano *et al.*, in press), showed high Phe level in cord blood like the previous patient, but plasma Phe markedly increased in the course of the first 24 h of life. The diagnosis of classic PKU was established by the biochemical findings, the family history and urinary pterins excretion (basal and after BH$_4$ load).

CONCLUSIONS

Our experience suggests that in newborns at risk of specific aminoacidopathies, plasma AA measurements during the first 24 h of life offer the opportunity for early diagnosis and treatment and, in addition, appear a valid alternative to prenatal diagnosis; the correct treatment can be started before the onset of clinical manifestations.

Further data are presented here (Table 1) concerning the quantitative pattern of AA in plasma from normal subjects during the first hours of life; these data are useful in assessing the importance of metabolic abnormalities observed in newborn patients.

REFERENCES

Caruso, U., Roncari. S., Scalisi, S. and Romano, C. Programma pilota per lo screening multiplo delle aminoacidopatie e per la verifica dello Screening Regionale PKU: aspetti critici. In Romano, C., Cerone, R. and Caruso, U. (eds.) *Aminoacidopatie. Clinica, Biochimica Diagnosi Precoce, Terapia*, International Symposium, Rapallo, 15–19 March 1984. Milupa Medical Service Publishing

Cerone, R., Caruso, U., Roncari, S. and Romano, C. Multiple screening for aminoacidopathies using TLC: results from a pilot program. 6th National Neonatal Screening Symposium, Portland, Oregon, 22–25 May 1988

Romano, C., Cerone, C., Caruso, U., Gandolfo, A. and Cotellessa, M. Maple Syrup Urine Disease (MSUD): prenatal diagnosis vs branched chain aminoacids levels during the first two days of life. *Perspect. Metab. Dis.* 6, (1985) 121–124

Romano, C., Cerone, R., Borrone, C., Scalisi, S., Caruso, U. and Gatti, S. Maternal hyperphenylalaninaemia: dietary treatment during the pregnancy. *J. Inher. Metab. Dis.* 9 suppl. 2 (1986) 225–226

Romano, C., Cerone, R., Gandolfo, M. T., Schiaffino, M-C., Zignego, G. and Caruso, U. Congenital malformations in the infant of a PKU mother. SSIEM 26th Annual Symposium, Glasgow, 1988, Abstract P23

J. Inher. Metab. Dis. 12 Suppl. 2 (1989) 315–317

Short Communication

Perinatal Diagnosis of Type 1c Glycogen Storage Disease

A. BURCHELL[1], I. D. WADDELL[1], L. STEWART[1] and R. HUME[2]
[1]*Department of Medicine, Ninewells Hospital and Medical School, University of Dundee, Dundee, DD1 9SY;* [2]*Department of Child Health, University of Edinburgh, Edinburgh, EH3 9EF, UK*

Hepatic glucose-6-phosphatase (EC 3.1.3.9) is a multicomponent system comprised of the glucose-6-phosphatase enzyme situated in the lumen of the endoplasmic reticulum and three transport proteins which facilitate movement of glucose-6-phosphate (T_1), phosphate and pyrophosphate (T_2), and glucose (T_3) between the cytosol and the lumen of the endoplasmic reticulum. A deficiency of any of these four proteins will impair both glucose-6-phosphate hydrolysis and hepatic glucose production.

Type 1c glycogen storage disease is an inborn error of metabolism caused by a deficiency of T_2, the phosphate/pyrophosphate transport protein of the hepatic microsomal glucose-6-phosphatase system. We recently developed a new microtechnique for the diagnosis of type 1c glycogen storage disease (Burchell *et al.*, 1988) and here we describe the first perinatal diagnosis of type 1c glycogen storage disease.

CASE REPORT

Mrs F. presented for a routine antenatal visit at 37 weeks gestation. Her pregnancy had been complicated by mild pre-eclampsia and growth retardation in twin 2. Non-stressed cardiotocography showed loss of beat-to-beat variation, late deceleration culminating in prolonged bradycardia. Emergency Caesarian section delivered a normally grown male infant (twin 1) with Apgar scores of 9 and 9 at 1 and 5 min.

Twin 2 was growth retarded, weighed 2.2 kg (3rd centile); OFC 37 cm (<3rd centile); and length 39 cm (<3rd centile) with Apgar scores of 1 and 4 at 1 and 5 min. At 15 min of age the infant was aglycaemic and a dextrose infusion of $25 \, mg \, kg^{-1} min^{-1}$ was required to maintain blood sugars of 2–3 mmol L^{-1}. After 6 h the glucose infusion was reduced to $7 \, mg \, kg^{-1} min^{-1}$ and satisfactory blood sugar was maintained.

Investigations gave the following results: glucose <0.5 mmol L^{-1}; lactate 18.3 mmol L^{-1}; insulin <5 mu L^{-1}; cortisol 638 nmol L^{-1}; thyroxine 70 nmol L^{-1}; TSH 35.5 mu L^{-1}; plasma amino acids within normal limits. The clinical course was complicated by convulsions, renal and cardiac failure, and the infant died at 39 h of age. Postmortem revealed no developmental abnormalities but a grade II

315

Journal of Inherited Metabolic Disease. ISSN 0141–8955. Copyright © SSIEM and Kluwer Academic Publishers, PO Box 55, Lancaster, UK.

intraventricular haemorrhage and some degree of cerebral softening. Karotype 46 XX.

METHODS

Microsomes were prepared from human liver biopsy samples as described in Burchell *et al.* (1987). Glucose-6-phosphatase, mannose-6-phosphatase and pyrophosphatase activities were assayed and calculated as in Burchell *et al.* (1988) and expressed as $\mu mol\,(mg\ microsomal\ protein)^{-1}\,min^{-1}$. Microsomes were disrupted with histone 2A (Blair and Burchell, 1988). Immunoblot analysis was carried out as in Countaway *et al.* (1988) using antibodies monospecific for T_2 (Waddell *et al.*, 1988).

RESULTS AND DISCUSSION

The results of the kinetic characterisation of the hepatic microsomal glucose-6-phosphatase system in twin 2 and five age-matched control cases are shown in

Table 1   Glucose-6-phosphatase activity in human liver microsomes

Case	Intact microsomes		Disrupted microsomes	
------	V_{max}	K_m	V_{max}	K_m
Glucose-6-phosphate as substrate				
Twin 2	0.06	7.0	0.23	1.9
Controls	0.10±0.01	2.9±0.8	0.26±0.05	0.7±0.1
Pyrophosphate as substrate				
Twin 2	0	—	0.08	1.2
Controls	0.05±0.02	4.3±1.1	0.16	0.5±0.1

Control values are the mean ±SEM of values obtained from five age-matched human liver samples. V_{max} is expressed as units $mg^{-1}\,min^{-1}$ and K_m as $mmol\,L^{-1}$.

Table 1. Disruption of microsomes removes the controlling influence of the translocases and the disrupted values are a direct measure of the glucose-6-phosphatase enzyme which was normal in twin 2 (see Table 1). The activity of glucose-6-phosphatase in intact microsomes with pyrophosphate as substrate is a measure of the combined rate of T_2 and the enzyme (see Burchell *et al.*, 1987, for a much more detailed explanation). In twin 2 this activity is completely absent showing that T_2 is completely deficient.

In order to obtain further information about the nature of the deficiency in twin 2, immunoblot analysis was carried out using monospecific antibodies to the 37 kDa T_2 protein. The immunoblots revealed that normal levels of the 37 kDa T_2 protein were present in hepatic microsomes isolated from twin 2. This strongly suggests that the deficiency is caused by a point mutation or a very small deletion which does not change the protein's electrophoretic mobility. The deficiency is therefore quite different to the only other case of type 1c glycogen storage disease in which immunoblot analysis has been carried out where the T_2 was found to be absent (Burchell *et al.*, 1988).

In the perinatal period definitive diagnosis of genetic deficiencies can be very difficult as the lack of enzyme activity or in this case transport capacity could be due either to an inborn error of metabolism or merely to a delay in the normal development pattern of the protein. In this case the finding that the levels of the T_2 protein were normal for gestational age means that twin 2 does have type 1c glycogen storage disease.

This is the first description of the perinatal diagnosis of type 1c glycogen storage disease and it is likely that this infant was hypoglycaemic *in utero* and that the heart rate abnormalities were related to this.

ACKNOWLEDGEMENT

This work was supported by grants from the Scottish Hospitals Endowment Research Trust to A.B. and R.H. and the British Diabetic Association to A.B.

REFERENCES

Blair, J. N. R. and Burchell, A. The mechanism of histone activation of the hepatic microsomal glucose-6-phosphatase system: a novel method to assay glucose-6-phosphatase activity. *Biochim. Biophys. Acta* 964 (1988) 161–167

Burchell, A., Jung, R. T., Lang, C. C., Bennet, W. and Shepherd, A. N. Diagnosis of type Ia and Ic glycogen storage disease in adults. *Lancet* 1 (1987) 1059–1062

Burchell, A., Hume, R. and Burchell, B. A new microtechnique for the analysis of the human hepatic microsomal glucose-6-phosphatase system. *Clin. Chim. Acta* 173 (1988) 183–192

Countaway, J. L., Waddell, I. D., Burchell, A. and Arion, W. J. The phosphohydrolase component of the hepatic microsomal glucose-6-phosphatase system is a 36.5-kilodalton polypeptide. *J. Biol. Chem.* 263 (1988) 2673–2678

Waddell, I. D., Lindsay, J. G. and Burchell, A. The identification of T_2 the phosphate/pyrophosphate transport protein of the hepatic microsomal glucose-6-phosphatase system. *FEBS Lett.* 229 (1988) 179–182

J. Inher. Metab. Dis. 12 Suppl. 2 (1989) 318–320

Short Communication

A 'Blood Spot' Androstenedione Radioimmunoassay Able to Detect Congenital Adrenal Hyperplasia

S. THOMSON[1], A. M. WALLACE[2] and B. COOK[2]

[1]*Neonatal Screening Unit, Department of Bacteriology, Stobhill General Hospital, and* [2]*Institute of Biochemistry, Royal Infirmary, Glasgow, UK*

Most neonatal screening programmes for congenital adrenal hyperplasia (CAH) are based on the measurement of 17-hydroxyprogesterone in blood eluted from filter paper samples (Pang *et al.*, 1988). Androstenedione (A4) measurement may offer greater potential as a diagnostic aid because it should also detect the second most common form of CAH, 11β-hydroxylase deficiency. Unfortunately, most A4 immunoassays are too insensitive to allow large-scale neonatal screening for CAH using filter paper blood spot samples. We describe below a sensitive radioimmuno-assay (RIA) able to measure A4 in blood spot samples with or without prior solvent extraction.

MATERIALS AND METHODS

Production and selection of radioimmunoassay reagents: A study of RIA reagents, all prepared 'in house', allowed selection of an androstenedione–carboxymethylox-ime (A4-3CMO) [^{125}I]iodohistamine label with an antiserum raised in a rabbit against A4-3CMO:bovine serum albumin (BSA) for full evaluation (Thomson, 1986).

Blood spot standards: Ethanol was evaporated from a volume of ethanolic A4 stock solution. The residue was taken up in, and diluted by, a whole blood matrix (charcoal-stripped serum:packed red blood cells; 1:1 by volume) to give a series of standards (5.5–525 nmol L^{-1}). Drops of each of these standard solutions were spotted onto filter paper and dried.

Direct (non-extraction) radioimmunoassay procedure: Phosphate buffer (0.1 mol L^{-1}; pH 7.4) containing 2.5 g BSA, 9 g sodium chloride and 0.25 mg merthiolate per litre was used throughout. A disc (5 mm in diameter) was punched from filter paper cards for both standards and samples and blood eluted overnight at 22°C into 50 μL buffer. Iodinated A4-3CMO (200 μL containing 10 000 cpm) was added followed by 200 μL antibody solution. All tubes were mixed and incubated for 2 h at 22°C. Precipitating antibody (400 μL) was added, the contents mixed and incubated overnight at 4°C and the tubes were then centrifuged for 1 h at 4°C and 3000 rpm. The supernatant was carefully aspirated and the precipitate (antibody-bound fraction) counted on a gamma counter.

318

Journal of Inherited Metabolic Disease. ISSN 0141–8955. Copyright © SSIEM and Kluwer Academic Publishers, PO Box 55, Lancaster, UK.

Extraction radioimmunoassay procedure: This was performed as outlined above, except that after elution of blood into buffer, steroid was extracted into 3 mL hexane:ether (4:1 by volume) and the solvent evaporated.

Blood spot specimens: Analysis of A4 was performed prospectively on Guthrie card blood spot samples from one infant with CAH, from infants born at term or prematurely or with respiratory distress syndrome and retrospectively from patients with CAH.

RESULTS AND DISCUSSION

The selected reagents produced a sensitive RIA suitable for measuring A4 in samples from blood spots on Guthrie cards. The sensitivity (and working range) of the blood spot extraction and direct RIAs were 42 pg per 5 mm disc (4–525 nmol L^{-1}) and 52 pg per 5 mm disc (5–300 nmol L^{-1}), respectively. Over these ranges the mean inter-assay precision was <10 and <16%, respectively, for the extraction and direct methods.

Cross-reaction studies indicated good specificity. The major cross-reacting steroids were 5α-androstane-3,17-dione (40%), 1,4-androstadiene-3,17-dione (43%), 5β-androstane-3,17-dione (6%) and 4-androstene-3,11,17-trione (5%). All other steroids tested showed a cross reaction of <0.5%.

Concentrations of A4 in specimens from neonatal blood spots are shown in Table 1. A4 concentrations were higher in the direct compared to solvent extraction

Table 1 **Androstenedione concentrations (nmol L^{-1}) in neonatal blood spot samples measured by direct RIA and following solvent extraction**

| | RIA method | |
	Extraction	Direct
Term: number	85	106
mean (range)	7.2 (UD–22)	15.7 (UD–88)
99% confidence limits	<18	<61
Premature: number	90	110
mean (range)	12.9 (UD–117)	30.3 (UD–175)
99% confidence limits	<84	<152
Stressed: number	18	11
mean (range)	26.4 (5–70)	60.9 (18–157)
99% confidence limits	<55	ID
21-hydroxylase deficiency: number	8[a]	1[b]
mean (range)	198 (80–>525)	107
11β-hydroxylase deficiency: number	1[a]*	ND
mean	91	ID

UD = undectable, ID = insufficient data for statistical analysis; ND = not determined.
[a]Retrospective analysis; [b]prospective analysis.
*This boy was diagnosed at age 4 after development of precocious puberty. Blood spot determination was performed retrospectively 12 years after sampling.

assay indicating possible interference from steroid conjugates that are not solvent extractable. Similar findings obtained earlier showed that 17-hydroxyprogesterone was higher in directly assayed samples than in samples determined after solvent extraction (Wallace *et al.*, 1986). Elevated A4 concentrations were found in some samples from infants born prematurely or suffering from respiratory distress syndrome. Grossly elevated concentrations were found in cases of 21-hydroxylase deficiency and in one case of 11β-hydroxylase deficiency. The case of 11β-hydroxylase deficiency remained undiagnosed until the age of 4 years when signs of precocious puberty became apparent. In this case measurement of A4 on a blood spot filter paper sample collected soon after birth was performed 12 years after sampling.

Our study suggests that neonatal screening for both 21-hydroxylase and 11β-hydroxylase deficiencies by measuring A4 in blood spots (direct screening assay followed by confirmation of elevated levels by measurement after solvent extraction) is possible using the reagents described above.

REFERENCES

Pang, S., Wallace, A. M., Hofman, L., Thuline, H., Dorche, C., Lyon, I. C., Dobbins, H., Kling, S., Fujieda, K. and Suwa, S. Worldwide experience in newborn screening for classical congenital adrenal hyperplasia due to 21-hydroxylase deficiency. *Pediatrics* 81 (1988) 866–874

Thomson, S. Studies on a novel androstenedione radioimmunoassay and its application to the neonatal detection of congenital adrenal hyperplasia. Fellowship Thesis, 1986, Institute of Medical Laboratory Sciences

Wallace, A. M., Beastall, G. H., Cook, B., Currie, A. J., Ross, A. M., Kennedy, R. and Girdwood, R. W. A. Neonatal screening for congenital adrenal hyperplasia: a programme based on a novel direct radioimmunoassay for 17-hydroxyprogesterone in blood spots. *J. Endocrinol.* 108 (1986) 299–308

J. Inher. Metab. Dis. 12 Suppl. 2 (1989) 321–324

Short Communication

Generalised Dicarboxylic Aciduria: A Common Finding in Neonates

M. Downing[1], P. Rose[1], M. J. Bennett[1], N. J. Manning[2] and R. J. Pollitt[2]
[1]*Department of Chemical Pathology and* [2]*University Department of Paediatrics, Children's Hospital, Sheffield S10 2TH, UK*

Inborn errors of organic acid metabolism presenting with sudden onset hypoglycaemia in association with infection or prolonged fasting have been shown to account for a proportion of sudden infant deaths (SID) (Howat *et al.*, 1985; Anonymous, 1986). In the most common of these disorders, medium-chain acyl-CoA dehydrogenase deficiency (MCADD; McKusick 20145), abnormal organic acids are excreted, including medium chain-length dicarboxylic acids (adipic, suberic and sebacic) and glycine conjugates of hexanoic and suberic acid (Gregersen *et al.*, 1983). While usually prominent only during hypoglycaemic attacks, these characteristic abnormal metabolites have been seen during the first week of life (Bennett *et al.*, 1987), probably reflecting the switch to fatty acids as an energy source that occurs soon after birth.

MCADD is inherited in an autosomal recessive mode (Coates *et al.*, 1985) with a one in four risk of recurrence in siblings of affected infants. We are, therefore, investigating the possibility that the examination of urinary organic acids could be used to detect MCADD in newborn siblings of children who have died suddenly without obvious cause.

MATERIALS AND METHODS

Random urine samples were collected onto cotton wool balls during the first five days of life from siblings of SID patients, along with similar samples from matched controls born on the same day in the same unit. Organic acids were extracted from 1 mL urine using ethyl acetate and diethyl ether after addition of an internal standard of heptadecanoic acid (75 μg). Trimethylsilyl derivatives were produced using BSTFA-pyridine and analysed by gas chromatography using capillary columns and a flame ionization detector. The identities of compounds were confirmed by gas chromatography-mass spectrometry.

Calibration curves for adipate and suberate were made by enriching normal urine. The standards were analysed as for sample urines. Sample concentrations were calculated as μmol (mmol creatinine)$^{-1}$.

Frequency histograms of adipate and suberate concentrations in subjects' urine showed obvious deviation from normality. Data were, therefore, normalized by the use of logarithmic values.

Journal of Inherited Metabolic Disease. ISSN 0141–8955. Copyright © SSIEM and Kluwer Academic Publishers, PO Box 55, Lancaster, UK.

RESULTS AND DISCUSSION

There have been several studies of urinary organic acids in newborns (Thompson *et al.*, 1977; Bjorkman *et al.*, 1976; Gregersen *et al.*, 1977; Alm *et al.*, 1978). Bjorkman and colleagues (1976) tentatively identified hydroxylated aliphatic dicarboxylic acids as a normal finding in urine in the first 24 h of life but to our knowledge there have been no further data published on this.

To date we have studied the urinary organic acid profile in the first 5 days of life in 180 subjects (147 siblings of cases of SID and 33 matched controls). Of these 37 (30 siblings and seven controls) showed varying amounts of hydroxylated dicarboxylic acids as part of a profile of 'moderate generalised dicarboxylic aciduria' (Figure

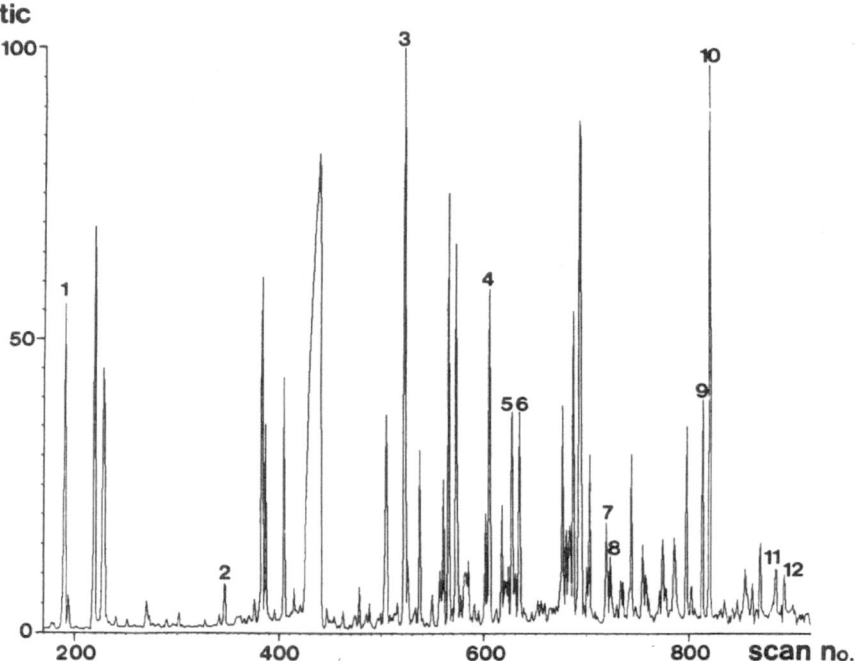

Figure 1 GC–MS total ion current trace showing moderate generalized dicarboxylic aciduria in a 1-day-old child. The peaks are: 1, 3-hydroxybutyric acid; 2, ethylmalonic acid; 3, adipic acid; 4, lactone of 3-hydroxyadipic acid; 5, octenedioic acid; 6, suberic acid; 7, 3-hydroxyoctenedioic acid; 8, 3-hydroxysuberic acid; 9, 3-hydroxysebacic acid; 10, internal standard; 11, 3-hydroxydodecenedioic acid; 12, 3-hydroxydodecanedioic acid

1). This profile usually included ethylmalonic, adipic, suberic and octenedioic acids as well as 3-hydroxy-adipic, suberic and sebacic acids. Glycine conjugates were not observed. The concentration of adipic acid ranged from 1.5–150 μmol (mmol creatinine)$^{-1}$ with a log mean ± 1 SD of 27 ± 2 μmol (mmol creatinine)$^{-1}$ while the concentration of suberic acid ranged from not detected to 81 μmol (mmol creatinine)$^{-1}$ with a log mean of 15 ± 2 μmol (mmol creatinine)$^{-1}$. These concentrations were comparable to those previously published. The median and logarithmic mean values were in good agreement, 26 and 27 μmol (mmol creatinine)$^{-1}$ for adipate and 16 and 15 μmol (mmol creatinine)$^{-1}$ for suberate, respectively. In general the highest excretions were seen in the day 1 samples.

In view of the 20% incidence of moderate generalized dicarboxylic aciduria and its equal distribution between suspect and control groups, we conclude that this is a harmless anomaly reflecting some immaturity of the fatty acid β-oxidation pathway.

This 'moderate generalized dicarboxylic aciduria' is clearly different to the profile during the first week of life in two affected siblings of known cases of MCADD. The first of these subjects was diagnosed prenatally (Bennet *et al.*, 1987) and urine analysed on the first day of life showed an adipate of 132 μmol (mmol creatinine)$^{-1}$ and a suberate of 214 μmol (mmol creatinine)$^{-1}$. Quantitation was not possible for the second subject but suberate gave a peak height more than twice that of adipate. In both cases hexanoylglycine was also present. The predominance of suberate over adipate in MCADD babies when clinically well was also observed by Gregersen *et al.* (1983).

We have recently diagnosed MCADD in a sibling of a SID case who unfortunately was not enrolled on our scheme. Urine was analysed at 6 weeks of age when the infant was well. The characteristic pattern was observed with an adipate of 5 μmol (mmol creatinine)$^{-1}$, a suberate of 21 μmol (mmol creatinine)$^{-1}$ (much lower concentrations than those seen in the first week of life in our prenatally diagnosed subject) and the presence of hexanoylglycine and suberylglycine. The diagnosis of MCADD was confirmed by a positive phenylpropionic acid load test*.

A further subject with a family history of an unidentified fatty acid oxidation defect also produced a recognisably abnormal profile.

We conclude from this study that neonates frequently show urinary organic acid profiles that would cause concern in older children. However, in looking for evidence of fatty acid oxidation defects in the neonatal period a qualitative assessment of the overall pattern is much more important than quantitation of individual metabolites.

ACKNOWLEDGEMENTS

We thank the Foundation for the Study of Infant Death for financial support (project no. 91) and the staff of the Sheffield Child Development Study for coordinating the sample collection. R.J.P. is a member of the external scientific staff of the MRC.

REFERENCES

Alm, J., Hagenfeldt, L. and Larsson, A. Concentrations of organic acids in the urine of healthy newborn children. *Ann. Clin. Biochem.* 15 (1978) 245–249

Anonymous. Sudden infant death and inherited metabolic disease. *Lancet* 2 (1986) 1073–1075

Bennett, M. J., Allison, F., Pollitt, R. J., Manning, N. J., Gray, R. G. F., Green,

A., Hale, D. E. and Coates, P. M. Prenatal diagnosis of medium-chain acyl-CoA dehydrogenase deficiency in a family with sudden infant death. *Lancet* 1 (1987) 440–441

Bjorkman, L., McLean, C. and Steen, G. Organic acids in urine from human newborns. *Clin. Chem.* 22 (1976) 49–52

Coates, P. M., Hale, D. E., Stanley, C. A., Corkey, B. E., Hall, C. L. and Cortner, J. A. Genetic deficiency of MCAD; studies in cultured skin fibroblasts and peripheral mononuclear leukocytes. *Pediatr. Res.* 19 (1985) 671–676

Gregersen, N.. Ingerslev, J. and Rasmussen, K. Low molecular weight organic acids in the urine of the newborn. *Acta Paediatr. Scand.* 66 (1977) 85–89

Gregersen, N., Kølvraa, S., Rasmussen, K., Mortensen, P. B., Divry, P., David, M. and Hobloth, N. General (medium-chain) acyl-CoA dehydrogenase deficiency (non-ketotic dicarboxylic aciduria): quantitative urinary excretion pattern of 23 biologically significant metabolites in three cases. *Clin. Chim. Acta* 132 (1983) 181–191

Howat, A. J., Bennett, M. J., Variend, S., Shaw, L. and Engel, P. C. Defects of metabolism of fatty acids in the sudden infant death syndrome. *Br. Med. J.* 290 (1985) 1771–1773

Thompson, J. A., Miles, B. S. and Fennessey, P. V. Urinary organic acids quantitated by age groups in a healthy pediatric population. *Clin. Chem.* 23 (1977) 1734–1738

NOTE ADDED IN PROOF

It transpires that a single urine specimen collected from this patient on the day of birth was passed as normal on examination by GC only. Dicarboxylic acids were present only in trace amounts.

J. Inher. Metab. Dis. 12 Suppl. 2 (1989) 325–328

Short Communication

Comparison of Urinary Acylglycines and Acylcarnitines as Diagnostic Markers of Medium-chain Acyl-CoA Dehydrogenase Deficiency

P. Rinaldo[1], J. J. O'Shea[1], S. I. Goodman[2], L. V. Miller[2], P. V. Fennessey[2], D. T. Whelan[3], R. E. Hill[3] and K. Tanaka[1]*

[1]*Department of Human Genetics, Yale University School of Medicine, New Haven, CT 06510, USA;* [2]*Department of Pediatrics, University of Colorado School of Medicine, Denver, CO 80262, USA;* [3]*Departments of Pediatrics and Pathology, McMaster University School of Medicine, Hamilton, Ontario L8N 3Z5, Canada*

At least eight inborn errors of mitochondrial fatty acid β-oxidation are currently known. In the span of the last few years, almost 200 patients suffering from one of these disorders have been diagnosed (Vianey-Liaud *et al.*, 1987), and some of them were initially mistaken as Reye's or sudden infant death syndrome. Since the prognosis of these patients can be greatly improved by treatment with available therapeutic measures, fast and accurate diagnosis of this group of diseases is crucial. In reality, however, the diagnosis has been difficult for many of these disorders (Editorial in *Lancet*, 1986).

Among the inborn errors of mitochondrial fatty acid oxidation, the incidence of medium-chain acyl-CoA dehydrogenase (MCAD) deficiency (McKusick 22274) is by far the highest (Vianey-Liaud *et al.*, 1987), and the vast majority of the cases mentioned above were affected with this disease. Until recently, the diagnosis of this disease by metabolite analysis has been difficult since no appropriate diagnostic markers were known. The diagnosis of MCAD deficiency has been possible only by acyl-CoA dehydrogenase assays. However, all these enzymatic assays are complex and time-consuming, and they are available only in a few laboratories. The need for fast and reliable methods, which are useful for the diagnosis of this dangerous and elusive disease of childhood, has been strongly advocated (Editorial in *Lancet*, 1986).

A few years ago, medium-chain acylcarnitines were detected in urine from a number of MCAD deficient patients during acute episodes using fast atom bombardment–mass spectrometry (FAB/MS) (Millington *et al.*, 1984), and have been considered by some investigators to be specific markers for the diagnosis of MCAD deficiency. However, the reliability of acylcarnitines as markers for MCAD

*Correspondence

Journal of Inherited Metabolic Disease. ISSN 0141–8955. Copyright © SSIEM and Kluwer Academic Publishers, PO Box 55, Lancaster, UK.

deficiency has not been systematically tested. Particularly, their excretion in asymptomatic patients has not been adequately studied.

Recently, we have accurately determined the amount of urinary *n*-hexanoyl-glycine (HG), 3-phenylpropionylglycine (PPG) and suberylglycine (SG) by gas chromatography–mass spectrometry (GC/MS) stable isotope dilution analysis in 54 urine specimens from 21 proved MCAD deficient patients and 99 specimens from appropriate controls, and demonstrated that HG and PPG are highly specific markers for MCAD deficiency, whereas SG was somewhat less specific (Rinaldo *et al.*, 1988).

In the present study, we compared the reliability of these two methods for the diagnosis of MCAD deficiency. We report here the result of a preliminary study of 12 MCAD deficient patients, three patients with glutaric aciduria type II (GAII)/ethylmalonic–adipic aciduria (EMA) and nine other controls. Thirty-four urine specimens from these children were analysed for both acylglycines and acylcarnitines using GC/MS stable isotope dilution analysis and FAB/MS, respectively.

MATERIALS AND METHODS

Samples: We analysed 18 urine specimens from 12 proved MCAD deficient patients, five specimens from three GAII or EMA patients and 11 samples from nine controls with dicarboxylic aciduria. All cases of MCAD deficiency and GAII/EMA were confirmed by MCAD assay (performed by Drs Daniel Hale and Paul Coates, Children's Hospital of Philadelphia; Coates *et al.*, 1985) or ETF/ETF dehydrogenase assay. Twelve of the MCAD deficiency samples were from eleven patients, who were clinically asymptomatic at the time of urine collection; four of them were under treatment with carnitine ($80–100\,mg\,kg^{-1}\,day^{-1}$). The remaining six urine specimens were from five patients, who were in acute stage of illness at the time of collection. Control urine specimens included four normal infants fed with medium-chain triglycerides-supplemented formula. Other controls were specimens from one patient with long-chain acyl-CoA dehydrogenase deficiency, two children with non-specific ketosis and two patients with recurrent episodes of hypoketotic hypoglycaemia. In the last two patients, long-, medium- and short-chain acyl-CoA dehydrogenase activities were normal in cultured fibroblasts.

Methods: HG, PPG and SG were quantitatively determined at Yale by the GC/MS stable isotope dilution method (Rinaldo *et al.*, 1988). Qualitative identification of urinary hexanoylcarnitine (HC) and octanoylcarnitine (OC) was performed at Denver in eight of the MCAD deficiency samples and all of the GAII/EMA and control specimens by FAB/MS according to the method of Roe *et al.* (1986). Acylcarnitine identification in the other MCAD deficiency samples was carried out at Hamilton by FAB/MS and collision activated decomposition mass analysed ion kinetic energy (CAD MIKE) analysis (Kondrat and Cooks, 1978) of the molecular ion fragmentation patterns (R. E. Hill, unpublished method).

Thirteen MCAD deficiency samples were first analysed for acylcarnitine excretion by FAB/MS or FAB/MS–CAD MIKE to determine their acylcarnitine profiles.

The remaining five were first tested for acylglycine using the stable isotope dilution analysis. In either case, the specimens were sent from the first laboratory to the second in a blind fashion, and the second analysis was performed with no knowledge of either the patients' diagnosis or the previous test results.

RESULTS

Urinary acylglycines: The stable isotope dilution analysis of HG, PPG, and SG was unambiguously diagnostic in all the MCAD deficiency samples (Table 1). As we demonstrated previously (Rinaldo *et al.*, 1988), the amounts of these acylglycines in urine from all the MCAD deficient patients were significantly higher than controls. They were smaller in asymptomatic patients than in those in acute episodes, but were not significantly different with or without prolonged L-carnitine treatment. The lowest values of HG, PPG and SG were five, three and six times higher than the mean of the respective control values. HG and SG were also increased in urine specimens from GAII and EMA patients. In contrast, PPG excretion in these samples was in the normal range. No false positive results were observed in any of the controls.

Table 1 **Diagnostic specificity of acylglycines and acylcarnitines urinary excretion in 12 MCAD deficient patients**

Clinical Conditions	No. of patients	No. of samples	Acylglycines[a] +	−	Acylcarnitines[b] +	−
Acute episodes	5	6	6	0	4	2
Asymptomatic periods						
without carnitine treatment	8	8	8	0	5	3
with carnitine treatment	3	4	4	0	2	2

[a]Diagnosis made by the quantitative determination of *n*-hexanoylglycine, 3-phenylpropionyl-glycine and suberylglycine using GC/MS stable isotope dilution: (+) positively identified; and (−) missed. A sample was considered (+) when the excretion of all three metabolites was at least 2 SD above the mean of the respective normal values.
[b]Diagnosis made by the qualitative identification of hexanoylcarnitine and octanoylcarnitine using FAB/MS: (+) positively identified; and (−) missed. Judgement of (+) was visually made when the height of HC and OC protonated ions at m/z 274 and 302, respectively, were clearly higher than the surrounding signal background.

Urinary acylcarnitines: Eleven of 18 urine specimens from MCAD deficient patients were unambiguously identified by FAB/MS detection of HC and OC, but the diagnosis was missed by this method in the remaining seven urine samples. In these negative FAB mass spectra, the protonated molecular ions of HC and OC were not significantly higher than the backgrounds. Negative results were also obtained in two of the six samples collected during acute episodes. Both of them were from one of the patients who did not excrete an increased amount of acylcarnitines when she was clinically asymptomatic. In all of the urine samples from GAII and EMA, a greatly increased amount of HC was detected. The amount of OC was also increased in all of the samples with a single exception. In most of the other control urine samples, HC and OC ions were not detectable. In one of the normal controls, a signal at m/z 302 (for octanoylcarnitine) was visible, but it was correctly judged negative, since its intensity was low.

DISCUSSION

Under the experimental protocol employed, the quantitative acylglycine determination using the stable isotope dilution method was more reliable than the qualitative acylcarnitine detection by FAB/MS, with or without CAD MIKE analysis, for the diagnosis of MCAD deficiency. While all of the 18 specimens from 12 MCAD deficient patients were accurately diagnosed by the acylglycine analysis, seven (from four patients) of these 18 specimens were missed by the acylcarnitine analysis by FAB/MS.

The apparent lower accuracy of urinary acylcarnitine identification is probably due to the fluctuating concentration of free carnitine that is available for acylation in patients' tissues. In contrast, the tissue glycine concentration is constantly maintained at much higher levels, ensuring its adequate supply for acylation. Thus, the urinary acylglycine excretion was significantly increased in all the MCAD deficiency samples, so that unambiguous diagnosis of MCAD deficiency was possible regardless of the patient conditions.

ACKNOWLEDGEMENT

We thank Drs Daniel E. Hale and Paul M. Coates for making their enzyme assay data available for this study. This work was supported by grants from NIH (DK29911) and March of Dimes (1-378). P.R. was supported in part by a James Hudson Brown–Alexander B. Coxe Fellowship from Yale University School of Medicine.

REFERENCES

Coates, P. M., Hale, D. E., Stanley, C. A., Corkey, B. E. and Cortner, J. A. Genetic deficiency of medium-chain acyl-coenzyme A dehydrogenase: Studies in cultured skin fibroblasts and peripheral mononuclear leukocytes. *Pediatr. Res.* 19 (1985) 671–676
Editorial. Sudden infant death and inherited disorders of fat oxidation. *Lancet* 2 (1986) 1073–1075
Kondrat, R. W. and Cooks, R. G. Direct analysis of mixtures by mass spectrometry. *Anal. Chem.* 50 (1978) 81A–92A
Millington, D. S., Roe, C. R. and Maltby, D. A. Application of high resolution fast atom bombardment and constant B/E linked scanning to the identification and analysis of acylcarnitine in metabolic disease. *Biomed. Mass Spectrom.* 11 (1984) 236–241
Roe, C. R., Millington, D. S., Maltby, D. A. and Kinnebrew, P. Recognition of medium chain acyl-CoA dehydrogenase deficiency in asymptomatic siblings of children dying of sudden infant death or Reye-like syndromes. *J. Pediatr.* 108 (1986) 13–18
Rinaldo, P., O'Shea, J. J., Coates, P. M., Hale, D. E., Stanley, C. A. and Tanaka, K. Medium chain acyl-CoA dehydrogenase deficiency: Diagnosis by stable isotope dilution measurement of urinary n-hexanoylglycine and 3-phenylpropionylglycine. *N. Engl. J. Med.* 319 (1988) 1308–1313
Vianey-Liaud, C., Divry, P., Gregersen, N. and Matthieu, M. The inborn errors of mitochondrial fatty acid oxidation. *J. Inher. Metab. Dis.* 10 Suppl. 1 (1987) 159–198

J. Inher. Metab. Dis. 12 Suppl. 2 (1989) 329–331

Short Communication – SSIEM Award

Aspartoacylase Deficiency: The Enzyme Defect in Canavan Disease

R. MATALON[1], R. KAUL[1], J. CASANOVA[1], K. MICHALS[1], A. JOHNSON[2],
I. RAPIN[2], P. GASHKOFF[1] and M. DEANCHING[1]
[1]*Department of Pediatrics, University of Illinois, Chicago, Illinois, USA 60612;*
[2]*Albert Einstein College of Medicine, NY, USA*

Spongy degeneration of the brain, Canavan disease (CD; McKusick 27190) is an autosomal recessive leukodystrophy (van Bogaert and Bertrand, 1967). Recently, Matalon *et al.* (1988) have reported three children with CD who had excessive amounts of *N*-acetylaspartic acid (NAA) in urine, blood and brain, and deficiency of aspartoacylase (EC 3.5.1.15) in cultured skin fibroblasts and brain. We have expanded our studies to other children with CD and patients with leukodystrophies other than CD. In addition, we have purified aspartoacylase from human and bovine brain and studied the distribution of aspartoacylase and NAA in brain.

MATERIALS AND METHODS

Twenty-one patients with CD were studied, 14 of whom had a confirmed diagnosis of spongy degeneration by brain biopsy or autopsy. Individuals with other leukodystrophies that were studied included two patients with Alexander's disease (confirmed by brain biopsy), three with metachromatic leukodystrophy, one with Krabbe's disease, one with adrenoleukodystrophy and three with undiagnosed leukodystrophies. Forty-two age-matched controls and sixteen obligate carriers were also studied. Aspartoacylase activity was determined as described previously (Matalon *et al.*, 1988) with slight modifications of the method of Hagenfeldt *et al.* (1987), using Tris buffer, pH 8.0. At the termination of the aspartoacylase reaction, 2-oxoglutarate, NADH, malate dehydrogenase and aspartate aminotransferase were added to each assay tube. The decrease of absorbance at 340 nm by the conversion of NADH to NAD indicated the amount of aspartic acid released by aspartoacylase (Hagenfeldt *et al.*, 1987).

N-Acetylaspartic acid was determined according to the method of Goodman and Markey (1981), using gas chromatography–mass spectroscopy of the silylated compounds (Matalon *et al.*, 1988). Cells from patients and controls were cultivated in Matalon's modified Eagle's medium (Gibco, Grand Island, NY) according to the method described by Matalon and Dorfman (1966). Aspartoacylase purification, localization of NAA and aspartoacylase activity were carried out on human and bovine brains.

Journal of Inherited Metabolic Disease. ISSN 0141–8955. Copyright © SSIEM and Kluwer Academic Publishers, PO Box 55, Lancaster, UK.

RESULTS AND DISCUSSION

Canavan disease is a serious neurodegenerative disease associated with hypotonia, megalencephaly, mental retardation and early death (van Bogaert and Bertrand 1967). The disease is prevalent among Ashkenazi Jews. Three variants of CD, congenital, infantile and late onset, have been reported. The enzyme defect in CD has recently been reported (Matalon *et al.*, 1988). However, a large sample of patients with CD was needed in order to ascertain the specificity of these findings to CD and not to other leukodystrophies. Of the twenty-one patients with CD that we studied, 14 had brain biopsy or autopsy confirming the findings of spongy degeneration of the brain. All individuals had excessive urinary NAA excretion, almost 200 times the amounts found in normal age-matched individuals or obligate carriers for CD (Table 1). The ten patients with leukodystrophies other than CD

Table 1   Estimation of *N*-acetylaspartic acid in urine and aspartoacylase activity in cultured skin fibroblasts

	N-Acetylaspartic acid (μmol/mmol creatinine)	Aspartoacylase (mU/mg protein)
Canavan disease	3068.2±1841.0 ($n = 21$)	0.030±0.019 ($n = 11$)
Obligate carriers (CD)	trace ($n = 16$)	0.117±0.042 ($n = 18$)
Controls, normal	trace ($n = 42$)	0.438±0.093 ($n = 28$)
Leukodystrophies:		
Alexander's disease	trace ($n = 2$)	NA
Metachromatic leukodystrophy	trace ($n = 3$)	NA
Krabbe's disease	trace ($n = 1$)	NA
Adrenoleukodystrophy	trace ($n = 1$)	NA
Unidentified leukodystrophies	trace ($n = 3$)	NA

NA = not available
Trace = less than 10 μmol/mmol creatinine

did not have increased levels of NAA in urine. The patients with Alexander's disease, who have megalencephaly similar to patients with CD, had normal levels of NAA. Levels of NAA in CD patients were also elevated in plasma (11.7 μmol/L). One sample of CSF from a CD patient contained 232 μmol/L of NAA, while, in a control sample, NAA was undetectable. Deficiency of aspartoacylase was found in all of our CD patients (Table 1). The levels of aspartoacylase in obligate carriers were less than 50% of the control values.

N-Acetylaspartic acid is a compound found in abundance in normal human brain (3.9 μmol/mg protein) and it is found at high levels in the CD brain (20.2 μmol/mg protein). The function of this compound is not understood. *N*-Acetylaspartic aciduria has been reported by Hagenfeldt *et al.* (1987) and Kvittingen *et al.* (1986). A brother and a sister with *N*-acetylaspartic aciduria were also presented at the symposium of the SSIEM at Sheffield in September 1987 (Divry *et al.*, 1988). In the case of Kvittingen, aspartoacylase was normal, while, in the case of Hagenfeldt, aspartoacylase was deficient. In the Divry presentation, no enzyme data were available. Our findings clearly establish a defect with a specific brain pathology.

Aspartoacylase was purified to homogeneity from human and bovine brain (Kaul, R. and Matalon, R. unpublished data). Based on SDS gel electrophoresis, we have established the molecular weight of this enzyme at 58 kDa. Sections of human brain showed that the enzyme activity is primarily in white matter, 1.25–1.42 mU/mg protein, while grey matter had less activity, 0.04–0.22 mU/mg protein. The substrate, NAA, is abundant in grey matter, 0.46 μmol/mg protein, while white matter contained 0.16 μmol/mg protein. A similar distribution was found in bovine brain, indicating similar function in both species. Based on these studies, CD can be diagnosed enzymatically, carriers can be identified and prenatal diagnosis should be possible for at-risk pregnancies. Further studies on aspartoacylase and NAA in the brain may aid in our understanding of the function of NAA.

REFERENCES

van Bogaert, L. and Bertrand, I. *Spongy Degeneration of Brain in Infancy*. North Holland, Amsterdam, 1967, pp. 3–132

Divry, P., Vianey-Liaud, C., Gay, C., Macabeo, V., Rapin, F. and Echenne, B. *N*-Acetylaspartic aciduria: report of three new cases in children with a neurological syndrome associating macrocephaly and leucodystrophy *J. Inher. Metab. Dis.* 11 (1988) 307–308

Goodman, S. I. and Markey, S. P. *Diagnosis of Organic Acidemias by Gas Chromatography–Mass Spectrometry*. Alan R. Liss, New York, 1981, pp. 3–24

Hagenfeldt, L., Bollgren, I. and Venizelos, N. *N*-Acetylaspartic aciduria due to aspartoacylase deficiency – a new etiology of childhood leukodystrophy. *J. Inher. Metab. Dis.* 10 (1987) 135–141

Kvittingen, E. A., Guldal, G., Borsting, S., Skalpe, I. O., Stokke, O. and Jellum, E. *N*-Acetylaspartic aciduria in a child with a progressive cerebral atrophy. *Clin. Chim. Acta* 158 (1986) 217–227

Matalon, R. and Dorfman, A. Hurler's syndrome: Biosynthesis of acid mucopolysaccharides in tissue culture. *Proc. Nat. Acad. Sci. USA* 56 (1966) 1310–1316

Matalon, R., Michals, K., Sebesta, D., Deanching, M., Gashkoff, P. and Casanova, J. Aspartoacylase deficiency and *N*-acetylaspartic aciduria in patients with Canavan disease. *Am. J. Med. Genet.* 29 (1988) 463–471

J. Inher. Metab. Dis. 12 Suppl. 2 (1989) 332–334

Short Communication

Iatrogenic Skin Lesions in Phenylketonuric Children due to a Low Tyrosine Intake

B. François[1,3], M. Diels[1] and M. de la Brassinne[2]
[1]*Dr L. Willems Institute, B3600 Diepenbeek;* [2]*Department of Dermatology;*
[3]*Department of Human Genetics, Liège University, B4000 Liège, Belgium*

There is now convincing evidence that early institution of a phenylalanine-restricted diet is effective in the prevention of severe mental deficits in patients with phenylketonuria (McKusick 26160). The usual treatment goal has been to achieve a strict control of serum phenylalanine (phe) levels below 600 μmol/L during early childhood. However, a gradual liberalization of the diet has been proposed thereafter to minimize the psychologic stress during school age. As a result of this situation, the phe levels rise up to 800–1000 μmol/L. In addition, there is some convincing evidence that the conversion of tyrosine (tyr) to melanin, dopamine and norepinephrine is decreased by high blood concentrations of phenylalanine (Nadler and Hsai, 1961). More recently, reports of the benefits of tyr supplementations, in preventing neurodysfunction following diet discontinuation, have stressed the central role of this amino acid in the treatment of phenylketonuric (PKU) patients (Güttler and Lou, 1986). On the other hand, various skin lesions, mainly xerosis and follicular hyperkeratosis, are frequently observed and seem to be related to a decrease in compliance in older PKU children (Fisch *et al.*, 1981). This study was therefore undertaken to examine (1) whether the tyrosine intake, under the condition of a more liberal diet, fits the daily requirement of the PKU patients and (2) whether there is any correlation between the tyrosine intake and the skin lesions.

METHODS

During the last two years, a group of 37 patients with classical phenylketonuria, aged 6–22 years old (mean 12±4 y), was regularly monitored at least twice a year, including clinical examination and evaluation of the nutritional intake. All patients remained on a diet with a phenylalanine intake less than 700–800 mg/day and supplementation of amino acids via a concentrated amino acids mixture: PKU2®, Maxamum®, or Aminogran®. Blood amino acids levels were monitored every 3 weeks on an amino acid analyser (LKB 4400). Skin lesions were systematically recorded and the patients were divided into two groups, according to the presence or absence of skin lesions. The amino acids content of a commercial amino acids mixture was also determined under various dilutions. 200 mg of powder was dissolved in 2, 10, 20 or 100 ml of a lithium buffer (pH 2.8, 0.2 mmol/L). 1 ml was further diluted in the same buffer and 60 μl was injected into the column.

Journal of Inherited Metabolic Disease. ISSN 0141–8955. Copyright © SSIEM and Kluwer Academic Publishers, PO Box 55, Lancaster, UK.

RESULTS AND DISCUSSION

All patients of group 1 ($n = 24$) displayed skin xerosis and perifollicular hyperkeratosis which has been demonstrated by skin surface biopsy to be of the orthokeratotic type (Figure 1). There is a good correlation between the presence of skin lesions and the plasma phe:tyr ratio. All but one of group 1 displayed a ratio higher than 10, and, by contrast, all patients of group 2 ($n = 13$) displayed a significant lower

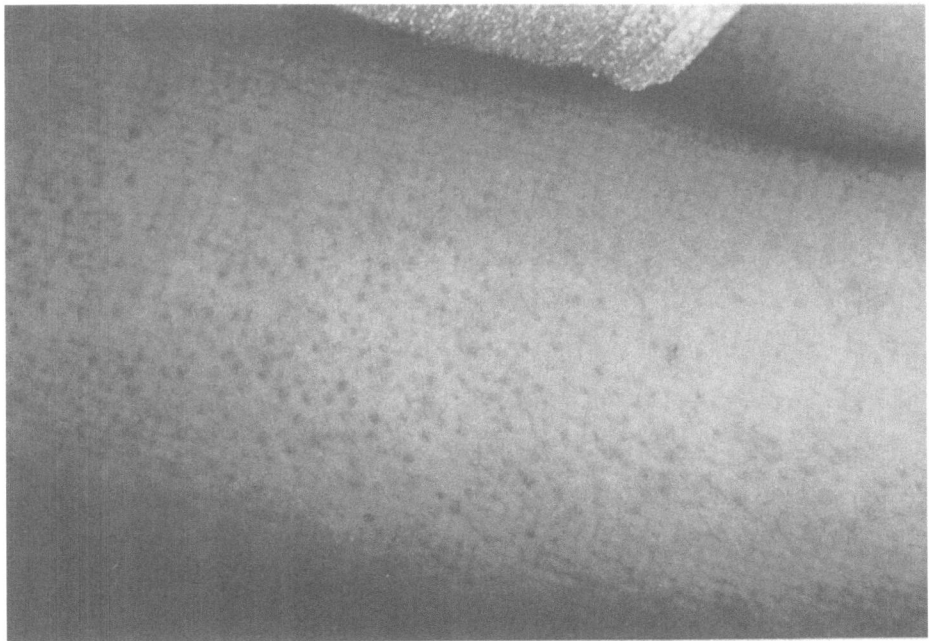

Figure 1   Follicular hyperkeratosis on the outer side of the arm

ratio ($p<0.005$). Careful examination of the home habits revealed that the patients received the amino acids mixture in a minimal volume of liquid (20% v/v). In those conditions, the concentration of 4 amino acids (aspartic acid, glutamine, cystine and tyrosine) are under the theoretical solubility rate in water. We found that 15% of the tyr is in solution with a dilution of 1/10 (29% for 1/50 and 38% for 1/100) and most of this amino acid remains in the bottom of the receptacle. A dilution of 1/500 would be necessary to bring all amino acids in solution. Taking into account these data and the difficulties for a PKU child to completely drink the amino acids mixture, we could estimate the real tyrosine intake in the group 1 patients at $18.8\pm6.9\,\mathrm{mg\,kg^{-1}\,day^{-1}}$ instead of $67.9\pm26.3\,\mathrm{mg\,kg^{-1}\,day^{-1}}$ as theoretically prescribed. These values are far below the RDS value for tyr. Although we still do not know the exact relationship between tyr and the skin lesions, they regressed after a 6-month supplementation of L-tyrosine tablets (30 mg/kg body weight).

These data suggest that the use of a highly concentrated amino acids mixture may not fit the daily requirement of PKU children due to the low solubility in liquid of some nutrients. We suggest that tyrosine blood levels, as well as the phenylalanine blood levels, should be monitored as part of the routine care of PKU children in addition to a careful examination of the skin to detect follicullar hyperkeratosis.

REFERENCES

Fisch, R., Tsai, M. and Gentry, W. Studies of phenylketonurics with dermatitis. *J. Am. Acad. Dermatol.* 4 (1981) 284–290

Güttler, F. and Lou, H. Dietary problems of phenylketonuria: effect on CNS transmitters and their possible role in behaviour and neurophysiological function. *J. Inher. Metab. Dis.* 9 (1986) 169–177

Nadler, H. L. and Hsia, D. Y. Y. Epinephrine metabolism in phenylketonuria. *Proc. Soc. Exp. Biol. Med.* 107 (1961) 721–722

J. Inher. Metab. Dis. 12 Suppl. 2 (1989) 335–338

Short Communication

Primapterinuria: A New Variant of Atypical Phenylketonuria

N. BLAU[1]*, H. CH. CURTIUS[1], TH. KUSTER[1], A. MATASOVIC[1], G. SCHOEDON[1], J. L. DHONDT[2], P. GUIBAUD[3], T. GIUDICI[4] and M. BLASKOVICS[5]

[1]*Division of Clinical Chemistry, Department of Pediatrics, University of Zurich, Steinwiestrasse 75, 8032 Zurich, Switzerland;* [2]*Laboratoire de Biochimie, University of Lille, Lille Cedex, France;* [3]*Centre d'Etude des Maladies Metaboliques, Hôpital Debrousse, Lyon, France;* [4]*Division of Genetics, Childrens Hospital, Los Angeles, USA;* [5]*Department of Pediatrics, Kaiser Permanente, Fontana, USA*

Primapterin (7-iso-biopterin) is a new pterin metabolite found recently in the urine of a child with mild hyperphenylalaninaemia (Dhondt *et al.*, 1988). Besides primapterin two other new 7-substituted pterins, namely 6-oxo-primapterin and anapterin (7-iso-neopterin), were also found in the patient's urine, however in much lower concentrations (Curtius *et al.*, 1988). In the meantime a second patient has been diagnosed with primapterinuria and transient hyperphenylalaninaemia (Blaskovics, personal communication). In both cases a tetrahydrobiopterin (BH$_4$) loading test normalized plasma phenylalanine levels after 4 to 6 h. In both patients the cerebrospinal fluid (CSF) neurotransmitter metabolites, 5-hydroxyindoleacetic acid and homovanillic acid were in the normal range and the activities of all enzymes of the BH$_4$ biosynthesis and regeneration (GTP cyclohydrolase I, 6-pyruvoyltetrahydropterin synthase, sepiapterin reductase and dihydropteridine reductase) were found to be normal. The neopterin to biopterin ratio of the patients' urine was significantly increased. Following oral tetrahydrobiopterin administration ($2\,\text{mg}\,\text{kg}^{-1}\text{d}^{-1}$) neopterin normalized and biopterin as well as primapterin increased about eight-fold in one of the patients. This finding suggests that primapterin is formed from biopterin by an isomerization reaction. However, the exact metabolic origin of primapterin and anapterin is still obscure.

MATERIALS AND METHODS

Pteridin standards were purchased from Dr B. Schircks Lab. (Jona, Switzerland), 7-iso-neopterin and 7-iso-biopterin were a gift from Professor H. Rembold, Munich, FRG. The respective tetrahydro compounds were prepared by catalytic hydrogenation with Pd/H$_2$. HPLC of pterins after oxidation with manganese dioxide was

*Correspondence: Dr Nenad Blau, Med. Chem. Abteilung, Universitäts-Kinderklinik, Steinwiesstrasse 75, 8032 Zurich, Switzerland.

Journal of Inherited Metabolic Disease. ISSN 0141–8955. Copyright © SSIEM and Kluwer Academic Publishers, PO Box 55, Lancaster, UK.

performed as described elsewhere (Niederwieser *et al.*, 1984). Electron impact spectra of trimethylsilyl derivatives were obtained with the triple stage quadrupole mass spectrometer, Finnigan MAT TSQ-70, at 70 eV as described previously (Kuster *et al.*, 1983).

RESULTS AND DISCUSSION

Structural information on three new 7-substituted pterins was obtained from the mass spectra of compounds isolated from the patient's urine and of reference substances (Kuster *et al.*, 1983). Analysis of urine samples by HPLC showed abnormal pterin patterns in the patient's urine. Primapterin and anapterin were present in very low concentrations in every human urine, whereas 6-oxo-primapterin was detected in the patient's urine only. Up to 7% of total biopterin (6 and 7 isomers) in the urine of controls was present as primapterin. In the urines of both patients with the new form of atypical phenylketonuria (PKU) the ratio between biopterin and primapterin was about 1:1, and biopterin was in the lower normal range (0.41 and 0.87 mmol (mol creatinine)$^{-1}$, respectively). Oxidation with iodine under acidic and alkaline conditions showed that about 50% of the total primapterin exists in tetrahydro form. In the urines of the mother, father, and two brothers of the patient P.P., primapterin was found to be 7.0, 3.8, 4.6, and 3.8%, respectively, of the sum of biopterin plus primapterin. In the second family very low primapterin concentrations were found in the parents' urine (up to 5%), whereas in the urine of the patient's brother, 46% of primapterin was found. This child, however, shows no clinical symptoms. The most interesting finding is that after tetrahydrobiopterin administration (2 mg kg^{-1}d^{-1}) in the patient J.S. biopterin as well as primapterin concentrations in the urine increased (Figure 1). Increase of neopterin at the age of 3 and 7 months was due to infections. The biopterin to primapterin ratio remains the same (between 0.9 and 1.6). The same increase in biopterin and primapterin was observed in the patient P.P. after phenylalanine loading. These results indicate that primapterin can be formed endogenously as well as from exogenously administered tetrahydrobiopterin, probably by an as yet unknown isomerization reaction. Involvement of the intestinal bacteria in the formation of primapterin from tetrahydrobiopterin was excluded by treatment of one child with neomycin. During a 2-day treatment concentrations of urinary primapterin and biopterin remained unchanged.

Since all enzyme activities were normal in both patients, in this form of atypical PKU there is probably no defect in tetrahydrobiopterin synthesis or regeneration. Although the neopterin to biopterin ratio was extremely high, in primapterinuria biopterin concentrations were not as low as in patients with pyruvoyltetrahydropterin synthase deficiency. Hyperphenylalaninaemia was corrected with a low protein diet and with BH$_4$, indicating that the defect might be at the cofactor side of the hydroxylation reaction. The reaction mechanism of 7-substituted pterins in phenylalanine hydroxylation is still unclear. Further investigations to localize the enzymatic defect are in progress.

J. Inher. Metab. Dis. 12 (1989)

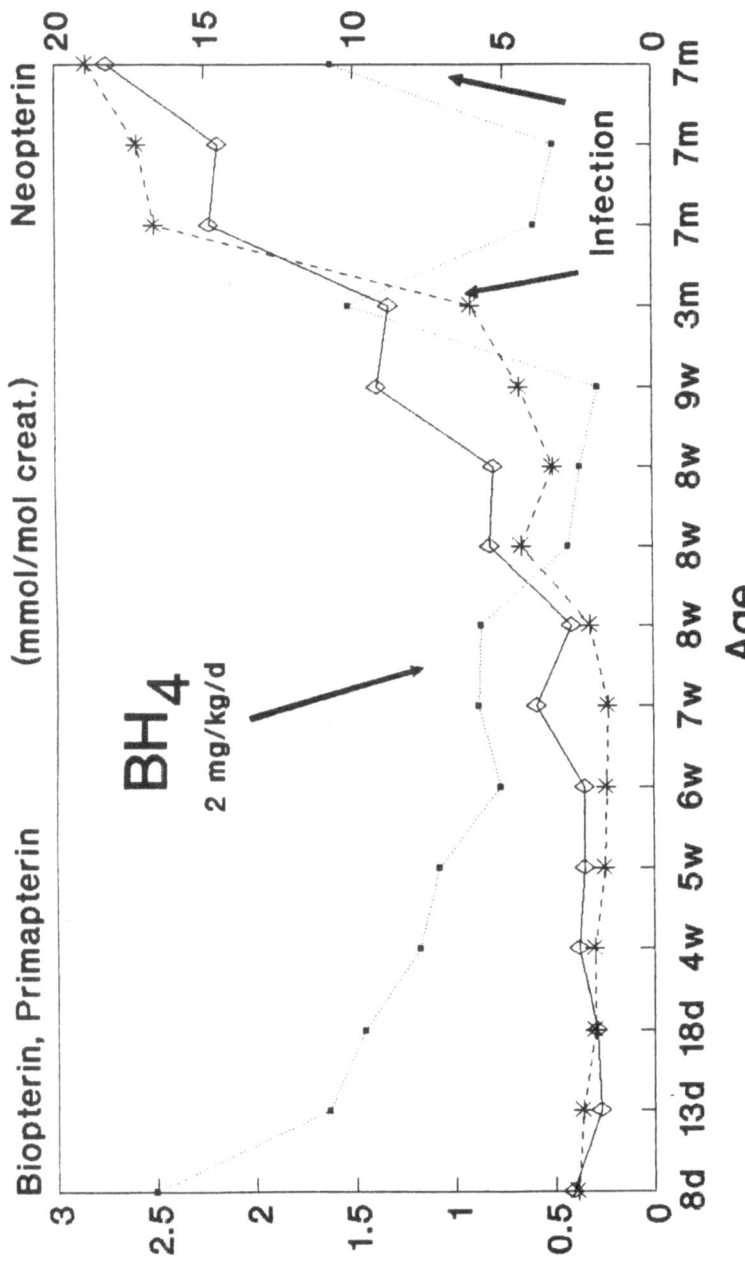

Figure 1 Neopterin (■), biopterin (◇), and primapterin (*) in the urine of patient J.S. before and during tetrahydrobiopterin therapy

ACKNOWLEDGEMENTS

We are grateful to W. Staudenmann for technical assistance. This work was supported by the Swiss National Science Foundation, project No. 3.395-0.86, and the Californian Department of Health Services, Genetics Disease Branch, project No. 87-91014.

REFERENCES

Curtius, H. Ch., Kuster, Th., Matasovic, A., Blau, N. and Dhondt, J. L. Primapterin, anapterin, and 6-oxo-primapterin, three new 7-substituted pterins identified in a patient with hyperphenylalaninemia. *Biochem. Biophys. Res. Commun.* 153 (1988) 715–721

Dhondt, J. L., Guiband, P., Rolland, M. O., Dorche, C., Andre, S., Forzy, G. and Hayte, J. M. Neonatal hyperphenylalaninaemia presumably caused by a new variant of biopterin synthetase deficiency. *Eur. J. Pediatr.* 147 (1988) 153–157

Kuster, Th. and Niederwieser, A. Gas chromatrography–mass spectrometry of trimethylsilyl pteridines. *J. Chromatogr.* 278 (1983) 245–254

Niederwieser, A., Staudenmann, W. and Wetzel, E. High-performance liquid chromatography with column switching for the analysis of biogenic amine metabolites and pterins. *J. Chromatogr.* 290 (1984) 237–246

J. Inher. Metab. Dis. 12 Suppl. 2 (1989) 339–342

Short Communication

Tyrosinaemia Type I: Orthotopic Liver Transplantation as the Only Definitive Answer to a Metabolic as well as an Oncological Problem

F. J. van Spronsen[1], R. Berger[1], G. P. A. Smit[1], J. B. C. de Klerk[2], M. Duran[2], C. M.A. Bijleveld[1], H. van Faassen[1], M. J. H. Slooff[3] and H. S. A. Heymans[1]

[1]*Department of Pediatrics, University Hospital of Groningen, 59 Oostersingel, 9713 EZ Groningen;* [2]*University Children's Hospital "Wilhelmina Kinderziekenhuis", 137 Nieuwe Gracht, 3512 LK Utrecht;* [3]*Department of Surgery, University Hospital of Groningen, The Netherlands*

Hereditary tyrosinaemia type I (McKusick 27670) is an autosomal recessive disorder, primarily caused by a deficiency of the enzyme fumarylacetoacetase (EC 3.7.1.2.) (Fallström *et al.*, 1979; Berger *et al.*, 1981), characterized by elevated concentrations of tyrosine, phenylalanine, methionine and α-1-fetoprotein (AFP) in plasma and increased urinary excretion of tyrosyl compounds, succinylacetone and δ-amino-levulinic acid. Its clinical picture consists of an acute and more chronic forms, all causing hepatocellular and renal tubular dysfunction. Dietary treatment has repeatedly been shown to decrease the renal tubular damage, but does not always prevent liver damage. Of patients with the acute form, 90% die before the age of 1 year (Mowat, 1987). In the chronic form, hepatocellular carcinoma (HCC) is known as a cause of death in about 35% of the patients (Weinberg *et al.*, 1976). However, there are no data about the risk for HCC in the acute form. In both forms, orthotopic liver transplantation (OLT) should be considered as the only definitive therapy so far.

In this study, it is the aim to develop a protocol for optimization of timing of OLT in tyrosinaemia type I. The study is based on a review of literature on OLT in tyrosinaemia type I and recent experiences with two of our Dutch patients.

CASE REPORTS

The first patient, RF, born in November 1978, has been described earlier (Berger *et al.*, 1981; Wadman *et al.*, 1983). During the first 9 years, the clinical course was uncomplicaeted. Growth and development were satisfactory. In 1985, noduli in liver were detected. AFP levels were elevated, but remained at the same level. Shortly after parental approval for a screening procedure for OLT, RF was admitted because of upper gastrointestinal bleeding. He died because of recurrent

Journal of Inherited Metabolic Disease. ISSN 0141–8955. Copyright © SSIEM and Kluwer Academic Publishers, PO Box 55, Lancaster, UK.

haemorrhagic problems. Post mortem, HCC with metastases in lung, haematotho-
rax with a primary bleeding locus probably in the vena azygos and intracranial
haemorrhage were found. From 1986 until his death (January 1988) no AFP was
measured, but stored heparin plasma samples, which had been preserved at −70°C,
were analysed afterwards. AFP showed a sharp continuous rise from about July
1986 onwards.

The second patient, JC, born in September 1985, presented at the age of 3
months with haemorrhagic problems in combination with gastrointestinal infections,
recurrent hypoglycaemias, disturbed liver function tests and ascites. Diagnosis was
established (JBC de K) at 1 year of age. In September 1987, she was referred to
our clinic for OLT because of recently detected noduli in liver, increasing in number
and volume on ultrasound and CT scanning. However, AFP remained at the same
level. Except for some minor haemorrhagic problems, the general condition of the
patient remained well until some months prior to OLT. Then she developed signs
of progressive liver failure, making OLT urgently necessary. OLT with reduced-
sized liver was performed in June 1988 and the patient is in good condition now.
The liver was full of noduli but HCC could not be detected.

RESULTS AND DISCUSSION

We reviewed the literature on OLT in tyrosinaemia type I. Until now, 9 cases with
tyrosinaemia type I, in which OLT has been performed, have been published in
detail (Table 1).

From Table 1, it should be concluded that, in the majority of cases, HCC was
the indication for OLT. However, in patients 2, 3 and 9, OLT was performed
because of liver failure. Furthermore, it is obvious that HCC does not develop in
the chronic form of tyrosinaemia type I only, but can also develop in the acute
form (patients 1 and 4). In fact, if treatment has been successful in preventing liver
failure, the risk for HCC in the acute form may even be higher.

Concerning the AFP levels, it may be concluded from Table 1 (patients 2 and
7) that an absolute elevated AFP level in itself has no predictive value for the
presence or development of HCC. Elevation could be due to continuous liver
damage in tyrosinaemia. The data of our patients suggest strongly that development
of HCC could, however, be predicted by a sharp rise of AFP, impossible to correct
by stricter dietary therapy. It should, however, be noted that AFP is not always
elevated in HCC. In patient 4, no elevated AFP level was reported.

In both forms of tyrosinaemia type I, liver noduli on ultrasound, combined with
a sharp rise of AFP, suggest the development of HCC. However, especially in the
acute form, in which development of progressive liver failure is so unpredictable,
it is disputable whether it is appropriate to withhold OLT until AFP shows a sharp
rise. Considering the data of Mowat (1987), it may even be necessary to perform
OLT in the first year of life. Although the idea exists that mortality due to OLT
in the first year is prohibitive, the data of Esquivel *et al.* (1987) and Gartner *et al.*
(1984) suggest that the survival rate of infants is comparable to that in older
children, while Otte *et al.* (1988) show that no significant difference exists between

Table 1 Orthotopic liver transplantation in tyrosinaemia type I

Patient no. with ref.	Onset of symptoms*	OLT*	AFP before OLT	Indications for OLT	HCC found in liver at time of OLT
1[1,2]	4/12	4	46 000	LF+HCC	+
2	3/12	2	10 000	LF+N	−
3	3/12	1 2/12		LF	−
4[3,4]	2/12	9 9/12	normal	HCC	+
5[4,5]	3	21	2 740	LF	−
6	1	2 6/12	>25 000	HCC	+
7	2 7/12	3 6/12	4 600		+
8		3	13 560		+
9[6,7]	6	23	normal	LF	−

LF, liver failure; *, age in years; AFP, α-1-fetoprotein in ng/ml; HCC, hepatocellular carcinoma; N, Noduli detected in liver
[1]Tuchman, M. *et al., J. Inher. Metab. Dis.* 8 (1985) 21–24
[2]Tuchman, M. *et al., J. Pediatr.* 110 (1987) 399–403
[3]Fisch, RO. *et al., J. Pediatr.* 93 (1978) 592–596
[4]Starzl, T. E. *et al., J. Pediatr.* 106 (1985) 604–606
[5]Van Thiel, D. J. *et al., J. Hepatol.* 3 (1986) 42–48
[6]Flatmark, A. *et al., Transpl. Proc.* 18 (1986) 67–68
[7]Kvittingen, E. A. *et al., J. Inher. Metab. Dis.* 9 (1986) 216–224

Clinical course: Patients 1 and 4 died because of metastases of HCC and metastases in combination with liver rejection, respectively. Patients 2, 3, 5–9 were alive for some weeks up to 3 years. They were in good health and without dietary restriction of phenylalanine, tyrosine and methionine. In patient 5, a right hepatic lobectomy was performed because of rontgenological evidence for hepatoma. Postoperatively, liver failure developed and successively OLT was necessary. No hepatoma was found. In patient 6, 1½ years after OLT a second OLT was performed because of rejection. Now the patient has been in good health for at least 2½ years

OLT with a total and a reduced-sized liver. Nevertheless, in tyrosinaemia type I, until more data are available, it seems appropriate to advocate elective OLT after the first year of life, but OLT should be considered before if necessary.

CONCLUSIONS

OLT should be considered in both forms of tyrosinaemia type I. The presence of noduli on liver ultrasound should arouse one's suspicion, while in combination with a sharp rise of AFP it strongly suggests the development of HCC. Concerning the acute form, elective OLT is advocated after the first year of life but should be considered before if necessary.

ACKNOWLEDGEMENTS

We thank Dr J. R. Markar and Dr F. van der Logt for the opportunity to study their patients, Dr A. Martijn for performing ultrasound of the liver and Dr A. M. Jonker and Dr A. Gouw for postmortem examination and examination of liver material in the patients.

REFERENCES

Berger, R., Smit, G. P. A., Stoker-de Vries, S. A., Duran, M., Ketting, D. and Wadman, .S. K. Deficiency of fumarylacetoacetase in a patient with hereditary tyrosinaemia. *Clin. Chim. Acta* 114 (1981) 37–44

Esquivel, C. O., Koneru, B., Karrer, F., Todo, S., Iwatsuki, S., Gordon, R. D., Makowka, L., Marsh, W. J. and Starzl, T. E. Liver transplantation before 1 year of age. *J. Pediatr.* 110 (1987) 545–548

Fallström, S. P., Lindblad, B., Lindstedt, S. and Steen, G. Hereditary tyrosinemia–fumarylacetoacetase deficiency. *Pediatr. Res.* 13 (1979) 78

Gartner, J. C., Zitelli, B. J., Malatack, J. J., Shaw, B. W., Iwatsuki, S. and Starzl, T. E. Orthotopic liver transplantation in children: two year experience with 47 patients. *Pediatrics* 74 (1984) 140–145

Mowat, A. P. Liver disorders in children: The indications for liver replacement in parenchymal and metabolic diseases. *Transplant. Proc.* 24 (1987) 3236–3241

Otte, J. B., Yandza, T., de Ville de Goyet, J., Tan, K. C., Salizzoni, M. and Hemptimnne, B. Pediatric liver transplantation: report on 52 patients with a 2 year survival of 86%. *J. Pediatr. Surg.* 23 (1988) 250–253

Wadman, S. K., Duran, M., Ketting, D., Bruinvis, L., van Sprang, F. J., Berger, R., Smit, G. P. A., Steimann, B., Leonard, J. V., Divry, P., Farriaux, J. P. and Cartigny, B. Urinary excretion of deuterated metabolites in patients with tyrosinaemia type I after oral loading with deuterated L-tyrosine. *Clin. Chim. Acta* 130 (1983) 231–238

Weinberg, A. G., Mize, C. E. and Worther, H. G. The occurrence of hepatoma in the chronic form of hereditary tyrosinemia. *J. Pediatr.* 88 (1976) 434–438

J. Inher. Metab. Dis. 12 Suppl. 2 (1989) 343–345

Short Communication

Lens Hexitols and Cataract Formation During Lactation in a Woman Heterozygote for Galactosaemia

M. Brivet[1], F. Migayron[1], J. Roger[2], G. Cheron[3] and A. Lemonnier[1]

[1]Laboratoire de Biochimie, Hôpital de Bicêtre 94275 Le Kremlin-Bicêtre Cedex;
[2]Service de Contactologie, Fondation Rothschild 75940 Paris Cedex 19;
[3]Départment de Pédiatrie, Hôpital Necker Enfants Malades 75730 Paris Cedex 15, France

The occurrence of cataracts in a healthy lactating woman, heterozygous for UDP glucose-hexose-1-phosphate uridyltransferase (GALT; EC 2.7.7.12) deficiency (McKusick 23040), may suggest a possible link to the enzymatic defect of galactose metabolism. As studies in rats (Ng et al., 1987) showed that prolactin accelerates galactose-induced cataractogenesis, i.e. aldose reductase mediated accumulation of galactitol in the lenses, our purpose was to determine the hexitol contents of the patient's lens tissue.

CASE REPORT

The proposita was healthy and only suffered from myopia, with good vision before her two pregnancies (left eye, corrected visual acuity $(-3.25):10/10$; right eye, corrected visual acuity $(-4):10/10$). She became pregnant at 26 years. The course of pregnancy and delivery was uncomplicated; nevertheless, the vision of both her eyes began to deteriorate. Two years later, in the third trimester of a second pregnancy, and during lactation, cataracts progressed very rapidly. At 1 month postpartum, she presented with bilateral posterior cortical cataract and visual acuity was $<1/10$ on both sides, necessitating surgery. Laboratory tests including blood fasting sugar, calcium and phosphorus in blood and urines, liver and kidney function tests were within normal limits. Erythrocyte activity of galactokinase (EC 2.7.1.6) (GALK) was normal, but GALT activity was in the heterozygous range. A Duarte variant was excluded by isoelectric focussing.

Neither child of the patient had ocular problems and never suffered from milk intolerance: GALT was within the heterozygous range for the first child and within the normal range for the second.

MATERIAL AND METHODS

Human lenses: The left tissue of the patient was analysed after cryoextraction. Control lenses were obtained at autopsy from individuals with no history of

343

Journal of Inherited Metabolic Disease. ISSN 0141-8955. Copyright © SSIEM and Kluwer Academic Publishers, PO Box 55, Lancaster, UK.

diabetes. One lens from a 4-year-old girl, homozygous for GALK deficiency, with bilateral anterior and posterior cortical opacities was also studied, after linear extraction. Samples were kept on ice for transport, and stored at −180°C.

Hexitols assays: Lens homogenates were divided into three parts for determination of: blank profile, myoinositol, and other hexitols (mannitol, sorbitol, galactitol) levels. Hexa-acetate derivatives were prepared according to Popp-Snijders *et al.* (1983). Different quantities of arabitol were used as internal standard. Derivatives were extracted into either 1 mL of chloroform for myoinositol determination, or into 100 μL of cyclohexane for other hexitol determinations. Capillary gas–liquid chromatography of hexa-acetates was performed essentially as described by Popp-Snijders *et al.* (1983).

RESULTS AND DISCUSSION

Myoinositol is the most abundant lens carbohydrate; its level can be 400-fold higher than other hexitol concentrations, thus we used two different solvents for the extraction of polyol derivatives:

(a) chloroform – all derivatives were found with a good recovery, but only myoinositol might be quantified, since minor hexitol peaks and the large peak of myoinositol overlapped;

(b) cyclohexane – myoinositol acetate was poorly extracted, whereas other hexitol derivatives were quantitatively found and might be measured (M. Brivet, F. Migayron, H. Offret and A. Lemonnier; in preparation).

The results of lens analyses are reported in Table 1. Galactitol was <3 nmol (g lens weight)$^{-1}$ (limit of detection) in the patient and control lenses, whereas a moderate level, 750 nmol (g lens weight)$^{-1}$, was observed in the GALK deficient lens. Myoinositol content was normal in the two cataractous lenses, compared to

Table 1 Levels of hexitols in lenses analysed

	Sex	Age (yrs)	Lens weight (mg)	Eye side	Myoinositol	Sorbitol	Galactitol
Próposita	F	28	155	L	13 500	64	<3
Controls	M	67	148.5	L	15 760	105	<3
	M	45	97	L	25 000	134	<3
			182.5	R	27 000	150	<3
	M	80	245.5	L	22 500	105	<3
			142.1	R	21 000	110	<3
GALK deficient girl	F	4	50.2	L	19 690	274	750

Hexitol levels are in nmol (g lens weight)$^{-1}$

Tomana *et al.* (1984) control values, but slightly decreased in the patient's lens, compared to our own controls. However the decrease in myoinositol is not sufficient to suggest breakdown of the permeability barrier as observed in mature cataract, and loss of galactitol by diffusion seems unlikely.

In a previous observation of rapidly progressing cataract in a lactating woman heterozygous for GALT deficiency, Avisar *et al.* (1982) showed modifications of the lens soluble protein pattern, as reported in galactose-fed rats (Ocken *et al.*, 1977). However, non-enzymatic galactosylation of proteins (Kador and Kinoshita, 1984) or impaired lens crystallin synthesis (Kador *et al.*, 1979), like galactitol accumulation, need high sugar concentration to occur. It is doubtful that these conditions may be encountered in lactating woman with partial GALT deficiency, since GALT is not a rate-limiting enzyme for the galactose pathway and only minimal amounts of endogeneous lactose may be hydrolysed to galactose. Thus we think that cataract formation in these patients is not related to partial GALT deficiency.

REFERENCES

Avisar, R. A., Schwartzman, S., Levinsky, H., Allalouf, D., Goldman, J., Ninio, A. and Savir, H. A case of cataract formation during the lactating period associated with galactose-1-phosphate uridyltransferase deficiency. *Metab. Pediatr. Syst. Ophthalmol.* 6 (1982) 45–48

Kador, P. F., Zigler, J. S. and Kinoshita, J. H. Alteration of lens protein synthesis in galactosemic rats. *Invest. Ophthalmol. Visual Sci.* 18 (1979) 696–702

Kador, P. F. and Kinoshita, J. Diabetic and galactosaemic cataracts. In *Ciba Foundation Symposium 106, Human Cataract Formation.* Pittman, London, 1984, pp. 110–131

Ng, M. C., Tsui, J. Y., Merola, L. O. and Unakar, N. J. Effect of prolactin on galactose cataractogenesis. *Ophthalm. Res.* 19 (1987) 82–94

Ocken, P. R., Fu, S-C J., Hart, R., White, J. H., Wagner, B. J. and Lewis, K. E. Characterization of lens proteins. I. Identification of additional soluble fractions in rat lenses. *Exp. Eye Res.* 24 (1977) 355–367

Popp-Snijders, C., Lomecky, M. Z. and de Jong, A. P. Determination of sorbitol in erythrocytes of diabetic and healthy subjects by capillary gas chromatography. *Clin. Chim. Acta* 132 (1983) 83–89

Tomana, M., Prchal, J. T., Garner, L. C., Skalka, H. W. and Barker, S. A. Gas chromatographic analysis of lens monosaccharides. *J. Lab. Clin. Med.* 103 (1984) 137–142

J. Inher. Metab. Dis. 12 Suppl. 2 (1989) 346–348

Short Communication

A Method for the Diagnosis of Glycogen Storage Disease Type Ib using Polymorphonuclear Leukocytes

N. Bashan, R. Potashnik, M. Phillip, Y. S. Shin[1] and S. W. Moses
Pediatric Research Laboratory, Soroka Medical Center, Beer-Sheva 84101, and Faculty of Health Sciences, Ben Gurion University of the Negev, Beer-Sheva 84105, Israel; [1]Children's Hospital, University of Munich, 8000 Munich 2, West Germany

Three variants of glycogen storage disease (GSD) type I have been described:

(1) A deficiency of microsomal liver phosphohydrolase in GSD 1a (Cori and Cori, 1952);
(2) Inactive glucose-6-phosphate (G6P) translocase in GSD Ib (Schaub and Heyne, 1983; Narisawa *et al.*, 1987); and
(3) A lack of a translocase for phosphate in GSD Ic (Nordlie *et al.*, 1983).

GSD Ib patients present, in addition to the clinical and metabolic features of GSD Ia, neutropenia and disturbances in neutrophil functions, such as reduction in random and direct cell migration, bactericidal activity and phagocytosis (Schaub and Heyne, 1983). Furthermore, a marked reduction in the activities of the hexose monophosphate shunt, glycolytic rates and 2-deoxyglucose transport in polymorphonuclear leukocytes (PMN) of GSD Ib patients has been reported (Bashan *et al.*, 1988). The metabolic deficiencies were attributed to a reduced glucose transport which leads to intracellular substrate limitation affecting both the hexose monophosphate shunt and anaerobic glycolysis.

In the homozygous state of GSD Ib, hepatic G6P-ase is present in normal amounts but its activity can be demonstrated only when the microsomal membranes are disrupted. This phenomenon has been coined an enhanced 'latency' of the enzyme within its natural membranous environment (Lange *et al.*, 1980). Thus, the availability of a fresh, unfrozen liver biopsy specimen is required for the enzymatic diagnosis of patients with GSD Ib. This paper presents a method of utilizing 2-deoxyglucose transport in PMN as a tool for the diagnosis of GSD Ib patients.

MATERIALS AND METHODS

Subjects: Subjects included 34 normal individuals ranging in age from 1 month to 40 years, 7 homozygotes for GSD Ib, aged from 6 months to 13 years, and 6 homozygotes for GSD Ia, aged from 2 months to 8 years. The diagnosis of GSD

346

Journal of Inherited Metabolic Disease. ISSN 0141–8955. Copyright © SSIEM and Kluwer Academic Publishers, PO Box 55, Lancaster, UK.

Ia and Ib in all patients was based on liver biopsies as described before (Lange *et al.*, 1980).

Human polymorphonuclear leukocytes were isolated as previously described (Bashan *et al.* 1988). The PMN cells were 95±5% pure and 91±8% viable. The average total recovery of PMN cells from whole blood was 75%.

2-Deoxyglucose transport: Uptake of 2-deoxyglucose was measured as described previously (Bashan *et al.*, 1988). Forty-five μl cell suspension in KRP was incubated for 15 min at 37°C in a 4.5 ml round-bottomed mini-scintillation vial. Uptake was initiated by adding 15 μl Krebs Ringer phosphate buffer containing 4 mmol/L [1-^{3}H]2-deoxyglucose (0.6 μCi) (Amersham). After incubation of 2 min at 37°C, uptake was stopped by adding 2 ml cold 0.85% NaCl containing 0.3 mmol/L phloretin. The samples were centrifuged at 3000 g for 3 min and the pellets were washed twice by centrifugation with 2 ml cold saline. The final pellets were counted for radioactivity in Instagel scintillation fluid.

RESULTS

Transport of 2-deoxyglucose in normal PMN clearly followed saturation type kinetics and yielded K_m and V_{max} of 0.6 mmol/L and 0.51±0.13 nmol min^{-1} (10^6 cells)$^{-1}$ respectively. 2-Deoxyglucose transport in PMN of cord blood and from individuals in different age groups (from 5 days to 40 years old) was the same.

Preservation of heparinized blood at 4°C resulted in a slow reduction of 2-deoxyglucose transport into PMN with a loss of 30% after 24 hours. Preservation of prepared PMN for 24 hours led to a 75% reduction in transport activity. In view of these findings, PMN preparations were examined within 2 hours and 2-deoxyglucose transport determined within 6 hours of blood collection.

The rates of 2-deoxyglucose transport in PMN of seven GSD Ib patients and six GSD Ia patients as compared with 34 controls are presented in Figure 1. In GSD Ib neutrophils, the rate was 0.13±0.03 compared with 0.51±0.17 and 0.61±0.26 nmol min^{-1} (10^6 cells)$^{-1}$ in neutrophils of controls and GSD Ia, respectively. The uptake of 2-deoxyglucose in PMN of GSD Ib patients was reduced to 30% even when neutropenia was not observed in those patients.

DISCUSSION

The present study clearly shows that homozygotes for GSD Ib can be detected by measuring 2-deoxyglucose transport in purified PMN leukocytes. No overlap between 2-deoxyglucose transport values of GSD Ib patients and those of control samples and GSD Ia patients was found. As, in preserved blood or leukocytes, transport activity is slowly reduced as a function of time, all measurements should be performed within 12 hours of drawing the blood sample.

Patients with fasting hypoglycaemia, lactic acidosis and hepatomegaly have to be tested for glycogen storage disease. Although neutropenia is frequently found in GSD Ib patients, its absence in some of these patients has also been described.

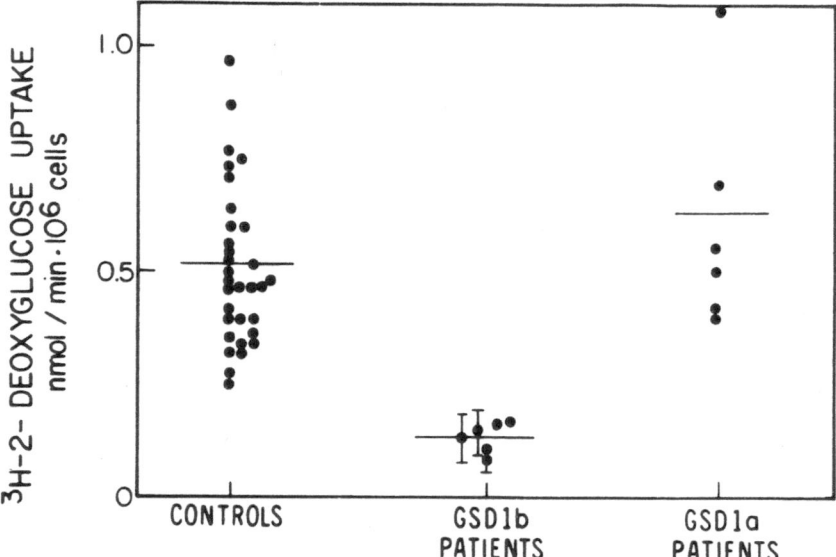

Figure 1 Scatter plot of [³H]2-deoxyglucose uptake by PMN of GSD Ib patients, GSD Ia patients and controls. Conditions for 2-DOG uptake as described in methods. In three patients, data are presented as the mean ±SD

Thus, neutropenia cannot be utilized as a critical criterion for differentiating between GSD Ia and Ib. 2-Deoxyglucose transport in PMN of GSD Ib patients (whether the patients are neutropenic or not) is reduced to about 30% of that in normal controls. Although the mechanism of the glucose transport disturbance is not yet clear, this method appears to be useful for establishing the diagnosis of GSD Ib but is not suitable for GSD Ia patients.

REFERENCES

Bashan, N., Hagay, Y., Potashnik, R. and Moses, S. W. Impaired carbohydrate metabolism of polymorphonuclear leukocytes in glycogen storage disease Ib. *J. Clin. Invest.* 81 (1988) 1317–1322

Cori, G. T. and Cori, C. F. Glucose-6-phosphate of liver in glycogen storage disease. *J. Biol. Chem.* 199 (1952) 661–667

Lange, A. J., Arion, W. J. and Beaudet, A. L. Type Ib glycogen storage disease is caused by a defect in glucose-6-phosphate translocase of microsomal glucose-6-phosphate system. *J. Biol. Chem.* 255 (1980) 8381–8384

Narisawa, K., Igarashi, Y. and Tada, K., Glycogen storage disease type Ib: genetic disorders involving the transport system of intracellular membrane. *Enzyme* 38 (1987) 177–183

Nordlie, R. C., Sukalski, K. A., Munoz, J. M. and Baldwin, J. J. Type Ic: a novel glycogenosis. *J. Biol. Chem.* 258 (1983) 9739–9744

Schaub, J. and Heyne, K. Glycogen storage disease type Ib. *Eur. J. Pediatr.* 140 (1983) 283–288

J. Inher. Metab. Dis. 12 Suppl. 2 (1989) 349–351

Short Communication

Familial NADH: Q_1 Oxidoreductase (Complex I) Deficiency: Variable Expression and Possible Treatment

F. A. Wijburg[1], P. G. Barth[1], W. Ruitenbeek[2], R. J. A. Wanders[1], G. D. Vos[1], S. L. B. Ploos van Amstel[1] and R. B. H. Schutgens[1]

[1]*Department of Pediatrics, University Hospital of Amsterdam (AMC), 1105 AZ Amsterdam, The Netherlands;* [2]*Department of Pediatrics, University Hospital Nijmegen, 6500 HB Nijmegen, The Netherlands*

NADH: Q_1 oxidoreductase (complex I; E.C. 1.6.99.3) deficiency (McKusick 31245), one of the more common respiratory chain defects, has been described in about 40 patients. Different clinical syndromes can be distinguished (DiMauro *et al.*, 1987). In neonates complex I deficiency can present as a multisystem disorder characterized by severe lactic acidosis, hypotonia, seizures and respiratory insufficiency. This type has been described in eight patients and seems usually to be fatal due to uncontrollable lactic acidosis and systemic complications. Results of treatment have been generally disappointing although some encouraging results were obtained (Arts *et al.*, 1983). We report a family in which we demonstrated complex I deficiency in two children while four others have a clinical history suggesting the same defect. We treated one infant with a multisystem disorder with severe congenital lactic acidosis. Initially treatment was by artificial respiration and peritoneal dialysis, subsequently by high doses of menadione. A remarkable recovery was observed.

PATIENTS

The sibs, seven sons (A–G), were born from healthy consanguineous (first cousins) Moroccan parents. A and B were born in Morocco. Both died within a few weeks after a period of tachypnoea. C has always been healthy and is now 7 years old. D died at 4 days from untreatable lactic acidaemia (lactate up to $24 \, \text{mmol L}^{-1}$, normal <2.0). Diagnosis was not made. E had congenital lactic acidaemia (up to $6.6 \, \text{mmol L}^{-1}$) during the first weeks of life. Symptomless cardiomyopathy was diagnosed on echocardiography and ECG. He completely recovered, had a normal development and is now 5 years old. At 4 years the diagnosis of complex I deficiency was made on muscle biopsy (see Table 1). F suffered from congenital lactic acidosis with lactate concentration up to $9.8 \, \text{mmol L}^{-1}$ in early life. He recovered spontaneously after a few weeks but died at 8 months in Morocco during a bout of gastroenteritis after a period of tachypnoea.

In patient G the blood lactate concentration at 24 h after birth was $27.8 \, \text{mmol L}^{-1}$.

349

Journal of Inherited Metabolic Disease. ISSN 0141–8955. Copyright © SSIEM and Kluwer Academic Publishers, PO Box 55, Lancaster, UK.

Table 1   Results of biochemical studies in patients E and G

| | Muscle | | | | Liver | | |
| | Patient | | Control | | Patient | Control | |
	E	G	Range	n	G	Range	n
Citrate synthase[a]	26	94	48–146	18	47	13–96	10
Cytochrome *c* oxidase[a]	92	219	73–284	39	213	14–108	11
Succinate: cyt. *c* oxidoreductase[b]	13	31	22–84	18	28	6–51	9
NADH: Q_1 oxidoreductase[c]	2.1	0.5	8.7–26	11	0	4.7–9.2	7

Values are expressed as: [a]milliunits $(mg\ protein)^{-1}$; [b]nmol cytochrome *c* reduced (mg protein)$^{-1}$min^{-1}; [c]nmol NADH oxidized (mg protein)$^{-1}$min^{-1}.

Lactate concentration in cerebrospinal fluid was also increased ($10.2\ mmol\ L^{-1}$). Bicarbonate infusions could not correct the acidosis and resulted in hypernatraemia. Artificial respiration was necessary because of respiratory insufficiency. Peritoneal dialysis with bicarbonate–glucose solution was started 14 h after birth. Blood lactate concentration decreased to $5\ mmol\ L^{-1}$ in 24 h and could be maintained at an acceptable level by prolonged intensive dialysis. Artificial respiration could be stopped after 4 days. At 21 days biochemical studies in muscle and liver biopsy material revealed the diagnosis complex I deficiency (see Table 1).

Therapy with riboflavin, thiamine, ascorbate, succinate and L-carnitine did not result in improvement. At 1 month of age dialysis had to be stopped because of catheter obstruction. Since then there have been recurrent episodes of lactic acidaemia (up to $18\ mmol\ L^{-1}$), which seemed to be provoked by restlessness or sustained crying and resulted in severe metabolic acidosis. Symptomless cardiomyopathy was diagnosed on echocardiography and ECG (left ventricular hypertrophy with septal enlargement). An EEG at 2 months was abnormal with signs of encephalopathy.

At 80 days, treatment with menadione (vitamin K_3) was started. Loading dosage was 10 mg i.m., followed by $2\ mg\ kg^{-1}\ day^{-1}$ orally. Temporary improvement was noticed but after 6 days the condition deteriorated and metabolic acidosis developed again. Then 10 mg menadione was given i.m. daily for 4 days, followed by $10\ mg\ kg^{-1}\ day^{-1}$ orally resulting in striking clinical and biochemical improvement with less tachypnoea and increased motor performance. Daily blood gas analysis showed normalization of pH and blood gas status. No further corrections with bicarbonate were necessary. The child could be discharged at the age of 4 months. EEG at 6 months was normal and ECG and echocardiography showed no progression of abnormalities. Only once, at 8 months, was readmission necessary when he developed temporary lactic acidaemia (up to $12\ mmol\ L^{-1}$) during a bout of gastroenteritis. He now is 14 months old and in good clinical condition showing normal development. Present medication: menadione $10\ mg\ kg^{-1}\ day^{-1}$, succinate $150\ mg\ kg^{-1}\ day^{-1}$ and L-carnitine $50\ mg\ kg^{-1}\ day^{-1}$.

BIOCHEMICAL STUDIES

The oxidation rates of labelled pyruvate and malate were decreased in the muscle tissue of both children. Measurement of respiratory chain activities with different substrates showed complex I deficiency in muscle and liver (Table 1, for methods see Fischer *et al.*, 1986). In line with the clinical presentation, the defect in muscle homogenate of patient E is milder. The relatively low activities of citrate synthase and succinate:cytochrome *c* oxidoreductase in patient E normalize after correction for the low yield of mitochondria in the $600 \times g$ supernatant.

DISCUSSION

We have obtained encouraging results in the treatment of a child affected by the severe neonatal form of complex I deficiency. Initially artificial respiration and prolonged peritoneal dialysis were necessary but subsequently a stable clinical condition resulted from treatment with menadione, succinate and carnitine. Psychomotor development is presently adequate for age. Menadione can act as an artificial electron acceptor and donor as it is able to bridge complex I. *In vitro* experiments revealed that menadione can restore respiration in mitochondria blocked by amytal, an inhibitor of complex I activity (Conover and Ernster, 1962). It has been shown to be effective in a patient with complex III deficiency (Eleff *et al.*, 1984). Menadione has been used in older patients with complex I deficiency resulting in subjective improvement with increased exercise tolerance in one patient (Land *et al.*, 1981) but with no improvement in other patients (Morgan-Hughes *et al.*, 1984). The dosage of menadione in those cases, however, was lower than the dosage we used. We conclude that menadione may be of value in the treatment of complex I deficiency presenting as a multisystem disorder with congenital lactic acidosis.

REFERENCES

Arts, W. F. M., Scholte, H. R., Bogaard, J. M., Kerrebijn, K. F. and Luyt-Houwen, I. E. M. NADH-CoQ reductase deficient myopathy: successful treatment with riboflavin. *Lancet* 2 (1983) 581–582

Conover, T. E. and Ernster, L. DT diaphorase. II Relation to respiratory chain of intact mitochondria. *Biochim. Biophys. Acta* 58 (1962) 189–200

DiMauro, S., Bonilla, E., Zeviani, M., Servidei, S., DeVivo, D. C. and Schon, E. A. Mitochondrial myopathies. *J. Inher. Metab. Dis.* 10 Suppl. 1 (1987) 113–128

Eleff, S., Kennaway, N. G., Buist, N. R. M., Darley-Usmar, V. M., Capaldi, R. A., Bank, W. J. and Chance, B. ^{31}P NMR study of improvement in oxidative phosphorylation by vitamins K_3 and C in a patient with a defect in electron transport at complex III in skeletal muscle. *Proc. Natl. Acad. Sci. USA* 81 (1984) 3529–3533

Fischer, J. C., Ruitenbeek, W., Gabreëls, F. J. M., Janssen, A. J. M., Renier, W. O., Sengers, R. C. A., Stadhouders, A. M., ter Laak, H. J., Trijbels, J. M. F. and Veerkamp, J. H. A mitochondrial encephalomyopathy: the first case with an established defect at the level of coenzyme Q. *Eur. J. Pediatr.* 144 (1986) 441–444

Land, J. M., Hockaday, J. M., Trevor Hughes, J. and Ross, B. D. Childhood mitochondrial myopathy with ophthalmoplegia. *J. Neurol. Sci.* 51 (1981) 371–382

Morgan-Hughes, J. A., Hayes, D. J., Clark, J. B. and Cooper, J. M. Mitochondrial myopathies. Results of exploratory therapeutical trials. In Folkers, K. and Yamamura, Y. (eds.), *Biochemical and Clinical Aspects of Coenzyme Q.* Vol. 4, Elsevier Science Publishers, Amsterdam, 1984, pp. 417–424

J. Inher. Metab. Dis. 12 Suppl. 2 (1989) 352–354

Short Communication

Mitochondrial Myopathies: Multiple Enzyme Defects in the Respiratory Chain

W. Ruitenbeek, J. M. F. Trijbels, J. C. Fischer, R. C. A. Sengers, A. J. M. Janssen and C. M. C. Kerkhof
Department of Pediatrics, University Hospital of Nijmegen, P.O. Box 9101, 6500 HB Nijmegen, The Netherlands

Approximately 100 patients suffering from disturbed energy metabolism of the skeletal muscle mitochondria have been reported in the literature. A malfunction of the respiratory chain was found in about two-thirds of these patients. NADH dehydrogenase and cytochrome *c* oxidase deficiencies have been most frequently reported, but the application of improved enzymatic techniques reveals that, in many patients, the defects in the respiratory chain are not restricted to a single enzyme deficiency. In this study the biochemical findings in six patients with representative defects in the respiratory chain of their skeletal muscle mitochondria are presented. Attention is focussed on the occurrence of the multiple defects.

PATIENTS AND METHODS

All six patients showed non-specific symptoms such as hypotonia, motor retardation and exercise-related complaints. Blood lactate concentration was elevated. Muscle biopsy was performed at ages between 5 days and 19 years. None of the patients used drugs known to interfere with the functioning of mitochondrial energy metabolism. Patients 2, 5 and 6 died before the third year of life. Case histories of patient 2, 4 and 6 have been published in detail (Sengers *et al.*, 1984; Fischer *et al.*, 1986; Böhles *et al.*, 1987, respectively), the case history of patient 3 is reported in this issue (Wijburg *et al.*, 1989; patient G).

Succinate:cytochrome *c* oxidoreductase, succinate dehydrogenase, and rotenone-sensitive NADH:O_2 and NADH:Q_1 oxidoreductase activities were measured according to Fischer *et al.* (1986). Other enzyme activities and the cytochrome contents were determined as described previously (Sengers *et al.*, 1984).

RESULTS

The results are summarized in Table 1. In patient 1, cytochrome *c* oxidase has the lowest residual activity of the measured mitochondrial enzymes. Deficiencies of the cytochromes aa_3 and *b* are the cause of the very low activity of cytochrome *c* oxidase and of succinate:cytochrome *c* oxidoreductase in patient 2. In patient 3 the diminished activity of NADH:O_2 oxidoreductase has been caused by a disturbance

Journal of Inherited Metabolic Disease. ISSN 0141–8955. Copyright © SSIEM and Kluwer Academic Publishers, PO Box 55, Lancaster, UK.

Table 1 Respiratory chain components in muscle mitochondria

Patient:	1	2	3	4	5	6
Cytochrome c oxidase	16	6	113	51	5	16
NADH:O_2 oxidoreductase	34	—	19	<1	6	<3
NADH:Q_1 oxidoreductase	37	—	3	<2	9	11
Succinate: cyt. c oxidoreductase	58	5	62	26	48	14
Succinate dehydrogenase	—	—	—	37	117	14
Cytochrome aa_3	—	7	—	—	<1	—
Cytochrome b	—	16	—	—	86	—
Cytochrome $c+c_1$	—	66	—	—	41	—
Citrate synthase	81	—	122	71	125	140

Activities are given as percentage of the mean of the control values (see Fischer *et al.*, 1986, and Sengers *et al.*, 1984, for absolute values for control muscles); — denotes not measured.

in NADH:Q_1 oxidoreductase (=NADH dehydrogenase). The activities of both NADH:Q_1 and succinate: cytochrome c oxidoreductase are reduced in patient 4, probably due to a disturbed microenvironment of coenzyme Q (Fischer *et al.*, 1986). A combined defect of cytochrome c oxidase and NADH:Q_1 oxidoreductase has been established in patient 5. In patient 6, the activities of all enzymes of the respiratory chain are clearly decreased, while the reference enzyme citrate synthase shows a high normal activity.

DISCUSSION

An increasing number of patients with a malfunction of the respiratory chain, resulting from diminished activity in more than one of its enzyme complexes, have been reported in the literature. A combined defect in NADH dehydrogenase and cytochrome c oxidase is found relatively frequently. Patient 5 is an evident example of this category. The results for patient 1 point to such a combination of defects rather than to an isolated cytochrome c oxidase deficiency. In most previously reported patients with cytochrome c oxidase deficiency the activities of other enzyme complexes of the respiratory chain have not been examined. Therefore, an additional defect, for example in NADH dehydrogenase, cannot be excluded in these patients.

The complexity of respiratory chain defects stresses the necessity of measuring the activity of at least one mitochondrial enzyme not involved in the respiratory chain (i.e. citrate synthase), in order to distinguish between a low number (or general activity) of mitochondria per gram muscle, and a disturbance restricted to the enzyme activities of the respiratory chain (see patient 6).

The molecular basis of the mitochondrial myopathies remains to be clarified. Primary mitochondrial myopathies are caused by mutations in the nuclear or mitochondrial genome of the muscle cells. Holt *et al.* (1988) showed that some patients with mitochondrial myopathy have two populations of DNA in the muscle mitochondria, one of them being deleted by several kilobases. Unfortunately, no clear relationship between the presence of mutant DNA and enzyme defects was established in these patients. Recently, Bolhuis *et al.* (1988) demonstrated the biosynthesis of an undersized protein, likely to be a subunit of NADH dehydrogenase, by the muscle mitochondria of patient 3. Application of immunochemical techniques to muscle tissue from patient 2 revealed diminshed concentration of not less than nine proteins from the complexes III and IV (Takamiya *et al.*, 1986). Some of the proteins lacking in this patient are encoded by mitochondrial DNA, others by nuclear DNA. One possible explanation of the multiple defects may be that the process of respiratory chain enzyme complex assembly is defective. Probably anchoring and assembling proteins (Hemmingsen *et al.*, 1988) are necessary for a correct post-translational assembly and membrane embedding of the oligomeric respiratory chain enzyme complexes. A disturbance in the system importing the proteins encoded by nuclear DNA can also be hypothesized.

Further investigations at both the DNA and protein levels should elucidate the complex aetiology of mitochondrial myopathies.

REFERENCES

Böhles, H., Singer, H., Ruitenbeek, W., Trijbels, J. M. F., Sengers, R. C. A., Ketelsen, U. P., Wagner-Thiessen, E. and Wick, H. Foamy myocardial transformation in a child with a disturbed respiratory chain. *Eur. J. Pediatr.* 146 (1987) 582–586

Bolhuis, P. A., Barth, P. G., Wijburg, F. A., Sinjorgo, K. M. C. and Ruitenbeek, W. Molecular basis of mitochondrial myopathies. *Lancet* 1 (1988) 884

Fischer, J. C., Ruitenbeek, W., Gabreëls, F. J. M., Janssen, A. J. M., Renier, W. O., Sengers, R. C. A., Stadhouders, A. M., Ter Laak, H. J., Trijbels, J. M. F. and Veerkamp, J. H. A mitochondrial encephalomyopathy: the first case with an established defect at the level of coenzyme Q. *Eur. J. Pediatr.* 144 (1986) 441–444

Hemmingsen, S. M., Woolford, C., Van der Vies, S. M., Tilly, K., Dennis, D. T., Georgopoulos, C. P., Hendrix, R. W. and Ellis, R. J. Homologous plant and bacterial proteins chaperone oligomeric protein assembly. *Nature* 333 (1988) 330–334

Holt, T. J., Harding, A. E. and Morgan-Hughes, J. A. Deletions of muscle mitochondrial DNA in patients with mitochondrial myopathies. *Nature* 331 (1988) 717–719

Sengers, R. C. A., Trijbels, J. M. F., Bakkeren, J. A. J. M., Ruitenbeek, W., Fischer, J. C., Stadhouders, A. M. and Ter Laak, H. J. Deficiency of cytochromes *b* and *aa₃* in muscle from a floppy infant with cytochrome oxidase deficiency. *Eur. J. Pediatr.* 141 (1984) 178–180

Takamiya, S., Yanamura, W., Capaldi, R. A., Kennaway, N. G., Bart, R., Sengers, R. C. A., Trijbels, J. M. F. and Ruitenbeek, W. Mitochondrial myopathies involving the respiratory chain: a biochemical analysis. *Ann. NY Acad. Sci.* 488 (1986) 33–43

Wijburg, F. A., Barth, P. G., Ruitenbeek, W., Wanders, R. J. A., Vos, G. D., Ploos van Amstel, S. L. B. and Schutgens, R. B. H. Familial NADH: CoQ oxidoreductase (complex I) deficiency: variable expression and possible treatment. *J. Inher. Metab. Dis.* 12 Suppl. 2 (1989) 349–351

J. Inher. Metab. Dis. 12 Suppl 2. (1989) 355–357

Short Communication

Familial Mitochondrial Complex I Deficiency with an Abnormal Mitochondrial Encoded Protein

P. G. Barth[1,2]*, P. A. Bolhuis[1], F. A. Wijburg[2], K. M. C. Sinjorgo[3], W. Ruitenbeek[4] and R. B. H. Schutgens[2]

Departments of [1]Neurology and [2]Pediatrics, University Hospital Amsterdam; [3]Department of Biochemistry, University of Amsterdam, 1105 AZ Amsterdam; [4]Department of Pediatrics, University Hospital Nijmegen, The Netherlands

PATIENTS

Six of seven male full sibs of Moroccan descent, consecutively indicated as A–G, had neonatal onset disease. Four (A, B, D, F) died, probably all from the same disorder. In four cases (D, E, F, G) neonatal onset lactic acidosis was documented. In cases E and G muscle biopsy was undertaken. A deficiency of NADH:Q_1 oxidoreductase (complex I) was revealed in both. A liver biopsy in case G revealed the same abnormality. Patient histories and data on the mitochondrial function studies in cases E and G are given by Wijburg *et al.* (1989).

METHODS

We investigated the mitochondrial DNA (mtDNA) in cultured muscle from case G by comparing the molecular weights of mitochondrially encoded protein subunits to controls. The mitochondrially encoded proteins were labelled in cell cultures of myoblasts and myotubes derived of the muscle biopsy from case G. Labelling of proteins encoded by mitochondrial DNA in myoblasts and myotubes was carried out according to a modification of the method described by Ching and Attardi (1982). RPMI 1640 medium was used containing 5% dialysed fetal calf serum and $0.1\,\mathrm{mg\,mL^{-1}}$ emetine. Methionine was omitted and after $1\,\mathrm{h}$ pre-incubation [^{35}S]methionine was added ($20\,\mathrm{mCi\,L^{-1}}$). The labelling period was $5\,\mathrm{h}$. Cells were washed in phosphate-buffered saline and dissolved in sample buffer with sodium dodecylsulphate (SDS) and β-mercaptoethanol. Electrophoresis of proteins was done under denaturing conditions on SDS-PAGE gradient gels of 12–20%. Radiolabelled markers were used for calibration. The proteins were labelled according the nomenclature used by Chomyn *et al.* (1985)

*Correspondence: P. G. Barth, Departments of Neurology and Pediatrics, University Hospital Amsterdam, AMC, Meibergdreef 9, 1105 AZ Amsterdam, The Netherlands.

Journal of Inherited Metabolic Disease. ISSN 0141–8955. Copyright © SSIEM and Kluwer Academic Publishers, PO Box 55, Lancaster, UK.

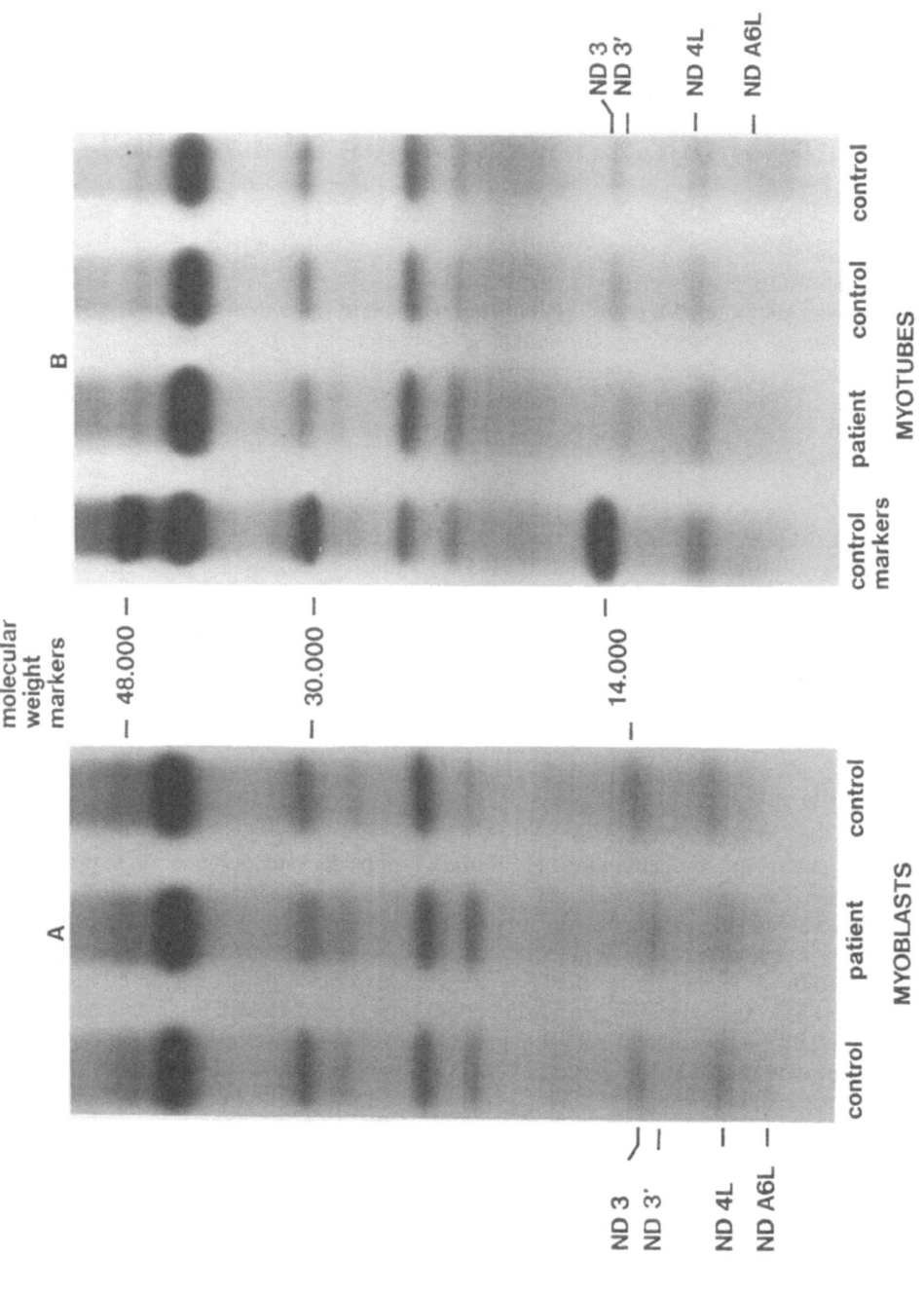

Figure 1 Electrophoresis of mitochondrially encoded proteins: (A) myoblasts; (B) myotubes with left lane control plus molecular weight markers. ND3, normal subunit of complex I; ND3', abnormal subunit

RESULTS AND DISCUSSION

Electrophoresis disclosed a shift in the molecular mass of one mitochondrially encoded protein with a mass of 13 100 Da compared to 13 700 Da in control cultures (Figure 1). The mutated protein was identified as ND3 according to Chomyn *et al.* (1985). The finding was made both in myotubes and in myoblasts.

The shift in the molecular mass of one mitochondrially encoded protein thus revealed in cultured muscle cells is indicative of a deletion of about 600 Da. The mutation was found in a protein which was identified by Chomyn *et al.* (1985) as subunit ND3 belonging to complex I. This finding is in accordance with the results of the mitochondrial respiratory chain studies in the present patient.

Polypeptide sequences belonging to complexes I, III, IV and V are in part encoded by mitochondrial DNA. Defects in mitochondrial DNA are inherited through maternal transmission. Proof of such inheritance however is difficult to obtain, and usually rests on pedigree studies (Egger and Wilson, 1983; Rosing *et al.*, 1985). But these are not always conclusive. A recent review summarises the evidence for mtDNA mutations as a cause of inherited human disorders (Poulton, 1988).

The findings in the present family illustrate that, at least in certain cases, it is possible to differentiate between genetic defects in mitochondrial and nuclear DNA, making use of altered molecular weight of the mitochondrial gene product. Such findings may have important implications for genetic counselling. Further studies are under way in muscle cell cultures and in cultured fibroblasts from other members of the present family.

REFERENCES

Ching, E. and Attardi, G. High resolution electrophoretic fractionation and partial characterization of the mitochondrial translation products from HeLa cells. *Biochemistry* 21 (1982) 3188–3195

Chomyn, A., Mariottini, P., Cleeter, M. W. J., Ragen, I., Matsuno-Yagi, A. *et al.* Six unidentified reading frames of human mitochondrial DNA encode components of the respiratory-chain NADH dehydrogenase. *Nature* 314 (1985) 592–597

Egger, J. and Wilson, J. Mitochondrial inheritance in a mitochondrially mediated disease. *N. Engl. J. Med.* 309 (1983) 142–146

Poulton, J. Mitochondrial DNA and genetic disease. *Arch. Dis. Child.* 63 (1988) 883–885

Rosing, H. S., Hopkins, L. C., Wallace, D. C., Epstein, C. M. and Weidenheim, K. Maternally inherited mitochondrial myopathy and myoclonic epilepsy. *Ann. Neurol.* 17 (1985) 228–237

Wijburg, F. A., Barth, P. G., Ruitenbeek, W., Wanders, R. J. A., Vos, G. D., Ploos van Amstel, S. L. B. and Schutgens, R. B. H. Familial NADH; Q_1 oxidoreductase (complex I) deficiency: Variable expression and possible treatment. *J. Inher. Metab. Dis.*, 12 Suppl. 2 (1989) 349–351

J. Inher. Metab. Dis. 12 Suppl. 2 (1989) 358–360

Short Communication

Peroxisomal Enzyme Deficiency in X-linked Dominant Conradi–Hünermann Syndrome

P. T. Clayton[1], D. Chester Kalter[2], D. J. Atherton[1], G. T. N. Besley[3] and D. M. Broadhead[3]

[1]*Institute of Child Health and Hospital for Sick Children, London WC1N 3JH;* [2]*St John's Hospital for Diseases of the Skin, London WC2H 7BJ;* [3]*Royal Hospital for Sick Children, Edinburgh EH9 1LF, UK*

The X-linked dominant Conradi–Hünermann syndrome (CHS-XD, McKusick 30295) is characterized by ichthyosiform erythroderma at birth giving way to whorled areas of hyperkeratosis, streaky follicular atrophoderma, cicatricial alopecia and coarse lustreless hair. The facies typically shows frontal bossing, a flattened nasal bridge and malar hypoplasia. Cataracts are common. Skeletal abnormalities include the transient punctate epiphyseal calcifications, asymmetric limb shortening and short stature. According to Happle (1981), CHS-XD can be readily distinguished from an autosomal dominant form of the Conradi–Hünermann syndrome (CHS-AD, McKusick 11865) because the latter does not produce whorled/streaky skin lesions or cataracts. Differentiation between CHS-XD and autosomal recessive rhizomelic chondrodysplasia punctata (RCP, McKusick 21510) presents no serious problem: patients with RCP have severe, symmetrical proximal limb shortening, marked psychomotor retardation, mild ichthyotic skin changes and they rarely survive beyond 2 years of age.

RCP is a peroxisomal disorder. Cultured fibroblasts show reduced activity of acyl CoA:dihydroxyacetone phosphate acyl transferase (DHAPAT, a peroxisomal enzyme involved in plasmalogen synthesis) and phytanic acid accumulates in the patient's plasma (Schutgens *et al.*, 1986). Reduced activity of DHAPAT in the fibroblasts of a female infant with Conradi–Hünermann syndrome was first reported by Holmes *et al.* in 1987. Although these authors referred to the condition as an autosomal dominant one, the patient described had 'swirls of hyperkeratotic skin' and she and her mother both had cataracts – features suggestive of CHS-XD.

This report describes another female infant with CHS and reduced activity of DHAPAT. The family history and clinical features both support the diagnosis of CHS-XD.

CASE REPORTS AND METHODS

The proband, V.S., was born with diffuse erythema and scaling. By 5 months a streaky and whorled pattern of erythema and pallor had become obvious. At 15 months examination revealed, in addition, sparse hair, frontal bossing, a flattened

358

Journal of Inherited Metabolic Disease. ISSN 0141–8955. Copyright © SSIEM and Kluwer Academic Publishers, PO Box 55, Lancaster, UK.

nasal bridge and malar hypoplasia. Length was below the third centile, developmental assessment indicated only mild delay, no cataracts were detectable and skeletal surveys at 6 months and 1 year showed no calcific stippling. White cell chromosomal analysis showed no evidence of a deletion or translocation. The steroid sulphatase activity in cultured skin fibroblasts was normal.

C.S., the mother of the proband, had also been born with a scaling erythroderma but this resolved spontaneously by 2 months. Patchy cicatricial alopecia had appeared in childhood and involved mainly the anterior scalp when she was examined. The surrounding hair was coarse and brittle. Her eyebrows and eyelashes were sparse. Examination of the skin of the anterior aspect of the forearms and the medial aspect of the knees revealed multiple patches and streaks of follicular atrophoderma. Also evident were bilateral asymmetric cataracts which had been present since her late teens and a mild degree of frontal bossing. Her adult height was 152 cm and her development had been normal.

C.S. gave the following family history: she had two normal sisters and two normal brothers but a third brother died at 24 weeks gestation. Her mother had no obvious features of CHS-XD but her maternal grandmother had been only 148 cm tall with shortened thighs and digits, bilateral cataracts, thick hair, thick nails and 'large pores'.

Skin biopsies were obtained from V.S. and C.S. for fibroblast culture. No attempt was made specifically to biopsy the area of a particular skin lesion. DHAPAT activity in the fibroblasts was assayed as described previously (Besley and Broadhead, 1987). Plasma phytanic acid, very long-chain fatty acids and bile acids were also assayed by established methods (Clayton *et al.*, 1987).

RESULTS

The activity of DHAPAT in cultured fibroblast from V.S. (Table 1) was reduced to a level similar that that seen in patients with RCP but not as low as seen in patients with absent peroxisomes (Zellweger syndrome). The activity of DHAPAT in fibroblasts from CS was at the lower limit of the normal range. Plasma phytanic acid, very long-chain fatty acids and bile acids were all normal in V.S.

Table 1   Activity of acyl CoA: dihydroxyacetone phosphate acyl tranferase (DHAPAT) in fibroblasts from control subjects, from patient V.S., her mother C.S., and patients with rhizomelic chondrodysplasia punctata, and Zellweger syndrome

	DHAPAT activity $(\text{nmol}(\text{mg protein})^{-1}\text{h}^{-1})$ $(\text{mean}\pm\text{SD})$
Patient V.S.	0.52 ± 0.03
C.S. (mother of V.S.)	1.30 ± 0.08
Rhizomelic chondrodysplasia punctata $(n=5)$	0.53 ± 0.11
Zellweger syndrome $(n=12)$	0.16 ± 0.11
Controls $(n=55)$	2.28 ± 0.70

DISCUSSION

Transmission of the disorder from mother to daughter through four generations, a complete absence of affected males, the unexplained death of a male foetus at 24 weeks gestation, and the physical signs in V.S. and C.S. all indicated CHS-XD. The biochemical findings in V.S. were similar to those found in patients with RCP in some respects (reduced activity of DHAPAT, normal very long-chain fatty acids, normal bile acids) but·differed in respect of the plasma phytanate concentrations (elevated in RCP but normal in V.S.). We conclude that reduced activity of DHAPAT in fibroblasts can occur as a result of carriage of the CHS-XD gene on one of the X-chromosomes. The fact that reduced activity of DHAPAT was not found in the fibroblasts from CS may be attributable to lyonization, the X chromosome carrying the CHS-XD gene being inactivated in many of the fibroblasts. Alternatively, the difference in ages may be important. Either way it is the same phenomenon as observed by Holmes *et al.* (1987) in a mother and daughter with Conradi–Hünermann syndrome.

REFERENCES

Besley, G. T. N. and Broadhead, D. M. Dihdroxyacetone phosphate acyl transferase deficiency in peroxisomal disorders. *J. Inher. Metab. Dis.* 10 Suppl. 2 (1987) 236–238

Clayton, P. T., Lake, B. D., Hall, N. A., Shortland, D. B., Carruthers, R. A. and Lawson, A. M. Plasma bile acids in patients with peroxisomal dysfunction syndromes; analysis by capillary gas chromatography – mass spectrometry. *Eur. J. Pediatr.* 146 (1987) 166–173

Happle, R. Cataracts as a marker of genetic heterogeneity in chondrodysplasia punctata. *Clin. Genet.* 19 (1981) 64–66

Holmes, R. D., Wilson, G. N. and Hajra, A. K. Peroxisomal enzyme deficiency in the Conradi–Hünermann form of chondrodysplasia punctata. (Letter) *N. Engl. J. Med.* 316 (1987) 1608

Schutgens, R. B. H., Heymans, H. S. A., Wanders, R. J. A., Van der Bosch, H. and Tager, J. M. Peroxisomal disorders: a newly recognised group of genetic diseases. *Eur. J. Pediatr.* 144 (1986) 430–440

NOTE ADDED IN PROOF

The DHAPAT activity in the fibroblasts from V.S. rose to $1\cdot5$ nmol $(\text{mg protein})^{-1}\text{h}^{-1}$ after prolonged culture of the cells. We speculate that the cells in which the normal X chromosome is active grow more rapidly and eventually comprise the majority of the population.

J. Inher. Metab. Dis. 12 Suppl. 2 (1989) 361–364

Short Communication

The Heterogeneity of Leber's Congenital Amaurosis

J. Aikawa[1], T. Noro[1], K. Tada[1], K. Narisawa[2] and T. Hashimoto[3]
Departments of [1]Pediatrics and [2]Biochemical Genetics, Tohoku University School of Medicine, 1-1 Seiryo-machi, Sendai 980; [3]Department of Biochemistry, Shinshu University School of Medicine, Matsumoto 390, Japan

Recent clinical and biochemical studies have revealed the existence of a 'peroxisomal disorder' originating in dysfunction of peroxisomes. In spite of intensive studies, the primary lesion of Zellweger syndrome is obscure (Aikawa *et al.*, 1987). Johan *et al.* (1986) reported peroxisomal dysfunction in a boy with neurological symptoms and amaurosis. In the patient's liver, electron microscopy did not show organelles that looked like peroxisomes in appearance and number. We report here four cases of Leber disease and the heterogeneity among them.

CASE HISTORIES

Case 1: A one-year-old girl is the first child of healthy unrelated parents. Pregnancy and delivery were normal. The birth weight was 2420 g. At 2 months old, she was diagnosed as having Leber's congenital amaurosis ophthalmologically and had a flat electroretinogram (ERG).

Case 2: a girl, was an older sister of case 3. Pregnancy and delivery were normal. The birth weight was 2250 g. After delivery, she had watery diarrhoea, resulting in failure to thrive. At admission to our hospital, she had hepatomegaly and pericarditis. Ophthalmologically she was diagnosed to have retinal dystrophy. In spite of intensive care, she died of heart failure.

Case 3: a 3½-year-old boy, had normal delivery. He had severe hypotonia, mental and physical retardation, convulsions and peripheral nerve disturbance. He had retinal pigmentary degeneration and flat ERG.

Case 4: a 3-year-old boy, had severe hypotonia and mental and physical retardation. He was diagnosed as having Leber's congenital amaurosis ophthalmologically. With CT scan and NMR–CT, demyelination was observed in mainly the occipital portion of the brain.

MATERIALS AND METHODS

Liver samples of cases 1 and 4 were obtained with needle biopsy. In case 3, open liver biopsy was performed. Urinary dicarboxylic acids were analysed with gas–

Journal of Inherited Metabolic Disease. ISSN 0141–8955. Copyright © SSIEM and Kluwer Academic Publishers, PO Box 55, Lancaster, UK.

liquid chromatography. Very long-chain fatty acids were extracted from the fasting serum and red blood cell membrane. VLCFA were analysed with gas–liquid chromatography (equipped with capillary column).

Bile acids in the serum and urine were extracted and analysed by gas–liquid chromatography. The liver specimens were subjected to electron microscopic study with diaminobenzidine.

For immunoblotting, the proteins were separated by sodium dodecyl sulphate–polyacrylamide gel electrophoresis (Laemmli, 1970). The proteins were transferred electrophoretically from the gel to nitrocellulose membranes (Towbin *et al.*, 1979) and the transferred proteins were visualized with first antibody and second peroxidase conjugated antibody.

RESULTS

In case 2, the specimens of liver, kidney, brain and so on were not obtained for biochemical analyses but histological examinations were made using autopsy specimens. The examinations revealed micronodullar cirrhosis in liver, subcortical microcysts in kidney and hypomyelination of white matter in brain.

Cases 1, 3 and 4 were diagnosed as Leber's congenital amaurosis ophthalmologic-ally. Case 1 had no elevated very long-chain fatty acids (VLCFA) in sphingomyelin fractions from serum and RBC membrane. Case 3 had elevated VLCFA in the sphingomyelin fraction from RBC membrane. Case 4 had elevated VLCFA in sphingomyelin fractions from serum and RBC membrane (Table 1). Phytanic acid, abnormal bile acids and dicarboxylic acids were undetectable in serum and urine from cases 1, 3 and 4.

In biopsied liver from cases 1, 3, and 4, we could recognize the bands of peroxisomal β-oxidation enzymes (acyl-CoA oxidase (EC 1.3.99.3), the bifunctional protein with enoyl-CoA hydratase (EC 4.2.1.17) and 3-hydroxyacyl-CoA dehydrogenase (EC 1.1.1.35) activities and 3-oxoacyl-CoA thiolase (EC 2.3.1.16)).

On electron microscopy with diaminobenzidine, we found peroxisomes in biopsied livers of cases 1, 3 and 4. We tried to estimate the number of peroxisomes in biopsied liver. The biopsied liver was embedded with Epon, treated with anticatalase antibody and horse radish peroxidase conjugated antirabbit IgG. We found a distinct decrease in the number of peroxisomes in biopsied liver of case 3 and histological examination revealed micronodullar cirrhosis.

DISCUSSION

Johan *et al.* (1986) reported a patient with biochemical findings similar to those in Zellweger syndrome but with a different clinical picture. The patient was diagnosed as having Leber's congenital amaurosis ophthalmologically. We have analysed four cases of Leber's congenital amaurosis. Case 1 had only ophthalmological disturbance. In case 2, the histological findings of the autopsied specimens were similar to those of Zellweger syndrome. Probably, case 2 had a severe type of Leber disease.

Table 1 Very long-chain fatty acids in sphingomyelin

	Serum sphingomyelin fraction					RBC membrane sphingomyelin fraction				
	Case 1	Case 2	Case 3	Case 4	Control ($\bar{x}$, n = 10)	Case 1	Case 2	Case 3	Case 4	Control ($\bar{x}$, n = 20)
$C_{24:0}/C_{22:0}$	0.71	—	0.936	0.81	0.45	2.14	—	2.30	2.51	2.50
$C_{24:1}/C_{22:0}$	0.31	—	0.540	0.49	0.30	1.77	—	1.81	1.90	1.45
$C_{26:0}/C_{22:0}$	0.05	—	0.188	0.31	0.03	0.04	—	0.46	0.38	0.06
$C_{26:1}/C_{22:0}$	0.03	—	0.135	0.10	0.05	0.03		0.51	0.29	0.07

In biopsied liver, we recognized the bands of peroxisomal β-oxidation enzymes by Western blotting. Since three peroxisomal β-oxidation enzymes were detected, cases 3 and 4 were thought to be different from pseudo-Zellweger syndrome (acyl-CoA oxidase deficiency) and pseudoneonatal adrenoleukodystrophy (3-ketoacyl-CoA thiolase deficiency). Furthermore, the liver in case 4 revealed peroxisomes normal in size and number. Case 3 had a decreased number of peroxisomes. The differences between case 3 and 4 at the enzyme level were unknown. These findings indicate a variety of heterogeneity in Leber's congenital amaurosis.

REFERENCES

Aikawa, J., Ishizawa, S., Narisawa, K., Tada, K., Yokota, S. and Hashimoto, T. The abnormality of peroxisomal membrane proteins in Zellweger syndrome. *J. Inher. Metab. Dis.* 10 Suppl. 2 (1987) 211–213

Johan, E. K., Bengt, F. K., Albrecht, R., Ingeman, B. and Jan, I. P. Peroxisomal dysfunction in a boy with neurologic symptoms and amaurosis (Leber disease): Clinical and biochemical findings similar to those observed in Zellweger syndrome. *J. Pediatr.* 108 (1986) 19–24

Laemmli, U. K. Cleavage of structural proteins during the assembly of the head of bacteriophage T₄. *Nature (London)* 227 (1970) 680–685

Towbin, H., Staehlin, T. and Gordon, J. Electrophoretic transfer of protein from polyacrylamide gels to nitrocellulose sheets. Procedure and some applications. *Proc. Natl. Acad. Sci. USA* 76 (1979) 4350–4354

J. Inher. Metab. Dis. 12 Suppl. 2 (1989) 365–368

Short Communication

Hurler–Scheie Phenotype Associated with Consanguinity

D. L. Davies[1], G. N. Dutton[2], J. Farquharson[3], R. W. Logan[3] and J. L. Tolmie[4]
Departments of [1]Medicine and [2]Ophthalmology, Western Infirmary, Glasgow G11 6NT; [3]Department of Biochemistry and [4]Institute of Medical Genetics, Royal Hospital for Sick Children, Glasgow, UK

Both Hurler(1H) and Scheie(1S) diseases (McKusick 25280) are caused by a deficiency of α-L-iduronidase (EC 3.2.1.76). To explain their widely different phenotypes McKusick *et al.* (1972) suggested that the abnormal genes H and S are allelic. A compound form was postulated (H/S) and at least 33 such cases have been reported (Roubicek *et al.*, 1985). Amongst such H/S compound cases the frequency of parental consanguinity should be no higher than in the general population. However, five instances of parental consanguinity amongst H/S cases have been reported suggesting a third allelic mutant. We describe a further case with H/S phenotype whose parents were related.

PATIENT

A 15-year-old girl, whose parents were first cousins once removed, presented with symptoms of tiring easily, stiff joints, frequent colds, breathlessness on exertion, post-exertional muscle stiffness, difficulty in wearing teenage skirts and poor eyesight. Past medical history included operations for congenital dislocation of hip (age 2 years), umbilical hernia (age 6) and grommets in both ears (age 8). Investigations elsewhere for mild 'spasticity' in the legs (age 10) had shown a normal CT scan of head, normal myelogram and slightly raised CSF protein content ($80\,mg\,dL^{-1}$). Menarche had occurred at the age of 11 years and her periods had been regular.

On examination (Figure 1) she had hypertelorism, a short neck, pixielike facies with receding chin and short stature (144 cm; −3 SD). Genital and axillary hair was sparse; breast development was normal. There was clinical evidence of aortic stenosis, hepatomegaly (down to level of anterior superior iliac spine), conductive deafness, lumbar lordosis, genu valgum and severe restriction of all movements of shoulders. Reflexes in the legs were brisk but there was no gross spasticity or muscle weakness and plantar reflexes were flexor. Sensation was intact. Blood pressure was 98/78. Corrected visual acuity was 6/12 (R) and 6/18 (L). Bilateral swelling of optic disc margins was present with a focal intra-retinal infiltrate present below the left disc. The cornea appeared clear.

365

Journal of Inherited Metabolic Disease. ISSN 0141-8955. Copyright © SSIEM and Kluwer Academic Publishers, PO Box 55, Lancaster, UK.

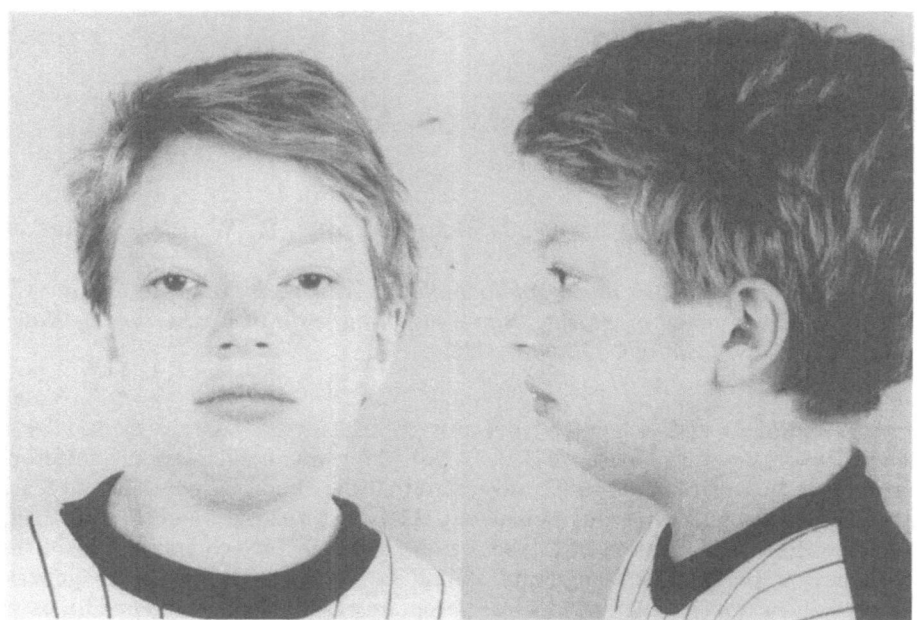

Figure 1 Appearance of a 15-year-old girl with α-L-iduronidase deficiency with a phenotype suggestive of the Hurler–Scheie syndrome

INVESTIGATIONS

Mucopolysaccharides: Urinary dermatan sulphate excretion (Duncan *et al.*, 1973) was increased whilst leukocyte enzyme studies and cultured skin fibroblasts (Hall and Neufeld, 1973, with reduction in sample size requirements) showed an absence of α-L-iduronidase activity using phenyl-α-iduronidide as substrate.

General biochemistry and haematology: Blood film was normal with no evidence of inclusion bodies. Serum electrolytes, blood urea, liver function tests, thyroid function, plasma active and inactive renin concentration, prolactin and pituitary–ovarian function were well within their respective normal ranges.

Radiology: Chest X-ray showed typical oar-shaped ribs. Skull views showed a J-shaped fossa and a very mild degree of platybasia. The humeral and femoral capital epiphyses appeared small in association with some underdevelopment of the glenoid fossa, acetabulum and iliac wings, the latter giving the appearance of 'flared' iliac crests. Lumbar spine showed some scalloping of anterior and posterior borders but no loss of height. The elbows, knees and hands were normal. CT scan of the brain now showed dilatation of lateral and 3rd ventricles but with normal 4th ventricle. Magnetic resonance imaging showed no evidence of a foramen magnum abnormality. Intracranial pressure monitoring was normal.

Opthalmology: Slit-lamp examination revealed bilateral fine peripheral granularity of the cornea compatible with the reduction in visual acuity. Fluorescein angiography showed late staining of the left disc and infiltrate, but the right eye was normal.

Heart: Echocardiography confirmed moderately severe aortic stenosis with a gradient of around 70 mmHg and evidence of mitral valve thickening with slightly impaired diastolic closure rate.

Intellectual assessment: (W.I.S.C.) Full scale IQ was assessed and compared with a previous school assessment. There was no overall change and she functioned within the average IQ range (IQ 92 at 13 years and 89 at 16 years). Of the verbal tests the comprehension subtest showed a particular gain (72 *vs* 90) perhaps due to learning strategies highlighted at school. Performance subtests, however, were worse (113 *vs* 91) reflecting increased physical difficulties and persistent poor retentive memory.

DISCUSSION

This 15-year-old girl with α-L-iduronidase deficiency has a phenotype suggestive of the Hurler–Scheie syndrome. The impish face, receding chin, mild mental and skeletal involvement, and severe heart disease correspond to phenotype I suggested by Roubicek *et al.* (1985). Corneal opacities were not suspected clinically but abnormal fine granularity was found on slit-lamp examination. The appearance of the optic discs was more suggestive of infiltration than papilloedema (intracranial pressure monitoring normal).

Biochemical differentiation between types 1H, 1H/S and IS has proved difficult (see Mueller *et al.*, 1984, and Roubicek *et al.*, 1985, for bibliography) although Fujibayashi *et al.* (1984) were able to distinguish between Hurler, Scheie and Hurler–Scheie intermediate case fibroblasts. Differences may exist between *in vitro* and *in vivo* enzyme activities. Recently, Whitley *et al.* (1987) have described a phenotypically normal obligate heterozygote for Hurler syndrome with very low levels of α-L-iduronidase activity with normal substrate affinity (K_m) but reduced catalytic activity (V_{max}); this may complicate prenatal diagnosis.

Presumably, to account for the extreme variability of phenotype ranging from apparent normality to full blown Hurler's syndrome, there may be a spectrum of mutations (variant normal and abnormal) affecting enzyme activity, subunit structure, post-translational processing and substrate specificity (Schuchman and Desnick, 1988). Until these mutations at the molecular level are better understood it remains difficult in any one case to distinguish 'genetic compounds' from homozygotes for mutations of intermediate severity.

REFERENCES

Duncan, D. M., Logan, R. W., Ferguson-Smith, M. A. and Hall, F. The measurement of acid mucopolysaccharides (glycosaminoglycans) in amniotic fluid and urine. *Clin. Chim. Acta* 45 (1973) 73–83
Fujibayashi, S., Minami, R., Ishikawa, Y., Wagatsuma, K., Nakao, T. and Tsugawa, S.

Properties of α-L-iduronidase in cultured skin fibroblasts from α-L-iduronidase deficient patients. *Hum. Genet.* 65 (1984) 268–272

Hall, C. W. and Neufeld, E. F. α-L-iduronidase activity in cultured skin fibroblasts and amniotic fluid cells. *Arch. Biochem. Biophys.* 158 (1973) 817–821

McKusick, V. A., Howell, R. R., Hussels, I. E., Neufeld, E. F. and Stevenson, R. E. Allelism, non-allelism and genetic compounds among the mucopolysaccharidoses. *Lancet* 1 (1972) 993–996

Mueller, O. T., Shows, T. B. and Opitz, J. M. Apparent allelism of the Hurler, Scheie, and Hurler/Scheie syndromes. *Am. J. Med. Genet.* 18 (1984) 547–556

Roubicek, M., Gehler, J. and Spranger, J. The clinical spectrum of α-L-iduronidase deficiency. *Am. J. Med. Genet.* 20 (1985) 471–481

Schuchman, E. H. and Desnick, R. J. Mucopolysaccharidosis Type 1 subtypes. *J. Clin. Invest.* 81 (1988) 98–105

Whitley, C. B., Gorlin, R. J. and Krivit, W. A non-pathologic allele (I^w) for low α-L-iduronidase enzyme activity *vis-à-vis* pre-natal diagnosis of Hurler syndrome. *Am. J. Med. Genet.* 28 (1987) 233–243

J. Inher. Metab. Dis. 12 Suppl. 2 (1989) 369–371

Short Communication

Detection of Fabry's Disease Carriers by Enzyme Assay of Hair Roots

C. E. Hatton, A. Cooper and I. B. Sardharwalla

Willink Biochemical Genetics Unit, Royal Manchester Children's Hospital, Pendlebury, Manchester, M27 1HA, UK

Fabry's disease (McKusick 30150) is an X-linked lysosomal storage disorder characterized by a deficiency of α-galactosidase (EC 3.2.1.22). In affected hemizygous males, tissue glycosphingolipid deposition causes extremity pain, angiokeratomous skin lesions and corneal opacities. Death usually occurs in mid-adulthood due to renal or cardiac failure. Female carriers of the disorder may show clinical symptoms, particularly corneal verticillata (Desnick and Sweeley, 1983).

Carrier detection is complicated by the phenomenon of random inactivation of the X chromosome during early embryonic development (Lyon, 1961). Thus carriers are a mosaic of normal and mutant cells in varying proportions and those with a higher proportion of normal cells may not show reduced enzyme activity in all tissues. Hair roots are clonal in origin, developing from three to four progenitor cells (Gartler *et al.*, 1971). It is probable that some roots will express only the normal or mutant allele, making this tissue suitable for carrier detection.

We report a method for detection of Fabry's disease carriers by assay of α-galactosidase activity in individual hair roots which has proved successful in identifying heterozygotes in the families studied to date.

METHODS

A minimum of 20 hair roots were plucked randomly from the scalp of each subject and trimmed just above the sheath. Individual roots were frozen and thawed five times in $60\,\mu L$ 0.1% Triton X-100 (Sigma). $40\,\mu L$ of extract was assayed for α-galactosidase activity by a 4-h incubation with $40\,\mu L$ $14\,\mathrm{mmol\,L^{-1}}$ 4-methylumbelliferyl-α-D-galactopyranoside (Koch-Light) in $0.1\,\mathrm{mol\,L^{-1}}$ sodium acetate buffer pH 4.8 containing $0.18\,\mathrm{mol\,L^{-1}}$ N-acetyl-D-galactosamine (Sigma).

Ten microlitres of extract were assayed for β-hexosaminidase (EC 3.2.1.30) activity by 30 min incubation with $20\,\mu L$ $6\,\mathrm{mmol\,L^{-1}}$ 4-methylumbelliferyl-N-acetyl-β-D-glucosaminide (Sigma) in $0.1\,\mathrm{mol\,L^{-1}}$ sodium citrate buffer pH 4.4.

Both incubations were carried out at 37°C and reactions terminated by addition of $2\,\mathrm{mL}$ $0.5\,\mathrm{mol\,L^{-1}}$ sodium carbonate/sodium hydrogen carbonate buffer pH 9.5. Fluorescence was determined using an Aminco Fluoro-colorimeter (excitation 360 nm, emission 450 nm). Hair root activities were calculated as $\mathrm{nmol\,h^{-1}}$ per root and expressed as a ratio of α-galactosidase/β-hexosaminidase (αgal/βhex).

Table 1 Hair root αgal/βhex ratios and leukocyte α-galactosidase activities of controls and families with a history of Fabry's disease

	αgal/βhex (mean ratio)	*No. of roots analysed*	*Less than ⅓ of mean (%)*	*Leukocyte α-galactosidase*[a]
		Hair roots		
Controls (n = 6)	0.030	>20	0–2.7	20–120
Family A:				
Proband P.L.	0.0006	34	—	0.3
Sister B.L.*	0.019	44	9	89
Sister M.T.*	0.022	37	5	53
Family B:				
Proband W.F.	ND		ND	1.2
Daughter, W.F.*	0.011	25	36	11.2
Niece K.L.*	0.016	40	20	ND
Sister G.B.*	0.011	21	38	5.5
Sister L.G.	0.032	39	2.5	ND
Family C:				
Proband M.M.	ND		ND	0.3
Mother S.M.*	0.021	39	13	17
Family D:				
Proband D.P.	ND		ND	0.6
Sister A.P.	0.033	35	0	ND
Family E:				
Proband P.M.	ND		ND	0.6
Aunt P.B.	0.053	26	0	33
Aunt S.D.	0.047	37	0	43
Family F:				
Aunt G.S.*	0.020	40	20	ND
Cousin E.S.	0.024	38	2.6	ND

* Subjects designated as heterozygotes.
[a] units of $\mu mol\,(g\ protein)^{-1}h^{-1}$.
ND = not determined.

Leukocyte α-galactosidase activity and protein content were measured as previously described (Cooper *et al.*, 1988) and activities expressed as $\mu mol\,(g\ protein)^{-1}h^{-1}$.

RESULTS AND DISCUSSION

Table 1 shows mean αgal/βhex ratios and the proportion of ratios below one-third of each individual's mean ratio in controls and six families with a history of Fabry's disease. Hair roots from an affected male (Family A, Proband P.L.) showed deficient α-galactosidase activity and normal β-hexosaminidase activity in all roots analysed. Controls showed 0–2.7% of ratios below one-third of their mean whereas family members designated as carriers showed a mixture of normal, intermediate and deficient ratios with 5–38% of values below the one-third level.

Carriers showed lower mean ratios than controls due to the presence of hair roots with deficient and intermediate α-galactosidase activity (Controls 0.034 ± 0.0148, $n = 11$; Carriers 0.017 ± 0.0046, $n = 7$). The α-galactosidase activity was related to a reference enzyme, β-hexosaminidase, in order to minimize variation due to differences in hair root morphology within and between individuals (Nwokoro and Neufeld, 1979). When results were expressed simply as $nmol\,h^{-1}$ per root carriers were indistinguishable from controls (data not shown).

The proband's daughter W.F. in Family B was the only obligate heterozygote examined. Six out of eleven other female members of Fabry's families tested were found to be carriers. The proband's mother S.M. in Family C showed a carrier distribution indicating that her son's disorder was not due to a new mutation.

All five affected males showed deficient α-galactosidase activity in leukocytes. However leukocyte α-galactosidase activity was decreased in only three of the five heterozygotes identified by hair root analysis, suggesting this tissue is unsuitable for carrier detection. Interestingly the proband's two sisters B.L. and M.T. in Family A were manifesting heterozygotes, presenting with corneal verticillata but showing normal α-galactosidase activity in leukocytes. This suggests that leukocyte activity may not reflect the degree of lyonization in other tissues.

In conclusion although hair root analysis is time consuming it appears to be a reliable technique for detection of carriers in families with a history of Fabry's disease.

REFERENCES

Cooper, A., Hatton, C., Thornley, M. and Sardharwalla, I. B. Human β-mannosidase deficiency: biochemical findings in plasma, fibroblasts, white cells and urine. *J. Inher. Metab. Dis.* 11 (1988) 17–29

Desnick, R. J. and Sweeley, C. C. Fabry's disease: α-galactosidase A deficiency. In Stanbury, J. B., Wyngaarden, J. B., Fredrickson, D. S., Goldstein, J. L. and Brown, M. S. (eds.). *The Metabolic Basis of Inherited Disease*, 5th Edn., McGraw-Hill Inc., New York, 1983, pp. 906–944

Gartler, S. M., Gandini, E., Hutchison, H. T., Campbell, B. and Zechhi, G. Glucose-6-phosphate dehydrogenase mosaicism: utilization in the study of hair follicle variegation. *Ann. Hum. Genet. London* 35 (1971) 1–7

Lyon, M. F. Gene action in the X–chromosome of the mouse. *Nature* 190 (1961) 372–373

Nwokoro, N. and Neufeld, E. F. Detection of Hunter heterozygotes by enzymatic analysis of hair roots. *Am. J. Hum. Genet.* 31 (1979) 42–49

J. Inher. Metab. Dis. 12 Suppl. 2 (1989) 372–374

Short Communication

Immunohistochemical Demonstration of GM$_2$-Ganglioside in the Central Nervous System of a 19-week-old Fetus of Tay–Sachs Disease

M. Taniike[1], K. Inui[1], Y. Hirabayashi[2], H. Tsukamoto[1], J. Nishimoto[1], M. Midorikawa[1], S. Okada[1] and H. Yabuuchi[1]

[1]*Department of Pediatrics, Osaka University Hospital, Osaka, 553 and*
[2]*Department of Biochemistry, Shizuoka College of Pharmacy, Shizuoka, 442, Japan*

Tay–Sachs disease (TSD, McKusick 27275) is an inherited neurodegenerative disorder due to the deficiency of β-hexosaminidase A (EC 3.2.1.52), which causes the accumulation of GM$_2$-ganglioside (GM$_2$) in the central nervous system (CNS) of the patients (O'Brien, 1983), but it remains unknown exactly when and where GM$_2$ begins to accumulate in the affected tissues. We have studied its distribution in the CNS of a TSD fetus and an age-matched control by an immunohistochemical method in conjunction with the distribution of sphingolipid activator protein (SAP)-1, myelin basic protein (MBP) and glial fibrillary acidic protein (GFAP).

MATERIALS AND METHODS

The brain and spinal cord of a 19-week-old fetus diagnosed prenatally as TSD and the spinal cord of a spontaneously aborted 19-week-old fetus were used in this study, with informed consent. Because the brain of the normal control fetus was damaged during delivery, only the spinal cord was used in this study. After fixation in Zamboni's fixative, the tissues were cut 20 μm thick on an LKB cryostat. The subsequent immunohistochemical procedures basically followed the indirect fluorescent method of Coons *et al.* (1941) or the peroxidase–antiperoxidase method of Sternberger *et al.* (1970).

Antibodies to SAP-1 and GM$_2$ was prepared in rabbit by Inui and Wenger (1983) and Higashi *et al.* (1987), respectively. Antibodies to MBP and GFAP were purchased from DAKO Corp., USA.

RESULTS AND DISCUSSION

The distribution of GM$_2$: In the normal spinal cord of the 19-week-old fetus, staining for GM$_2$ was not significant at the thoracic level. However, in the TSD fetus GM$_2$ was recognized in the motor neurons in the anterior horn of the spinal

Journal of Inherited Metabolic Disease. ISSN 0141–8955. Copyright © SSIEM and Kluwer Academic Publishers, PO Box 55, Lancaster, UK.

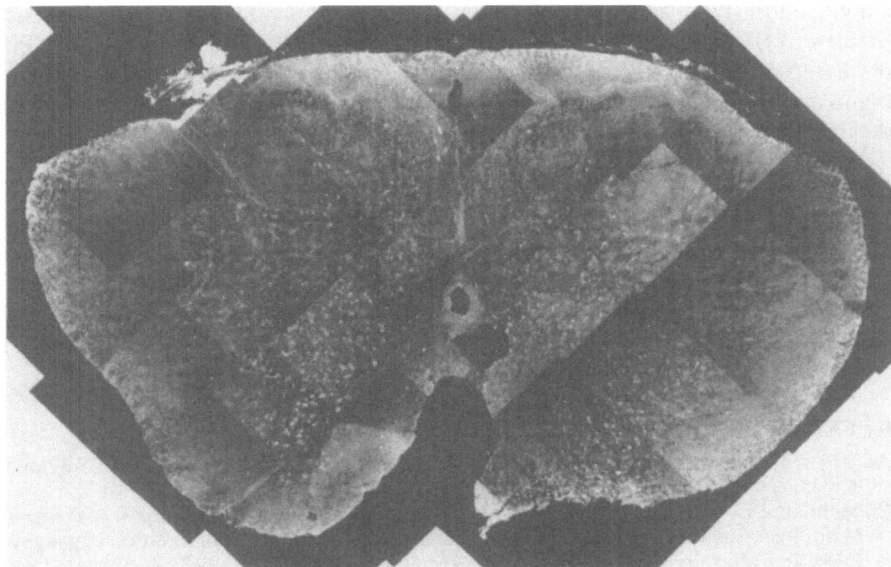

Figure 1 The indirect immunofluorescent staining for GM_2 of the spinal cord of the 19-week-old TSD fetus. The significant fluorescence was recognized in the neurons of the anterior horn

cord (Figure 1), the neurons of the motor nucleus in the midbrain, and the neurons of the thalamic nucleus. But GM_2 was not recognized in the cerebellum nor in the cerebrum. The staining pattern shows the accumulation of GM_2 in the neurons of the phylogenetically older areas of the CNS. Adachi *et al.* (1974) observed GM_2 storage in TSD electron microscopically in the form of loosely packed membranous cytoplasmic bodies in the brain stem, even as early as 12 weeks of gestation in TSD fetuses. In the present study accumulation of GM_2 in neurons of the 19-week-old fetus was demonstrated directly by the immunohistochemical method for the first time. This immunological staining method is very useful for examining the distribution pattern of GM_2 during the differentiation of the CNS.

The distribution of MBP, GFAP and SAP-1: The staining patterns of MBP and GFAP were not different between the control and affected fetus, which confirms normal light microscopic findings in the affected fetuses. On the other hand, the distribution pattern of SAP-1 was different. In the normal control fetus, SAP-1 was present mainly along the fibres in the anterior and posterior funiculus of the spinal cord, suggesting some role of the protein in the myelination process along with sulphatide metabolism. In the affected fetus, the strongest stain for SAP-1 was found in the motor neurons in the anterior horn of the spinal cord, the neurons of the motor nucleus in the midbrain and the neurons of the thalamic nucleus. Its localization was almost the same as that of GM_2. This protein is known to bind GM_2 (Wenger and Inui, 1984) and to increase in content in the brain of GM_2

gangliosidosis (Inui and Wenger, 1983). This is probably the reason why the staining pattern of SAP-1 was almost the same as that of GM_2. The hydrolysis of GM_2 is mediated by GM_2 activator (SAP-3) and the enzyme β-hexosaminidase A (Conzelmann and Sandhoff, 1978). So it is also important to know its distributional changes during the pathological process in TSD.

In this study, we directly demonstrated accumulation of GM_2 in neurons in the phylogenetically older areas of the TSD fetus by the immunohistochemical method. It is easier to survey wide areas of tissues by this method than by an electron microscopical study. Recently antibodies to various sphingolipids have been made. It is very important to examine the distribution patterns of sphingolipids in the CNS of patients with sphingolipidoses using these antibodies and further to follow changes of localization of sphingolipids during the differentiation of human CNS.

REFERENCES

Adachi, M., Schneck, L. and Volk, B. W. Ultrastructural studies of eight cases of fetal Tay–Sachs disease. *Lab. Invest.* 30 (1974) 102–112

Conzelmann, E. and Sandhoff, K. AB variant of infantile GM_2 gangliosidosis: deficiency of a factor necessary for stimulation of hexosaminidase A-catalyzed degradation of ganglioside GM_2 and glycolipid GA_2. *Proc. Natl. Acad. Sci. USA* 75 (1978) 3979–3983

Coons, A. H., Creech, H. J. and Jones, R. N. Immunological properties of an antibody containing a fluorescent group. *Proc. Soc. Exp. Biol. Med.* 47 (1941) 200–202

Higashi, H., Hirabayashi, Y., Hirota, M., Matsumoto, M. and Kato, S. Detection of ganglioside GM_2 in sera and tumor tissues of hepatoma patients. *Jpn. J. Cancer Res.* 78 (1987) 1309–1313

Inui, K. and Wenger, D. A. Concentration of the activator protein for sphingolipid hydrolysis in liver and brain samples from patients with lysosomal storage diseases. *J. Clin. Invest.* 72 (1983) 1622–1628

O'Brien, J. S. The gangliosidoses. In Stanbury, J. B., Wyngaarden, J. B., Fredrickson, D. S., Goldstein, J. L. and Brown, M. S. (eds.), *The Metabolic Basis of Inherited Diseases* 5th Edn., McGraw-Hill, New York, 1983, pp. 945–969

Sternberger, L. A., Hardy, P. H. Jr., Cuculis, J. J. and Meyer, H. G. The unlabelled antibody–enzyme method of immunohistochemistry. Preparation and properties of soluble antigen–antibody complex (horseradish peroxidase–antihorseradish peroxidase) and its use in identification of spirochaetes. *J. Histochem. Cytochem.* 18 (1970) 315–333

Wenger, D. A. and Inui, K. Studies on the sphingolipid activator protein for the enzymatic hydrolysis of GM_1 ganglioside and sulfatide. In Brady, R. O. and Barranger, J. A. (eds.), *The Molecular Basis of Lysosomal Storage Disorders*, Academic Press, New York, 1984, pp. 61–78

J. Inher. Metab. Dis. 12 Suppl. 2 (1989) 375–378

Short Communication

Visualization of the Sugar Moiety in Lymphoid Cell Lines from Fabry's Disease by Lectin Binding

A. LAGERON[1], A. NEGRE[2] and R. SALVAYRE[2]
[1]*INSERM U.55, 184, Rue du Faubourg St-Antoine, 75012-Paris;* [2]*INSERM U.101, Hôpital Purpan - 31059 - Toulouse, France*

Glycosphingolipid storage due to α-galactosidase deficiency (EC 3.2.1.22) charac-terizes the X-linked inherited Fabry's disease (McKusick 30150). Accurate sugar moiety visualization obtained in kidney patients by lectin binding (Faraggiana *et al.*, 1981; Lageron, 1987) prompted us to apply the same method to cell cultures. We chose to work on lymphoid cell lines (LC) obtained by Epstein–Barr virus transformation of lymphocytes, material often used in the study of genetic disease (Glade and Beratis, 1976), with the aim of determining what the lectin-binding method could bring to the knowledge of cell culture storage compared to other histochemical methods and whether modifications of the storage could be brought about by changes in the lipids in the culture medium.

MATERIAL AND METHODS

Lymphoid cell lines were obtained from two male patients (A, B) suffering from Fabry's disease and two normal controls (C, D). Cells were cultured for either 3 or 8 days without medium renewal in RPMI 1640 (Intermed, France) with:

(a) fetal calf serum (10%) (FCS) (Gibco, Grand Island, NY, USA);

(b) human low-density lipoprotein (LP) (100 mg of apolipoprotein B mL^{-1}) prepared in our laboratory by sequential ultracentrifugation; or

(c) ultroser HY (2%) (US) (IBF, France).

Cells were then centrifuged, rinsed twice with PBS and cytocentrifuged onto slides. A 15-minute formalin vapour fixation was performed immediately, followed by two washings. Smears thus obtained were stained by α-amylase–PAS or bound to one of the following HRP lectins (Sigma St-Louis, Mo, USA) (0.25 mg mL^{-1}): *Bandeiraea simplicifolia* (BSA), *Arachis hypogaea* (PNA), *Glycine max* (SBA), *Triticum vulgaris* (WGA), which are specific respectively for α-galactose, lactose, galactosamine, glucosamine and neuraminic acid. Binding to SBA and WGA was tested only in LC cultured in FCS medium. Peroxidase activity was revealed using 3,3-diaminobenzidine (Sigma) and H_2O_2. Control of binding specificity was performed using appropriate sugars (0.2 mol L^{-1}).

Journal of Inherited Metabolic Disease. ISSN 0141–8955. Copyright © SSIEM and Kluwer Academic Publishers, PO Box 55, Lancaster, UK.

We have also checked α-galactosidase deficiency in LC cells: 15 and 8% for patients A and B, respectively, of the normal average (subjects C and D).

RESULTS

Cells from 3-day cultures generally exhibited weak storage patterns so the results are reported for 8-day cultures in the same medium.

PAS positivity after α-amylase digestion occurred only in some LC from A and B subjects as intracytoplasmic vacuoles or as diffuse staining located in the nucleus indentation corresponding to the location of the Golgi apparatus.

BSA binding was seen in almost all LC from A and B cultured in FCS as rings lining vacuoles (Figure 1a). These vacuoles, often numerous, were scattered throughout the cytoplasm and a slight diffuse positivity occurred in the Golgi apparatus of some cells. Cells cultured in LP-enriched medium exhibit the same pattern but with increased and enlarged vacuoles. In contrast, in LC from US medium, the size and number of vacuoles decreased and they were mainly located along the plasma membrane. No binding was seen in cells from C or D controls except around rare vacuoles on some cells cultured in LP medium.

PNA binding disclosed an aspect of hairy binding lining plasma membranes (Figure 1b). In some cells, vacuoles could also be seen gathered at a cell pole or in the nucleus indentation. The same pattern occurred in LC from FCS or LP cultures with a slight increase of the number of vacuoles in the latter case while only scattered vacuoles were seen in cells from US medium. In controls, only slight binding underlined part of the plasma membrane. Binding of both BSA and PNA was inhibited by D-galactose in cells of Fabry patients.

SBA binding featured as scattered rings only in cells from patients A and B; it was totally inhibited by N-acetyl-galactosamine.

WGA binding was seen only on Fabry cells as small scattered vacuoles. This binding was not inhibited by N-acetyl-glucosamine but totally disappeared with acetyl neuraminic acid indicating a sialo-compound.

DISCUSSION

This study underlines several points:

(a) Lectin binding enables visualization of the sugar moiety of the storage material in lymphoid cell lines from Fabry's disease. It discloses much more storage than the PAS method; nevertheless the glycolipid overload was obvious only after an 8-day culture without medium renewal.

(b) The results obtained are totally in agreement with previous ultrastructural and biochemical analyses performed in one of our patients showing typical patterns of glycolipid storage on the same material (Bes *et al.*, 1984).

(c) Variations in lipid in the medium induce expected changes in the lipid-laden cells: LP-enriched medium produces the greatest storage, the LDL being the

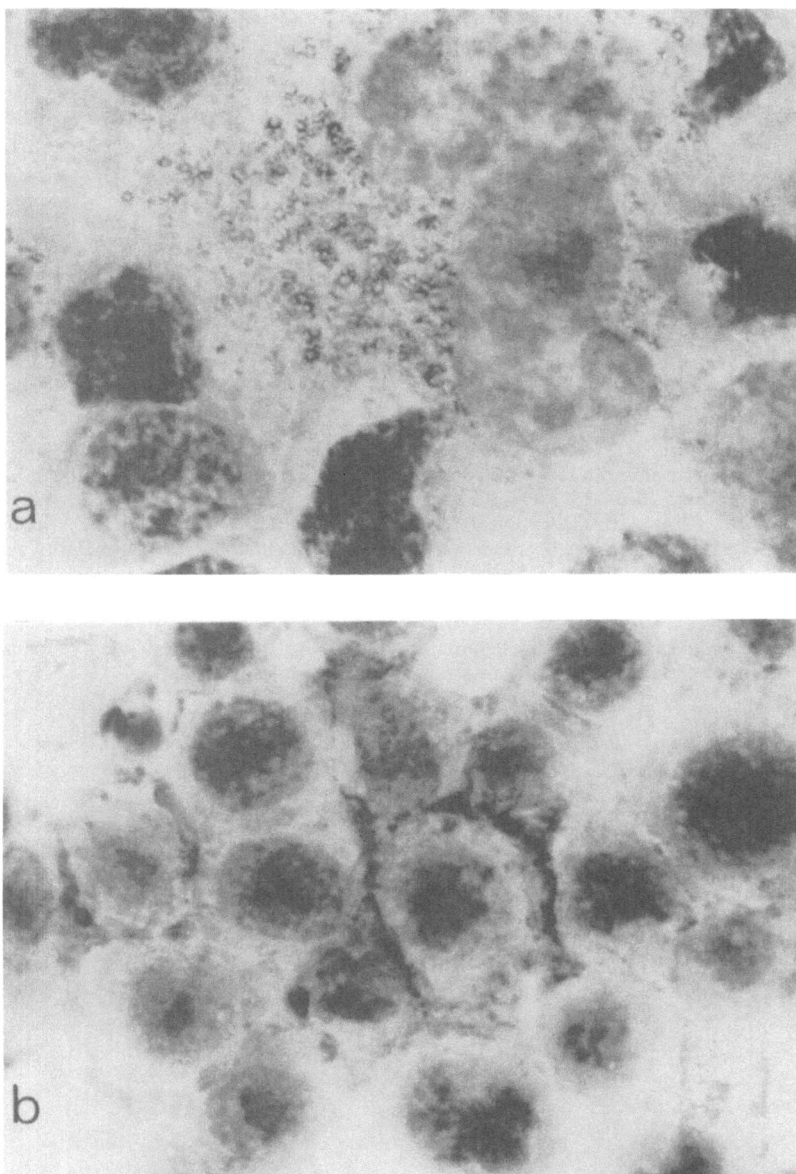

Figure 1 Lymphoid cells from patient A cultured in FCS medium (×900): (a) BSA binding showing rings around numerous vacuoles scattered throughout the cytoplasm; (b) PNA binding visualizing mainly hairy patterns along some plasma membranes and some cytoplasmic vacuoles

normal carrier of plasmatic glycolipids; cells from US medium, on the contrary, show less storage; in these conditions the lipid material may be partially derived from dead cells in the 8-day cultures.

(d) Some binding of lectins such as BSA, specific for α-galactose residues, are consistent with an overload in Fabry's tissues mainly constituted of tri- and digalactosylceramides but, this study also demonstrates the presence of sialo-compounds, galactosamine and lactosyl terminal sugars. The latter, visualized by PNA binding, are particularly interesting in regard to their appearance as a hairy pattern lining the plasma membrane, a pattern not seen in control cells. Their precise composition and their significance remain to be established.

REFERENCES

Bes, J. C., Salvayre, R., Caratero, C., Maret, A., Icart, J., Soleilhavoup, J. P. and Planel, H. Ultrastructural findings on an Epstein–Barr virus-transformed lymphoid cell line from a Fabry patient. *Biol. Cell* 47 (1983) 247–250

Faraggiana, T., Churg, J., Grishman, E., Strauss, L., Prado, A., Bishop, D. F., Schuchman, E. and Desnick, R. J. Light and electron microscopic histochemistry of Fabry's disease. *Am. J. Pathol.* 103 (1981) 247–262

Glade, P. R. and Beratis, N. G. Long-term lymphoid cell lines in the study of human genetics. *Progr. Med. Genet.* 1 (1976) 1–48

Lageron, A. Characterization by lectin binding of the sugar moiety of glycocompounds stored in inherited diseases. *Histochem. J.* 19 (1987) 419–425

J. Inher. Metab. Dis. 12 Suppl. 2 (1989) 379–382

Short Communication

Identification of Intact Dolichol-linked Oligosaccharides in the Brains of Patients with Ceroid-Lipofuscinosis (Batten's Disease)

N. A. HALL and A. D. PATRICK
Department of Clinical Biochemistry, Institute of Child Health, 30 Guilford Street, London WC1N 1EH, UK

Ceroid-lipofuscinosis (CL) (Batten's disease) is an inherited neurodegenerative disorder characterized by the accumulation of tertiary lysosomes containing a storage material. The underlying primary biochemical abnormality has yet to be discovered. However, very marked increases in phosphorylated dolichol (P-dolichol) levels have been found in brain from all four forms of the human disease (Hall and Patrick, 1985; Pullarkat, 1987; Hall and Patrick, 1987; Wolfe *et al.*, 1988), and in a canine form of CL (Keller *et al.*, 1984). We have also found that P-dolichol is highly concentrated in purified storage bodies from an ovine form of CL (unpublished observations).

The solubility properties of the P-dolichol in CL brain imply that it is present largely in the form of dolichyl pyrophosphoryl oligosaccharides (Dol-PP-O) (Hall and Patrick, 1985). These components are extracted by chloroform/methanol/water (1:1:0.3; referred to as 1103) and release their carbohydrate chains on mild acid hydrolysis. Analysis reveals up to ten different oligosaccharides; the predominant components being $Man_5GlcNAc_2$, $Man_6GlcNAc_2$, $Man_7GlcNAc_2$ and $Hex_{10}GlcNAc_2$ (Hall and Patrick, 1988a and b). In this report we confirm that P-dolichol accumulates as Dol-PP-O in CL tissues by identifying high levels of intact Dol-PP-O in extracts of CL brain.

MATERIALS AND METHODS

Brain was obtained at postmortem from two cases of juvenile CL (JCL) (aged 21 and 22 years), two cases of late-infantile CL (LICL) (both aged 5 years), and two disease controls (congenital heart disease and Hunter disease; aged 12 and 13 years, respectively). Lipid extractions were carried out at room temperature using silanised glassware: each extraction consisted of mixing for 30 min on a rotary mixer, followed by centrifugation at $230 \times g$ to separate the phases. Homogenates ($0.5 \, g \, mL^{-1}$ in water) were extracted first with 40 volumes of chloroform/methanol (2:1), and then with a further 20 volumes. The residue was extracted with a mixture of chloroform (3.75 vol.), methanol (2.5 vol.) and water (1.25 vol.) and, after extraction and separation of phases, the lower phase plus interfacial pellet was washed twice with 2.5 volumes of methanol/water (1:1). The composition of the lower phase plus

379

Journal of Inherited Metabolic Disease. ISSN 0141–8955. Copyright © SSIEM and Kluwer Academic Publishers, PO Box 55, Lancaster, UK.

interfacial pellet was adjusted to chloroform/methanol/water (1103) by the addition
of methanol and water. The residue was then extracted twice with 1103 (5 volumes).
Pooled 1103 extracts were dried under nitrogen at 40°C and redissolved in 1103.

Extracts were loaded onto Merck HP-TLC Silica gel 60 plates, and developed
in butanol/acetic acid/water (2:1:1.5). After drying, lipids were located by exposure
to iodine vapour. Sugars were located (after the iodine had evaporated) by spraying
with orcinol (50 mg) dissolved in 10% sulphuric acid (5 mL) and acetone (20 mL),
followed by heating at 110°C. Radioactivity was located by spraying with EN[3]-
HANCE (NEN) and exposing the plates against Kodak X-omat XAR-5 film at
−70°C. Gel filtration was carried out on Lipidex LH 60 (50 × 1.2 cm) eluted with
1103, collecting 2 mL fractions.

P-Dolichol was assayed as described previously (Hall and Patrick, 1987). Oligosaccharides were released from P-dolichol and analysed as described (Hall and
Patrick, 1988a). Synthetic radioactive Dol-PP-O labelled with [³H]glucose was
prepared as described previously (Hall and Patrick, 1988a). Lipid weights were
determined gravimetrically.

RESULTS AND DISCUSSION

Analysis of P-dolichol in CL brains demonstrated that at least 60% of extractable
P-dolichol was in the 1103 extract. In one JCL case where weights of extracts were
determined, Dol-PP-O contributed 12% of the dry weight of the 1103 extract. A

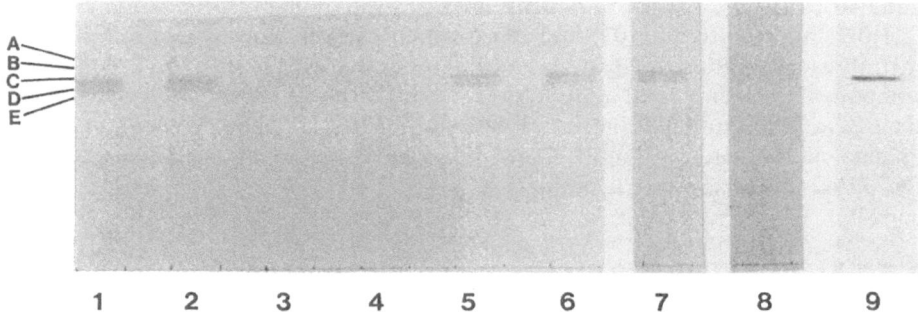

Figure 1   TLC separations of 1103 extracts of brain. 1103 extracts of brain from cases of
JCL (lanes 1 and 2), controls (lanes 3 and 4), or LICL (lanes 5 and 6), were separated by
TLC. Each channel contains extract from 6 mg of tissue. Lipid was detected by iodine vapour
(lanes 1–6). Lanes 7 and 8 show lanes 5 and 4 from the same plate stained with orcinol.
Lane 9 shows fluorography of synthetic [³H]Dol-PP-O separated on the same plate

separation of 1103 extracts from six different brains is shown in Figure 1. Two
bands (labelled D and E) were detected with iodine in all four CL brains but were
present at much reduced levels in the two control brains. Three faint faster migrating
bands (labelled A–C) were detected in all six brains. Detection of sugars on the
same plate located bands D and E in all four CL cases. Lane 9 contains synthetic

[³H]Dol-PP-O (predominantly $Glc_3Man_9GlcNAc_2$-PP-Dol). This is revealed as a single band which comigrates with band E.

These results suggest that bands D and E may be Dol-PP-O. Firstly, band E comigrates with an authentic Dol-PP-O standard. Secondly, both bands are present at much higher levels in CL cases than in controls. Thirdly, their staining properties indicate that they contain both lipid and carbohydrate.

The bond between dolichyl pyrophosphate and oligosaccharide in Dol-PP-O is extremely acid labile (Behrens and Tabora, 1978). We therefore investigated the susceptibility of bands D and E to mild acid hydrolysis. Hydrolysis of the 1103 extract from JCL brain resulted in the complete elimination of bands D and E and the release of oligosaccharide and of a lipid, most of which comigrated with dolichyl monophosphate after TLC.

To investigate why Dol-PP-O appeared to be separated into two bands after TLC, a 1103 extract of brain from a JCL case was fractionated by gel filtration.

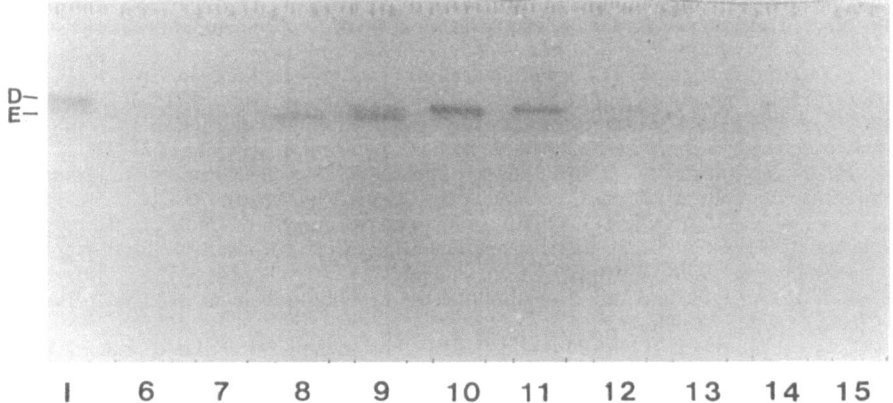

Figure 2 Lipidex LH60 separation of the 1103 extract of brain from a juvenile CL case. A 1103 extract from a JCL brain was separated on a Lipidex LH60 column (50 × 1.2 cm) eluted with 1103 collecting 2 mL fractions. The initial sample (I) and aliquots of fractions 6 to 15 were separated by TLC. Lipid was detected with iodine, though a similar pattern could also be revealed by staining with orcinol. The void volume was at fraction 7, with a low molecular weight marker (Rhodamine 6B) eluting at fraction 18

TLC separations of the fractions containing bands D and E are shown in Figure 2. Both bands elute close to the void volume. However, band E elutes in slightly earlier fractions than band D. Assays of P-dolichol indicated that it was largely present in fractions 8–11. In a separation of synthetic [³H]Dol-PP-O, radioactivity eluted mainly in fractions 8 and 9. TLC analysis of oligosaccharides liberated by mild acid hydrolysis from successive fractions showed high molecular weight oliogosaccharides predominantly in fractions 8 and 9 and the lower molecular weight oligosaccharides in fractions 10 and 11. These results demonstrate that separation on Lipidex LH 60 fractionates Dol-PP-O on the basis of the length of the oliogosaccharide chain. They imply that TLC also fractionates Dol-PP-O on the basis of size, and that molecules with longer oligosaccharide chains (band E) have lower mobilities than those with shorter oligosaccharide chains (band D).

We conclude that the TLC method described here is effective in separating Dol-PP-O. It has enabled us to demonstrate the presence of intact Dol-PP-O in brain from CL patients. The accumulation of Dol-PP-O in CL may be related to the primary metabolic defect in this disorder.

ACKNOWLEDGEMENT

The support of the MRC is gratefully acknowledged.

REFERENCES

Behrens, N. H. and Tabora, E. Dolichol intermediates in the glycosylation of proteins. In Ginsburg, V. (ed.) *Methods in Enzymology*, Vol. 50, Academic Press, New York, 1978, pp. 402–435

Hall, N. A. and Patrick, A. D. Dolichol and phosphorylated dolichol content of tissues in ceroid-lipofuscinosis. *J. Inher. Metab. Dis.* 8 (1985) 178–183

Hall, N. A. and Patrick, A. D. Accumulation of phosphorylated dolichol in several tissues in ceroid-lipofuscinosis (Batten disease). *Clin. Chim. Acta* 170 (1987) 323–330

Hall, N. A. and Patrick, A. D. Accumulation of dolichol-linked oligosaccharides in ceroid-lipofuscinosis (Batten disease). *Am. J. Med. Genet.* Suppl. 5 (1988a) 221–232

Hall, N. A. and Patrick, A. D. Analysis of dolichol-linked oligosaccharides in brains from patients with Batten's disease. *Biochem. Soc. Trans.* 16 (1988b) 1031–1032

Keller, R. K., Armstrong, D., Cram, F. C. and Koppang, N. Dolichol and dolichyl phosphate levels in brain tissue from English Setters with ceroid lipofuscinosis. *J. Neurochem.* 42 (1984) 1040–1047.

Pullarkat, R. K. Dolichols and phosphodolichols in aging and in neurological disorders. *Chem. Script.* 27 (1987) 85–88

Wolfe, L. S., Gauthier, S. and Durham, I. Dolichols and phosphorylated dolichols in the neuronal ceroid-lipofuscinoses, other lysosomal storage diseases and Alzheimer disease. Induction of autolysosomes in fibroblasts. In Zs.-Nagy, I. (ed.), *Lipofuscin-1987: State of the Art*, Elsevier, Amsterdam, 1988, pp. 389–411

J. Inher. Metab. Dis. 12 Suppl. 2 (1989) 383–385

Short Communication

Study of Pathogenesis in Twitcher Mouse, an Enzymatically Authentic Model of Human Krabbe's Disease

K. Inui, J. Nishimoto, M. Taniike, M. Midorikawa, H. Tsukamoto, S. Okada and H. Yabuuchi
Department of Pediatrics, Osaka University, Fukushima-ku, Osaka, 553, Japan

Krabbe's disease (globoid cell leukodystrophy; McKusick 24520) is a genetic neurological disorder due to an enzymic deficiency of galactosylceramidase. The disease is conceptually a lysosomal storage disorder but galactosylceramide (Galcer), the natural substrate of the deficient enzyme, apparently does not accumulate despite the genetic catabolic block (Suzuki and Suzuki, 1983). Recently, accumulation of galactosylsphingosine (Galsph) was demonstrated in nervous system in human Krabbe's disease (Svennerholm *et al.*, 1980) and its animal model (twitcher mouse) (Igisu and Suzuki, 1984). The Galsph, also a substrate of galactosylceramidase, has a cell toxicity which resulted in cell dysfunction. However, the reason why Galcer accumulation does not occur and how Galsph was made still remain unclear. To answer these questions, *in vivo* synthesis of Galcer and Galsph in a sciatic nerve culture and *in vitro* enzymic activities for synthesis of Galcer and Galsph in spinal cord were examined.

MATERIALS AND METHODS

Twitcher mice were a generous gift from Dr Kobayashi, Kyushu University (Fukuoka, Japan) and the genetic status of each mouse was identified by assays of galactosylceramidase activity in the clipped tail (Kobayashi *et al.*, 1982).

In vivo study: About 1 cm of sciatic nerve was excised from mice at different ages and directly cultured in Eagle's minimum essential medium and 10% fetal calf serum containing [³H]galactose (10 μCi mL⁻¹). After washing with phosphate-buffered saline, the sciatic nerve was homogenized with 0.2 mL distilled water and lipid was extracted with 1 mL of chloroform–methanol (2:1). The lower lipid layer was analysed by HPTLC and radioactivity was visualized by exposing the plate to X-ray film (Kodak X–OmatAR) after spraying the plate with enhancer (New England Nuclear). Each spot was identified by comigration with standard lipids by two-dimensional TLC and hydrolysis by specific enzyme or mild acid. The amount of each lipid was calculated after scraping off each spot and measuring the radioactivity. In some experiment, Galsph was added with [³H]galactose to investigate the effect on the synthesis of Galcer.

Journal of Inherited Metabolic Disease. ISSN 0141–8955. Copyright © SSIEM and Kluwer Academic Publishers, PO Box 55, Lancaster, UK.

In vitro study: Spinal cord at different ages was taken and homogenized with distilled water, 20 times the wet weight. Then the homogenate was centrifuged at $800 \times g$ for 10 min and the supernatant was used as enzymic source. UDP-galactose: ceramide galactosyltransferase (GalcerTase) activity was assayed by the method of Neskovic *et al.* (1986) with slight modification. UDP-galactose: sphingosine galactosyltransferase (GalsphTase) was assayed as follows: 10 µg sphingosine was sonicated in 30 µL of $0.5 \, \text{mol} \, \text{L}^{-1}$ Tris–HCl (pH 8.0) and 10 µL of $0.1 \, \text{mol} \, \text{L}^{-1}$ $MgCl_2$ by bath-type sonicator at 60°C for 10 min, then enzyme source and UDP-[^{14}C]galactose (10 nmol) were added and incubated in 0.1 mL total volume for 20 min at 37°C. The reaction was stopped by adding 1 mL of chloroform–methanol (2:1) and 0.15 mL of 5% ammonia solution. The work-up procedure was the same as the method for GalcerTase assay.

RESULTS AND DISCUSSION

In vivo study: In normal mouse sciatic nerve culture, over 60% of the radioactivity of the lipid extract was Galcer and the synthesis of Galcer per mg protein was increased about two-fold from the 1st week of age to the 3rd week of age (Figure 1). On the other hand, the percentage of radioactivity in the lipid extract in the affected mice was decreased and the synthesis per mg protein was also reduced with age to 15% of control at 4 weeks of age (Figure 1). There was no increase of Galcer synthesis in the affected mice. Reciprocally, the synthesis of ceramide hexosides was increased with age, which is probably due to the constituents of globoid cells. Galsph synthesis was not detected by autoradiogram of a 1-day [^{3}H]galactose pulse; but the experiment with a 7-day pulse, gave radioactivity corresponding to the Galsph fraction on silica gel column chromatography about two times higher than control. To examine the effect of Galsph on the synthesis of Galcer, Galsph was added to the culture medium up to a concentration of $300 \, \mu\text{g} \, \text{mL}^{-1}$ but no effect on the synthesis of Galcer was found.

In vitro study: The activity of GalcerTase is highest at 3 weeks in normal mouse spinal cord but the activity in the affected cord was about 30% of control. The activity of GalsphTase is lower than control after 2 weeks of age and about 40% that in normal mice after 3 weeks of age. Galsph did not influence the activity of GalcerTase *in vitro*.

From the *in vivo* study, it is evident that the synthesis of Galcer was increased after 2 weeks of age in normal mice but no increase was found in the affected mice. This may be one of the reasons for the absence of accumulation of Galcer in the affected mice. *In vitro* GalcerTase activity was maintained at about 40% of control at 4 weeks of age, but it does not seem to reflect the *in vivo* synthesis of Galcer. Increased myelination does not occur after birth in the affected mice. The origin of Galsph is not clear in this experiment. In the 7-day pulse experiment the amount of Galsph in the affected mouse was two times higher than control, probably indicating reduced metabolism of Galsph. A Galsph spot was not detected on the TLC plate in a preliminary feeding experiment of sphingosine-labelled Galcer to

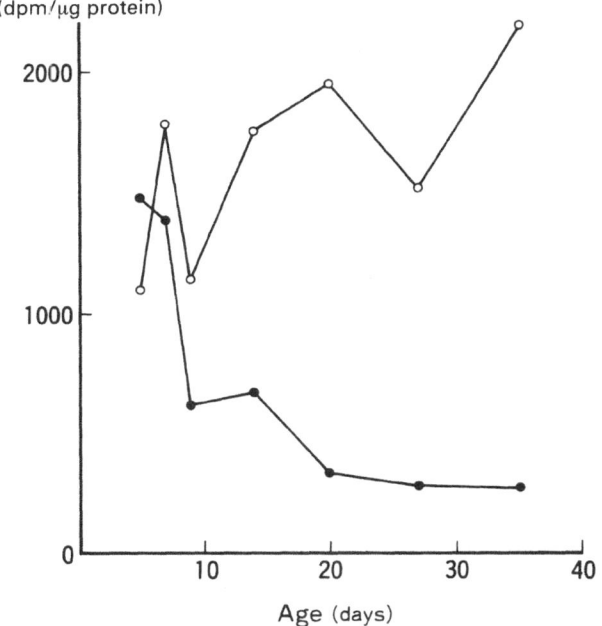

Figure 1   Change of net galactosylceramide synthesis with age. At different ages sciatic nerve was excised and cultured directly for 1 day with [³H]galactose and lipid then extracted and analysed as described in Methods. Radioactivity of galactosylceramide was calculated from the percentage of radioactivity and total radioactivity of lipid extract. The radioactivity was expressed as dpm (mg protein)⁻¹: (○) control; (●) affected

the culture medium of sciatic nerve or skin fibroblasts from Krabbe's disease. Probably Galsph is made through a synthetic pathway that is not via the breakdown of Galcer. This *in vivo* study using a sciatic nerve reflects the metabolic disturbances in the affected mice well, so this is a good method for studying the pathogenesis in twitcher mouse.

REFERENCES

Igisu, H. and Suzuki, K. Progressive accumulation of toxic metabolite in a genetic leukodystrophy. *Science* 224 (1984) 753–755

Kobayashi, Y., Nagara, H., Suzuki, K. and Suzuki, K. The twitcher mouse: Determination of genetic status by galactosylceramidase assay on clipped tail. *Biochem. Med.* 27 (1982) 8–14

Neskovic, N. M., Roussel, G. and Nussbaum, J. L. UDP-galactose: Ceramide galactosyltransferase of rat brain: A new method of purification and production of specific antibodies. *J. Neurochem.* 47 (1986) 1412–1418

Suzuki, K. and Suzuki, Y. Galactosylceramide lipidosis: Globoid cell leukodystrophy (Krabbe's disease). In: Stanbury, J. B., Frederickson, D. S., Goldstein, J. L. and Brown, M. S. (eds.) *The Metabolic Basis of Inherited Disease*, McGraw-Hill, New York, 1983, pp. 857–880

Svennerholm, L., Vanier, M-T. and Manson, J-E. Krabbe disease: a galactosylsphingosine (psychosine) lipidosis. *J. Lipid Res.* 21 (1980) 53–64

J. Inher. Metab. Dis. 12 Suppl. 2 (1989) 386–388

Short Communication

Nuclear Magnetic Resonance Brain Study in a Case of Wilson Disease

R. Longhi[1], E. Riva[1], A. Rottoli[1], R. Valsasina[1], P. Pinelli[2] and M. Giovannini[1]

[1]5th Department of Pediatrics and [2]1st Department of Neurology, University of Milan, Ospedale S. Paolo, via A. di Rudinì 8, 20142 Milano, Italy

CLINICAL CASE

BR was referred to us at the age of 13 years because of slowly progressing neurological signs that had started two years earlier. Symptoms had been dyspnoea, sialorrhoea, ataxic unco-ordinated movements and choreic head and arm tremors. The child appeared excessively emotional. The intelligence quotient was good. Slight hepatomegaly and Kayser–Fleisher rings were found. Wilson disease was suggested by clinical findings and laboratory test results (cupraemia 46 μg dL^{-1} (normal range 65–165); cupruria 348 μg day^{-1} (normal, <80); ceruloplasminaemia 7 mg dL^{-1} (normal 15–60) and generalized aminoaciduria). The hepatic copper concentration (483 μg g^{-1} dry tissue; normal, <55) confirmed the diagnosis.

Nuclear magnetic resonance (NMR) scanning of the brain had shown extensive involvement of the pontine and brainstem trunk white substance and of the basal ganglia and cerebellum (in terms of increased NMR signal). A cortico-subcortical area presented uneven alterations in the left frontal region.

Therapy was started with penicillamine (600 mg day^{-1}), zinc sulphate (200 mg day^{-1}) and vitamin B$_6$ (150 mg day^{-1}), but, after five months, there was slight worsening of the neurological symptoms. Repeated NMR showed accentuation of the cortical lesions and extension to both frontal lobes. Nevertheless, at a later visit, almost one year from the start of therapy, the boy presented definitely improved motor co-ordination: his writing had become more precise and he walked more easily. Eighteen months after the start of therapy, when neurological symptoms and clinical and laboratory findings all pointed to improvement, the child suffered oculocephalogyric crises on the right, which responded immediately to barbiturates. NMR brain scan (Figure 1) confirmed the definite regression of the brainstem and pontine alterations, but showed that a zone of poroencephaly had formed in the left frontal region, the cause of these crises. Electroencephalogram (EEG) during the crises had, in fact, shown a sharp wave pattern in the left posterior frontal zone. For 1–2 seconds before the crises, the amplitude of the tracing decreased (burst suppression).

Journal of Inherited Metabolic Disease. ISSN 0141–8955. Copyright © SSIEM and Kluwer Academic Publishers. PO Box 55, Lancaster, UK.

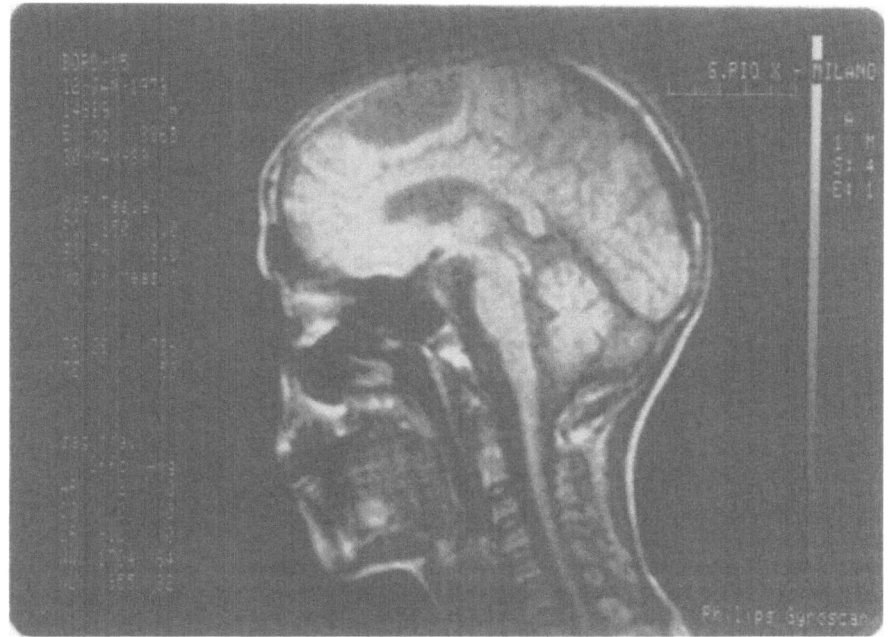

Figure 1   Sagittal scan: a zone of poroencephaly has formed in the frontal region

DISCUSSION

In this one case, NMR investigation showed up aspects of Wilson disease that have already been widely described but are still not clear. It is acknowledged that, despite correction of the copper metabolic disorder, only a small proportion of patients with the mixed hepatocerebral picture, probably under 25%, attains complete functional recovery. Lesions observed in the NMR tracing as a diminution or increase in the signal intensity may be caused by copper accumulation, by ischaemic-type phenomena, by demyelination, oedema or atrophy (Lukes *et al.*, 1983).

The multiple lesions shown up by NMR in this boy, involving the basal ganglia and the midbrain, are those seen most frequently in this disease (Starosta-Rubinstein *et al.*, 1987). The subcortical white substance lesions are not rare and often distributed in frontal lobes (Starosta-Rubinstein *et al.*, 1987). Lesions of the cerebellum and of the mesencephalic tegmentum are the cause of the ataxic symptoms, tremors and dysmetria, while lesions the striatum and caudate nuclei underly the choreic movements. The frontal lobe alterations found in the patient described here only gave rise to patent symptoms 18 months after the start of therapy, when oculocephalogyric crises occurred.

It is conceivable that the initial worsening was linked to excessive mobilization of copper from tissue deposits (Brewer *et al.*, 1987; Starosta-Rubinstein *et al.*, 1987) or imbalances in the concentrations of other trace elements (Pfeiffer and

Camo, 1988). The delayed onset of convulsive crises, however, was very likely related to the severe atrophic-degenerative lesions clearly detectable in the right and left frontal regions on NMR. The exact pathogenesis of these lesions is still much debated. Probably, sponge-like destruction of tissue is the result of abnormal vascular permeability secondary to alteration in the encephalon's energy metabolism or to degeneration of the astrocytes (Lindenberg, 1982). More extensive lesions may result in small cystic cavities, or areas of poroencephaly (Le Fort *et al.*, 1988).

In the light of these considerations, it is difficult to establish a prognosis for our patient, since the brain lesions do not appear to be caused directly by copper deposition. They therefore respond poorly, at least directly, to the chelating action of penicillamine. Only by clarifying the primary defect underlying Wilson disease shall we be able to shed light on the many problems it still poses.

REFERENCES

Brewer, G. J., Terry, C. A., Aisen, A. M. and Hill, G. M. Worsening of neurologic syndrome in patients with Wilson disease with initial penicillamine therapy. *Arch. Neurol.* 44 (1987) 490–493

Lindenberg, L. Tissue reaction in the grey matter of the central nervous system. In Haymaker, W., Adams, R. D. and Thomas, C. (eds.) *Histology and Histopathology of the Nervous System*, Springfield, Illinois, 1982, pp. 1085–1091

Le Fort, D., Deleplanque, B., Louiset, P., Pautrizel, B. and Loiseau, P. Maladie de Wilson: demonstration de lesions corticales et de la substance blanche par IRM. *Rev. Neurol.* 144 (1988) 365–367

Lukes, S. A., Aminoff, M. J., Crooks, L., Kaufman, L., Mills, C. and Newton, T. H. Nuclear magnetic resonance imaging in movement disorders. *Ann. Neurol.* 13 (1983) 690–691

Pfeiffer, C. C. and Camo, B. Wilson's disease. *Arch. Neurol.* 45 (1988) 247

Starosta-Rubinstein, S., Young, A. B., Kluin, K., Hill, G., Aisen, A. M., Gabrielsen, T. and Brewer, G. J. Clinical assessment of 31 patients with Wilson disease. Correlations with structural changes on magnetic resonance imaging. *Arch. Neurol.* 44 (1987) 365–370

J. Inher. Metab. Dis. 12 Suppl. 2 (1989) 389–392

Short Communication

Vitamin C Treatment in Menkes' Disease: Failure to Affect Biochemical and Clinical Parameters

C. J. de Groot[1], F. A. Wijburg[1], P. G. Barth[1], P. A. Bolhuis[2],
W. Peelen[3], N. G. G. M. Abeling[1] and C. J. A. van den Hamer[4]
[1]*Department of Pediatrics and* [2]*Department of Neurology, University Hospital of
Amsterdam (AMC), 1105 AZ Amsterdam, The Netherlands;* [3]*Department of
Pediatrics, St. Jansdal Hospital, Harderwijk, The Netherlands;* [4]*Interuniversitair
Reactor Institute (IRI), Delft, The Netherlands*

Menkes' disease (kinky hair disease, McKusick 30940) is an X-linked recessive disorder characterized by progressive neurological degeneration, hypothermia, seizures, growth retardation, abnormal hair and abnormalities of the major arteries, with death usually within the first 3 years of life (Menkes *et al.*, 1962; Danks *et al.*, 1972). There is an abnormal distribution of copper with low serum, cerebrospinal fluid (CSF), brain and hepatic copper levels but increased copper concentration in kidney, muscle and gut. Cultured fibroblasts show an abnormal accumulation of copper but reduced levels of lysyl oxidase, a copper-containing enzyme (Royce *et al.*, 1980). Decreased activities of other copper-dependent enzymes, such as cytochrome *c* oxidase, tyrosinase and dopamine-β-hydroxylase, explain many of the clinical symptoms. An abnormal metallothionein gene regulation in response to copper has been found (Leone *et al.*, 1985), but the basic defect has yet to be identified.

Results of treatment have been disappointing. Parenteral copper administration did not result in improvement. There is one report of clinical and biochemical improvement in a patient with Menkes' disease due to vitamin C therapy (Ueki *et al.*, 1985). We attempted to treat a patient with copper infusions and vitamin C and report the results.

PATIENT AND TREATMENT

The patient is the third son of healthy, unrelated parents, the sibs are healthy. In the first months of life there were recurrent episodes of hypothermia and recurrent infections. At the age of 4 months he had severe convulsions. Menkes' disease was diagnosed on the peculiar hair, the low serum copper ($0.7\,\mu mol\,L^{-1}$, normal: 10.2–26.0) and ceruloplasmin levels ($<0.07\,g\,L^{-1}$, normal: 0.15–0.60), and a decreased intestinal absorption of ^{64}Cu. The diagnosis was confirmed by the demonstration of abnormal accumulation of ^{64}Cu in cultured fibroblasts (N. Horn, J. F. Kennedy Institute, Glostrup, Denmark). Blood and CSF lactate levels were elevated (2.84

389

Journal of Inherited Metabolic Disease. ISSN 0141–8955. Copyright © SSIEM and Kluwer Academic Publishers, PO Box 55, Lancaster, UK.

and 2.70 mmol L^{-1}, normal: <2.0 and <2.3, respectively). Dopamine-β-hydroxy-lase (which catalyses conversion of dopamine to norepinephrine) activity in serum was very low (<1U, normal >3.0).

At 5 months of age copper infusion therapy was started with 825 µg copper

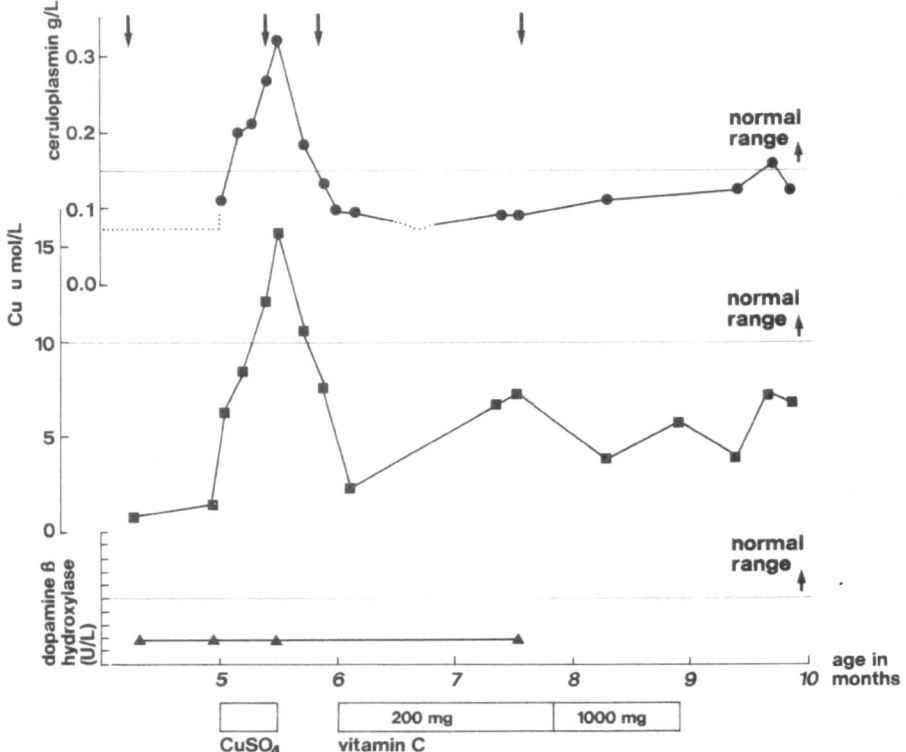

Figure 1 Serum copper, ceruloplasmin and dopamine-β-hydroxylase concentration during copper and vitamin C treatment. The arrows indicate the days CSF copper level was measured, respectively, 0.02, 0.04, 0.02 and 0.02 µmol L^{-1} (normal: 0.48–0.80)

sulphate every other day for 14 days (Figure 1). Serum copper and ceruloplasmin levels were measured at regular intervals. CSF copper concentration and serum dopamine-β-hydroxylase activity were measured during normalization of the serum copper level.

At 6 months of age a trial with vitamin C (ascorbate) was started. Initial dosage was 200 mg day^{-1}, orally. After 6 weeks the dosage was increased to 1000 mg day^{-1} (Figure 1). Serum copper and ceruloplasmin levels, CSF copper level and serum dopamine-β-hydroxylase activity were measured during vitamin C treatment.

RESULTS

Copper infusion resulted in normalization of serum copper and ceruloplasmin levels within 2 weeks. CSF copper level and the activity of dopamine-β-hydroxylase in serum, however, remained unchanged and extremely low (Figure 1). CSF lactate level remained elevated during the copper infusion therapy. The clinical condition of the child did not improve.

Vitamin C treatment seemed to result at first in an increase of serum copper and ceruloplasmin levels but normalization was not achieved. Increasing the dosage did not result in further increase. Subsequent cessation of vitamin C administration did not result in a decrease of copper and ceruloplasmin concentrations. CSF copper level and the activity of dopamine-β-hydroxylase did not change during vitamin C treatment.

DISCUSSION

Vitamin C administration was tried by Ueki *et al.* (1985) resulting in increased serum copper and ceruloplasmin levels and improvement of the clinical condition. This was explained on the basis of *in vitro* studies which showed vitamin C to prevent the binding between copper and metallothionein (Evans *et al.*, 1970). Furthermore vitamin C may play a role in intestinal copper absorption (Disilvestro and Harris, 1981). We failed to demonstrate a clear effect of vitamin C on the biochemical or clinical condition in our patient. The effect observed by Ueki *et al.* may be spurious, representing only the normal fluctuation of copper and ceruloplasmin levels in patients with Menkes' disease.

Furthermore, our results confirm that copper infusion in patients with Menkes' disease does not result in clinical or biochemical improvement. Normalization of serum copper does not result in an increase of the activity of the copper-dependent enzyme dopamine-β-hydroxylase, which can be explained by the abnormal accumulation of copper in the affected cells, without the cell being able to use this unusual amount of copper for normal cellular metabolic functions.

The inability to increase CSF copper concentration, despite normalization of serum copper level, demonstrates another reason for the therapeutic failure. Because the brain copper level will remain extremely low, no improvement of the activity of brain cytochrome *c* oxidase or dopamine-β-hydroxylase can be expected. Failure to normalize the copper CSF level was also reported by Grover *et al.* (1981), who observed very low dopamine-β-hydroxylase activity in CSF. The decreased activity of these enzymes is held responsible for part of the cerebral manifestations of the disease. The cause of the inability of copper to cross the blood–brain barrier in Menkes' disease may be the expression of the defect in the endothelial cells in the brain, resulting in copper accumulation and decreased copper transport out of the cells, similar to the situation found in the gut and kidney.

REFERENCES

Danks, D. M., Campbell, P. E., Stevens, B. J., Mayne, V. and Cartwright, E. Menkes' kinky hair syndrome: an inherited defect in copper absorption with widespread effects. *Pediatrics* 50 (1972) 188–201

Disilvestro, R. A. and Harris, E. D. A postabsorption effect of ascorbic acid on copper metabolism in chicks. *J. Nutr.* 111 (1981) 1964-1968

Evans, G. W., Majors, P. F. and Cornatzer, W. E. Ascorbic acid interaction with metallothionein. *Biochem. Biophys. Res. Commun.* 41 (1970) 1244–1247

Grover, W. D., Henkin, R. I., Schwartz, M., Brodsky, N., Hobdell, E. and Stolk, J. M. A defect in catecholamine metabolism in kinky-hair disease. *Ann. Neurol.* 12 (1982) 263–266

Leone, A., Pavlakis, G. N. and Hamer, D. H. Menkes' disease: abnormal metallothionein gene regulation in response to copper. *Cell* 40 (1985) 301–309

Menkes, J. M., Alter, M., Steigleder, G. K., Weakley, D. R. and Sung, J. H. A sex-linked recessive disorder with retardation of growth, peculiar hair and focal cerebral and cerebellar degeneration. *Pediatrics* 29 (1962) 764–779

Royce, P. M., Camakaris, J. and Danks, D. M. Reduced lysyl oxidase activity in skin fibroblasts from patients with Menkes' syndrome. *Biochem. J.* 192 (1980) 579

Ueki, Y., Narazaki, O. and Hanai, T. Menkes disease: is vitamin C treatment effective? *Brain Dev.* 7 (1985) 519–522

J. Inher. Metab. Dis. 12 Suppl. 2 (1989) 393–396

Short Communication

Copper Histidinate Therapy in Menkes' Disease: Prevention of Progressive Neurodegeneration

G. Sherwood[1], B. Sarkar[2], and the late A. Sass Kortsak[2]

[1]*Metabolic Diseases Center, Baylor University Medical Center, Dallas, TX, USA;* [2]*Department of Biochemistry & Pediatrics, The Hospital for Sick Children, Toronto, Ontario, Canada*

Menkes' disease (MD) is an X-linked inherited disorder of tissue copper distribution that invariably results in death with severe progressive neurodegeneration by the age of three years (Danks, 1986). Parenteral therapy with various copper salts, commenced either before or after neurological impairment develops, has never been convincingly shown to result in significant cessation, reversal, or prevention of the devastating neurodegenerative progression (Garnica, 1984).

We report most favourable neurological outcomes in two unrelated boys with classical MD in whom subcutaneous copper histidinate therapy was begun within weeks of birth and continued through to their present ages of 12 and 2 years respectively.

CASE HISTORIES

Case 1 (MF)

Four years after a previous sibling had died with severe neurodegeneration associated with confirmed classical MD, MF was born in November 1976, at 36 weeks gestation weighing 2.4 kg. At three days of age, his serum copper (Cu) and caeruloplasmin (CRP) levels were 70 µg/dL and 9 mg/dL, declining to 15 µg/dL and 3 mg/dL respectively by day 15 of life. He exhibited moderate lethargy, hypothermia and pili torti. Serum Cu and CRP levels remained unchanged with oral copper chloride, up to 1500 µg Cu/day, but did increase to the normal ranges with intravenous copper sulphate, up to 650 µg/day. At three months of age, subcutaneous copper histidinate, up to 650 µg/day, was substituted and serum Cu and CRP remained normal. Urinary Cu excretion increased from 47 µg/day pretreatment to 200 µg/day post-treatment. At 12 months of age, supranormal serum Cu and CRP levels were attained and the dose of Cu was reduced to 250 µg/day, whereupon, low normal levels of serum Cu and CRP were maintained.

Multiple three-day Cu balance studies were conducted. With no Cu treatment, a net Cu deficit of about 100 µg/day was found. With 650 µg Cu/day, a net Cu retention of about 200 µg/day was found. With 250 µg Cu/day, a net Cu retention

393

Journal of Inherited Metabolic Disease. ISSN 0141–8955. Copyright © SSIEM and Kluwer Academic Publishers, PO Box 55, Lancaster, UK.

of about 100 μg/day was found. Skeletal muscle Cu content was 10 times normal. While continuing to receive 250 μg Cu/day, 250 mg D-penicillamine also was administered daily. Urinary Cu excretion increased by 100 μg/day, thus limiting net Cu retention and concern about potential systemic Cu toxicity.

During the first 3 years of life, he showed poor growth and recurrent severe infections. Psychomotor development progressed, but lagged by 6–9 months. Nevertheless, he eventually approached the 3rd percentile for height and weight and the 50th percentile for head circumference. At about 3 years of age, remarkable gains were made – he learned to walk, talk, ride a tricycle and climb stairs, limited only by moderate global hypotonia. He attends regular school in age-appropriate grades. He is of low average intelligence, is excused from physical activities, has a delightful personality, many friends, and a good sense of humour. He never has had seizures and his EEG/BSEPs are normal.

From age 3 to 8 years, the Cu histidinate treatment maintained his serum Cu and CRP in the normal range. His Cu excretion was 100 μg/day, increasing to 250 μg/day with alternate month D-penicillamine. Over the following 1–2 years, his serum Cu and CRP levels declined below the normal ranges. His urinary Cu excretion declined to 25 μg/day, increasing only to 100 μg/day with D-penicillamine. There was no discernible change in growth and development except for a gradual decrease in exercise tolerance. He preferred to crouch rather than stand. Significant orthostatic hypotension was documented which has not been improved by increasing his Cu dose to 500 μg/day, even though normalization of serum Cu and CRP levels had been achieved.

He is inconvenienced by dry ichthyotic-like skin, bilateral radial head dislocations that limit manual dexterity, chronic persistent diarrhoea with nocturnal soiling, orthodontic problems, and nasal polyps. He has no evidence of gastrointestinal or genitourinary diverticulae, vascular aneurysms, or any increased tortuosity of cerebral vessels over or above that evident in early life.

Case 2 (RH)

RH presented at two weeks of age with severe hypothermia and lethargy. He had sparse hair and eyebrows, palpable occipital wormian bones, unusual facial appearance and umbilical/inguinal herniae. He was born in September 1986 at 35 weeks gestation weighing 2.15 kg, with no previous family history of MD. His serum Cu and CRP levels were 19 μg/dL and 5 mg/dL respectively. Subcutaneous copper histidinate, providing 450 μg Cu/day, was commenced at four weeks of age. Within two weeks, his serum Cu and CRP were increased to 80 μg/dL and 20 mg/dL respectively.

During the early months of life, he underwent uneventful reparative surgery for herniae and pyloric stenosis. He suffered recurrent respiratory and urinary tract infections. Cystograms revealed two massive bladder diverticula with left ureteric reflux and early calyceal blunting. He received antibiotic prophylaxis and intermittent bladder catheterization. Developmentally, he sat unsupported at 9 months, crawled at 13 months and took his first independent steps at 18 months of age. His height, weight and head circumference have been at the 10th and 50th percentiles respectively since six months of age. He has never suffered seizures and his EEG is normal.

After having received 450 μg Cu/day for 12 months, his serum Cu and CRP levels became supranormal. A reduction in the Cu dose of 250 μg/day has resulted in serum Cu and CRP levels of 82 μg/dL and 31 mg/dL, respectively. Unfortunately, poor bladder and bowel habits have prevented conduct of adequate Cu balance studies.

Additional cases

In 1979 and 1984, two further unrelated cases of classical MD presented at the respective ages of five and four months. Both already were markedly development- ally delayed and suffered recurrent seizures. Both were treated with subcutaneous copper histidinate therapy, providing 500 μg Cu/day for periods of six months. During these times, considerable neurological regression occurred. Between 10 and 12 months of age, serum Cu and CRP levels attained the supranormal range, whereupon therapy was discontinued. Both infants died before three years of age.

FORMULATION FOR COPPER HISTIDINATE

Dissolve 106 mg cupric chloride (anhydrous) and 244.4 mg L(+)-histidine in 70 ml 1 mol/L NaCl at room temperature. Adjust the pH to the 7.38–7.40 range with 0.2 mol/L NaOH, whereupon the colour changes from blue to clear, and then adjust the volume to 100 ml with 1 mol/L NaCl. Transfer to vented, sterile, dark glass vials via a 0.22 μ multipore filter and store in a refrigerator. The suggested shelf life is two months. The final copper concentration is 500 μg/mL.

DISCUSSION

The neurological outcomes in these early-diagnosed cases of classical MD appear to be considerably better than in any previously reported cases.

Copper histidinate is most probably the form in which Cu crosses the blood– brain barrier (Hartter and Barnea, 1988). Presumably, in untreated MD, systemic sequestration of Cu reduces the serum copper histidinate pool, thus limiting Cu availability to the brain for incorporation into key enzymes during the early months of life (Prohaska, 1987). Parenteral copper histidinate, but not Cu in other forms, appears to replete that pool, which normally accounts for only 1% of the total serum Cu content. However, in order to observe the desired clinical effects, this therapy must be commenced at least before two months of age and preferably sooner.

The amount of Cu required to maintain normal serum Cu and CRP levels appeared to take a sharp decline at about 12 months of age, suggesting that the process of postnatal distribution of copper among various tissues is most active during the first year of life.

Normal Cu and CRP levels were maintained at the expense of appreciable daily net Cu retention. The potential for systemic Cu toxicity existed, but this never became clinically overt. Augmentation of urinary Cu excretion with intermittent D-penicillamine therapy limited that potential hazard, but the necessity for this adjunctive therapy is unclear.

The appearance of orthostatic hypotension occurred at an age when the dopamine/norepinephrine ratio normally declines. Norepinephrine deficiency, due to reduced Cu-dependent dopamine hydroxylase activity, is suspected as a cause of the hypotension, and this is being investigated (Man In't Veld *et al.*, 1987).

Experience with our two cases, together with preliminary unpublished reports of three other cases subsequently treated with copper histidinate by others, indicates that the severe neurodegeneration of MD can be prevented. The coexisting connective tissue abnormalities are inconvenient, but manageable in most cases. Copper histidinate therapy should be seriously considered in early-diagnosed cases.

REFERENCES

Danks, D. M. Of mice and men, metals and mutations. *J. Med. Genet.* 23 (1986) 99–106

Garnica, A. D. The failure of patenteral copper therapy in Menkes' kinky hair syndrome. *Eur. J. Pediatr.* 142 (1984) 98–102

Hartter, D. E. and Barnea, A. Brain tissue accumulates ^{64}copper by two ligand-dependent saturable processes. *J. Biol. Chem.* 263 (1988) 799–805

Man In't Veld, A. J., Cook, C. M., Giles, W. B., Connelly, A. and Thompson, R. S. Congenital dopamine hydroxylase deficiency. *Lancet* 1 (1987) 183–187

Prohaska, J. R. Functions of trace elements in brain metabolism. *Physiol. Rev.* 67 (1987) 858–901